MARCUCCI'S HANDBOOK O

Medical
Eponyms

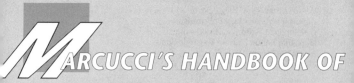

MARCUCCI'S HANDBOOK OF

MEDICAL EPONYMS

Lisa Marcucci, M.D.

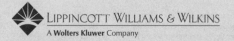

LIPPINCOTT WILLIAMS & WILKINS
A **Wolters Kluwer** Company

Editor: Elizabeth A. Nieginski
Editorial Director: Julie P. Scardiglia
Development Editor: Martha Cushman
Managing Editor: Marette Magargle-Smith
Artist: Christopher Wikoff
Marketing Manager: Aimee Sirmon

Photographs provided by Codman & Shurtleff, Inc.

Library of Congress Cataloging-in-Publication Data
Marcucci, Lisa.
    Marcucci's handbook of medical eponyms / Lisa Marcucci.
        p. ; cm.
    ISBN 0-7817-2368-X
    1. Medicine—Dictionaries. 2. Eponyms—Dictionaries. I. Title: Handbook
of medical eponyms. II. Title.
    [DNLM: 1. Eponyms—Dictionary—English. 2. Terminology—
Dictionary—English. W 13 M3234m 2002]
    R121 .M348 2002
    610′.3—dc21
                                                                    2001038393

The publishers have made every effort to trace the copyright holders for bor-
rowed material. If they have inadvertently overlooked any, they will be
pleased to make the necessary arrangements at the first opportunity.

We'd like to hear from you! If you have comments or suggestions regarding
this Lippincott Williams & Wilkins title, please contact us at the appropriate
customer service number listed below, or send correspondence to **book_com-
ments@lww.com**. If possible, please remember to include your mailing ad-
dress, phone number, and a reference to the book title and author in your
message. To purchase additional copies of this book call our customer service
department at **(800) 638-3030** or fax orders to **(301) 824-7390**. International
customers should call **(301) 714-2324**.

02 03
1 2 3 4 5 6 7 8 9 10

DEDICATION

To Joey, Cath, Danny, Sooz, and Andy

CONTENTS

PREFACE

Despite many attempts to eliminate them, the use of medical eponyms continues to flourish, mostly because doctors (including this author!) love to see their names in print. Even though eponyms are here to stay, they can be difficult and confusing to remember, especially when used as quiz questions on rounds.

This handbook of eponyms is not intended to be definitive. By providing two or three of the most salient features of each entry, it is intended to be used as a quick review by medical personnel at all levels of training, as well as a reference tool for professionals in other fields. Included are the most commonly used eponyms as well as a selection of more obscure and specialty-specific eponyms.

To reflect recent changes in medical usage, the nonpossessive form of each eponym is listed, except for a few entries (e.g., Ringer's lactate) for which the possessive form is still more common. Also included (but noted as misnomers) are some terms that are commonly, but inaccurately, thought to be eponyms (e.g., Angelman syndrome).

As an aid to the reader, this book includes an appendix that lists the proper names for each entry in alternate order. Although the commonly used pulmonary artery catheter is typically known as the Swan-Ganz catheter, Dr. Ganz may have preferred the name Ganz-Swan catheter! This appendix allows readers to locate the desired information quickly, even if they can remember only one of two or more proper names. Another appendix provides a list of selected eponyms by subject matter. This appendix is especially useful for quick perusal and cramming the night before a new rotation begins.

My goal for this book is to provide readers with the reference on eponyms I wish I had available to me during my training. I hope that readers will find this book helpful, easy to use, and interesting. I welcome reader suggestions for future editions, including both new eponyms and ideas for improving the presentation of the information.

Lisa Marcucci, M.D.

ACKNOWLEDGMENTS

I would like to extend my thanks to Les Gundry for allowing me unlimited access to the Pew Medical Library at the Bryn Mawr Hospital. Thanks also to David Keller, DO, who lent me his textbooks and made several helpful suggestions. Special thanks to Mike Williams, MD, who agreed to review my manuscript and returned his helpful comments in a timely manner.

Finally, I want to give my most heartfelt thanks and appreciation to Karla Schroeder. Her patience, encouragement, and attention to detail were instrumental in getting this manuscript to publication.

Aagenaes syndrome:
Recurrent jaundice and progressive leg edema, with development of liver fibrosis and cirrhosis; rare condition with early childhood onset (esp. Norwegian descent) resulting from idiopathic paucity of interlobular bile ducts. Treatment is liver transplantation.

Aaron sign: Epigastric or sternal tenderness on palpation over McBurney point; occurs in appendicitis.

Aarskog syndrome (Aarskog-Scott syndrome, facial-digital-genital syndrome): Short stature, hypoplastic maxilla, overriding "shawl" scrotum, cryptorchidism, hypospadias, wide-set eyes, small hands, and droopy eyelids; rare condition with variable heredity.

Aase-Smith syndrome:
Anemia, with triphalangeal thumb, mild growth retardation, narrow shoulder girdle, ventricular septal defect, and variable hepatosplenomegaly; rare congenital condition. Treatment is repeat blood transfusions in 1st year of life; anemia improves with age.

Abadie sign: Spasm of superior levator muscle in thyroid-related exophthalmus.

Abadie sign: Insensibility to pain when Achilles tendon is palpated vigorously; can be seen in locomotor ataxia or tabes dorsalis (neurosyphilis).

Abbe apertometer: Device used to measure numerical and angular apertures of objective or condenser.

Abbe apparatus: Microscope substage used to achieve oblique lighting; has rack-and-pinion design for displacement of iris diaphragm.

Abbe condenser (illuminator): Microscope lens system that focuses and condenses light on object being studied.

Abbe flap: "Lip switch," regional full-thickness flap (including skin and labial mucosa) used to reconstruct medial defects of opposite lip, esp. bilateral cleft. 2nd stage procedure is required to detach lip pedicle. Best results are obtained when lower lip is used to reconstruct upper lip.

Abbe law of diffraction:
Equation is $D = 0.5\lambda/NA$, where D is diffraction, λ is wavelength of monochromatic light or shortest of mixed wavelengths, and NA is numerical aperture of condenser or objective.

Abbe limit: Limit of resolution in diffraction-limited microscope.

Abbe operation: Lateral anastomosis of small intestine using catgut rings.

Abbe ring: Early surgical device composed of multiple turns of catgut used in intestinal anastomosis.

Abbe string method: Incision of esophageal stricture performed by passing string from mouth to stomach and using a sawing motion.

Abbe test plate: Series of cover slips of several different thicknesses coated with silver and scored with lines, which are placed on microscopic slide for lens calibration; used to test microscopic objectives for chromatic and spherical aberrations.

Abbé-Zeiss apparatus (counting chamber, Thoma-Zeiss chamber): Instrument for counting RBCs in blood sample.

Abbey salt: Mixture of tartaric acid, magnesium sulfate, sodium bicarbonate, and sugar; used as laxative.

Abbot paste: Analgesic mixture of morphine, arsenic trioxide, and creosol; used to kill nerve roots of teeth.

Abbott approach (Abbott-Carpenter approach, Brackett-Osgood technique, Putti technique): Surgical approach to posterior knee using curvilinear incision over popliteal fossa. Medial sural cutaneous nerve is located between heads of gastrocnemius muscle, traced to its origin at tibial nerve, and kept under visualization throughout procedure to reduce risk of injury. Dissection of tibial nerve reveals common peroneal nerve proximally and popliteal vessels anteromedially.

Abbott artery: Infrequently occurring arterial branch off proximal descending aorta that must be ligated and divided in subclavian flap aortoplasty for coarctation of aorta.

Abbott method: Treatment for curvature of spine; overcorrects spinal defect and uses plaster cast and jacket for immobilization.

Abbott stain: Solution of Löffler alkaline methylene blue, nitric acid, and eosin; stains spores blue.

Abbott tube: See Miller-Abbott tube.

Abbott-Fisher-Lucas procedure: 2-stage technique for hip fusion in absence of femoral head, failed femoral prosthesis, or infected trochanteric mold arthroplasties. Stage 1, anterior femoral approach (acetabular cavity debrided and deepened, greater trochanter denuded and seated into acetabulum using wide abduction, and bilateral spica cast applied); stage 2, transverse osteotomy just distal to lesser trochanter (femur adducted and spica cast reapplied bilaterally with patient immobilization).

Abbott-Gill osteotomy: Procedure used to correct for abnormal bone growth in leg. Medial approach involves metallic fixation of epiphysis and metaphysis in proximal tibia and distal femur. Lateral approach involves metallic fixation of epiphysis and metaphysis in proximal tibia and fibula.

Abbott-Lucas technique: Posterior approach for dislocation of lateral scapula and shoulder.

Abbott-Rawson tube: Double-lumen tube placed in stomach to allow infusion and aspiration of fluid.

Abbott-Saunders-Bost arthrodesis: Wrist arthrodesis using cortical bone grafts.

Abderhalden test: Early test for pregnancy involving detection of antibodies produced when small amounts of chorionic villi are released into maternal serum.

Abderhalden-Kauffman-Lignac syndrome: Renal rickets with cystinosis.

Abegg rule: All atoms have 8 valences.

Abel bacillus: *Klebsiella pneumoniae* (subspecies *ozaenae*); gram-negative bacterium found in nasal secretions of patients with atrophic rhinitis.

Abercrombie degeneration: Amyloid degeneration.

Abernethy fascia: Subperitoneal areolar tissue overlying psoas muscle; separates external iliac artery from iliac fascia.

Abernethy operation: Ligation of external iliac artery through incision made from 1 in.

above anterior superior iliac spine to 1 in. above Poupart ligament.

Abernethy sarcoma: Well-circumscribed fatty tumor, usu. found on trunk.

Abeshouse triad: Flank discomfort, palpable mass, downward displaced kidney on radiography; associated with congenital benign adrenal cysts. Treatment is surgical removal.

Abney effect: Visual disappearance of brightness of object based on time-delay and object contours that occurs when surface of large object is suddenly lit; brightness is first sensed in middle of object and then toward periphery.

Abney law: Mixture of colors has same luminance as sum of luminances of individual colors.

Abouker stent complex: Metal tracheostomy tube wired to Silastic stent that remains in tracheal lumen; used in pediatric laryngotracheal reconstruction.

Abraham-Pankovich technique (V-Y repair): Surgical repair for neglected rupture of calcaneal tendon. Patient is placed in prone position with tourniquet on thigh. S-curve incision is made from mid-calf to lateral side of calcaneal tendon, sural nerve is retracted laterally, and inverted V-incision is made over central aponeurosis. Arms of incision are 1.5 × length of tendon defect (defect is measured with knee in 30° of flexion and ankle in 20° of plantar flexion). Flap is then pulled distally and sutured into place.

Abrahams sign: Dullness to percussion over acromion process; occurs when TB affects lung apex.

Abrahams sign: Tenderness resulting from palpation at spot midway between 9th right costal margin and umbilicus; occurs in cholelithiasis.

Abram modification: Variation of Glenn shunt using a superior vena cava–to–pulmonary artery anastomosis. Proximal pulmonary artery is not ligated and inferior vena cava remains intracardiac.

Abrams needle: Percutaneous biopsy (cutting) needle.

Abrams reflex: Myocardial contraction when skin of precordial area is irritated.

Abrams reflex: Increase in lung volume when chest wall skin is irritated.

Abrams test: Used to detect lead in urine; positive if mixture of ammonium oxalate, metallic magnesium, and iodine forms precipitate on magnesium rod.

Abrams treatment: Percussion of spine to diagnose aortic aneurysm.

Abrams-Griffiths nomogram: Plot of bladder detrusor pressure against flow rate; used to evaluate bladder outlet obstruction during micturition.

abreuography: Photofluorography.

Abrikossoff tumor (myoblastoma): Pink-gray nodular tumor found in mouth (esp. tongue) or vulva; usu. benign (3% malignant). Onset occurs at 30–50 years of age. Condition affects both sexes equally. Treatment is excision.

accessory ligament of Henle (lateral) [temporomandibular ligament]: Strong fibrous connective tissue band running from zygomatic process of temporal bone to posterolateral condyloid neck of mandible; partially fuses with anterior joint capsule.

accessory ligament of Henle (medial) [sphenomandibular ligament]: Thin fibrous connective tissue band running from angular spine of sphenoid bone to mandibular lingula and temporomandibular joint.

accessory portal system of Sappey: Small collateral arteries and veins formed in perihepatic tissues in cirrhosis.

Ace-Colles fixator: See Colles fixator.

Ace-Fischer frame: See Fischer frame.

Achalme bacillus: See Welch bacillus (*Clostridium perfringens*).

Achard syndrome: Variant of Marfan disease, with joint laxity in hands and feet only and with mandibulofacial dysostosis.

Achard-Thiers syndrome (diabetic bearded woman syndrome): Virilizing disorder characterized by voice changes, hypertrichosis of face, acne, enlarged clitoris, obesity, hypertension, small breasts, and abdominal striae. Condition is typically seen in postmenopausal women; cause is hyperplasia of adrenal cortex and increased 11-oxysteroids and androgens. Control is adrenalectomy.

Achenbach syndrome: Spontaneous severe pain and hand hematoma after straining or rapid temperature change; etiology unknown. Condition is more common in women.

Achilles bulge sign (heel–cord sign): Positive for ankle instability when leg is pushed backward, foot is pulled forward, and Achilles tendon bulges.

Achilles reflex (jerk): Contraction of calf muscles when Achilles tendon is percussed; considered deep tendon reflex.

Achilles squeeze test: Positive for Achilles tendon rupture if no plantar flexion of ankle occurs when calf is squeezed.

Achilles tendon: Combined tendon of soleus and gastrocnemius muscles that inserts on back of heel.

Achterman-Kalamachi classification: Scheme for description of congenital fibular hemimelia. Type 1A, more-distal-than-normal proximal tibia and more-proximal-than-normal distal tibia; type 1B, severely shortened fibula (30%–50%) with lack of articulation with ankle joint; type 2, absence of fibula with pronounced tibial bowing.

Achúcarro stain: Tannin silver stain used for connective tissue. Stains astrocytes violet to gray, neurofibrils black, and other structures reddish; forerunner of Hortega stain.

Ackerman syndrome (taurodontism): Single root canal with fused pyramidal molar root, juvenile glaucoma, sparse body hair, variable syndactyly, and hyperpigmented finger joints; rare congenital condition.

Acosta disease: Acute onset of mountain sickness.

Acree-Rosenheim test: Indicates proteins present if violet color appears when sulfuric acid is added to solution to be tested.

Acrel ganglion: Ganglion appearing on wrist extensor tendons.

Adair Dighton syndrome: Type 1 (mild) osteogenesis imperfecta.

Adam apple: Laryngeal prominence formed by ventral edges of thyroid cartilage.

Adam operation: Corneal incision used to draw iris into tight circle.

Adam operation: Osteotomy of hip joint secondary to ankylosis; neck of femur is divided within capsule.

Adam operation: Procedure to correct deviated nasal

septum; flattened forceps is used to straighten cartilage forcibly.

Adam operation: Procedure to correct Dupuytren contracture, esp. when bands extend distally onto fingers; palmar fascia is resected in multiple places through subcutaneous incision.

Adam operation: Procedure to correct ectropion; triangular resection of full-thickness lower lid is made with reapproximation of free edges.

Adam operation: Modification of Cripps operation; vertical incision is made external to epigastric artery.

Adamantiades-Behçet syndrome: See Behçet syndrome.

Adamkiewicz cell: Nerve cell that lies deep to neurilemma of medullated nerve fibers; stains yellow with safranin.

Adamkiewicz reaction: Test for presence of proteins; positive if mixture of sulfuric acid, acetic acid, and sample produces brown-violet color.

Adams clasp: Arrow tooth clasp with undercuts for mesial, buccal, and distal proximal surfaces of tooth.

Adams saw: Instrument with long handle and short blade; used in osteotomies.

Adams suspension wires: Supports used to secure midface bone fragments in repair of osteotomies/trauma. Overzealous tightening causes midface retrusion postoperatively.

Adams test (forward bending test): Method used to diagnose direction and severity of vertebral rotation in scoliosis. Patient stands with feet together and knees straight and bends at hips with palms held together. Positive result (viewed from behind) is 1 side of thorax higher than other.

Adams test: Used to measure fat content in milk. Known volume is dried on filter paper, extracted in Soxhlet apparatus, and weighed.

Adams-Foley disorder: Asterixis; caused by hypercapnia, drowsiness, and hepatic and toxic encephalopathy.

adamsite: Diphenylamine chlorarsine.

Adams-Kershner disease: Term for chronic interstitial pneumonia; originated in 1940s.

Adams-Oliver syndrome: Congenital absence of legs, ulcerated scalp lesions, bony skull defects, and variable absence of fingers and hands.

Adams-Stokes syncope (Adams-Stokes attacks; Morgagni-Adams-Stokes syncope): Cardiac arrest and syncope due to abnormal pacemaker activity; seen with ventricular fibrillation and infranodal AV block.

Adams-Stokes syndrome: Bradycardia and heart block in setting of seizures.

Adams-Victor-Mancall syndrome (central pontine myelinosis): Progressive facial and oral weakness and emotional lability, sometimes resulting in flaccid quadriplegia and "locked-in" state. Onset occurs in adulthood; condition affects alcoholics and persons with nutritional depletion. Associated disorders are Wernicke encephalopathy, Wilson disease, organ transplantation, diabetes, amyloidosis, and leukemia. Treatment is adequate nutrition, thiamine, and correction of electrolyte abnormalities.

Addis count: Quantity of RBCs, WBCs, and casts in 12-hour urine collection; indicator of severity and progression of chronic glomerulonephritis. Method mostly used in suspected subclinical pediatric renal diseases.

Addis test (method): Measurement of urine specific gravity after consumption of dry diet for 24 hours.

Addis test: Knee flexion to 90° by prone patient; used to detect unequal tibia and femur lengths.

Addison anemia: See Biermer disease.

Addison disease: Adrenocortical insufficiency from primary causes (autoimmune condition, bilateral hemorrhage, TB, fungal infection) or secondary causes (ACTH suppression by iatrogenic corticosteroid administration). Both causes result in cortisol deficiency with hypoglycemia, hypotension, anorexia, vomiting, atrophic gastritis, weight loss, malaise, abdominal pain, inability to react to stress, and sometimes skin hyperpigmentation. With primary causes only, aldosterone deficiency leads to hyperkalemia, hyponatremia, volume depletion, acidosis, and azotemia. Patients undergoing surgery or invasive procedures must receive stress-dose steroids (typically hydrocortisone 100–300 mg perioperatively, tapered over next 1–5 days).

Addison keloid: Focal fibrosis of muscle fascia, subcutaneous fat, and skin in extremities; occurs unilaterally in young individuals.

Addison line (transpyloric line): Imaginary line running horizontally through midpoint between sternoxiphoid junction and umbilicus (or midway between symphysis pubis and suprasternal notch). It crosses spine at L1 level when patient is upright and at pylorus when patient is horizontal.

Addison pill: See Guy pill.

Addison planes: Imaginary planes marking anatomic boundaries of abdomen and thorax. 5 horizontal planes run through the sternal jugular notch and the upper border of symphysis pubis, with transtubercle, transpyloric, and transthoracic lines (bottom to top) spaced equally between them. 5 vertical planes are comprised of 2 planes passing through each anterior superior iliac spine, 1 median plane, and 2 lateral sagittal planes (each bisecting the space between iliac spine and median plane).

Addison point: Midpoint of epigastrium.

Addison-Hunter disease: See Biermer disease.

Addison-Schilder disease: See Siemerling-Creutzfeldt disease.

Addison-Scholz disease: See Siemerling-Creutzfeldt disease.

Addisonian crises (Bernard-Sergent syndrome): Stress-related altered mental status (e.g., from trauma, infection, surgery), fatigue, vomiting, fever, abdominal pain, hypotension, and collapse, which characterize acute episodes of Addison disease. Treatment is IV fluid and hydrocortisone.

Adelaide scale: Pediatric coma scale used for infants and young children with limited verbal abilities.

Aden fever (disease): Dengue fever.

Aden ulcer: Sloughing of necrotic tissue caused by Old World cutaneous leishmaniasis.

Adie syndrome (Holmes-Adie disease, Markus disease, tonic pupil, Weill-Reys disease): Absent tendon reflexes (esp. patellar) and unilateral slowness in pupillary accommodation and convergence; initial complaint is visual blurring or appearance of unequal pupils. Condition is harmless autosomal dominant disorder that is more common in women. Cause is postsynaptic parasympathetic denervation and probable lesion in ciliary ganglion.

Adie syndrome (partial) [Argyll-Robertson nonluetic syndrome]: Adie syndrome with normal deep tendon reflexes.

Adie-Critchley syndrome (Fulton syndrome): Forced grasping of object with affected hand when object moves. When object touches affected hand, patient grabs it and cannot release it. Cause is tumor in superior contralateral frontal lobe (area 6).

Adler reaction: Used to indicate presence of blood if mixture of benzidine, alcohol, acetic acid, hydrogen dioxide, and sample produces blue-green color.

Adler test: Very sensitive test for occult blood in urine and feces if addition of benzidine (carcinogenic), hydrogen peroxide, and acetic acid to sample produces blue color; used infrequently.

Adler theory: Cause of neurosis is psychological compensation for social or physical inferiority complex.

Adlerian psychology (individual psychology): Approach that maintains major issues to be resolved in life involve social adjustments, occupation, and love. Emphasis is on ego rather than libido; major feature of neurosis is feeling of inferiority arising from frustrated drive for superiority.

Adonis: Genus of herbs with cardiac properties; largely indigenous to Europe.

Adrian mixture: Solution of sodium chloride, iron chloride, and H_2O; causes hemostasis when applied topically.

Adson hemostatic forceps: Locking forceps with ring-handles and fine, straight, or curved tips; used to grasp small bleeding vessels before suture ligation or cautery.

Adson maneuver: Somewhat imprecise test for scalenus anticus syndrome; positive if arm is held in dependent position and radial pulse is obliterated when head is turned toward ipsilateral shoulder during inhalation. Bruit also may be heard in supraclavicular fossa with cool, blue hand. Maneuver sometimes described as turning head toward contralateral shoulder.

Adson maneuver (modified): Ipsilateral arm elevation and Valsalva maneuver, causing obliteration of pulse.

Aebi-Etter-Coscia fixation: Cervical fusion for fractured dens of C2; uses screws placed via anterior approach.

Aeby division: Early categorization of bronchial branches of lung based on topographical relation to pulmonary artery. Eparterial branch, found only in right lung, rises above where pulmonary artery crosses mainstem bronchus; hyparterial branches arise below.

Aeby plane: Imaginary surface passing through nose to base of skull perpendicular to median plane.

African coast fever (Rhodesian fever): Fatal, tick-transmitted disease of African cattle; caused by *Theileria parva.*

African siderosis: Iron overload found in black populations in southern Africa, which is caused by cooking in iron pots and drinking homemade beer with high iron content.

African sleeping sickness (African trypanosomiasis): Disease characterized by peculiar pain syndrome, neuropsychiatric symptoms, and meningoencephalitis, which leads to increasing somnolence and death, esp. in West African type. East African type has more acute course and usu. leads to death secondary to myocarditis. Vector is tsetse fly *Glossina.*

African swine fever: Fatal, tick-transmitted viral disease of pigs in Africa, Brazil, and southern Europe.

African tapeworm: *Taenia saginata;* common human pathogen.

African tick fever: Relapsing fever seen in humans; pathogen is *Borrelia duttonii.*

African tick typhus (Indian tick typhus, Marseilles fever, Mediterranean spotted fever): Acute febrile illness with lymphadenopathy and rash; often mistaken for clinical signs and symptoms of acute HIV infection. Cause is *Rickettsia conorii*. Incubation period before onset of fever is 5–7 days.

African trypanosomiasis: See African sleeping sickness.

Afzelius disease (erythema chronicum migrans, Lipschutz disease, Lyme disease): Early description (1921) of pathognomonic skin lesion of Lyme disease caused by *Borrelia* spirochetes via bite of *Ixodes* tick; usu. occurs as 1st sign of infection but occasionally accompanied by arthritis and meningeal symptoms.

Agnell rule: Patients with Wilms tumor are considered cured following tumor resection after disease-free interval of 9 months plus age in months.

Agnew splint: Long splint with pelvic support bands and foot piece for lower extremity; designed to support full weight of torso.

Agostini reaction (test): Glucose present in urine if addition of gold chloride and potash with heating produces red color.

Ahlback changes: Descriptions of arthritic degeneration of knee seen on anterior-posterior radiographs. Grade 0, normal; grade 1, narrowing of joint space; grade 2, obliteration of joint space; grade 3, minor bone attrition; grade 4, moderate bone attrition; grade 5, severe bone attrition; grade 6, subluxation.

Ahlfeld sign (breathing movements): Irregular, localized contractions of gravid uterus occurring after 3rd month of pregnancy.

Ahumada-Del Castillo syndrome: Deficient gonadotropin secretion, causing amenorrhea and galactorrhea.

Aicardi syndrome: Mental retardation, spasmodic seizures, dorsal vertebral defects, characteristic EEG findings, malformed or absent corpus callosum, "bat-wing" 3rd and 4th ventricles, abnormal corneas and retina, and microphthalmos. In males, condition is lethal in utero; in females, it usu. manifests in 1st few months of life but occasionally develops as late as adolescence.

Aicardi-Goutieres syndrome: Calcification of basal ganglia and CSF lymphocytosis; marked by progressive mental retardation, spastic quadriplegia, and encephalopathy, leading to death. Onset occurs in infancy.

Aich metal: Alloy of zinc and iron.

Aiello test: Used to indicate presence of tryptophan in CSF if mixture of hydrochloric acid, formaldehyde, sodium nitrate, and specimen produces purple color.

Aiko-Okamato rat: Most commonly used animal model of essential hypertension; esp. useful in study of alterations of Ca^{2+} metabolism.

air of Hales: Carbon dioxide.

Aitken classification: System for description of congenital hip abnormalities. Type A, shortened femur and absent femoral neck (hip joint appears formed on radiograph); type B, severe proximal femoral shaft deformity with rudimentary femoral head and pseudoarthrosis; type C, small tufted proximal femur, absent femoral head, and shallow acetabulum; type D, absence of proximal femoral shaft, femoral head, and acetabular hypoplasia.

Aitkin operation: Double cervical incision for dystocia resulting from narrow pelvis.

Åkerlund deformity: Deformity of duodenal bulb caused by ulcer.

Akin procedure: 1st toe osteotomy (proximal phalanx) for bunion treatment.

Al-Ghorab procedure: Surgical correction of priapism performed under local anesthesia. 2-cm transverse incision is made on dorsal surface of penis just distal to coronal ridge, distal tip is then pulled forward to expose bulging corporal bodies, 5-mm section (including septum) is then resected and blood is allowed to drain, and dorsal skin is reapproximated with chromic sutures.

Alagille syndrome: Odd facies with high prominent forehead and deep-set eyes, chronic cholestasis and paucity of interlobular bile ducts, butterfly-shaped vertebral arches, peripheral pulmonary stenosis, renal failure, and hepatic failure in children. Supportive measures are ursodeoxycholic acid and phenobarbital; eventually liver transplantation is required.

Alajouanine syndrome: Bilateral paralysis of CNs VI and VII, strabismus, and talipes equinovarus; rare congenital condition.

Alajouanine-Foix syndrome: See Foix-Alajouanine syndrome.

Åland disease: See Forsius-Eriksson syndrome.

Alanson amputation: Circular amputation of an extremity with cone-shaped stump.

Albarran disease: Presence of *Escherichia coli* (*Bacillus coli communis*) in urine.

Albarran gland: Portion of median prostate lobe underlying rounded elevation at neck of bladder.

Albarran test: Evaluation of renal insufficiency based on principle that after known quantity of fluid is given, greater destruction of nephrons means less secretion by kidney.

Albee fusion (Albee-Delbet operation): Fusion of spinous processes, facets, and lamina in lumbar spine; uses posterior approach.

Albee operation: Surgical fusion of hip joint. Upper edge of femoral head and edge of the acetabulum are resected, and 2 surfaces are approximated.

Albee procedure: Vertebral body fusion using small bone grafts; used to treat spinal TB.

Albers-Schönberg disease (type 1) [osteopetrosis]: Increased bone density and thickness throughout body ("chalk bones, thick bones, marble bones"), which encroaches on skull foramina, resulting in optic atrophy; rare autosomal recessive condition. Cause is disorder of macrophage colony-stimulating factor.

Albers-Schönberg disease (type 2): See Buschke-Ollendorff disorder.

Albert achillodynia: Pain in distal heel cord.

Albert disease (Schanz disease): Achilles tendon bursitis, sometimes accompanied by calcification. Causes include trauma and ill-fitting shoes.

Albert disease: See Swediauer disease.

Albert operation: Fusion of knee by resection of articular ends of tibia and femur and approximation of exposed surfaces.

Albert position: Radiographic positioning technique that places patient in semirecumbent position; used to visualize superior borders of pelvis.

Albert suture: Modification of Czerny suture; initial row of stitches placed through all layers of intestine wall.

Albert stain: Mixture of toluidine blue, methyl green, and iodine, which stains diphtheria metachromatic granules black, bars green-black, and rest of organism green.

Albert-Lindner bone sectioning: Procedure used to prepare bone for histologic examination for alkaline phosphatase. Bone fragments are fixed in alcohol, treated with tropical ester wax, and coated with celluloid before being cut.

Albini nodules: Small nodules located on free edge of heart valves in some infants.

Albinus muscle: Risorius muscle; action is to pull mouth laterally. Origin is masseter fascia, insertion is skin at corners of mouth, and innervation is by buccal branch of facial nerve.

Albinus muscle: Middle scalene muscle; elevates 1st rib and bends neck laterally. Origin is C2–C6 transverse process, and insertion is superior border of 1st rib.

Albrecht bone (basiotic bone): Fetal bone lying between basioccipital and basisphenoid bone.

Albright anemia: Anemia and osteitis deformans in setting of hyperparathyroidism.

Albright disease (Albright-McCune disease, Albright-McCune-Sternberg syndrome): Polyostotic fibrous dysplasia, endocrine dysfunction, short stature, irregular brown skin pigmentation (usu. café-au-lait,) and precocious puberty; condition usu. occurs in females.

Albright hereditary osteodystrophy: Mental retardation, short stature, oval facies, brachydactyly, heterotopic calcification, shortened metatarsals, and pseudohypoparathyroidism. Cause is defective parathyroid thyroid hormone receptor on adenyl cyclase.

Albright solution: Mixture of 140 g citric acid, 75 g sodium citrate, and 25 g potassium citrate in 1 L of H_2O; used in renal tubular acidosis.

Albright syndrome: See Forbes-Albright syndrome.

Albright-Chase resection: See Darrach procedure.

Albright-Hadorn syndrome: Term for hypokalemia in setting of osteomalacia, renal tubular acidosis, and variable paralysis; originated in 1940s.

Alcian blue: Dye used in electrophoresis to stain and distinguish sulfomucins from other mucins, sulfated polysaccharides, and glycoproteins.

Alcock canal: Anatomic space which allows passage of pudendal vessels and nerve through lateral separated fibers of obturator fascia.

Alder sign: Indicates that source of pelvic pain is uterine or adnexal if pain decreases in intensity when patient is placed in lateral decubitus position.

Alder-Reilly anomaly: Hereditary occurrence of azurophilic granules in leukocytes in mucopolysaccharidoses; seen in Hunter, Hurler, and Maroteaux-Lamy syndromes. Condition is clinically benign when it occurs as isolated event. Granules stain dark purple with Wright-Giemsa stain.

Alder-Reilly granules: Acid mucopolysaccharide deposits most commonly seen in neutrophils in Hunter, Hurler, and Maroteaux-Lamy syndromes.

Aldor method: Test for proteinuria.

Aldrich syndrome: See Wiskott-Aldrich syndrome.

Aldrich-Mees lines: See Mees lines.

Aleppo boil (button, disease, evil, pustule, ulcer; Bagdad boil, cutaneous leishmaniasis, Lahore sore): Successive formation of papule, tubercle, scab, and circumscribed ulcer on facial cheeks and mouth angle; condition most commonly occurs in persons living on Mediterranean coastline.

Aleutian disease: Multiple myeloma-type illness found in minks.

Alexander disease (factor VII deficiency, proconvertin deficiency): Clinical syndrome similar to hemophilia but less severe, with normal PT. Frequency is 1/500,000.

Alexander disease (leukodystrophy): White matter demyelination associated with presence of Rosenthal fibers, esp. in frontal lobes, with seizures, spasticity, macrocephaly, and psychomotor retardation; usu. manifests by 6 months of age. Brain biopsy is required for definitive diagnosis.

Alexander disease: Recurrent pericardial effusions, eventually progressing to constrictive pericarditis due to calcifications; adolescent onset.

Alexander hearing loss: Congenital aplasia of organ of Corti and ganglion cells of basal coil.

Alexander law: Ability to accentuate nystagmus by moving eyes in direction of "jerky" correcting movement and to dampen it by looking in opposite direction.

Alexander method: Theory that physical diseases can be ameliorated through conscious control of psychophysical functions, providing ability to coordinate and integrate entire organism.

Alexander paste: Early treatment for burns using mixture of olive oil, ichthyol, and wool-fat.

Alexander position: Radiographic patient positioning technique using anterior-posterior and lateral projections in imaging acromioclavicular articulations (good for detecting shoulder subluxation or dislocation).

Alexander technique: Method that uses release of muscle tension as central strategy in relearning simple tasks of daily living (e.g., breathing, speaking, eating).

Alexander view: Radiographic patient positioning technique using lateral view of scapula with shoulders hunched forward.

Alexanderism (agriothymia ambitiosa): Overriding urge or obsession to conquer nations.

Alezzandrini syndrome: Unilateral visual loss followed by (months to years later) ipsilateral loss of skin pigmentation on face (vitiligo) and poliosis; usu. associated with eventual bilateral perceptive deafness. Onset occurs in adolescence or early adulthood.

Alfidi syndrome (renal-splanchnic steal syndrome): Occlusion of celiac axis, eventually leading to renal-based hypertension.

Alfraise test: Iodine indicator; positive if mixture of hydrochloric acid, starch, and potassium nitrate is boiled, and blue color develops when it is added to the sample.

Alfven instability: Electromagnetic instability that occurs near ion cyclotron frequency in mirroring devices used in radiobiology.

Alfven velocity: Phase velocity of Alfven wave.

Alfven waves: Transverse electromagnetic waves that originate parallel to lines of magnetic force in plasma substance.

Alibert disease (false keloid, Hawkin disease): Hypertrophic scar forming 3–4 weeks after skin wounding. Treatment is systemic steroids, radiotherapy, intradermal injection, and retinoic acid.

Alibert disease: See Aleppo boil.

Alibert disease: Scleroderma.

Alibert-Bazin disease (Auspitz syndrome, mycosis fungoides, Vidal-Brocq syndrome): Cutaneous T-cell lymphoma; more common in men, with usual onset in 5th–7th decade.

Alibert keloid: True keloid.

Alibert-Bazin disease: Arthritis and psoriasis.

Alice in Wonderland syndrome (Todd syndrome): Occurrence in some conditions (e.g., drug intoxication, febrile illness, schizophrenia) of abnormal mental status, with hallucinations (esp. Lilliputian) and depersonalization.

Alius-Grignaschi anomaly: Myeloperoxidase deficiency in neutrophils and monocytes; causes increased infection rate (esp. candidiasis). Condition is generally benign in absence of other immunologic defects. Frequency of partial or complete congenital defect is 1/2000.

Allan-Herndon syndrome: Loss of ability to hold head erect, ataxia, athetosis, mental retardation, muscle atrophy, joint contractures, elongated facies, and large ears; X-linked disorder that manifests at 6 months of age.

Allemann syndrome: Association of club fingers with duplication of urogenital system; also occurs with variable facial asymmetry and motor neuropathy.

Allen cards: Series of handheld cards with pictures of common items (birthday cake, boat, telephone) drawn at varying distances; used to test vision in verbal children.

Allen intestinal anastomosis clamp: Locking clamp with long jaw length (57 mm), straight tips, and ring-handles. Tips have longitudinal serrations and 1×2–teeth configuration.

Allen maneuver: Test for scalenus anticus syndrome; positive if radial pulse is obliterated when head is turned toward ipsilateral, which is flexed at elbow, extended horizontally, and rotated externally.

Allen paradoxic law: The more sugar administered, the higher the sugar utilization in normal patients (opposite occurs in diabetics).

Allen reaction (test): Used to indicate presence of phenol; positive if mixture of sample, hydrochloric acid, and nitric acid turns bright red.

Allen stirrups: Attachable, padded leg supports for operating room table; used to place patient in lithotomy position.

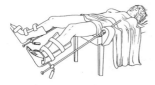

Allen stirrups

Allen test (radial compression test): Used to assess patency of ulnar artery and arterial arches of hand; performed by having patient clench fist (causing skin on palm to blanch) and occluding radial and ulnar artery with firm pressure. Prompt return of pink tone of skin after releasing clenched fist and removing occlusion of ulnar artery indicates patent flow through ulnar artery and arches.

Allen treatment: Starvation treatment for diabetes.

Allen-Brown criteria: Standards used in diagnosis of Raynaud phenomenon.

Allen-Doisy test: Estrogen-like substances present in laboratory animals that have cornified epithelial cells in vaginal secretions.

Allen-Doisy unit: Smallest amount of estrogen that causes cornification and desquamation in vaginal epithelia of spayed rats or mice.

Allen-Hines syndrome: Onset of progressive fat deposition and fluid accumulation in buttocks and legs, usu. out of proportion to total body fat deposition. Condition is benign except for cosmetic concerns.

Allen-Masters syndrome (universal joint syndrome): Enlargement and engorgement of uterus combined with lacerations in fascial tissue layers of broad, cardinal, and uterosacral ligaments, allowing cervix to move independently in all directions with variable presence of 3rd-degree retroversion. Associated symptoms include pain, dyspareunia, pelvic pain, backache, and headache. Controversy exists regarding diagnosis and prevalence of this clinical syndrome.

Allgrove syndrome (addisonian–achalasia syndrome, 3A syndrome): Achalasia, alacrima, and glucocorticoid deficiency, with congenital absence of zona fasciculata and congenital defective tear formation. Associated symptoms include mild mental retardation, ataxia, sensory disturbances, and optic atrophy. Onset of Addison disease begins at 2 years of age, and onset of achalasia occurs during school years. Heredity is autosomal recessive.

Allingham plug: Device to control rectal hemorrhage.

Allingham ulcer: Anal fissure.

Allis method: Technique for manual reduction of posterior hip dislocation. Patient lies in supine position with pelvis stabilized by assistant. Hip and knee are flexed to 90°, slightly adducted, and internally rotated; upper traction is then applied at proximal calf.

Allis sign: Loosening of fascia running from greater trochanter to iliac crest; occurs in femoral neck fractures.

Allison operation: Antireflux operation performed through abdominal incision, using anatomic repair of lax gastroesophageal junction.

Allison syndrome: Demineralization occurring after prolonged disuse or immobilization (e.g., casting, space flight). Treatment is calcium enrichment and gradual exercise.

Allison-Millar classification: Description of diagnosis of multiple sclerosis as probable, early, or possible.

Allis-Thoms tissue forceps (nontoothed): Forceps used for grasping soft tissue.

Allman classification: System for describing location of clavicle fractures. Group 1, middle third; group 2, distal to coracoclavicular ligament (frequent nonunion); group 3, proximal third (rare nonunion).

Allport A-S reaction study: Psychological test that assesses patient's functioning in everyday life for ascendancy versus acquiescence traits.

Allport-Vernon-Lindzey study of values: Updated version of Allport-Vernon study.

Allport-Vernon study of values: Early version of psychological test that assesses person's interest in theoretical, religious, social, aesthetic, political, and economic ideas.

Almeida disease: Paracoccidiomycosis.

Alouette amputation: High-leg amputation with outer flap rotated to greater trochanter and inner flap rotated outward.

Alper test: Used to indicate presence of albumin in urine; positive if addition of hydrochloric acid and mercury succinimide forms white, cloudy mixture.

Alpers disease: Progressive cerebral poliodystrophy with convulsions, spasticity, ataxia, visual loss, dementia, growth retardation, and stunted brain growth; occasionally marked by cirrhosis late in disease. Condition is autosomal recessive and results in loss of middle cell layers in cerebrum and cerebellum ("walnut brain"). Onset occurs in infancy.

Alpers-Huttenlocher syndrome: Diffuse degeneration of cerebral tissue, causing dementia, spasticity, myoclonus, and seizures; may also be marked by liver cirrhosis and hemorrhagic anemia. Death results from status epilepticus. Condition is autosomal recessive; familial onset is at 1–2 years of age. Etiology is unknown; some patients show glutathione oxidase deficiency.

Alport syndrome (Dickinson syndrome): Craniofacial abnormalities, variably detached retinas, exophthalmos, glaucoma, cone-shaped eye lens, hemorrhagic nephritis, mild thrombocytopenia, cataracts, and high-frequency nerve deafness. Renal failure occurs in 2nd–3rd decade of life. Condition is autosomal dominant or X-linked recessive and is more severe in males. Cause is genetic defect of type 4 collagen, resulting in deficiency in basement membrane collagen.

Alsberg angle (angle of elevation): Angle of cephalad apex in Alsberg triangle.

Alsberg triangle:
Approximate equilateral triangle with apex cephalad; formed by imaginary lines running through long axis of femoral neck, base of femoral head, and long axis of femoral head.

Alström syndrome:
Congenital blindness or severely impaired vision secondary to defect in cones, deafness, baldness, nystagmus, acanthosis nigricans, obesity, male hypogonadism, diabetes insipidus (vasopressin-resistant), and renal failure. Laboratory abnormalities include hypertriglyceridemia, hyperuricemia, and aminoaciduria. Autosomal recessive condition most commonly seen in Netherlands and Sweden.

Altamira disease: Diffuse ecchymosis and petechiae, hemorrhagic skin lesions, mucosal bleeding, moderate painless lymphadenopathy, thrombocytopenia, and low RBC count. Nonnative population in Altamira region of Brazil is affected. Cause is injection of bile from black fly bite. Treatment is prednisone and IV glucose.

Altemeier procedure:
Surgical correction of rectal prolapse using circumferential incision in perineum distal to dentate line. Redundant bowel is pulled down, its blood supply is ligated and resected, and free ends of bowel wall and mucosa are sutured together and everted.

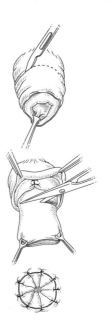

Altemeier procedure

Althausen test: Used to determine rapidity of intestinal absorption. Sugar is administered orally, with blood sampling for galactose done at routine intervals.

Altherr syndrome: See Meyenburg-Altherr-Uehlinger syndrome.

Altmann granule: Any granule that binds readily with fuchsin.

Altmann stain: Combination of potassium bichromate, osmic acid, acid fuchsin, and picric acid used to visualize liver tissue; mixture stains fat droplets blue or black and mitochondria red.

Altmann-Gersh stain: Technique used in preparing histologic specimens by rapidly freezing and then dehydrating in a vacuum.

Alton giant: Reference to specific male individual who suffered from extreme gigantism caused by hypersecretion of growth hormone and deficiency of gonadotropin; patient died in his early 20s at height of 280 cm.

Alzheimer cells: Enlarged astrocytes with prominent nuclei occurring in hepatic coma and hepatolenticular degeneration.

Alzheimer disease: Progressive dementia that increases in prevalence with age, with usu. subtle, insidious onset; early stages are marked by memory loss for recent events and mood change. Histopathology shows neurofibrillary tangles, neurites, and neuronal cell death. Brain biopsy is required for definitive diagnosis.

Amapari virus: Arenavirus in Tacaribe lineage B complex; causes severe hemorrhagic disease. Host is rodent.

Amato body: Pale-blue staining neutrophil cytoplasmic clumps seen in scarlet fever, diphtheria, and pneumonia; similar to Döhle inclusion bodies.

American hookworm: *Necator americanus;* parasitic intestinal nematode found in humans and other mammals.

American tarantula: *Eurypelma hentzii;* bite is poisonous to humans.

American trypanosomiasis: See Chagas disease.

Ames demonstration: Highlights concept that physical properties of objects and spaces often conflict with unconscious assumptions of them (e.g., distorted room, aniseikonic lens).

Ames test: Method for determining potential mutagenicity of substance; uses special strains of *Salmonella typhimurium* incubated on histidine-lacking medium, as well as rat liver microsomes and substance to be tested. Colony growth indicates mutagenicity and likely carcinogenicity.

Amici disk (Amici line, Dobie line, intermediate disk, Krause membrane): Thin dark line seen in center of I band on longitudinal section of striated muscle. Distance between Amici lines equals sarcomere length.

Amies medium: Agar that contains charcoal, sodium thioglycolate, sodium chloride, potassium chloride, calcium chloride, and magnesium chloride; used for transporting anaerobic organisms.

Amish albinism: Yellow-colored corneas.

Ammon fissure: Pear-shaped cleft found in embryo sclerae.

Ammon horn: Early term for hippocampus.

Ammon operation: Blepharoplasty with use of a cheek flap.

Ammon operation: Method for creating new orifice leading into lacrimal sac.

Ammon operation: Surgical technique for epicanthus removal. Narrow strip of skin is removed with undermining of epicanthal flaps and primary closure.

amniotic infection syndrome of Blane: Fetal sepsis due to swallowing of contaminated intrauterine contents.

Amoss sign: Indicates presence of back pain when patient rises from supine to sitting position with hands placed well behind body for support.

Ampere postulate (law): Relationship between electric current and resulting magnetic field; concept is important in nuclear magnetic imaging.

Amplatz coronary catheter: Thin, J -shaped device placed into femoral vascular system; used to inject dye during coronary angiography.

Amplatz dilators: Instruments used for mechanical dilation of ureters or percutaneous access tract to kidney. Set includes 8F catheter, which is passed over guidewire, and sequentially larger dilators (up to 30F–36F), which are placed until desired caliber is reached.

Amplatz sheath: Instrument placed percutaneously into kidney collecting system after Amplatz dilator has enlarged ureter; allows further access to collecting system and tamponades tract.

ampulla of Thoma: One of multiple small terminal dilations in splenic pulp.

ampulla of Vater: Slightly dilated portion of distal common bile duct that terminates in papilla-type opening on posterior medial wall of 2nd part of duodenum/pancreatic duct junction. Tumors here manifested by jaundice; weight loss and dull, achy abdominal pain.

Amsler chart: Graphic diagram used to detect defects in central visual field, which can be used to monitor severity of macular degeneration. Series of grids and

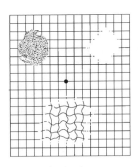

Amsler chart

parallel lines is placed 35.5 cm from patient, and missing areas and distorted areas are used to test for scotomata and metamorphopsia, respectively.

Amsler marker: Type of caliper used to mark spot for cautery in Gonin operation.

Amspacher-Messenbaugh osteotomy: Distal humeral incision to correct cubitus varus and rotation deformity of elbow.

Amsterdam criteria: Standards that describe risk of developing hereditary nonpolyposis colon cancer. Only 1 of following need be true for risk to be considered high: 3 relatives with colon cancer (2 of 3 1st-degree relatives); 1st-degree relative who develops colon cancer before 50 years of age; occurrence of colon cancer in 2 generations.

Amsterdam dwarf: Short stature associated with de Lange syndrome.

Amstutz-Wilson osteotomy: Surgical procedure to correct congenital coxa vara.

Amussat operation: Transverse abdominal incision used to expose colon.

Amussat valves: Posterior urethral valves.

Amussat valves: Spiral folds of mucosa in cystic duct.

Anagnostakis operation: Surgical technique for repair of entropion.

Anagnostakis operation: Surgical technique for removal of ingrowing eyelashes.

Ancell disease (Ancell-Spiegler disease, turban tumors): Multiple small scalp lesions, usu. benign cylindromas. Condition is autosomal dominant and more common in females. Onset occurs in childhood.

Andermann syndrome (Charlevoix syndrome): Agenesis of corpus callosum with mental and growth retardation, progressive motor neuropathy, paraparesis, and seizures. Condition is congenital, with both autosomal recessive and X-linked forms.

Andernach ossicles (wormian bones): Small bones found in sutures of skull, most commonly in fontanelles and lambdoid suture.

Andersch and Gibson test: Quantitative test for fibrinogen in blood.

Andersch ganglion: Inferior or petrosal ganglion of CN IX, which carries both sensory and motor fibers; lies in lower part of jugular foramen and is connected to superior cervical ganglion by fine nerve strand.

Andersch nerve: Tympanic nerve originating from Andersch ganglion; carries sensory and parasympathetic fibers to tympanic cavity, ear canal, mastoid air cells, and parotid gland.

Anders disease: See Dercum disease.

Andersen disease: Type 4 glycogen storage disease with

accumulation of abnormal glycogen, resulting in cirrhosis; caused by deficiency of branching enzyme 1, 4-glucan and 1, 5-glucan-6-glucosyl transferase in liver and muscle (primarily). Condition manifests in infancy as failure to thrive.

Andersen syndrome: Vitamin A deficiency, bronchiectasis, and pancreatic cystic fibrosis.

Anderson disease (familial osteodysplasia): Congenital hypoplasia of midface, abnormal mandible (decreased bigonial width and widened angle), large ears, hypertension, and kyphoscoliosis; autosomal recessive condition.

Anderson disease (hypobetalipoproteinemia): Low levels of β apoproteins in blood; intestinal wall becomes engorged with fat-containing enterocytes. Condition is marked by severe diarrhea in infancy and variable growth retardation and mild mental retardation. Serum shows low levels of HDL, LDL, and tocopherol. Treatment is restriction of dietary fats with supplementation of fatty acids and vitamins A and E.

Anderson grind test (medial-lateral grind test): Used to detect meniscus injuries of knee. Patient lies supine, and examiner lifts leg to be tested and alternately places knee under flexion and valgus stress and extension and varus stress. Positive result is "grinding" sensation felt with examiner's opposite hand when placed over anterior knee being tested.

Anderson phenomenon: Presence of RBCs on microscopic examination of stools in amebic dysentery.

Anderson procedure: External fixation to effect tibial lengthening in unequal leg lengths.

Anderson procedure: Reconstruction of hypopharynx and cervical esophagus using bilateral, rectangular flaps.

Anderson-Adson scalp retractor: Instrument used in plastic surgery.

Anderson-D'Alonzo classification: Descriptive system for C2 odontoid fractures. Type 1, avulsion fracture of tip; type 2, fracture running to edge of vertebral body; type 3, extension into cancellous bone of vertebral body.

Anderson-Fowler procedure: Use of wedge osteotomy of distal lateral calcaneus, tibial bone graft, wedge osteotomy of medial cuneiform, and capsulotomy of talonavicular joint to treat pes planus.

Anderson-Hutchins procedure: Insertion of bone pins and subsequent casting to stabilize tibial fractures.

Anderson-Pindborg syndrome: Congenital growth retardation, permanent hair loss starting at 1 year of age, hypoplasia of face and variable optic atrophy, pectus excavatum, polycystic kidneys, umbilical hernia, and glaucoma.

Greatly shortened life span; autosomal recessive condition.

Andes disease: Altitude sickness caused by overly rapid ascent to high altitude.

Andogsky disease: Chronic eczema in neck, flexor areas, elbows, and knees; onset in childhood, with bilateral cataracts beginning in 3rd decade. Associated conditions include asthma, uveitis, and keratoconjunctivitis. Severe cases may progress to leonine facies.

Andrade indicator: Positive for acid-producing organism if sample grown in a solution of acid fuchsin glucose, sodium hydroxide, and peptone produces purple-red color.

Andrade syndrome: Familial amyloid polyneuropathy found most commonly in persons of Portuguese descent; marked by abnormal transthyretin with methionine substituted for valine at position 30 of prealbumin molecule. Amyloid deposits occur in spinal nerve roots, autonomic ganglia, and peripheral nerves.

Andrade-MacNab procedure: Cervical occiput fusion via anterior approach.

André Thomas sign: Exaggeration of claw effect seen in claw–hand deformity due to low ulnar nerve palsy. Wrist flexion magnifies claw effect when attempts are made to extend finger.

Andre Thomas sign: Indication of cerebellar lesion if during performance of finger-to-nose test, patient's arm rebounds when asked to raise arm above head and then allow it fall onto their head.

Andre Thomas sign: Pinching trapezius muscle causes piloerection cephalad to spinal cord lesion.

Andresen appliance: Functional orthodontic activator.

Andrew syndrome: Recurring pustular eruptions on palms and soles.

Andrews maneuver: See Brandt-Andrews maneuver.

Andrews procedure: Iliotibial band tenodesis; used to treat anterior cruciate ligament laxity.

Andrew-Minneapolis hemoglobin: Type of high-oxygen affinity that produces erythrocytosis; lysine molecule in β 144(HC1) position is replaced by asparagine.

Andy Gump deformity: Facial profile with "weak chin" due to loss of soft and hard tissue in floor of mouth and anterior mandible; occurs most commonly after loss of anterior mandible following ablative cancer surgery.

Anel probe: Very small-diameter probe used to intubate lacrimal ducts.

Angelchik device: Horseshoe-shaped Silastic band placed around distal esophagus through abdominal incision;

used to keep distal esophagus intra-abdominal to correct gastroesophageal reflux disease.

Angelman syndrome ("happy puppet syndrome"): Jerky movements of arms and legs, uncontrollable laughing, enlarged tongue, and speech difficulties; onset in early childhood. Cause is defect on chromosome 15 inherited from mother. Eponym is misnomer.

Angelucci syndrome: Flushing palpitations and excitable demeanor in setting of vernal conjunctivitis and photophobia; symptoms are usu. worse in springtime. Severity decreases as patient ages.

Anger camera: Scintillation camera used to form image of radionuclide distribution. Radiation interacts with large sodium iodide crystal, which produces light pulses that are converted to image on cathode ray tube.

Anghelescu sign: Test for vertebral body disease; positive if patient is unable to lift spine off flat surface while placing weight on head and heels.

Angle classification: System that describes dental occlusion. Class 1 (normal), mesiobuccal cusp of 1st maxillary molar fits into mesiobuccal groove of 1st mandibular molar; class 2, mesiobuccal cusp of 1st maxillary molar is closer to dental midline than mesiobuccal groove of 1st mandibular molar; class 3, mesiobuccal cusp of 1st maxillary molar is distal to mesiobuccal groove of 1st mandibular molar.

angle of Boogaard: Basal angle of skull on midsagittal radiographic view; normal value is $118°–147°$.

angle of His: Anatomic area formed by junction of distal esophagus and cardia of stomach. If "acuteness" of angle is maintained, gastroesophageal reflux disease is unlikely.

angle of Louis (sternal angle): Cartilaginous disk forming joint between cephalad and caudal sternal bones, which is felt as transverse ridge beneath skin at level of 2nd rib.

angle of Ludwig: See angle of Louis.

angle of McRae: Normal basal angle of skull $(120°–140°)$ on midsagittal view.

angle of Rolando: Angle formed by central sulcus and superomedial border of brain; average is approximately $72°$.

Ångström law: Light wavelengths absorbed by substance are identical to that given off when object is luminous.

angstrom unit: 1/10000 micron; technically defined in terms of red line wavelength of cadmium.

Anitschkow myocytes: Enlarged mesenchymal cells found in cardiac muscle in rheumatic fever.

Ann Arbor classification: Staging system used in Hodgkin disease. Stage 1, nodal involvement in 1 region only; stage 2, nodal involvement in 2 or more regions on same side of diaphragm; stage 3, nodal involvement on both sides of diaphragm (spleen counts as lymph node); stage 4, disseminated involvement of extranodal organs (liver, lung, brain), with or without lymph node involvement; subtype A, no night sweats, fever, weight loss or pruritus; subtype B, presence of night sweats, fever, weight loss, or pruritus.

Anrep effect (homotropic autoregulation): Positive inotropic effect seen with acute increase in aortic pressure (independent of heart muscle fiber length).

Ansbacher effect: Optical illusion demonstrated by placing illuminated arc at edge of rotating disk; arc appears shorter as disk rotates faster.

Ansbacher unit: Dosage unit of vitamin K.

Anstie test: Used to indicate toxic alcohol level in urine if mixture of urine, potassium dichromate, sulfuric acid, and urine produces green color.

Anthony stain: Placement of histologic specimen in milk smear, crystal violet, and copper sulfate to distinguish bacterial capsule (unstained) from cell (deeply colored).

Antigone complex: Sacrifice of person's own life for sake of loved one; usu. love is nonsexual in nature (e.g., siblings).

anti-Monson curve (reverse curve): Development of flat or grooved occlusal surfaces when excessive tooth wear eliminates cusps; slope of mandibular teeth becomes tilted facially rather than lingually.

Anton disease: Blindness in patients who insist they can see; such denial of physiologic state is regarded as hallucinatory. Other features include confabulation and sensation on contralateral side as stimulus.

Anton syndrome (Anton-Babinsky syndrome): Condition usu. seen in patients with dense hemiplegia of left side who deny contiguity of that side; occurs in some patients with brain damage who are unaware of their mental (esp. abstraction) or physical impairment. Cause is lesion in superior parietal cerebral cortex. If lesion extends into adjacent frontal, temporal, or occipital lobes, syndrome may be associated with hallucinations, blunted affect, or abnormal space perception.

Anton test: Used to identify *Listeria monocytogenes;* culture specimen is injected into rabbit conjunctiva to determine pathogenicity.

Antoni patterns A and B: Description of cellular arrangements found in schwannomas (neurilemmoma). A, tightly packed, spindle-shaped cells with eosinophilic cytoplasm and indistinct cell membranes and oval-shaped nuclei that have palisading configuration (Verocay bodies); B, more disorganized cell arrangement in mucoid matrix, which is more similar to neurofibroma.

antrum of Willis: Dilated prepylorus portion of stomach.

anus of Rusconi: Blastopore.

Anzio effect: Role of psychological readiness in patients to experience and report improvement in pain and symptoms. In World War II, Allied soldiers wounded in Anzio, Italy, apparently responded significantly better to treatment than did civilians, who were trapped in battle area and could not escape war. For soldiers, injury meant return to safety at home, with improvement allowing increased activities in noncombat setting.

Apathy medium (gum syrup medium): Water-soluble medium used for mounting histology specimens; contains cane sugar, acacia, thymol, and distilled H_2O.

Apert syndrome: Type 1 acrocephalosyndactyly; characterized by congenital premature closing of skull sutures with peaked head, fusion of 2nd–5th fingers with 1 common nail, mental retardation, cleft palate or highly arched and constricted palate, acne of forearms, and defects of hair shafts. Inheritance is both sporadic and autosomal dominant.

Apert-Crouzon syndrome: Type 2 acrocephalosyndactyly; characterized by facial features typical of Crouzon syndrome with severe hypoplasia of maxilla and fusion of 2nd–4th fingers. Condition is autosomal dominant.

Apert-Gallais syndrome: See De Crecchio syndrome.

Apgar score: System used to assess newborn infant's adaptation to extrauterine environment at 1 and 5 minutes postbirth. Five characteristics—color (**a**ppearance), heart rate (**p**ulse), muscle tone (**g**rasp), respiratory effort (**a**irway), and reflex irritability (**r**eflex)—are scored on scale of 0–2 and added. Best possible score is "10 and 10."

Apley law: The recurrent abdominal pain is experienced the greater the distance from umbilicus greater the chance of organic etiology.

Apley scratch test: Used as initial screen for gross abnormalities of shoulder motion. Patient's arms are abducted with palms and backs of hands together, and patient then moves arms around back in attempt to scratch contralateral shoulder.

Apley sign: Method for distinguishing ligament from meniscus injuries. Prone patient flexes knee, and examiner pushes and pulls to elicit tibial rotation. Pain during compression is likely meniscal, and pain during pulling is likely ligamentous.

Apley test: Evaluation of meniscal injury to knee, in which patient lies prone with knee flexed to 90°. Positive result is pain in knee when examiner distracts and compresses knee joint.

apophysis of Ingrassia: Minor wing of sphenoid bone, which articulates with frontal bone and partially forms orbital roof and anterior cranial fossa floor.

apophysis of Rau: Slender anterior process of malleus running anteriorly and inferior to petrotympanic fissure.

apparatus of Goormaghtigh: Juxtaglomerular cells.

Appolito suture: See Gély suture.

Appunn lamella: Early device composed of thin strip of metal with disk attached to end; measures hearing sensitivity for low-frequency sounds.

Appunn tonometer: Early device used in acoustic research that could produce multiple sounds 4 cycles apart over 2–3 octaves.

Apt test: Method for differentiating maternal from neonatal blood in which supernatant from centrifuged sample is mixed with sodium hydroxide. Maternal blood with hemoglobin A changes from pink to yellow; neonatal blood with hemoglobin F remains pink.

aqueduct of Cotunnius: Small opening connecting vestibule of inner ear to posterior petrous part of temporal bone; anatomic space is traversed by arteriole, venule, and endolymphatic duct.

aqueduct of Sylvius (midbrain aqueduct): Anatomic space connecting 3rd and 4th brain ventricles.

Arakawa test (reagent): Used to detect peroxidase in milk.

Aran law: Basilar skull fractures result from trauma forces that traverse shortest circle.

Aran-Duchenne disease: Weakness and atrophy of limbs and trunk with fasciculation of affected muscles, which usu. begins in small muscles of hands or less frequently upper arm/shoulder muscles and slowly progresses to legs; X-linked recessive condition. Disorder is marked by degeneration of anterior horn cells of spinal cord, elevated creatinine kinase, and cardiomyopathy. Course is occasionally benign, with prolonged survival.

Arantius ligament: Fibrous cord in liver, representing embryonic remnant of fetal ductus venosus.

Arantius nodule (Bianchi nodule, Morgagni nodule): Small nodular mass at edge of semilunar valve on aorta and pulmonary arteries.

Arantius ventricle: Terminal depression of median sulcus as it leads into central canal in floor of 4th ventricle.

arc of Riolan: Short arterial loop running from root of superior mesenteric artery to inferior mesenteric artery or 1 of its branches; condition is frequently and inaccurately described as marginal anastomosis at left colic flexure. Condition occurs in 7% of individuals. Reimplantation during aortic aneurysm surgery should be considered.

arcade of Frohse: Aponeurotic proximal border of superficial part of supinator muscle in forearm. Posterior interosseus nerve runs beneath this structure, and deep radial nerve runs through adjacent tunnel.

arcade of Struthers: Fibrous portion of distal medial triceps; may cause entrapment of ulnar nerve.

arch of Corti: Anatomic structure formed by rows of inner and outer pillar cells in organ of Corti.

Archer disease: Supravalvular aortic stenosis; marked by cyanosis in infancy, unequal pulses on left and right neck and arms, and systolic murmur. Condition is more common in males. Treatment is surgery.

Archetti test: Method for detection of caffeine or uric acid, which uses boiling mixture of potassium ferricyanide, nitric acid, and H_2O added to sample; if either substance is present, blue precipitate forms.

Archibald sign: Dimpling of skin over shortened 4th and 5th fingers when skin is clenched; occurs in Albright hereditary osteodystrophy.

Archimedes principle: Body placed in liquid is buoyed up by force equal to weight of displaced liquid.

Arctic anemia: Microcytic anemia that eventually progresses to normocytic; caused by chronic exposure to cold environment.

area of Laimer: Anatomic area on outside of posterior wall of esophagus where scanty longitudinal muscles form V shape on circular esophageal muscle fibers.

Argand burner: Oil or gas burner with air supplied by inner tube.

Argentinian hemorrhagic fever: Chills, fever, myalgia, hemorrhage, neurologic deficits, and leukopenia; caused by Junin arenavirus. Transmission probably occurs via contact with infected rodent urine.

Argonz-Del Castillo syndrome: See Del Castillo syndrome.

Argyll Robertson pupils: Bilateral, small, irregular pupils responsive to accommodation but nonresponsive to light stimulation. Condition is seen in CNS syphilis and occasionally in alcoholic avitaminosis and encephalitis. Vision is normal.

Arias syndrome: See Crigler-Najjar syndrome type 2.

Arias-Stella phenomenon (effect, reaction): Endometrial changes characterized by enlarged epithelial cells with irregular, hypertrophic nuclei in luminal part of cells and foamy, vacuolated cytoplasm; seen in trophoblastic disease or ectopic or intrauterine pregnancy. Condition may also occur in patients taking oral contraceptives.

Aries-Pitanguy mammaplasty: Surgical technique that provides moderate reduction of breast tissue.

Arieti-Gray disease: Multiform angiosis and aneurysms of circle of Willis, intracerebral vessels, and aorta; causes mental deficiency and seizures.

Arion sling: Mechanical device used to aid in eyelid closure when orbicularis function is impaired; silicon band is placed in pretarsal space that encircles eyelids.

Aristotle illusion (anomaly experiment; tactile diplopia): Illusion produced by crossing 2nd and 3rd fingers and placing thin rod between fingertips; tactile sensation is of 2 rods touching skin.

Arizona hinshawii: Organisms infrequently found in mycotic aneurysms.

Arizona support: Suspension device with adjustable anterior thigh pad for lower leg fractures.

Arkin disease: See Bayford-Autenrieth condition.

Arkless-Graham syndrome (acrodysostosis, Maroteaux-Malamut syndrome): Uncommon congenital growth retardation with eventual loss of joint mobility, mental deficiency, hypogonadism, middle ear infections, brachycephaly, and hypoplastic maxilla; mostly occurs in children of older parents. Etiology is unknown.

Arloing-Courmont test: See Widal test.

Arlt disease: Contact infection (can be congenital) of external eye causing tearing, eyelid edema and spasm, photophobia, mucous discharge, conjunctival blebs, and corneal scarring and opacities. Cause is *Chlamydia trachomatis, Lymphogranuloma venereum,* or *Bartonella.* Treatment is topical antibiotics and tetracycline.

Arlt operation: Surgical replacement of eyelashes in trichiasis.

Arlt sinus: See sinus of Maier.

Arlt-Davidsen syndrome: Seizures, brownish hypoplastic teeth, and cataracts.

Armanni-Ebstein kidney (nephropathy): Marked by glycogen-containing cells in straight portion of proximal convoluted tubercle; condition sometimes occurs in diabetes, esp. if untreated.

Armendares syndrome: Congenital retinitis pigmentosa, craniosynostosis, eyelid ptosis, scant eyebrows, microcephaly, single palmar crease, stubby fingers, and dwarfism; intelligence is normal.

Armstrong acromionectomy: Procedure most useful in surgical treatment of supraspinatus syndrome or bursitis. Patient is placed in lateral decubitus position, and saber-cut incision is made over acromioclavicular joint. Periosteum is incised lateral to acromioclavicular joint and retracted medially, and acromion is divided with separation of deltoid muscle and with division of acromioclavicular and coracoacromial ligaments. This allows inspection and excision of bursa tissue.

Armstrong procedure: Surgical removal of acromion to correct rotator cuff impingement.

Arnason syndrome: Early onset of cerebral hemorrhage; associated with amyloid deposits in cerebral vessels. Condition is autosomal dominant condition and occurs in Icelandic families.

Arndt-Gottron syndrome (scleromyxedema): Diffuse papular lesions with underlying skin thickening, which limits movement of finger and facial features; onset in 3rd–5th decade.

Arneth count: Classification of neutrophils with differing nuclear lobes. Percentages in normal blood smear: 1 lobe, 5%; 2 lobes, 35%; 3 lobes, 41%; 4 lobes, 17%; 5 lobes, 2%. "Shift to left" involves higher percentage of 1-lobed nuclei and usu. represents bacterial infection. "Shift to right" involves higher percentage of multilobed

nuclear and indicates folic acid or vitamin B_{12} deficiency.

Arneth group: Whispering pectoriloquy, bronchial murmur, and bronchophony seen in lung hepatization.

Arnold bodies: Erythrocyte fragments.

Arnold brace: Posterior back support with molded sacroiliac piece and rigid scapular thoracic harness.

Arnold bundle: Frontal cerebropontine tract arising in cortex of frontal lobe, which traverses anterior internal capsule and medial cerebral peduncle base and terminates in gray substance of pons.

Arnold canal: Opening in petrous temporal bone traversed by auricular branch of vagus nerve.

Arnold ganglion (otic ganglion): Motor and sensory ganglion of mandibular nerve; lies in zygomatic fossa below foramen ovale.

Arnold head: Parietal bone bossing, small skull, maxillary hypoplasia, and coarse facial features.

Arnold ligament: Small fibrous band running from body of incus to tympanic cavity roof and just posterior to superior malleolar ligament.

Arnold nerve: Auricular branch of vagus arising from superior vagal ganglion and traversing stylomastoid foramen; receives branch from petrosal ganglion of CN IX and supplies part of tympanic membrane, external acoustic meatal floor, and cranial surface of auricle.

Arnold neuralgia: Reflex cough with pain in suboccipital area radiating to neck or shoulder. Palpation in posterior ear area causes tenderness due to irritation (e.g., friction, temperature changes) of auricular branch of CNX.

Arnold Pick syndrome: Inability to fix gaze on objects in visual field; associated with central atrophy.

Arnold-Chiari malformation (type I) [Celand-Arnold-Chiari malformation, adult-type]: Abnormality of occipital bone, medulla, and cerebellum with hydrocephalus; cerebellar tonsils extend down into upper cervical canal (below foramen magnum).

Arnold-Chiari malformation (type II): Cerebellar tonsils extend farther down spinal canal than in type I; narrowed 4th ventricle also extends below foramen magnum. Upper cord has dorsal hump, displacing cervical nerve roots. Condition is associated with stridor, respiratory dysfunction, and cor pulmonale; it occurs in children and with hydrocephalus and myelomeningocele.

Arnold-Chiari malformation (type III): Cerebellum herniates into widened cleft of upper cervical spine; rare condition seen with meningocele.

Aronson-Prager procedure: Percutaneous pin fixation for pediatric supracondylar fracture.

Arrhenius acid: Substance that increases H^+ concentration and lowers pH when mixed with aqueous solution; also reacts with alkali to form salts, produces sour taste, and turns litmus paper red.

Arrhenius equation: Expression describing effect of temperature on reaction rate constant. Equation is $k = Ae^{-\Delta E}a/RT$, where k is rate constant, R is gas constant, A is frequency factor constant, T is absolute temperature, e is base of natural logarithms (ΔE_a), and ΔE_a is activation energy.

Arrhigi point: ECG electrode site; 2–3 cm to left lateral side of 7th thoracic vertebra.

Arroyo sign (asthenocoria): Sluggish pupillary light reflex; seen in hypoadrenal states.

Arruga procedure: Surgical correction of detached retina using sutures placed in ring around lesion to mechanically tack retina in place. Risks are higher-than-normal rates of cataract formation and scleral erosion.

arterial circle of Vieussens: Area in pulmonary conus section of heart in which small branches of right coronary artery anastomose with left coronary artery branches.

arteries of Mueller: Helicine arteries in penis; engorgement during sexual arousal causes erection.

artery of Adamkiewicz: Branch of anterior spinal artery that supplies thoracolumbar core (T5–conus); poses risk with repair of abdominal aortic aneurysm. Ligation causes paraplegia/paraparesis (anterior spinal syndrome).

artery of Huebner (recurrent artery of Huebner, medial striate artery:) Arterial branch off anterior cerebral artery just before entry into circle of Willis.

artery of Percheron: Posterior thalamosubthalamoparamedian artery.

artery of Zinn: See Zinn circle.

Arthur point scale of performance tests: Intelligence test for children using picture assembly, form boards, and block and stencil design; useful in non-English speaking and deaf patients.

Arthus reaction: Edema, hemorrhage, and necrosis at injection site of antigen in already sensitized patient, resulting in antigen–antibody complexes, complement, anaphylatoxins, aggregated neutrophils, lysosomal enzymes, and permeable vessel walls; mediated primarily by antibodies, rather than T cells.

Arthus-type phenomenon: Type 3 hypersensitivity reaction initiated by antigen–antibody complexes.

Asboe-Hansen disease: Congenital eosinophilia, bullae, and pigment dermatitis; can occur as 1st phase of Bloch-Sulzberger syndrome.

ascending veins of Rosenthal: Large superficial cerebral veins at base of brain, which drain into sagittal and cavernosus sinuses on inferior surface of frontal sinus; into straight sinus on occipital lobe; and into transverse and superior petrosal sinuses on temporal lobe surface.

Asch operation: Early 20th-century surgical technique for correction of abnormal septum using fracture and repositioning.

Asch situation: Experimental test of social conformity. Patient is placed in situation in which correct judgment is deemed incorrect by group of tester's confederates, thus putting pressure on patient to conform.

Ascher disease: Congenital double lip associated with nontoxic thyroid gland enlargement.

Ascher glass-rod phenomenon: Sign of glaucoma; positive when aqueous humor enters conjunctival vessel when glass rod compresses recipient vessel, and negative when blood enters into conjunctival or subconjunctival vessel when glass rod compresses recipient vessel.

Ascher syndrome (Laffer-Ascher syndrome): Recurrent eyelid swelling followed by atrophy of skin and subcutaneous tissue of eyelid and lip and gum thickening. Treatment is plastic surgery.

Ascherson membrane: Thin casein layer surrounding milk globules.

Aschheim-Zondek test: Early, widely used pregnancy test; based on ability of human chorionic gonadotropin in urine of pregnant woman to induce ovulation in experimental animals.

Aschner inverted phenomenon (reflex): Increase in heart rate when eyes are compressed.

Aschner phenomenon (reflex): Decreased heart rate when eyes are compressed; normal slowing is 5–13 beats/min.

Aschoff node (Aschoff-Tawara node): AV node located in right atrium between coronary sinus opening and tricuspid valve; composed of Purkinje fibers that receive electrical impulses from sinoatrial node before distributing them to ventricles. Blood supply is right coronary artery.

Aschoff nodule (body): Histiocytic granuloma formed in response to fibrinoid swelling and necrosis of perivascular connective tissue. Histiocytes phagocytize fibrinoid material, forming microscopic giant cells; end stage is connective tissue scar with fibroblasts and collagen deposition that is susceptible to formation of additional Aschoff nodules and scarring. Condition occurs esp. in heart and sometimes in rheumatic fever joints.

Ascolli test (reaction): Method for detecting anthrax infection that uses precipitin test with antiserum and tissue extract.

Aselli gland: Collection of lymph nodes at root of mesentery.

Ash system: Grading scheme for transitional cell carcinoma. Grade 1—usu. pedunculated, soft pink, delicate, frond-like papillary structures with central fibrovascular core, transitional cells almost identical to normal, with few mitoses; grade 2—more solid consistency than grade 1, more crowding and layering of cells, with enlarged nuclei and scattered mitoses; grade 3—sessile, cauliflower-type form, frequent ulceration and necrosis, with common mitoses; grade 4—sessile, necrotic, ulcerated, widely invasive, pronounced cellular atypia and pleomorphism, with frequent mitoses.

Ashby method (differential agglutination technique): Earliest reliable test for measuring RBC survival after transfusion; non-O blood type patient was given O cells and phlebotomized at routine intervals to measure O-cell decline. Method has largely been computerized and now used only for research purposes.

Asherman syndrome: Intrauterine fibrous adhesions that obliterate the uterine cavity; often caused by endometrial curettage.

Asherson disease:
Dysfunction of upper esophageal sphincter; marked by dysphagia, coughing, and defect of cricopharyngeal muscle relaxation (worse after consumption of liquids as opposed to solids). Condition is associated with bilateral recurrent laryngeal nerve injury or poliomyelitis affecting pharynx. Treatment is cricopharyngeal sphincter dilatation or (in severe cases) cricopharyngeal myotomy.

Ashkanazy cells: Large epithelial cells marked by oxyphilic changes; typically found in Hashimoto disease.

Ashman phenomenon:
Abnormal ventricular contraction causing a shortened cardiac cycle; associated with atrial arrhythmias.

Ashhurst classification:
System used to describe ankle fracture/sprains. *External rotation injuries* —1st degree, transsyndesmotic fibula fracture [1st degree (alternate), anterior tibiofibular ligament rupture]; 2nd degree, deltoid ligament rupture [2nd degree (alternate), medial malleolus avulsion]; 3rd degree, distal tibial and fibula fracture with external rotation. *Abduction injuries* —1st degree, transverse medial malleolus fracture; 2nd degree, deltoid ligament rupture or medial malleolus fracture with distal fibula fracture; 3rd degree, distal tibia fracture with lateral displacement of medial malleolus. *Adduction injuries* —1st degree, fibular malleolus avulsion; 2nd degree, fibular malleolus avulsion with vertical tibial shaft fracture; 3rd degree, supramalleolar fracture of fibula and tibia with medial displacement. *Long-axis compression fractures* —1st degree, marginal fracture of distal tibial plate; 2nd degree, comminuted tibial plafond fracture; 3rd degree, Gosselin V-fracture or T-Y fracture.

Ashhurst sign: Widening of overlap of fibula and distal anterior tubercle seen on radiography in ankle diastasis.

Asian cobra: *Naja naja;* highly venomous hooded snake found from India to Philippines.

Ask-Upmark kidney:
Segmental spongiform hypoplasia of kidney marked by transverse indentations with dilations of underlying calices; usu. affects girls. Treatment is segmental resection, if possible, or medical management of hypertension and associated retinopathy occasionally requires kidney transplantation.

Askin tumor: Malignant, small, round-cell tumor resembling neuroblastoma with rosette-like structures; usu. occurs on chest wall.

Asnis procedure: Placement of cannulated screw for fixation of slipped capital femoral epiphysis.

Asnis screw: Cannulated screw with reversed thread; used in hip fractures.

Asperger syndrome:
Primarily European term for childhood condition closely

resembling schizoid personality disorder; marked by unusual interest in electronics wiring diagrams and collecting of objects. Autistic-like social interaction problems are characteristic; patients often have rapid, bizarre vocal intonations and overdeveloped skill or mental ability in 1 area.

Aspinall progressive tests: Series of clinical maneuvers performed by examiner on patient in both sitting and lying positions to assess vertebral artery pathology.

Aspinall transverse ligament test: Used to detect hypermobility of atlantoaxial articulation of spine. Supine patient flexes head, and examiner supports occiput with hand and applies anterior force to atlas (test should be performed with extreme caution). Positive result is sensation of pain or "lump in throat" as atlas moves toward esophagus.

Assézat triangle: Facial triangle formed by imaginary lines running through points on nasion, and basion, and the alveolar point.

Assmann disease: Aseptic necrosis of 1st metatarsal head.

Astler-Coller classification: 1954 modification of Kirklin classification of colorectal tumor, using C1 as lesion limited to bowel wall with positive lymph nodes and C2 as penetrating into pericolonic fat with positive lymph nodes.

Astler-Coller classification (modified): Most common system used today to describe colorectal cancer. A, mucosal involvement only; B1, invasion into muscularis; B2, invasion into serosa; B3, invasion into adjacent organs; C, lesions identical to those in B but with lymph node involvement.

Åström-Mancall-Richardson syndrome (progressive multifocal leukoencephalopathy): Central and peripheral demyelination with hemiparesis, blindness, aphasia, and dementia. Associated disorders include infectious (Papovaviridae), neoplastic, or granulomatosis conditions. Death usu. occurs within 1–2 years of onset.

Astrup method: Evaluation of acid–base physiology using standard bicarbonate (24.5 mEq) and base excess values.

Astwood test: Sucking, chewing, and swallowing movements after stimulation of lips; seen in diffuse cerebral disease.

Atkin syndrome: Small mouth, cleft lip, cerebral cysts, heart defects, deformed ears, webbed neck, and split hands and feet; congenital condition with X-linked inheritance.

Atkins-Wolff procedure: Resection of milk duct to treat chronic discharge in lactating breast.

Atkinson block: Technique used to achieve retrobulbar

anesthesia before cataract surgery. Injection is made into orbicularis oculi muscle cone with eye in supranasal position to cause akinesia of muscle.

Atlanta brace:
Foot–ankle–knee orthosis used in Legg-Calvé-Perthes disease; allows walking without crutches.

atrophoderma of Pasini and Pierini: Atrophic, blue-brown plaques developing on trunk; seen most commonly on backs of young women. Condition resolves slowly over several months.

Aub-Dubois table: Table giving average rates of metabolism for individuals of different ages.

Auberger blood group: Serum protein occurring in 80% of Caucasians.

Aubert diaphragm: Device used to control amount of light present in experiments involving vision testing. Presence of 2 overlapping leaves with notches cut out means that different-sized square apertures can be formed.

Aubert phenomenon: Illusion that vertical line on empty background is tilted in opposite direction when observer tilts head to 1 side.

Aubert-Fleischel paradox: Illusion that moving object moves faster when observer focuses on background rather than object.

Audouin microsporon: *Microsporum audouini;* ringworm fungus that is common cause of childhood tinea capitis.

Audry syndrome: Hyperostosis of feet and hands, coarse facies, and digital clubbing.

Auenbrugger sign: Epigastric bulging due to pericardial effusion.

Auer classification: System for describing DNA histograms in carcinoma.

Auer rod (body): Oblong inclusion found in myeloid or monocytic leukemia cells, which stain azurophilic and produce positive reaction with peroxidase and acid phosphatase; seen in acute myelogenous leukemia (5% of cases), rarely in refractory anemia, and never in lymphocytic leukemia or in normal individuals.

Auerbach plexus (myenteric plexus): Parasympathetic ganglion cells found in connective tissue between muscle layers in esophagus, jejunum, and ileum; supplies motor function to muscle layers and secretory stimulus to mucosa.

Aufranc-Turner prosthesis: Modification of Charnley hip prosthesis; uses larger femoral head for increased stability.

Aufrecht sign: Soft respiratory sound heard over jugular fossa occurring in tracheal stenosis.

Auger effect: Process by which atom existing in electron-capture excited state returns to ground state. As electron moves from outer orbital to vacant orbital, emitted photon is absorbed by another electron in same atom and then ejected from atom.

Auger electron: Particle ejected from atom during Auger effect.

Aujeszky disease: Pseudorabies.

Auspitz sign: Positive when scratching causes punctate bleeding points in skin lesion; suggestive of psoriasis.

Auspitz syndrome: See Alibert-Bazin disease.

Aussage test: Method used to measure ability to recount previously made observations with accuracy.

Austin Flint murmur: Diastolic murmur occurring in marked aortic insufficiency (regurgitation); relatively short and faint and lacks opening "snap." Sound is best heard at apex; it is often confused with murmur of mitral stenosis. Cause is interference with ventricular filling due to regurgitant jet.

Austin Flint respiration: Hollow sound similar to that of air being blown over mouth of open bottle; occurs in pneumothorax, lung cavities caused by bronchiectasis and TB, and in effusions causing lung collapse.

Austin Moore arthroplasty: Reconstruction of hip joint using Austin Moore prosthesis.

Austin procedure: Chevron-shaped osteotomy of distal 1st metatarsal; used to correct bunion.

Austin syndrome: Disorder caused by deficiency in 1 or more of following enzymes; steroid sulfatase, arylsulfatase A and B, galactosamine-6-sulfatase, iduronate-2-sulfatase, or heparan sulfatidase; marked by mental deterioration, blindness, scaly skin, demyelination and neurologic deficits, and organomegaly. Onset is in early childhood, with death occurring in childhood.

Australian antigen: Hepatitis B surface antigen.

Australian octopus: *Hapalochlaena maculosa;* bite causes serious neurotoxicity by blocking sodium conduction. Complete paralysis and death occurs within minutes; if breathing is supported, neurotoxicity usu. resolves within 6–10 hours.

Australian tick typhus (Queensland typhus): Spotted fever caused by *Rickettsia australis.*

Austrian school of psychology (Graz school of psychology): Designation used to describe group of psychologists living and working in Austro-Hungary in late 1800s. Tenets included idea of mental processes as key psychological phenomenon; members promoted importance of sensory processes in scientific observation.

Austrian syndrome:
Pneumococcal pneumonia and meningitis in chronic alcoholism.

Auth device (Rotablator):
Diamond-studded, football-shaped burr (uses a "rotating over the wire" mechanism) that causes abrasive effect and effects atheroblation of intra-arterial plaque. Disadvantages are larger-than-desired fragments and nonexpandability, requiring complementary angioplasty.

autoeroticism: Sexual thoughts or acts that are initiated by the self; includes masturbation.

Avellino dystrophy: Granular corneal dystrophy with amyloid and hyaline deposits in stroma; usu. occurs centrally. Condition is autosomal dominant.

Avellis syndrome (Avellis-Longhi syndrome, jugular foramen syndrome): Ipsilateral paralysis of soft palate, larynx, and pharynx with contralateral loss of temperature and pain sensation; seen after thrombosis of vertebral artery or brainstem lesion. Ipsilateral Horner and contralateral corticospinal tract paralysis may result from involvement of spinothalamic tract, nucleus ambiguus, and bulbar nucleus of accessory nerve.

Avogadro law: Gases at equal volume, temperature, and pressure theoretically contain same number of molecules.

Avogadro number
(constant): 6.02246×10^{23};
number of particles in 1 mole of substance.

Axenfeld-Rieger anomaly
(Axenfeld syndrome): Strands of iris attached to a prominent and anteriorly displaced Schwalbe ring in eye. 50%–60% of affected patients develop glaucoma, usu. as juveniles. Condition may be autosomal dominant or sporadic.

Axenfeld-Schürenberg paralysis: Unilateral CN III paralysis; "relaxed" phase (mydriasis, upper lid ptosis, and abduction) cycles with "spastic" phase (myosis, upper lid lifting, and adduction). Condition manifests from birth to 1 year.

Ayala index: Calculation of intracerebral pressure as [(closing lumbar pressure $\times$ 10)/opening pressure] after 10 ml have been removed; poor correlation with clinical signs.

Ayer test: Positive result is equal pressures in cisterna magna and lumbar punctures in normal patients after correctly performed spinal block.

Ayerza disease: Polycythemia vera with chronic dyspnea, bronchitis, cyanosis, bone marrow hyperplasia, and hepatosplenomegaly; seen with pulmonary artery stenosis.

Ayerza-Arrillaga disease
(Ayerza syndrome): Pulmonary artery hypertension that may be associated with aneurysms in pulmonary artery. Possible causes are syphilitic obliteration of pulmonary artery and bronchopulmonary infection; condition may be congenital.

Ayoub-Shklar method: Uses acid fuchsin and aniline blue-orange G solution to stain keratin red, connective tissue deep blue, and prekeratin orange.

Ayre T-piece: 1930s pediatric anesthesia airway; early prototype for modern pediatric breathing systems.

Azimuth resolution (elevation resolution): Ability to determine spatial distance between 2 objects emitting or reflecting sound; important when describing ability of ultrasound beam to differentiate between 2 closely positioned objects. Determination is made by slice thickness of plane perpendicular to ultrasound transducer and beam, height of beam, and shape and size of transducer. Value is always less than axial resolution of beam.

Aztec ear (Cagot ear): Earlobe with missing lower part (tubercle).

Azua disease: Fever, infectious erythema, and exanthema, with thrombocytopenic purpura and variable hemolysis; caused by infection with human parvovirus B19. Condition affects mostly children.

Azzopardi-Salvadori classification: Histologic description of phyllodes tumors; uses benign, borderline malignant, and malignant designations.

Baastrup syndrome (Michotte syndrome): Development of vertebral joint degenerative disease with bony bridges forming between adjacent osteophytes.

Babbitt metal: Dental alloy.

Babcock operation: Saphenous vein stripping used for treatment of varicose veins. Long probe with an acorn-shaped tip is inserted into vein and then withdrawn, bringing vein with it.

Babcock sentence: Patients of normal intelligence and recall should be able to hear and repeat without error, "One thing a nation must have to become rich and great is a large secure supply of wood."

Babcock test: Used to determine milk fat content.

Babcock tissue forceps:
Instrument used to grasp internal organs.

Babès tubercle (node, nodule): Cell aggregation found around dead neurons in medulla and spinal ganglia; occurs in rabies and other encephalitis diseases.

Babès-Ernst bodies: Granules of polyphosphate in bacterial protoplasm (esp. *Corynebacterium diphtheriae*) that stain blue with methylene.

Babesia: Protozoa that causes malaria-like condition in cattle, sheep, and horses; can infect humans.

babesiosis: Protozoal infection causing fever, chills, myalgia, and hemolytic anemia; can occur as coinfection with Lyme disease. Vector is deer tick. Definitive diagnosis is detection of basket-shaped intraerythocyte parasites. Condition leads to severe and often fatal infections in splenectomized patients. Treatment is pentamidine, chloroquine phosphate, or increasingly, Mepron or Malarone.

Babinski pronator phenomenon: See Strümpell reflex.

Babinski reflex (phenomenon, sign, test): Dorsiflexion of 1st toe with flaring of other toes when sole of foot is stroked with rigid object; normal finding in infants with decreasing strength of response up to 2 years of age. Reflex is also seen in upper motor neuron disease and sometimes in severe intoxication and postictal states.

Babinski reinforcement sign: Patient sits on table with both legs dangling freely. When flexed fingers of one hand are pulled against other, extension of paretic leg occurs; seen in unilateral paralysis of leg.

Babinski sign: Positive for S1 pathology if ipsilateral Achilles reflex is diminished or absent.

Babinski sign: Positive if absence of palpable and visible platysma muscle contraction occurs when grimacing or opening mouth forcibly; seen in corticospinal hemiparesis and ipsilateral peripheral facial nerve lesions.

Babinski thigh reflex:
Patient lies supine with legs together and arms folded on abdomen. Attempts to rise to sitting position cause flexion of thigh and lifting of leg and heel off flat surface; seen in patients with unilateral paralysis of lower extremity.

Babinski-Fröhlich syndrome (Fröhlich dystrophy): Slipped capital femoral epiphysis.

Babinski-Nageotte syndrome: Ipsilateral paralysis of soft palate, pharynx, and larynx with loss of taste on posterior 1/3 of tongue, Horner syndrome, and contralateral spastic hemiplegia; also with loss of contralateral tactile and proprioceptive sensation as well as pain and temperature sensation of face. Causes include partial or total occlusion of vertebral artery and branches secondary to scattered, multiple lesions in the medullary pyramid and sensory tracts, reticular formation, and cerebellar peduncles.

Babinski-Vaquez syndrome: Development of cardiac and arterial pathology along with abnormal quadriceps and triceps reflexes, meningoencephalitis, and Argyll Robertson pupils; seen in late-stage syphilis.

Babinsky syndrome: Early 1900s term for cerebellar ataxia associated with multiple sclerosis.

Babinsky-Weil test: Performed by having patient with eyes shut walk fowards and backwards in a straight line several times. Positive result is bendung to one side when moving forward and to other side when moving backward; indicates labyrinthine disease.

Babkin reflex: Pressure on palms causes mouth to open; occurs in infants.

Baccelli sign (aphonic pectoriloquy): Whisper detectable over chest when patient with large pleural effusion speaks.

Bachman test: Method for diagnosis of trichinosis with intradermal skin test. Powdered trichina larvae antigen is injected; small, white swelling that develops 15 minutes later indicates past or current infection.

bacille Calmette-Guérin (BCG): see Calmette-Guérin bacillus.

Backhaus towel clamp: Sharp-tipped, perforating, ring-handle surgical instrument used to fasten drapes on sterile field.

Badelon classification: System used to describe pediatric lateral condylar fractures of humerus. As visualized on radiographs Type 1, nondisplaced fracture visible on one view only; type 2, easily visible fracture with minimal displacement; type 3, fracture with displacement > 2 mm visible on all views; type 4, displacement with complete separation.

Bado classification: System used to describe ulnar fractures with radial head dislocation. Type 1, ulnar diaphysis with anterior angulation and dislocation of head of radius; type 2, ulnar diaphysis with posterior angulation and dislocation of head of radius; type 3, ulnar metaphysis with anterolateral or lateral dislocation of head of radius; type 4, proximal radius and ulnar fracture with anterior dislocation of head of radius.

Baehr-Löhlein lesion: Focal embolic glomerulonephritis.

Baelz disease (Puente disease, Volkmann cheilitis, von Baelz disease): Pain, tenderness, and slight enlargement of lower lip; Volkmann variant includes suppuration with crusting. Condition is seen in Ascher disease (congenital double lip); etiology is unknown. Degeneration to squamous cell carcinoma occurs in 20%–30% of cases.

Baer cavity: Groove located beneath blastoderm.

Baer law: Features common to group of animals at an earlier embryologic stage develop earlier than features that distinguish animals (which develop later in maturation process).

Baer point: Anatomic location in right iliac fossa slightly medial to McBurney point and anterior to right sacroiliac joint. Pain and tenderness at this point indicate spasm and tenderness in right iliac muscle; pressure that elicits reaction indicates infection or sprains of right sacroiliac ligament.

Baerman test: Technique used to isolate nematode larvae, esp. *Strongyloides.* Specimen is rinsed with H_2O over fine mesh that is connected to rubber collecting tube; organisms migrate from soil or feces sample and collect in tube.

Bäfverstedt syndrome: Lymphocytoma cutis.

Bageshaw chemotherapy (modified): 2nd-line treatment protocol for metastatic trophoblastic neoplasm when 1st–line drug resistance develops; consists of 8-day course of hydroxyurea, dactinomycin, vincristine, methotrexate, cyclophosphamide, and folic acid (with drug holidays on days 6 and 7).

Baghdad boil: See Aleppo boil.

Bailey-Cushing disease: Poor balance, altered coordination (in absence of frank ataxia), headache, and vomiting caused by midline cerebellar lesion (e.g., medulloblastoma, vascular lesion) or chronic alcoholism.

Bailey-Dubow technique: Method used to correct osteogenesis imperfecta of long bones. Multiple osteotomies are performed, elongating medullary rod is placed through segments, and spica cast is used until osteotomies have healed.

Bailey-Gibbon rib contractor: Ratchet-action instrument used to reapproximate ribs after chest surgery before tying sutures.

Bailey-Williamson forceps: Obstetrical forceps.

Baillarger sign: Unequal-sized pupils occurring in paresis.

Baillarger stripes (bands, lines, striae): Two areas of white substance strata found in anterior central gyri and medial surface of occipital lobe; formed from coalesced short association fibers.

Baillarger syndrome: See Frey syndrome.

Bain circuit: See Mapleson D circuit.

Bainbridge reflex: Increase in heart rate caused by increased distention of or increased pressure of right atrium or large systemic veins.

Bairnsdale ulcer: See Buruli ulcer.

Bakamjian flap: Deltopectoral fasciocutaneous flap swung up to face; used to close large soft tissue defects caused by trauma or cancer resection.

Bake dilator: Instrument used to dilate common bile duct.

Baker anastomosis: Side-to-end bowel anastomosis performed when significant differences in lumen size occur in low anterior resection of rectosigmoid.

Baker calcium: Histologic formol-based fixative used on phospholipids.

Baker cyst (popliteal cyst): Inflammation of synovium (semimembranous-gastrocnemius bursa) behind the knee, which manifests with pain and swelling; best seen and palpated with standing. Condition can be isolated or occur in osteoarthritis or rheumatoid arthritis; rarely becomes infected. Treatment is aspiration and instillation of steroid–anesthetic mixture.

Baker resection: Anterior resection of rectosigmoid (usu. for carcinoma) via midline incision; uses double-layer, hand-sewn, side-to-end bowel anastomosis. Care must be taken to avoid injuring ureters bilaterally.

Baker Sudan black method: Technique used to detect Golgi bodies in cells. Tissue is fixed in formalin, rinsed with potassium dichromate, sectioned, rinsed with Sudan black B, rinsed in alcohol, and stained with alum carmine. Golgi bodies stain blue, cytoplasm light gray, chromatin pinkish-red, and Golgi vacuoles clear.

Baker test (extraction test): Removal of phospholipids from histologic sections using pyridine.

Baker test: Staining procedure using acid hematin and histologic sections; stains phospholipids bluish-black, mucin blue to brown, and galactolipids pale-to-dark blue.

Baker tube: Long intestinal tube inserted directly into jejunum and passed distally at laparotomy via opening of jejunal wall; useful for stenting bowel or decompressing greatly distended bowel.

Baker velum: Prosthesis used to close defect in cleft palate.

Baker-Gordon phenol peel (formula): Chemical skin peel for face to improve cosmesis; uses 3 ml 88% liquid phenol, 8 drops liquid soap, 3 drops croton oil, and 2 ml H_2O.

Baker-Rosenbach syndrome (Klauder disease): Erysipeloid occurring after skin contact with marine animals (e.g., spiny fish, crabs, mollusks). Causative agent is *Erysipelothrix rhusiopathiae* .

Baker-Winegrad syndrome (FDPase deficiency): Fructose-1,6-diphosphatase deficiency causing acidosis, hyperventilation, and refractory hypoglycemia, which often results in seizures and coma; autosomal recessive condition occurring in infants after infection, severe stress, or prolonged fasting. Normal development and life span are possible with early diagnosis.

Bakes dilators: Set of 9 thin, easily bendable metal "plungers" used to dilate common bile duct or measure orifice size; bullet-shaped tips with diameter ranging from 3–11 mm.

Bakody sign: Positive if relief of headache symptoms occurs when patient places arm or hand of affected side on top of head; usu. indicates pathology at C4–C5.

Balamuth buffer solution: Dipotassium phosphate in distilled H_2O.

Balamuth medium: Egg yolk, saline, distilled H_2O, balamuth buffer solution, liver extract, and stool specimen; used to grow *Entamoeba histolytica*.

balanitis of Zoon: Skin disorder marked by "cayenne pepper"—type plaques of the glans penis found most commonly in uncircumcised elderly men. Rare condition represents lymphoplasmacellular infiltrates of unclear etiology. Treatment is topical cortisone or gentamicin and circumcision.

Balbiani body (nucleus): Nucleus of embryonic yolk.

Balbiani chromosome: Giant chromosome found in certain fly species containing large number of chromatids; used in genetics research because of easily mapped chromosome banding.

Balbiani rings: Area of Balbiani polytene chromosome

(e.g., *Diptera*) in which RNA transcription occurs.

Baldwin figure: Illusion in which line is drawn connecting small square drawn at 1 end with large square at other end. Perpendicular line is drawn bisecting first line, making length of 2 halves of line connecting boxes appear unequal.

Baldy-Webster operation: See Webster flap.

Balfour abdominal retractor: Instrument placed on either side of inner abdominal wall and pulled "open" to retract tissues laterally for exposure of peritoneal contents. Solid blade

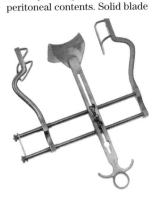

Balfour abdominal retractor

is used to retract bladder and pelvic contents.

Balfour bodies: *Aegyptianella pullorum;* parasites found in blood of fowl.

Balint syndrome: Visual inattention with inability to scan visual field and grasp object;

usu. due to bilateral occipital or parietal lesions.

Balkan cross adder (European viper, Iberian cross adder): *Vipera berus;* only venomous snake in Northern Europe. Bite causes tissue necrosis and hemorrhage but is rarely fatal. Reptile is usu. confined to high altitudes when found in southern and central Europe. Color ranges from gray-brown to black.

Balkan myoclonus (Eldridge disease): Light-sensitive myoclonic epilepsy with worsening of symptoms on wakening; autosomal recessive condition with childhood onset. Treatment is valproic acid; phenytoin is never used because of symptom aggravation and possible death.

Balkan nephropathy (Danubian nephropathy, Yugoslavian nephropathy): Atrophy of kidney cortex with interstitial fibrosis and amyloid changes on histology; high association with transitional cell carcinoma of upper tracts/renal pelvis. Renal failure develops over 5–10 years. Etiology is unknown but likely environmentally related.

Balke-Ware protocol: Exercise tolerance test protocol; used in decreased cardiac reserve or disability.

Ball disease: Increased viscosity of blood in brain in acute leukemia; potentially fatal condition.

Ball valves: Mucosal membrane folds that connect caudal edges of anal columns.

Ballance sign: Palpable tender mass in left upper quadrant; due to splenic hematoma.

Ballance sign: Right flank resonance occurring in splenic rupture when patient lies in left lateral decubitus position.

Ballantyne disease (Clifford disease, Runge disease): Condition found in newborns. Marked by prolonged gestation (> 39 weeks), decreased alertness, low birth weight, and increased respiratory distress; skin, nails, and cord often stain greenish. Cause is likely placental insufficiency.

Ballantyne-Smith disease: Abnormal amniotic structure surrounding limbs; leads to severe malformations of distal extremities.

Ballard disease (μ heavy chain disease): Presence of μ-protein with hypogammaglobulinemia and pathologic fractures due to skeletal infiltration of lymphocytes, plasma cells, or reticular cells; usu. seen in association with chronic lymphocytic leukemia, non-Hodgkin lymphoma, amyloidosis, and Bence Jones protein. Treatment is cyclophosphamide and chlorambucil.

Baller-Gerold syndrome: Craniosynostosis involving coronal suture; marked by tilted forehead, high nasal bridge, dysplastic ears, absent/hypoplastic radius with malformed ulna, hip dislocation, hypoplastic 3rd/4th toes, and occasional mental retardation; autosomal recessive condition.

Ballet sign: Loss of external eye movement; seen in Graves disease and some psychiatric conditions.

Ballotment sign: Positive for triquetrolunate dissociation if pain, significant laxity, or crepitus occurs when lunate and triquetrum are stabilized with examiner's hand and then displaced dorsally and volarly over each other with pressure.

Baló disease: Severe variant of MS with demyelination developing in concentric pattern in CNS tissue; death usu. occurs several months to 2–3 years after onset.

Balser-Fitz disease: Acute (often hemorrhagic) pancreatitis.

Bamatter syndrome (Walt Disney syndrome): Short stature, senile skin changes, multiple skeleton deformities and fractures, and corneal opacities; X-linked or autosomal recessive condition of unknown etiology.

Bamberg disease: Jerky movements during ambulation caused by irritation of spinal cord motor cells, results in clonic muscle spasms.

Bamberg disease: See Concato disease.

Bamberger albuminuria: Spillage of albumin and RBCs into urine; sometimes seen in advanced, prolonged anemia.

Bamberger area: Cardiac dullness in left intercostal area; suggests pericardial effusion.

Bamberger sign: Indicator of pericardial effusion if patient has decreased breath sounds at angle of scapula, which disappear when patient leans forward.

Bamberger sign (allochiria): Positive if sensation is felt in one extremity when contralateral extremity is stimulated.

Bancroft filariasis: Infection with *Wucheria bancrofti*; causes elephantiasis and lymphangitis. Vectors are *Culex*, *Aedes* (Pacific islands), and *Anopheles* mosquitoes. Condition occurs in central Africa, Asia, and Australia, including Pacific islands.

Bancroft sign: Positive for thrombosis of deep vein calf veins with tenderness of anteropositive but not lateral compression of calf. Occurs in 1/3 of cases.

Bancroft worm: *Wuchereria bancrofti*; thread-like nematodes with blunt ends. Female adult worms measure 65–100 mm $\times$ 0.2–0.3 mm.

band of Schreger: Light striae seen when passing light through longitudinal section of dried tooth; corresponds to twisting of enamel rods in outer portion of tooth.

Bandrowski base: Type of quinoediimine reported to cause anaphylactic reaction.

Banff classification: System used to describe rejection for kidney transplants, with 6 diagnostic categories: acute rejection, chronic rejection, hyperacute rejection, normal histology, borderline changes and changes not related to rejection. *Acute rejection:* grade I, moderate interstitial infiltrate with tubulitis but no vascular changes; grade II, moderate to severe interstitial infiltrate with severe tubulitis and possible mild to moderate intimal arteritis; grade III, severe intimal arteritis with fibrinoid necrosis, infarcts, interstitial hemorrhage (severity of interstitial infiltrate is irrelevant). *Chronic rejection:* grade I, mild interstitial fibrosis with tubular atrophy; grade II, moderate intertitial fibrosis with tubular atrophy; grade III, severe interstitial fibrosis and tubular atrophy and loss.

Bang bacillus: *Brucella abortus* .

Bangle body (angulated body): Filamentous type inclusion; seen in cytoplasm of spindle-shaped cells in granular cell tumors under transmission electron microscopy.

Bankart fracture: One fragment that splinters off anterior-inferior part of glenoid fossa; seen in anterior shoulder dislocation.

Banker-Victor-Adams disease: Congenital muscular dystrophy with contractures of proximal muscles and trunk and mental retardation; progresses to death by 2nd decade.

Bankhart (Bankart) lesion (Perthes-Bankhart lesion): Detached anterior-inferior glenoid labrum, with possible presence of bony fragments.

Bankhart (Bankart) lesion (reversed): Detached posterior rim of labrum from glenoid.

Bankhart (Bankart) skid: Spoon-shaped retractor used in orthopedic surgery to retract humeral head away from glenoid cavity.

Banki syndrome: Short metacarpal bones, thin diaphysis, and fusion of cuneiform and lunate bones.

Banks-Dervin rod: Type of spinal instrumentation used to treat scoliosis; involves rod placed across several vertebrae with oblique spinal process screwed to contralateral lamina.

Bannayan syndrome (Bannayan-Riley-Smith syndrome, Bannayan-Zonana syndrome, Ruvalcaba-Myhre-Smith syndrome): Symptom complex marked by multiple lipomas and/or hemangiomas in CNS, as well as macrocephaly and variable mental and developmental deficits; autosomal dominant condition.

Bannister disease (Milton disease, Quincke disease): Increased permeability of capillaries in subcutaneous or submucosal tissues, causing giant wheals. Hereditary form has more visceral involvement and impairment of C1 esterase inhibitor.

Bannwarth syndrome (Garin-Bujadoux-Bannwarth syndrome): Neurologic sequelae (e.g., meningitis, encephalitis, polyneuropathy) following Lyme borreliosis (*Borrelia burgdorferi* infection); occurs in 10%–20% of untreated infections.

Banti disease: Anemia, leukopenia, and splenomegaly.

Banti syndrome: Anemia caused by portal hypertension from intrahepatic or extrahepatic sources. Splenectomy temporarily alleviates anemia but does not affect portal hypertension.

Bantler syndrome: Diffuse skin pigment lesions (e.g., café-au-lait spots, ephelides) and hemangiomas in small bowel. Treatment is surgical excision.

Bantu haplotype (Central African haplotype): 1 of 4 major gene clusters on chromosome 11 characteristic sickle cell disease; has 6 base deletion.

Bantu siderosis: See African siderosis.

Barach-Davidson tent: Early 1900s device used to administer oxygen; delivery, humidity, and temperature of inhaled gas are controlled by running oxygen through ice bath.

Bar syndrome: Presence of bacteria in urine, gallbladder, and appendix during pregnancy; leads to abdominal pain.

Baraitser syndrome: Mental retardation, obesity, macrocephaly, and macrosomia; X-linked condition.

Baraitser-Burn syndrome: Type 4 Mohr-Mejewski syndrome; manifested by severe tibial dysplasia.

Barakat syndrome: Hypoparathyroidism, deafness, and renal failure; autosomal recessive condition.

Bárány chair: Early apparatus used to rotate patient to test dizziness and vestibular sensitivity.

Bárány maneuver (Dix-Hallpike maneuver): Technique used to detect positional vertigo, specifically to distinguish peripheral positional nystagmus vs. central positional nystagmus. Patient sits close to end of table, turning head 45° to 1 side. Examiner quickly places patient in reclining position while supporting head and shoulders, with turned head hanging over table edge for 30 seconds. Patient reports any symptoms and examiner notes presence and timing of nystagmus.

Bárány pointing test: Positive for brain lesion if when pointing to object with eyes both open and closed, the patient repeatedly points inaccurately but in fixed manner only when the eyes are closed.

Bárány syndrome: Positional vertigo caused by cupulolithiasis of posterior semicircular canal; marked by periodic unilateral headache, ipsilateral intermittent deafness, vertigo, and tinnitus. Condition is most commonly seen in elderly men; first presents on morning awakening. Diagnosis involves Bárány maneuver. Disorder is not corrected by inducing nystagmus.

Bárány test (caloric test): Warm-water irrigation of normal ear, causing rotatory nystagmus toward irrigated ear; cold water irrigation causes rotatory nystagmus away from irrigated ear.

Barbados lily: *Atropa belladonna.* All parts of belladonna plant are highly toxic; consumption of 2–3 of black-colored berries by children may be fatal. Plant contains atropine, alkaloids (1-hyoscyamine, tropane, scopolamine); roots contain scopolamine and scopoletin.

Barbeau disease: Muscle dystrophy affecting swallowing and speech (pharyngeal muscles) and eye movements.

Barber disease (psoriasis): Relapsing–remitting psoriasis occurring on limbs (thenar eminences and heels) with scaling, itching, and pustule formation. Treatment is aspirin, steroids, and tetracycline.

Barbour-Stoner-Kelly medium: Substance used to grow spirochetes that cause tick-borne relapsing fever.

Barcoo rot: Australian term for diphtheritic desert sore occurring in desert areas; caused by *Corynebacterium diphtheriae* infection. Condition starts with papules that progress to pustules and then chronic ulcers.

Barcroft apparatus: Manometer used to investigate a small tissue sample or blood sample.

Bard disease: Lung metastasis due to gastric carcinoma.

Bard sign: Used to distinguish congenital vs. acquired nystagmus. In congenital form, frequency of eye oscillations decreases as examiner's finger is moved back and forth. In acquired form, frequency of oscillations increases.

Bard-Pic disease: See Courvoisier sign.

Bardet-Biedl syndrome: Congenital vision loss progressing to blindness, mental retardation, underdeveloped genitalia, polydactyly, glomerulonephritis, liver fibrosis, and obesity; differs from Laurence-Moon syndrome because of lack of paraplegia.

Barfurth law: Initial regeneration after skin wounding occurs perpendicular to incision.

Barkan operation (goniotomy): Method for treatment of glaucoma; uses surgical opening of Schlemm canal.

Barker pills: Medication used as postpartum laxative in early 1900s.

Barker point: Anatomic location for trephine in drainage of temporosphenoid lobe; lies 1.25 in. above and behind external middle auditory meatus.

Barkhof criteria: Standards used to distinguish between small vessel disease and MS lesions on MRI. For suspicion of MS, 3 lesions must be present, with 2 of the following: areas of abnormal signal ≥ 6 mm, abnormal areas bordering ventricles, and abnormal areas in infratentorial region.

Barkman reflex: Contraction of rectus muscle on same side after stimulation of skin below nipple.

Barkow ligament: Fibrous tissue that connects plantar surfaces of cuneiform bones.

Barkow ligament: Fibrous tissue used to secure posterior and anterior surfaces of elbow joint.

Barlow sign (test): Used to detect unstable and potentially dislocatable hip in newborns; positive if movement of head of femur occurs when thumb pressure is applied to lesser trochanter and index finger pressure is applied to greater trochanter.

Barlow syndrome: Mitral valve prolapse.

Barlow syndrome (Cheadle-Moeller-Barlow syndrome): Scurvy occurring in infants; marked by easy bruising of skin and gums, enlarged heart, and partially healed fracture sites. Treatment is vitamin C with good results.

Barlow syndrome: Scurvy in setting of rickets.

Barmah forest virus: Alphavirus transmitted by mosquito genera *Aedes*, *Culex*, and *Anopheles;* occurs in Australia. Virus causes clinical symptoms that mimic epidemic febrile polyarthritis.

Barnard approach: Extrapleural or extraperitoneal technique used to incise and drain abscesses; avoids contamination of body cavity.

Barnard snake (Australian collared snake): *Glyphodon barnardi;* venomous but relatively harmless snake in New Guinea. Reptile generally avoids human contact.

Barnard-Scholz syndrome: Retinitis pigmentosa in setting of progressive weakness of eyelid and ocular muscles; also seen with heart block; hearing loss; and muscle weakness in face, neck, and shoulders.

Barnes curve: Imaginary half-circle running with concavity pointed dorsally and center lying at sacral promontory.

Barnes dystrophy: Atrophy of peroneal muscles and myotonia of thigh muscles; rare autosomal dominant condition.

Barnes syndrome: Stenosis of larynx, bell-shaped thorax, and short stature; autosomal dominant condition.

Barnes-Crile hemostatic forceps: Fine, curve-tipped, ring-handle, locking forceps placed on small vessels to control bleeding before suture ligation or cautery.

Barnett-Bourne nitrate:
Acetic alcohol–silver fixative used to highlight bile pigment in liver parenchyma, in focal hemorrhages.

Barnett-Seligman dihydroxydinaphthyl disulfide method: Staining technique used to demonstrate disulfide and sulfhydryl groups; pink turns to dark blue.

Barnett-Seligman indoxyl esterase method: Staining technique used to highlight lipase, esterases, and cholinesterases; produces purple color by causing hydrolysis.

Barr body: Condensed X chromosome in nondividing cells, which is cytologic marker for female cells; always 1 less in number than X-chromosomes [e.g., 1 Barr body in XXY male (Klinefelter syndrome)].

Barr body test: Pre-1970 procedure used to count number of Barr bodies; now largely supplanted by karyotyping.

Barraquer operation: Surgical method of eye lens removal by suctioning; used in cataract treatment.

Barraquer-Simons syndrome (Höllander disease, Mitchell disease type 2, Simond syndrome, Smith syndrome): Symmetric loss of facial subcutaneous fat with associated mental retardation and glomerular nephritis. Condition is sometimes accompanied by fat loss from upper limbs and trunk; no fat loss occurs below umbilicus. Onset occurs in childhood.

Barré sign: Patient is placed prone. Both knees are flexed to 90° and then released by examiner; a paretic leg will fall to table. Result is seen with unilateral leg paresis due to pyramidal tract lesion.

Barré sign: Slow iris contraction with loss of brain functioning.

Barré syndrome (Deiter nucleus syndrome): Vertigo, unsteady gait, and lateropulsion. Likely etiology is lesion in lateral vestibulospinal pathways with sparing of superior Deiter nucleus connections.

Barré-Liéou syndrome (Bartschi-Rochain syndrome, cervical migraine, Kuhelendahl syndrome, Schuetzenberger syndrome): Arthritis of 3rd and 4th cervical disks, resulting in CN V and CN VIII irritation; marked by eye pain, headaches, tinnitus, and vertigo. Vasomotor disturbance of face is caused by irritation of sympathetic plexus around vertebral artery.

Barré-Masson syndrome (angiomyoneuroma): Well-demarcated, blue-red masses of vascular channels occurring in conjunction with glomus cells on distal extremities; may or may not be painful. Condition is present at birth up to early adulthood. Treatment is excision.

Barrett adenoma:
Macroscopic polypoid form of
mucosal dysplasia in esophagus.

Barrett esophagus
(epithelium): Metaplasia of
distal esophageal mucosa from
squamous cell to columnar-type
cell; associated with impaired
functioning of esophageal body
and lower esophageal sphincter.
Cause is gastroesophageal
reflux disease. Condition is
considered premalignant and is
not reversible with
fundoplication. Indication for
esophageal resection includes
high-grade dysplasia on random
biopsy taken during 2 separate
endoscopies.

Barrett ulcer: Ulceration in
columnar epithelium of Barrett
esophagus; has tendency to
perforate or bleed. Male-to-
female ratio is 3:1. Treatment is
antacids, H_2-receptor
antagonists, omeprazole,
metoclopramide (Reglan),
bethanecol, and lifestyle
modifications.

Barron banding: Placement
of rubber bands on hemorrhoids
as initial manual decompression
treatment.

**Barroso-Moguel-Costero
silver method:** Staining
technique used on carotid body
tumors to highlight argentaffin
cells, which appear black on
light violet background.

Barrow syndrome: Congenital
heart defect, congenital limb
abnormalities, midline capillary
hemangiomas, sloping forehead,
and prominent nose bridge;
occurs only in males.

Barsky operation: Method of
repairing cleft hand with
missing middle central ray; 2nd
and 4th fingers are surgically
reapproximated.

**Barsony-Teschendorff-
Polgar syndrome:** Diffuse
esophageal spasms secondary to
irregular contractions of
peristaltic waves; results in
dysphagia and regurgitation.

Bart disease: Epidermolysis
with congenital absence of skin
over legs and aplastic or
hypoplastic nails; autosomal
dominant condition associated
with blistering and bullae.

Bart hemoglobin: Found in
homozygous form of α-
thalassemia; has 4 gamma
chains, which result in
aggregation of excess globin
chains that have greatly
increased affinity for oxygen.
Presence causes fetal death in
utero or shortly after birth.

Barth disease: Congenital
skeletal muscle degeneration,
dilated cardiomyopathy, and
growth retardation; also with
neutropenia. This X-linked
recessive condition leads to
death in 1st few years of life.

Barthel index: Current
modification of system to
evaluate patient's functional
ability on long-range basis;
points are assigned in 15
domains based on intact,
limited, help-dependent and
absent abilities. System assesses
capacity for eating and drinking,
transfers, grooming, bathing,
incontinence, dressing, and
walking. Index correlates

significantly with placement after discharge and recovery from stroke.

Barthel-PULSES index (BPI): Combination of scores on Barthel and PULSES indices, which measure level of physical dependence after injury or disability; BPI = Barthel score $\times$ 10 $\times$ 6/PULSES score.

Barthelemy disease: Acne occurring in clusters with thick patches of pustules covered with red, moist scabs; usu. seen with exposure to bromine.

Bartholin abscess: Purulent collection in Bartholin (vulvovaginal) gland; typical presentation is erythema, swelling, and tenderness in lower part of labium minus. Treatment is application of heat until fluctuant and then incision at mucocutaneous border between vagina and vulva; margins may be marsupialized with interrupted chromic sutures. Antibiotics are given if cellulitis or systemic symptoms occur.

Bartholin cyst: Blockage of mucous ducts draining Bartholin glands; can form painful mass in labium minus. Small asymptomatic cysts may be followed conservatively if no suspicion of malignancy exists.

Bartholin duct: Largest of minor sublingual ducts that open alongside submaxillary duct; usu. originates from anterior part of gland.

Bartholin duct: Single canal draining each Bartholin gland opening onto floor of vestibule between vaginal orifice and hymenal attachment.

Bartholin glands: Paravaginal glands with openings lying posterior and on either side of vaginal opening; orifices are often not discernible on visual exam.

Bartlett tube: Device used to collect samples in bronchoalveolar brush or aspirate sampling; reduces contamination of specimen.

Barton bandage: Figure-of-8 bandage placed around head to support lower jaw both inferiorly and anteriorly.

Barton forceps: Obstetrical forceps using sliding lock; useful when infant's head is in occiput transverse position.

Barton fracture: Breakage of distal radius with displacement of radial carpal joint; part of articular cartilage is displaced upward and backward onto dorsal surface of radius.

Barton operation: Method of correcting ankylosis by removing V-shaped piece of bone.

Barton tongs: Instrument that uses pins inserted into skull to provide cervical traction.

Barton traction handle: Instrument used with Barton forceps.

***Bartonella* anemia:** See bartonellosis; anemia may be present until after splenectomy.

Bartonella: Single species (*B. bacilliformis*), gram-negative aerobic coccobacillus with polar flagella; causes bartonellosis. Bacillus lives in and on RBCs; best visualized with Giemsa stain.

Bartonellaceae: Family in Rickettsiales, containing gram-negative bacteria *Bartonella* and *Grahamella* .

bartonellosis (Carrión disease, Oroya fever): Severe hemolytic anemia with fevers followed by hemangioma-type skin lesions; also with hepatosplenomegaly, jaundice, and lymphadenopathy with variable centrilobular necrosis and splenic infarction. Cause is *Bartonella* infection; vector is sand fly. Condition is found in Ecuador, Peru, and Colombia. Treatment is streptomycin, penicillin, or chloramphenicol.

Bartshci-Rochain syndrome: See Barré-Liéou syndrome.

Bartsocas-Papas syndrome: Congenital winged skin flap in popliteal fossa, low birth weight, microcephaly, cleft palate, mental retardation and bicornuate uterus; autosomal recessive condition.

Bartter syndrome (congenital hypokalemic alkalosis, juxtaglomerular cell hyperplasia): Decreased blood pressure, renal potassium wasting, increased renin production, and metabolic alkalosis with chloride reabsorption defect; indistinguishable from diuretic abuse. Autosomal dominant condition usu. occuring in children and adolescents; sometimes found in persons born prematurely or with polyhydramnios, with possible mental retardation and dwarfism. Cause is secondary hyperaldosteronism. Treatment is prostaglandin inhibitors and potassium-sparing diuretics.

Baruch sign: Inability to lower body temperature after immersion in 75° F bath; classically seen in typhoid fever.

Basan syndrome: Congenital skin milia, bullae on feet and hands, and tapered fingertips; autosomal dominant condition.

Bascom closure: Surgical treatment for pilonidal cyst. Buttocks are pushed together and marked at point of contact and then taped apart. Unhealed tract is then incised via triangular resection off midline. Skin flaps are then raised out to previously marked lines and then reapproximated after tape is removed. Procedure is performed on outpatient basis with 3%–4% recurrence rate.

Basedow disease (goiter, syndrome): Exophthalmus due to hyperthyroidism; marked by loss of normal convergence.

Basedow goiter: Enlarged thyroid that becomes hyperfunctional after stimulation by iodine administration.

Basham mixture: Iron and ammonia acetate solution.

Bashaw device: Cervical spine immobilizer; uses pillow harness (Velcro straps and polyethylene foam) fastened to spine board and then to head.

Basmajian principle: Subluxation of humeral head out of downward-tilted glenoid fossa; often seen in hemiplegia.

Bass syndrome: Congenital absence of middle phalanges, with absent toenails and hypoplastic articular cartilage.

Bassen-Kornzweig syndrome (abetalipoproteinemia): Metabolic disease caused by absence of plasma lipoproteins (β -lipoproteins) with relative density ≤ 1.062; marked by neuromuscular abnormalities, ataxia, malabsorption, decreased vitamin A, degeneration of retinal pigments, and acanthocytes in blood. Condition is autosomal recessive, with onset at 6–16 years of age.

Basset operation: Technique in radical vulvectomy for resection inguinal lymph nodes.

Bassini herniorrhaphy (operation): High ligation of hernia sac with suturing of conjoined tendon and internal oblique muscle to inguinal ligament; alternately described as approximating transversus abdominis to Poupart ligament. Spermatic cord remains in anatomic location. In females, internal ring is closed, and round ligament is ligated.

Bastedo sign: Pain and tenderness in right lower quadrant when colon is distended; seen in chronic appendicitis.

Bastian law (Bastian-Bruns law): Loss of lower tendon reflexes in complete transection of spinal cord above lumbar level.

Bastyr formula: See Robert formula (modified).

Batchelor plaster: Spica cast used to treat hip dysplasia in infants; holds hip in internal rotation but allows other movement.

Bateman drops: Tincture of opium and gambir.

Bateman syndrome: Purpura on forearm and back of hands in elderly people receiving corticosteroids; leaves residual brownish pigmentation on resolution.

Batson plexus: Spinal cord venous plexus formed by internal and external venous plexuses; allows hematogenous brain metastases of prostate cancer.

Batten disease (ceroid lipofuscinosis): Universally fatal juvenile condition marked by mental retardation, progressive loss of vision, molar abnormalities, and seizures, with onset usu. by 10 years of age. Cause is 1 or more of 23 different mutations isolated to chromosome 16, p11.2–12.1. Disorder may be diagnosed by biopsy in tissue other than brain.

Batten-Turner syndrome: Benign congenital muscular dystrophy, with muscle weakness more pronounced in proximal muscle group; onset in early childhood of frequent falling and stumbling and delay in motor milestones. Serum shows increase in aldolase, LDH, and AST (SGOT).

Battey bacillus:
Mycobacterium intracellulare; causes pulmonary lymph node infection in children and tubercular infection in adults. Bacterium does not hydrolyze polysorbates (Tween 80).

Battle operation: Rarely used technique for removing appendix; rectus muscle is retracted intact.

Battle sign: Ecchymosis of mastoid region; indicates basilar skull fracture.

Battle-Jalaguier-Kammerer incision: Vertical incision of skin and subcutaneous tissue in midline.

Battstrom procedure: Type of C1–C2 spinal fusion using acrylic cement.

Baudet latent period: Asymptomatic interval of several days to weeks between blunt abdominal injury and delayed splenic rupture; occurs in 10%–15% of cases.

Bauer disease: Shortened middle bone of 5th finger associated with clinodactyly; more common in females.

Bauer reaction: Modification of periodic acid–Schiff reaction using chromic acid as oxidizer; also part of Gridley stain for fungus.

Bauhin valve: Ileocecal valve.

Baumann angle: Angle formed by imaginary line running tangential to epiphyseal border of lateral distal metaphysis and line running perpendicular to long axis of humerus if viewed on anterior-posterior radiographic view of distal humerus. Normal value is 70°–75°; > 75° suggests cubitus varus.

Baumé scale: Method allowing calculation of specific gravity of fluids at a baseline temperature of 60°; specific gravity = 145/(145—n), where n = Baumé scale reading.

Baumgartner method: Technique for measurement of platelet aggregation when exposed to subendothelium of rabbit aorta.

Baumgartner needle holder: Locking needle holder used in suturing.

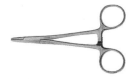

Baumgartner needle holder

Baxter formula: See Parkland formula.

Bayes rule: Principle used to compute likelihood of 1 event happening given that another event has occurred; useful when evaluating immunoassay data reduction analyses.

Bayes theorem: Principle that determines predictive value of positive test result; uses sensitivity and specificity of clinical trials. Outcome varies with prevalence rate and whether test is for screening or diagnosis.

Bayford-Autenrieth condition (Arkin disease): Abnormal subclavian artery origin with subsequent mechanical compression of esophagus; seen esp. in coarctation of aorta. Treatment is surgery.

Bayle disease: Paralytic dementia.

Bayley scale of infant development: Method used to screen for mental and motor skills from birth to 30 months of age; should not be used in physically handicapped children.

Bayliss effect: Increased muscle contraction and resistance; seen with elevated perfusion pressure and increased vascular smooth muscle stretch.

Bazelon syndrome: Variant of Lesch-Nyhan syndrome occurring in females; marked by self-mutilation of hands and lips, mental retardation, and hyperuricemia. Choreoathetosis is absent.

Bazex syndrome (paraneoplastic acrokeratosis): Congenital follicular atrophoderma ("multiple ice pick marks") on hands and feet and multiple basal cell carcinomas developing on face; also with segmental twists in hair shafts (pili torti). Condition occurs in adolescence.

Bazex-Griffith syndrome: Paraneoplastic syndrome with psoriasis-like lesions developing on extremities, ears, and nose, and diffuse cervical and submaxillary lymph node enlargement; seen most commonly in men with neoplasms of upper respiratory tract.

Bazin disease: Vasculitis seen in *Mycobacterium tuberculosis;* marked by multiple large brownish nodules commonly seen on back of legs.

Bazzana syndrome: Progressive otosclerosis causing deafness and contraction of visual field.

Beale cells: Cells found in cardiac ganglia, which have 2 processes with distinctive morphology of having 1 wrapped around the other.

Beals syndrome: Short stature, elongation of ear lobe, elbow joint dysplasia, masculine torso, and shortened metacarpals; autosomal dominant condition.

Beals-Hecht syndrome: Congenital kyphoscoliosis, micrognathia, abnormal external ear, long limbs, and multiple joint contractures; absence of eye and cardiovascular defects are absent.

Bean syndrome: Multiple, small, blue subcutaneous nodules that may be tender to palpation; also marked by melena, anemia, nocturnal pain, hyperhidrosis, hemangioma of eye, and neurologic deficits. Condition is autosomal dominant, with onset in first few years of life.

Beard disease (neurasthenia): Insomnia, fatigability, vague aches, loss of interest in surroundings, irritability, depressed mood, and GI distress.

Beare-Stevenson cutis gyratum (Beare-Dodge-Nevin syndrome): Congenital wide-set eyes; cleft palate; cloverleaf skull; acanthosis nigricans; bifid scrotum; and cutis gyratum of palms, soles, facial skin, axilla, and perineum.

Bearne-Künkel-Slater syndrome (lupoid hepatitis): Autoimmune chronic active hepatitis marked by hepatomegaly, liver fibrosis, ascites, variceal bleeding, fever, and hirsutism; seen in females with usu. onset at puberty. Treatment is steroids, immunosuppression, and (in advanced cirrhosis) liver transplantation. Condition commonly recurs in transplanted organs.

Beau lines: Transverse grooves in fingernails appearing several weeks after acute, severe illness. Defects grow out with nail and disappear over 2–3 months.

Beaumés sign: Retrosternal pain of angina pectoris.

Beaver method: Technique used to count *Ascaris* or *Trichuris* egg infestation of feces. Fecal samples are diluted with saline and viewed with photoelectric light meter.

Beccaria sign: Painful throbbing in posterior skull during pregnancy.

Bechterew bundle (Helweg bundle): Spino-olivary fasciculus.

Bechterew nucleus: Superior nucleus of vestibular nerve; located in midbrain.

Bechterew sign: Popliteal space numbness seen in syphilitic tabes dorsalis.

Bechterew sign: Condition seen in patients with motor disturbances, most commonly corticospinal tract abnormalities or hemiparesis. The examiner flexes patient's arms at the elbow passively and raises them to shoulder level and then allows them to fall. In normal patients, arms "float" for 1–2 seconds and then drop. In those with corticospinal tract lesions, arms remain "floating" for longer time and descend more slowly. In those with flaccid paralysis and psychogenic etiologies, arms drop precipitously.

Bechterew syndrome: Ankylosing spondylitis.

Bechterew test: Used to detect sciatica in seated patient. Positive result is inability to extend legs both straight because of pain, even with ability to extend legs one at a time.

Bechterew-Mendel reflex (tarsophalangeal reflex): Tapping on cuboid or external cuneiform bone that produces flaring and dorsiflexion of 2nd and 3rd or 5th toes; seen in central lesions of motor nervous system.

Beck Depression Inventory: Self-administered questionnaire that assesses presence of signs and symptoms of depression.

Beck paste: Bismuth subnitrate and sterile petrolatum; injected therapeutically into chronic tuberculous cavities and sinuses of skin.

Beck syndrome: Occlusion of anterior spinal artery, usu. due to thrombosis; symptoms vary depending on site of lesion.

Beck triad: Hypotension, distended neck veins, and distant heart sounds; seen in pericardial tamponade.

Beck-Ibrahim syndrome: Chronic fungal infection of oral mucosa and skin with paronychia, crusted lesions, and change of hair color to white with alopecia. Infantile form (autosomal recessive) is associated with myeloperoxidase and ferritin abnormalities and dwarfism. Adult form has sporadic inheritance. Treatment involves antifungals.

Becke line: Narrow band of light that may appear when viewing specimen through microscope; most noticeable when specimen has both solid and liquid phase and when microscope tube is being adjusted. Band of light usu. is seen on outside of specimen.

Becker disease: Dilated cardiomyopathy.

Becker joint: Foot or ankle prosthesis using double-stopped (pin-and-spring) ankle joint.

Becker muscular dystrophy: Muscle disease similar to Duchenne muscular dystrophy, but with less severe symptoms and later onset (childhood to early adulthood); X-linked recessive condition. Muscle pain with exercise is prominent; disorder is also marked by pseudohypertrophy of calves with global muscle atrophy and moderate rise in serum creatinine. Condition is also associated with color blindness. Defect involves dystrophin. Incidence is 1 in 50,000 live male births. Death in 4th decade is usu. of cardiac nature.

Becker nevus: Benign pigmented hamartoma seen most commonly on shoulders of adolescent boys, usu. with hair growth in hamartoma within 1 year of onset.

Becker phenomenon: Pronounced pulsation in retinal arteries in Graves disease.

Becker test: Technique used to detect presence of alkaloid picrotoxin. Fehling solution is mixed with solution to be tested; positive result occurs with heating if Fehling solution is reduced.

Becker test: Used to detect presence of astigmatism. Patient examines sets of 3 lines on test card and determines which is blurred.

Becker-Lennhoff index: See Lennhoff index.

Becker-Reuter syndrome: Benign brown macules appearing on neck or forearms of female infants.

Beckmann apparatus: Device used to determine molecular weight of sample by dissolving it in pure liquid and noting change in boiling or freezing point.

Beckmann thermometer: Instrument that can detect small changes in temperature by using large bulb and small-bore stem.

Beckwith-Wiedemann syndrome (EMG syndrome): Congenital omphalocele, visceromegaly, macroglossia, microcephaly, umbilical hernia, and cryptorchidism, with 10%–20% risk of tumor development (e.g., nephroblastoma, adrenocortical tumors, hepatoblastoma); autosomal recessive condition. Serum shows hypoglycemia and polycythemia. Treatment is zinc glucagon, diazoxide, and surgical correction of omphalocele and partial tongue resection.

Béclard amputation: Hip disarticulation with closure of wound using posterior flap fashioned first at level of hip joint.

Béclard hernia: Femoral hernia that passes through saphenous opening.

Béclard nucleus: Oral-shaped ossification center occurring in lower epiphyseal cartilage in late fetal development.

Béclard sign: Onset of femur ossification in fetus.

Beclard triangle: Anatomic area bounded by greater horn of hyoid bone, posterior belly of digastric muscle, and posterior border of hyoglossus muscle.

Becquerel (Bq): Unit of radioactivity; 1 curie = 3.7×10^{10} Bq.

Bednar aphthae: Excoriated hard palate over pterygoid plates in infant's mouth; probably due to sucking pressure.

Bednar tumors: Melanin-containing dermatofibrosarcoma protuberans lesions; appear as noncircumscribed, multinodular areas most usu. on legs and trunk. Lesions are locally aggressive and require complete excision.

Bedson test: Used to detect presence of apomorphine; positive if brown color appears when potassium hydroxide is added to boiling solution to be tested.

Beemer syndrome: Dense bone, odd facies, hydrocephalus, thrombocytopenia, and cardiac defects (double-outlet right ventricle); congenital autosomal recessive condition.

Beemer-Langer syndrome (short rib syndrome): Narrowed thorax, bowed limbs, cleft upper lip, ascites, and hydrops; congenital autosomal recessive condition. Death occurs in perinatal period.

Beer law (Beer-Bouguer-Lambert law): Amount of light absorbed by solution is proportional to wavelength of light, solute, solvent, concentration and path length of light; basis of pulse oximetry.

Beer operation: Cataract removal using flap.

Beery test (Developmental Form Sequence Test): Used to measure visual–motor integration by testing ability to copy geometric forms of increasing complexity.

Beery-Buktenica developmental test: Used to assess visual–motor skills in children of 2–16 years of age through ability to copy geometric shapes; individual's performance is measured against standard age norms.

Beevor sign: Positive is upward movement of umbilicus caused by weakness of lower abdominal muscles when neck is flexed against resistance to forehead; implies T10–L1 lesion.

Beevor sign: Loss of ability to inhibit antagonistic muscle action in motor paralysis.

Beger procedure: Duodenum-preserving proximal pancreat-ectomy with Roux-en-Y drainage of body and tail of pancreas; used for resection of inflammatory mass at head of pancreas in chronic pancreatitis. 80% of patients have total pain relief.

Begg appliance (technique): Bracket-and-light-wire device used to tip tooth crowns; horizontal buccal tubes anchor molars.

Behçet syndrome (Adamantiades-Behçet syndrome, Gilbert syndrome, Halushi-Behçet syndrome, Touraine disease): Chronic inflammatory disorder with recurrent oral and genital ulcerations, uveitis, arthritis, vasculitis, and GI symptoms; may be marked by presence of smooth muscle antibodies.

Condition is most common in young Japanese men.

Behnken unit: Amount of x-ray exposure in 1 cc of air at 18° C and 760 mm Hg of pressure; equal to 1 electrostatic unit.

Behr pupil: Contralateral dilation of pupil occurring in optic tract pathology.

Behr syndrome: See Rochon-Duvigneaud syndrome.

Behr syndrome: Ataxia, spasticity, optic atrophy, and mental retardation; autosomal recessive condition with onset from birth to 6 months of age.

Behr syndrome: Progressive atrophy and degeneration of central retina with pigment changes in macular area.

Behring law: Blood transfusion from immunized person to previous unimmunized person renders receiving patient immune for a specific antigen

Beigel disease: Fungal infection of hair follicles (tinea nodosa).

Beighton disease: Osteogenesis imperfecta type IV, with normal color sclerae, opalescent teeth, osteoporosis, and wormian bones; joint hypermobility is lacking in this autosomal dominant condition. Cause is defect in collagen metabolism.

Békésy audiometry: Early test used to investigate CN VIII disorders. Patient pushes button that decreases tone and then releases button when tone is no longer heard.

Bekhterer-Strümpell syndrome: Type of senescent vertebral ankylosis.

Bekhterev arthritis: Ankylosing spondylitis.

Bekhterev deep reflex: Positive if dorsal flexion of toes, foot, knee, and hip occur when toes and foot are passively flexed in plantar direction; seen in corticospinal tract lesions.

Bekhterev nucleus (superior vestibular nucleus): Small collection of nerve cells lying above lateral vestibular nucleus.

Bekhterev reflex (Geigel reflex, hypogastric reflex): Positive if lower abdominal muscle contracts when inner thigh is stroked.

Bekhterev reflex: Positive if facial muscle contracts when ipsilateral nasal mucosa is tickled.

Bekhterev reflex (paradoxical pupillary reflex): Pupil dilation when light is shone into eye; can be seen occasionally in tabes dorsalis.

Bekhterev sign (Bechterew sign): Paralysis of automatic facial movements, with voluntary movement remaining intact.

Bekhterev test: Positive for sciatica if patient sitting on flat surface cannot extend both legs at same time; patients with sciatica are usu. able to extend 1 leg at a time.

Bell muscle (ureteric bridge): Muscle fibers located in bladder trigone between ureteric orifices.

Bell nerve (external respiratory nerve): Long thoracic nerve carrying motor fibers originating from C5–C7; supplies serratus anterior muscle.

Bell palsy: Most accurately described as idiopathic facial paralysis caused by a lower motor neuron lesion of CN VII; usu. preceded by viral prodrome involving stiffness and pain along facial nerve distribution. Condition causes ipsilateral paralysis of side of face, including inability to close eyelids or raise eyebrows and occurrence of flattened nasolabial fold. Improvement usu. occurs within 4–6 months, with resolution by 12 months. Term is commonly used inaccurately to describe facial paralysis seen in diabetes, Lyme disease, MS, and sarcoidosis.

Bell phenomenon: Bilateral eyelid closure and upward eye deviation with corneal irritation; mediated by brainstem reflex. Condition may also occur with normal eyelid closure.

Bell phenomenon: Superior and lateral deviation of ipsilateral eye when attempting to close lid in Bell palsy.

Bell-Dally dislocation: Nontraumatic dislocation of C1 vertebrae.

Bell-Magendie law: Early elucidation that motor functions are located in ventral spinal cord and sensory functions in posterior spinal cord.

Bellini ducts (tubules): Collecting ducts, which allow passage of urine from calyx to renal pelvis; rare site of carcinoma with highly aggressive activity.

Bellini ligament: Section of articular capsule of hip that extends to greater trochanter.

Belsey operation (Belsey-Mark IV): Antireflux operation performed through chest; uses 270° anterior gastric wrap and posterior plication of crura. 2 layers of plicating sutures are placed between distal esophagus (muscle layer) and gastric fundus (seromuscular layer), and diaphragmatic sutures are placed at 4, 8, and 12 o'clock positions.

Bence Jones albumosuria: Presence of albumose in urine due to sarcomatous disease; usu. occurs with associated softening of bones.

Bence Jones cylinders: Gelatinous bodies containing contents of seminal vesicles (Trousseau-Lallemand bodies).

Bence Jones proteins: Light-chain protein fragments, with molecular weights of 25,000–50,000 d, seen in urine in multiple myeloma and Waldenström macroglo-bulinemia; when heated they coagulate at 40°–60° C and redissolve at 80°–100° C. Fragments are also detected as narrow monoclonal bands between alpha-2 and gamma-globulins on serum protein electrophoresis and by sulfosalicylic acid precipitate. They are filtered by glomerulus and reabsorbed by tubule cells, causing injury.

Bencze syndrome: Submucosal cleft palate, strabismus, amblyopia, and facial asymmetry.

Bender test (Gestalt Motor Test): Used to measure ability to copy 9 geometric forms of increasing complexity freehand. Test also evaluates organic brain disease, neurologic maturity, motor perception, and personality dynamics; used in persons > 5 years of age.

Benditt hypothesis: Smooth muscle cells in atherosclerotic plaques are benign tumors. Reasoning is based on monoclonal origin of smooth muscle cells seen in some patients.

Benedict reagent: Alkaline copper sulfate solution used in Benedict test for glucose.

Benedict solution: Cupric sulfate–containing reagent used to detect reducing substances in urine both qualitatively and quantitatively. Positive result is color change from blue to yellowish pink on heating (qualitative test). Reagent titrates addition of potassium thiocyanate and ferrocyanide until pink color disappears (quantitative test).

Benedict test: Technique used to detect presence of glucose if red, green, or yellow precipitate forms. 125 g of potassium thiocyanate, 200 g of sodium carbonate, and 200 g of potassium (or sodium) citrate are dissolved in 800 ml boiling H_2O. Solution is cooled, filtered, mixed with 100 ml H_2O containing 18 g cupric acid, and diluted to 1 L. Finally, 10 drops of test sample are added.

Benedict-Roth spirometer: Closed-circuit instrument used to determine oxygen consumption over time; used to calculate basal metabolism. Each liter of oxygen consumed represents 4.825 calories.

Benedikt syndrome: Injury to tegmentum of midbrain with variable structural injury to CN III (ipsilateral palsy), spinothalamic tract (contralateral loss of pain and temperature sensation), medial lemniscus (contralateral loss of joint position), superior cerebellar peduncle (contralateral ataxia), and red nucleus (contralateral chorea).

Bengston method: Modification of Macchiavello stain that colors rickettsial bacteria red and others blue.

Benin haplotype: 1 of 4 major gene clusters on chromosome 11 for sickle cell disease; marked by sequence changes of −369 (C→ G) and −309 (A→ G).

Bennett angle: Radiographic angle seen on horizontal view of jaw; formed by sagittal plane and line of advancement of condyle during lateral mandibular movement.

Bennett fracture (boxer fracture): Avulsion of thumb metacarpal at intra-articular surface; usu. bone fragments stay attached in ligaments. Fracture manifests with pain and swelling; may be caused by severe traction of abductor pollicis longus muscle.

Bennett method: Positive for presence of sulfhydryl groups when mercury orange produces red color after applied to histologic specimen.

Bennhold Congo red stain: Material that stains amyloid pinkish-red, elastic tissue red, and nuclei blue.

Benninghoff arcades: Orientation of collagen fibers in articular cartilage. Fibers run at right angles to surface deep in cartilage and curve to run parallel with surface closer to articular surface.

Bensley aniline–acid fuchsin–methyl green method: Technique used to stain mitochondria maroon, zymogen granules red, and nuclei green; also stains alpha pancreatic islet cells red and beta islet cells green.

Bensley osmic dichromate fluid: Potassium dichromate, osmium tetroxide, and acetic acid used to stain cytoplasmic structures.

Bensley safranin acid violet: Material used to distinguish types of pancreatic islet cells with neutral stains.

Benson disease: Condition marked by crystals of calcium

stearate or polynitrile precipitating as irregularly shaped bodies in vitreous of eye. Vision impairment is negligible; occurs in elderly.

Benton test (visual retention test): Used to measure short-term memory for geometric configurations in different spatial arrangements.

bentonite: Aluminum silicate–type earth that holds 12 times its weight in water; used as laxative, antibody detection test, and skin base.

bentonite flocculation test: Used to detect antibodies against rheumatoid factor, DNA, and *Trichinella*. Positive if flocculation occurs when known antigens are absorbed by bentonite and then exposed to sera.

Berant-Berant syndrome: Sagittal synostosis and fusion of radius and ulna.

Bérard ligament: Fibrous tissue that suspends pericardium and attaches to 3rd and 4th thoracic vertebrae.

Berardinelli-Seip syndrome: Fatty liver, hepatomegaly, hyperlipidemia, acanthosis nigricans, and nonketotic insulin-resistant diabetes mellitus; autosomal recessive condition.

Béraud valve: Mucosal membrane fold sometimes present at junction of nasolacrimal duct and lacrimal sac.

Berdon syndrome (megacystic microcolon

syndrome): Decreased peristalsis of GI tract and urinary retention; caused by degeneration of smooth muscle in intestinal wall. Onset occurs in infancy or childhood; more prevalent in females.

Berendes-Bridge-Good disease: Congenital chronic severe granulomatous disease marked by increased infections in all tissues. Inflammatory masses develop throughout body and may compress internal organs. Pathogens include *Staphylococcus aureus*, *Candida albicans*, *Serratia marcescens*, and *Salmonella*. Cause is inability to activate neutrophils to respiratory burst. Palliative treatment with steroids, antibiotics, gamma-interferon, and bone marrow transplantation.

Berg chelate removal method: Staining technique used to demonstrate inorganic triphosphatases.

Berger disease (Berger-Hinglais disease): Mesangial proliferative glomerulonephritis caused by deposition of IgA complexes; marked by repeated macroscopic hematuria and sometimes associated with upper respiratory infections. Onset is in adolescence or early adulthood. 50% of patients who receive kidney transplants experience recurrence.

Berger operation: Radical arm amputation.

Berger rhythm: EEG wave pattern or rhythm generated

from the occipital area; fully developed by 10 years of age. Frequency is 10 cycles/sec with amplitude of 10–75 mV.

Berger sign: Elliptical pupil occurring in tabes dorsalis and some paralytic conditions.

Berger space: Potential space within Wiegert ligament in eye; continuous with Cloquet canal.

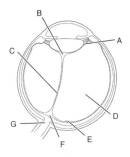

A. Weigert ligament
B. Berger space
C. Cloquet canal
D. Vitreous base
E. Fovea
F. Space of Martegiani
G. Peripapillary

Berger space

Berger syndrome: Idiopathic muscle weakness and paresthesias in legs.

Berger-Goldberg disease (Hardero porphyrinuria): Congenital increased serum level of coproporphyria; hepatomegaly, jaundice, and photosensitivity (developing in childhood); normal life span.

Bergey classification: System for categorization of bacteria based on Gram stain, morphology, metabolism, order, family, genus, and species.

Bergkvist system: Grading scheme for transitional cell carcinoma ranging from grade 0–grade IV.

Bergman sign: Radiographic finding in urology. Ureter distal to blockage due to neoplasm is dilated, and ureter distal to blockage due to stone is collapsed.

Bergman triad: Altered sensorium, dyspnea, and petechiae (usu. on chest wall/axilla); seen in fat emboli.

Bergmann fibers: Neural processes originating in molecular layer of cerebellum and radiating to pia.

Bergmeister papilla (congenital vein): Periarterial sheathing of intravitreous hyaloid artery by glial cells during fetal development; usu. completely regresses before birth, but remnants may be found as triangular structure on nasal side of disk.

Bergonié-Tribondeau law: Radiation sensitivity varies inversely with cell differentiation and directly with reproductive ability.

Bergstrand disease: Osteoid lesion developing as a partially calcified rounded bone nodule; lacks inflammatory component. Condition causes pain at site (worse at night). Onset occurs at 10–25 years of age. Treatment is excision.

Berk-Sharp technique:
Technique of genetic mapping in which single-strand DNA is hybridized with mRNA and then subjected to restriction mapping. DNA strand that is not merged with mRNA is removed using S1 nuclease.

Berk-Tabatznik syndrome:
Cervical kyphosis, hemivertebral wedging, short fingers, optic atrophy, and spastic quadriparesis.

Berke operation:
Modification of Blaskovics operation for correction of upper eyelid ptosis; skin incision is made to allow for resection of excess levator muscle.

Berke operation: Modification of Motais operation for correction of upper eyelid ptosis; eyelid is tacked to superior rectus muscle.

Berke-Reese modification:
Variation of Krönlein operation for lateral orbitotomy; uses transverse skin incision from lateral canthus of eye toward ear, allowing for resection of lateral orbital bone.

Berkefeld filter: Bacterial filter made of diatomaceous earth. Comes in V (coarse), N (normal), and W (fine) pore sizes. Most bacteria filter out with V pore.

berkelium: Artificially occurring radioactive element; atomic number is 97, most stable isotope is Bk-247, and half-life is 1.4×10^3 years.

Berlin blue: See Prussian blue.

Berlin blue reaction:
Bichromic stain; uses nuclear fast red to stain nuclei red and calcium ferrocyanide to stain hemosiderin and iron blue.

Berlin disease: Mottled skin, stunted growth, hypodontia, hypotrichosis, and mental retardation; autosomal recessive condition.

Berlin disease: Retinal pallor caused by trauma. Treatment is corticosteroids, diuretics, and vitamin A.

Berlin disease: Blindness caused by nonocular head trauma; due to peripheral nerve fiber necrosis in intracanalicular or intracranial portions of CN II.

Berlock disease: Dark-brown pigmentation developing in susceptible patients after light exposure of skin that has been in contact with furocoumarin.

Berman oropharyngeal airway: Device with open channels on both sides and a central support.

Bernard duct: See Santorini duct.

Bernard glandular layer: Cell layer lining pancreatic acini.

Bernard procedure: Method of cheek advancement flap used for lip reconstruction, specifically to resect lesion on middle part of lower lip. Nasolabial triangles are removed, and buccal mucosa, muscle, and skin are advanced to reconstruct lower lip.

Bernard puncture: Method of inducing glycosuria in experimental animals by puncturing a site on floor of 4th ventricle.

Bernard syndrome (Claude Bernard syndrome): Lesion (tumor, infection, and aneurysm) in central sympathetic nerve fibers; causes ipsilateral increase in sweating, lacrimation, and eyelid retraction, along with decreased blinking.

Bernard-Sergent syndrome: See Addisonian crisis.

Bernard-Soulier syndrome: Defect in glycoprotein receptor, which results in decreased platelet adhesion through inability to bind von Willebrand factor. Onset occurs in infancy with epistaxis, purpura, and prolonged bleeding time. Platelets are enlarged and megakaryocytes are increased in number.

Bernhardt sign (Bernhardt-Roth sign, Roth sign): Pain on anterior lateral thigh; caused by injury to external cutaneous nerve.

Bernheim syndrome: Right ventricular failure due to obstruction by hypertrophied left ventricle; marked by pulmonary congestion and enlarged liver. Condition causes bulging of septum and impaired emptying of right atrium. Treatment is same as for hypertension and heart failure.

Bernoulli distribution (binomial distribution): Probability distribution that describes likelihood of various combinations of 2 alternate outcomes in series of independent trials. Computation involves expansion of binomial $(p + q)^N$, where N is number of independent trials, p is probability of 1 outcome alternative, and q is probability of other alternative $(q = 1 - p)$.

Bernoulli effect: Description of air flowing through tubes of different diameters; pressure in narrower spaces is less than in wider spaces.

Bernoulli effect: Method of humidification in which small droplets are produced when gas is passed rapidly across narrow, fluid-filled orifice.

Bernstein test: Confirmatory test for gastroesophageal reflux disease; positive if symptoms occur with placement of dilute hydrochloric acid into esophagus.

Berthsen methylene violet: Weakly basic stain used in MacNeal tetrachrome stain.

Bernuth hemophilia: Hemophilia occurring with sporadic inheritance pattern.

Berry circle: Instrument for testing stereoscopic vision. Patients view series of different charts that contain drawings of circles.

Berry ligament: Fibrous attachment of posterior thyroid gland to the trachea.

Berteil projection: Special radiographic view for visualization of inferior orbital fissure, with forehead placed on plate on tabletop 15° off incline with 20° extension of neck.

Berthelot reaction: Berthelot reagent mixed with ammonia to form deep-blue product; used in colorimetric stains for urea and ammonia.

Berthelot reagent: Hypochlorite–phenol alkaline solution.

Bertin bones: Sphenoidal turbinal bones.

Bertin columns (renal columns): Inner portion of kidney cortex; runs inward between pyramids to reach bottom of sinus.

Bertin ligament (anterior ileofemoral ligament, Bigelow ligament, Y-ligament): Fibrous connective tissue running on anterosuperior border of hip joint from lower area of anterior-inferior iliac spine to intertrochanteric edge of femur; forms anterior part of capsule covering femoral neck. Ligament acts to resist hyperextension of hip joint.

Bertol method: Technique used to assess hip dysplasia in newborn infants; compares distance from horizontal acetabular line to top of femoral physis with distance from superior medial femoral shaft to medial wall of acetabulum. Normal value is > 2.

Bertolotti syndrome: Symptoms of sciatica caused by progressive scoliosis and sacralization of 5th lumbar vertebrae.

Bertrand pneumotaxic guide: Early stereotactic guide used in brain surgery.

Besnier prurigo (diathetic prurigo): Alternating exacerbations of asthma and localized, lichenized lesions with pruritus; most common sites are knees, elbows, wrists, and face. Etiology is unknown; condition usu. follows infantile atopic dermatitis. 80% of patients have increased IgE.

Besnier prurigo of pregnancy: Small crusty papules developing in 3rd trimester of pregnancy; most commonly found on extensor areas of limbs and occasionally on upper trunk.

Besnier-Boeck disease: Sarcoidosis.

Bessauds-Hilmand-Augier syndrome: Sexual infantilism and intestinal polyposis.

Bessey-Lowry-Brock unit: Measure of acid or alkaline phosphatase activity (1 L of serum that hydrolyzes 1 mmol of p-nitrophenylphosphatase at 37° C in 1 hour).

Best carmine stain: Alcohol and ammonia solution of carmine that stains glycogen red in cytoplasm of hepatocytes; used to visualize liver tissue.

Best disease (vitelliform macular dystrophy): Congenital macular degeneration of eye.

Initial vitelline lesion progresses to irregular pigmentation and yellowish masses.

Bethea sign: Decreased unilateral thoracic expansion; detected by having examiner place fingertips on corresponding ribs bilaterally and noting excursion when patient takes deep breath.

Bethesda system: Method developed in 1988 to clarify competing terminology systems for cervical intraepithelial neoplasm. Grades: normal, benign cellular changes, atypical squamous cells of undetermined significance, low-grade squamous intraepithelial, and high-grade squamous intraepithelial.

Bethesda unit: Measure of inhibitor activity to factor VIII; 1 unit equals amount needed to inactivate 50% of factor VIII in a 2-hour period.

Bethke-Kleihauer test (Bethke stain): Stain used on maternal blood to investigate possible fetomaternal hemorrhage. Dark cells from retained hemoglobin F are fetal in origin, and light cells from acid eluting hemoglobin A are maternal in origin.

Bethlem myopathy (Bethlem-Wijngaarden myopathy): Slowly progressive limb girdle weakness; autosomal dominant condition with onset in infancy. Contractions of fingers, elbows, and ankles also occur; proximal muscles are more involved than distal ones. Death can occur from perforation of intestinal ulcers.

Bettley syndrome: Crusting blisters of the skin and ulceration of oropharyngeal cavity and intestinal tract; rare condition with unknown etiology and variable inheritance patterns.

Betz cells: Large pyramidal ganglion cells found in cerebral layer 5 of the motor area of cerebral gray matter.

Betz cell area: See Brodmann area 4.

Beukes dysplasia: Pain in hips in childhood progressing to crippling disability by young adulthood, with absence of extraskeletal manifestations; autosomal dominant condition. Radiographs show flattened and irregular femoral capital epiphyses.

Bevan incision: Vertical incision parallel to outer border of rectus muscle; used for access to upper abdominal quadrants.

Bevan operation: Surgical technique for positioning undescended testicle into scrotum.

Bezold abscess: Suppurative collection located deep to superior attachment of sternocleidomastoid muscle; associated with mastoid tip perforation and infection.

Bezold ganglion: Collection of cell bodies in interatrial septum.

Bezold sign: Swelling below mastoid apex seen in mastoiditis.

Bezold-Jarisch reflex: Bradycardia and hypotension caused by stimulation of left ventricle chemoreceptors by some alkaloid and antihypertensive drugs.

Bezredka bilivaccine: Highly effective killed oral cholera vaccine developed in 1920s; unfortunately, fell into disuse because diarrhea produced by added bile salts mimicked diarrhea of cholera and caused panic in recipients.

Bhattacharyya-Connor syndrome (phytosterolemia): Atherosclerosis of coronaries and large arteries, hemolytic anemia, recurrent arthralgias, xanthelasma, and tendon xanthomas; rare autosomal recessive condition with onset in childhood. Cause is increased absorption of sitosterol with tissue accumulation. Death is common in 2nd–3rd decade due to coronary artery disease. Treatment is low dietary intake of plant sterols, cholestyramine, and neomycin.

Bial reagent: Solution of 25 drops of 10% ferric chloride, fuming hydrochloric acid, and 1.5 g of orcinol; indicates pentose in urine if green color develops when reagent is added to sample.

Bianchi nodule: See Arantius nodule.

Bianchi syndrome: Expressive alexia, hemianesthesia, and temporary hemiplegia; usu. caused by lesion in left parietal lobe.

Bianchi valve: See Häsner valve.

Biber-Haab-Dimmer dystrophy (Bucklers dystrophy, Haab-Dimmer dystrophy, lattice dystrophy): Progressive discrete grayish threads in cornea (between Bowman membrane and epithelium); onset in early adulthood. Cause is hyaline degeneration. Condition leads to gradual reduction in vision.

Bichat fissure (great fissure of cerebrum): Fissure that runs between ventral surface of cerebral hemispheres and dorsal diencephalon; formed by "folding back" of cerebral hemispheres during embryonic development.

Bichat ligament: Lower part of posterior sacroiliac ligament.

Bick procedure: V -shaped full-thickness eyelid resection performed at lateral margin; used to correct involutional ectropion. Medial edge of resection is attached to lateral canthal tendon stump.

Bickel ring: See Waldeyer tonsillar ring.

Bickel-Fanconi syndrome: Growth retardation, hepatomegaly, rickets (not responsive to vitamin D), and tubulopathy. Etiology likely involves glycogen storage abnormality; onset in 1st year of life.

Bickers-Adams syndrome: Hydrocephalus with spasticity, severe mental retardation, abnormally flexed thumb, and short 1st metacarpal; congenital X-linked condition caused by stenosis of aqueduct of Sylvius. Females are carriers with below-average intelligence.

Bickerstaff syndrome: Migraine symptoms (e.g., visual loss, visual field scintillation, dysarthria, vertigo, ataxia, paresthesias of digits, vomiting due to basilar artery constriction); often occurs in young women at menses.

Bidder ganglion: Collection of cell bodies on cardiac nerves at lower end of atrial septum.

Bidder organ: Anterior segment of gonad in male toad.

Bidwell ghost: Purkinje after-image.

Biebrich scarlet red: Stain used for connective tissue, sex chromatin, and basic protein; also component of Shorr stain.

Biebrich scarlet–picroaniline blue: Material that stains erythrocytes orange-red, muscle pink, mucus pale blue, and connective tissue and basement membrane blue; when used with iron hematoxylin, stains nuclei black.

Biederman sign: Indicator of syphilis if anterior pillars of throat appear dusky red instead of pink.

Biedl syndrome: See Laurence-Moon-Biedl syndrome.

Bielschowsky method: Uses diamine silver, silver nitrate, acidic gold chloride, and sodium thiosulfate; stains reticular fibers brown-black and collagen fibers gray-purple.

Bielschowsky test (head tilt test): Used to confirm superior oblique muscle (CN IV) palsy; positive if when patient is asked to straighten head, eye on opposite side deviates. If weakness exists, patient will tilt head away from affected side to overcome tendency of eye to extort on straight-ahead gaze.

Bielschowsky-Jansky syndrome (Bielschowski syndrome, Dollinger-Bielschowsky syndrome): Loss of mental functioning, visual loss, seizures, and ataxia; associated with demyelination and cerebromacular degeneration. Onset occurs at 3–4 years of age.

Bielschowsky-Lutz-Cogan syndrome (Lhermitte syndrome): Internuclear ophthalmoplegia; caused by any lesion affecting medial longitudinal fasciculus. Condition leads to unilateral or bilateral palsy on conjugate lateral gaze.

Biemond syndrome: Congenital absence of pain sensation; physical and mental development usu. normal otherwise; occasionally associated with seizures, auditory aphasia, anhidrosis, and oligophrenia.

Biemond syndrome: Mental retardation, dwarfism, hypospadias, iris colomba, obesity, hydrocephalus, and polydactyly; autosomal recessive condition.

Biemond syndrome: Nystagmus, strabismus, ataxia, mental retardation, and shortened metacarpal and metatarsals.

Bienstock bacillus: *Clostridium putrificum.*

Bier amputation: Leg amputation with bone flap

fashioned from tibia and fibula proximal to stump.

Bier block anesthesia: Regional limb anesthesia produced by IV injection of local anesthetic; used in conjunction with extremity tourniquet. Compression prevents systemic effects of anesthesia and provides bloodless operative field.

Biermer disease (Addison anemia, Addison-Hunter disease, Biermer-Ehrlich disease, Lebert disease): Pernicious anemia with paresthesias, GI complaints, painful mouth, ataxia, and stomach carcinoma. Adult type has global gastric acid secretion deficiency and gastric atrophy; congenital type has deficiency of intrinsic factor only.

Biernacki sign: Numbness in ulnar nerve distribution; seen in tabes dorsalis and general paresis.

Biesenberger mammaplasty: Technique for reduction of breast tissue; uses transposition of nipple via excision of lateral part of breast with rotation of pedicle containing the breast.

Bietti keratopathy (Labrador keratopathy): Appearance of opacities (oil-like droplets) that arise in horizontal line in periphery of cornea and eventually coalesce to form band; caused by excessive eye exposure to UV radiation and severe environment (e.g., Eskimos). Treatment is excision.

Bietti retinopathy: Tapetoretinal degeneration marked by crystalline deposits in all layers of retina; also with varying degrees of choriocapillaris, esp. in posterior pole.

Bietti syndrome: Slowly progressive corneal degeneration, retinal degeneration, bowing of Descemet membrane, and loose connective tissue replacing stroma; may cause night blindness and loss of peripheral vision. Condition is common among elderly in China.

bifurcate deep ligaments of Arnold (bigeminate ligaments): Fibrous connective tissue running from plantar surface of base of metatarsal bones to plantar surface of cuneiform and cuboid bones.

Bigelow ligament: See Bertin ligament.

Bigelow operation: Lithotripsy for treatment of kidney calculi.

Bigelow septum: Anatomic plane of extra-hard bone in femoral neck.

Biglieri syndrome: Congenital defect in 17-hydroxylase with variable defect in 17,20-lyase activity; marked by female genotype with amenorrhea, lack of secondary sexual development, muscle weakness, paresthesias in extremities, and hypertension. Condition results in decreased levels of cortisol, androgens, and estrogens.

Bignami-Marchiafava disease (Bignami disease): Focal necrosis of corpus callosum; usu. thought to occur secondary to chronic alcoholism.

Bikele sign: Resistance to elbow extension when arm is elevated, flexed at elbow, and externally rotated; suggests meningeal irritation or brachial plexus neuritis.

Bilderbeck disease (acrodynia, Selter disease, Swift disease, Swift-Feer disease): Pink discoloration as well as swelling and pain in toes and fingers; also with failure to thrive, photophobia, listlessness, and reddish rash on nose and cheeks. Condition occurs in infancy and early childhood; most cases caused by mercury intoxication.

Bilginturan syndrome: Arterial hypertension and short fingers; autosomal dominant condition.

Bilhaut-Cloquet procedure: Surgical repair of congenital duplicated thumb (Wassel type I and II). Technique involves fusing slightly more than half of each small thumb with resection of remaining tissue.

Billings method: Birth control method using abstinence of intercourse during high periods of fertility; high failure rate. Basis is awareness of vaginal "wetness" to predict upcoming ovulation.

Billroth cords: Diffuse strands of lymphatic tissue found in red pulp of spleen between venous sinuses; form spongy network spread on underlying scaffolding of reticular connective tissue. Cords serve as anatomic microfilter and also remove foreign material.

Billroth disease: Bladder cancer caused by chronic *Schistosoma haematobium* infection. Treatment is radical anterior pelvic exenteration.

Billroth disease: Fluid accumulation under scalp caused by skull fracture and arachnoid tear. Treatment is conservative in absence of infection.

Billroth I procedure: Distal gastrectomy with gastroduodenal reconstruction;

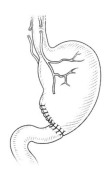

Billroth I procedure

operation of choice for type I gastric ulcer.

Billroth II procedure: Distal gastrectomy with gastrojejunal reconstruction; less physiologic than Billroth I procedure. If patients complain of constant, burning epigastric pain unrelieved by vomiting postop, alkaline reflux gastritis or stomal obstruction with

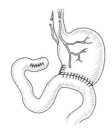

Billroth II procedure

marginal ulceration should be suspected.

Billroth-von Winiwarter disease: See Buerger disease.

Bimler appliance (stimulator): Removable orthodontic device that stimulates muscle activity to effect tooth movement.

Binder syndrome (maxillonasal dysostosis): Congenital flat, vertical nose and crescent-shaped nostrils, hypoplasia of premaxillary area, absent nasal spine, flat chin, and relative mandibular prognathism; normal sense of smell. Frontal sinuses are usu. absent.

Binet age: Mental age corresponding to age in years of child with normal level of intelligence; used to measure intelligence level of persons with abnormal mental development.

Binet test (Binet-Simon test): Method of testing mental capacity and mental age of children; involves asking series of questions and comparing results obtained with normal children at various ages.

Bing sign (reflex): Used to determine direction of plantar response by pricking dorsum of big toe (direction of movement of big toe); performed when patient voluntarily withdraws from plantar stroking, thus eliminating its usefulness. Response is seen in corticospinal tract lesions.

Bing test: Used to distinguish conductive and sensorineural hearing deficits. When vibrating tuning fork is held to mastoid process and ear canal is alternately open and occluded, increase and decrease in loudness is detected with normal hearing and impaired sensorineural hearing. No difference is discerned with impaired conductive hearing.

Bing-Neel syndrome (neuropsychiatric Waldenström macroglobulinemia): Anorexia, profound weight loss, pallor, generalized asthenia, lymphadenopathy, convulsions, hemorrhage, encephalopathy, stroke, coma, and disseminated spinal lesions; poor prognosis, with death occurring 6–12 months after onset of neurologic symptoms.

Binswanger encephalopathy: Dementia due to subcortical demyelinization and lacunar infarcts caused by arteriosclerosis of small arteries in white matter; slowly progressive condition. Typical onset is 50–60 years of age.

Biot breathing (sign): Apneic periods interspersed with several identical breaths; occurs with increased intracranial pressure.

Birbeck granules: Rod-shaped organelles found in Langerhans cells; contain central striation and sometimes resemble tennis racket on cross-section. Function is unknown.

Birch-Jensen syndrome: Congenital malformation of unilateral or bilateral hands and occasionally feet, with characteristic "lobster claw" defect. Condition is associated with other somatic malformations.

Bird sign: Area of dullness with absence of breath sounds; seen in hydatid disease of lung.

Birnbaum syndrome: Variation of Huntington chorea with presence of cerebellar atrophy.

Birsch-Hirschfield syndrome: Idiopathic hypertrophy of parotid gland causing parotitis; occurs in elderly.

Birt-Hogg-Dube syndrome: Multiple, small, yellow-white papules on face; associated with hidradenomas and achrocordans. Condition is autosomal dominant.

Bischoff myelotomy: Treatment of severe spastic hypertonia by surgically interrupting reflex arc in spinal cord, which is partially severed through lateral funiculus on 1 side and from middle of cord to gray matter on opposite side.

Bishop deformity (benediction hand): Wasting of hypothenar and interosseous muscles and 2 medial lumbrical muscles of hand; due to ulnar nerve palsy. Eponym is misnomer.

Bishop score: Measurement used to assess risk of preterm delivery based on digital exam; factors evaluated are position of cervix in relation to vagina, cervical consistency, station of fetal head, extent of cervical dilation, and extent of cervical effacement.

Biskra button: See Aleppo boil.

Bismarck brown: Group of basic synthetic azo dyes that are nondiffusable in aqueous solution; used to demonstrate nuclei in fat cells and stain mucin and cartilage (esp. tracheal and fetal tissue) yellow-brown. Common types are brown R (dark-brown solid) and brown Y (black-brown powder).

Bismuth classification: System used to describe injuries to extrahepatic bile ducts. Level 1, damaged common bile duct with intact hepatic stump > 2 cm; level 2, damaged common bile duct with intact hepatic stump < 2 cm; level 3, high stricture with intact duct confluence; level 4, damaged duct confluence; level 5, injury to right sectorial ducts.

Bitot breathing: Ataxic breathing marked by irregular pattern; shallow and deep breaths are interspersed with short periods of apnea. Condition is often associated with medullary brain damage.

Bitot spots: Superficial white flecks formed on conjunctiva; seen in vitamin A deficiency and other conditions.

Bitter syndrome:
Hemihypertrophy of face (starting from birth), with sebaceous nevus in trigeminal and upper cervical area; occurs in infants whose mothers received thalidomide. Condition is also associated with dwarfism and other anomalies of brain, eyes, and mouth.

Bittner virus (agent): Retrovirus (RNA) that causes breast tumors in mice.

Bittorf reaction: Highly suggestive of presence of renal calculi if firm palpation of testes or abdominal wall overlying ovary produces ipsilateral kidney or flank pain.

Bixler syndrome (Harper dwarf): Dwarfism (occurring in females only) with psychomotor retardation, deafness, microstomia, cleft palate and nose, hypertelorism, atrial septal defects, and ectopic kidneys.

Bixler-Antley syndrome: Variant of Erdheim syndrome, with addition of ectopic pigment layer of iris in anterior surface of iris.

Bjerrum scotoma: Loss of vision largely encircling fixation point; originates near blind spot.

Bjerrum screen (tangent screen): Apparatus used with campimeter to evaluate field of vision; has large, black scrollable background with central point for fixation.

Bjoerck disease (Cassidy syndrome, Hedlinger disease, Scholtze disease, Thorson-Bjoerck disease): Carcinoid syndrome; usu. metastasis are present. Diarrhea, weight loss, flushing, asthma, pellagra-like rash, hepatomegaly, and ascites occur. Systemic signs and symptoms are caused by tumors derived from amine precursor uptake and decarboxylation (APUD) cells. Urine shows high levels of 5-hydroxy-3-indoleacetic acid (5-HIAA). Treatment is excision of primary lesion and metastasis if possible, plus somatostatin, octreotide, and methysergide.

Bjork flap: Tracheal flap sewn to skin to ensure tracheostomy remains patent.

Bjork-Shiley valve: Tilting-disk type mitral valve prosthesis; requires chronic anticoagulation.

Björnstad syndrome: Deafness and segmental twists in hair shafts (pili torti); autosomal recessive condition.

Bjornstad-Crandall syndrome: Sensorineuronal hearing loss in association with segmental twists in hair shafts (pili torti) and deficiency of growth and follicle-stimulating hormones; severity of brittleness of hair correlates with degree of deafness. Condition produces secondary hypogonadism.

Björnström algesimeter: Instrument for measuring skin sensitivity to pain.

Black formula (Pignet formula): Used to assess overall vigor and strength of adult man. Equation: $F = (W + C) - H$, where W is weight (lb.), C is chest circumference (in. at full inspiration), and H is height (in.). $F > 120$ is considered very strong and < 80 very weak.

Black reagent: Solution of 100 ml H_2O, 0.4 g ferrous chloride, and 5 g ferric chloride.

Blackburne ratio
(Blackburne-Peel ratio): Value determined by flexing knee to $30°$ and dividing distance from inferior patellar surface to tibial condylar surface by height of weight-bearing part of patella. Normal value: 0.8.

Blackett-Healy position:
Radiographic patient positioning technique using anterior-posterior view to image subscapularis insertion at lesser tuberosity.

Blackett-Healy position:
Radiographic patient positioning technique using posterior-anterior view to image teres minor insertion onto humerus.

Blackfan-Diamond syndrome (Joseph-Diamond-Blackfan syndrome, Kasnelson disease): Congenital normocytic and normochromic RBC anemia, growth retardation, low birth weight, pallor, and failure of sexual maturation. Treatment is chronic blood transfusions (significant long-term sequelae) and bone marrow transplantation.

Blainville ear: Asymmetrical ears.

Blair incision: Incision starting at middle of border of mandible and running to middle of medial edge of ear lobe; used in facial surgery (e.g., when transposing branch of facial nerve to contralateral side).

Blair-Brown operation:
Method for repairing cleft palate; uses lateral flap sized to 1/2 length of lip.

Blalock-Hanlon operation:
Palliative technique for transposition of great vessels using surgically created atrial septal defect.

Blalock-Taussig procedure:
Operation performed by connecting subclavian artery to a branch of the pulmonary artery via graft; used to correct systemic cyanosis due to congenital pulmonary artery stenosis. Injury to thoracic duct may occur, causing chylothorax.

Bland-Garland-White syndrome: Anomalous origin of left coronary artery from pulmonary artery, resulting in no clinical sequelae at birth but development of myocardial ischemia as infant. If inadequate coronary artery circulation occurs, lesion progresses to death; otherwise symptoms improve, with development of left heart dilatation, mitral insufficiency, arrhythmias, and coronary artery steal syndrome.

Blandin ganglion: Collection of parasympathetic neurons lying superior to deep part of submandibular glands and on lateral surface of hyoglossus muscle.

Blandin glands (Nuhn glands): Anterior seromucous lingual glands located on inferior tongue surface on either side of frenulum; can become obstructed in children, causing mucocele under tongue.

Blaskovics operation: Method for correction of upper eyelid ptosis; conjunctival approach is used to remove excess tarsus and levator muscle.

Blatin sign: Vibratory sensation or thrill felt when examiner places cyst (classically described as hydatid) under tension.

Blatt syndrome: Congenital deformities of eyelid, face, orbit, and skull; autosomal dominant condition with meningocele, wide-set eyes, absent meibomian glands, and distichiasis (skin tags).

Blaud pill: Ferrous carbonate pill.

Blauth classification: System used to describe congenital hypoplasia of thumb: grade I, minor hypoplasia; grade II, adduction contracture of 1st web with normal skeletal articulations; grade III, significant hypoplasia of tendons and articulations; grade IV, vestigial uncontrolled digit (floating thumb); grade V, total absence.

Bledsoe brace: Adjustable locking knee brace used to restrict range of motion after repair of tibial plateau fractures and anterior cruciate ligament injuries.

Blegvad-Haxthausen syndrome: Anetoderma occurring in association with osteogenesis imperfecta; lesions appear as thin, translucent skin with grayish, ovoid patches.

Blencke syndrome: Pain in heel area, worsened by walking; caused by ischemic necrosis of epiphysis.

Blessig cyst (lacunae, spaces): Variable development of anatomic spaces at edges of retina close to ora serrata; vision usu. not impaired.

Blessig groove: Area in embryo eye corresponding to retina.

Blessig-Iwanoff syndrome: Degeneration of retina due to cystic accumulation of glycosaminoglycan in outer plexiform layer; individual cysts eventually coalesce, causing retinal detachment. Condition may be asymptomatic or present with acute vision loss.

Blinks effect: Transient increase in photosynthesis noted when ambient energy shifts from long to shorter wavelength.

Blix diagram: Representation of total and passive tension of muscle; used to evaluate exercise in developing muscle strength and endurance. Graph plots percent of maximum tension on ordinate and percent of resting length on abscissa.

Bloch equations: Mathematical description of motion for macroscopic magnetization vector, including T1 and T2 relaxation time and effects of precession about magnetic field (static and radiofrequency); important in nuclear MRI.

Bloch-Sulzberger syndrome:
Hyperpigmented lesions in band, splatter, or whorl pattern following development of bullous-verrucous lesions on skin; associated with optic atrophy, epilepsy, spastic paralysis, deafness, mental retardation, stunted bone growth, dental abnormalities, and localized atrophic alopecia. Condition has X-linked inheritance and onset is at birth or in early infancy. Death usu. occurs at early age.

Blocksom vesicotomy:
Surgical procedure of bladder diversion in children. A 2–3-cm transverse incision is made halfway between pubis and umbilicus; rectus, fascia, and skin are retracted; blunt dissection of peritoneum is performed. Urachus is then transected and brought up into incision. Procedure can be reversed at later date.

Blom-Singer device: Used to produce speech in postlaryngectomy patients; has 1-way valve surgically placed between posterior wall of trachea and through anterior wall of cervical esophagus. To speak, patient forces air into esophagus by occluding tracheal stoma.

Bloom syndrome: Congenital dwarfism, malformed teeth and photosensitivity, with resulting butterfly telangiectatic erythema primarily on face but also on hands and forearms; associated with increased risk of leukemia and lymphoma and chromosomal breaks and rearrangements. Condition is autosomal recessive; 50% of patients have Jewish ancestry.

Bloom-Richardson grade:
Histologic grading system for breast carcinoma. Grade 1, well-differentiated; grade 2, moderately differentiated; grade 3, poorly differentiated.

Blount disease: Aseptic necrosis of medial tibial condyle; can cause bowlegs.

Blücher shoe: Firm, rigid shoe used in ankle–foot prosthesis; allows for ease in taking device on and off.

Blumberg sign (rebound tenderness): Tenderness occurring after examiner presses and quickly releases anterior abdominal wall; seen in peritoneal inflammation and acute abdomen.

Blumenau nucleus: Lateral part of cuneate nucleus.

Blumenbach clivus: Bony area from foramen magnum to dorsum sellae in the posterior cranial fossa.

Blumenbach process:
Uncinate process of ethmoid bone; extends inferiorly and posteriorly from ethmoid labyrinth.

Blumensaat line:
Radiographic line used in assessing height of patella on lateral plain film; runs parallel to superior part of intercondylar notch.

Blumenthal lesion: Small artery proliferative lesions found in diabetes mellitus.

Blumer shelf: Metastatic tumor occurring in rectovesical or rectouterine pouch; palpable on rectal exam.

Boari flap procedure: Method for ureteral implantation into bladder in setting of long ureteral injury (up to 12 cm). Diseased or damaged ureter is replaced by using bladder wall flap fashioned around catheter and closed in 2 layers (running mucosal and interrupted muscularis); usu. performed in combination with psoas hitch of bladder.

Boas algesimeter: Early instrument used to measure epigastric pain sensitivity, with spring-loaded weights placed over area. Tolerance in gastric ulcer: 1–2 kg; normal tolerance (no pathology): 9–10 kg.

Boas point: Tenderness to left of T12 vertebra; occurs in gastric ulcer.

Boas sign: Right subscapularis pain; occurs in cholelithiasis.

Boas-Oppler bacillus: *Lactobacillus* species; sometimes occurs in gastric secretions in gastric carcinoma.

Bobath method of exercise: Theory of exercise and muscular training for inpatients with cerebral palsy; stresses need for prior inhibition of hypertonia and neurodevelopmental sequence training (simple activities progressing to more complex ones). Reflex facilitation of postural activities are used.

Bochdalek duct: See His canal.

Bochdalek ganglion: Structure located at junction of anterior and middle branches of superior dental plexus; surrounds roots of upper teeth.

Bochdalek hernia (foramen, gap): Posterolateral defect in developing pleuroperitoneal fold; most common type of congenital diaphragmatic hernia (1/2200 live births) and more prevalent in males. Cause is failure of fusion of pleuroperitoneal canal. Condition is often diagnosed on chest radiograph; 88% occur on left side.

Bock ganglion (carotid ganglion): Collection of cells in internal carotid plexus; located in cavernous sinus.

Bock nerve: Pharyngeal nerve; originates from posterior pterygopalatine ganglion, traverses pharyngeal canal with pharyngeal branch of maxillary artery, and supplies mucosal membrane of posterior pharynx.

Bodal test: Used to test for color perception using series of different colored blocks.

Bodansky unit: Amount of alkaline phosphatase needed to liberate 1 mg of phosphate ion from glycerol 2-phosphate at 37° C in 1 hour.

Bodian method: Stain for argyrophilic matter and nerve fiber, which uses formalin fixative, copper–protargol solution, hydroquinone–sodium sulfate solution, gold chloride, sodium thiosulfate, and oxalic acid; stains nerve fibers and nuclei black on blue background.

body of Luys syndrome:
Lesion (e.g., tumor, hemorrhage, granuloma) occurring in body of Luys (subthalamic nucleus), causing acute contralateral violent involuntary movements of arm and leg; may remit spontaneously or progress to death in several weeks.

Boeck-Drbohlar-Locke medium: Buffered eggs, serum, and rice powder; used to culture amebae.

Boerhaave syndrome:
Esophageal rupture approx. 5 cm above gastroesophageal junction; caused by forceful vomiting or retching. Condition is classically described as occurring after large meal but also may occur after childbirth, defecation, and heavy lifting. It is usu. diagnosed late because of relative rarity and requires emergent surgical repair. Patients present with severe retrosternal pain and little or no bleeding.

Boerjeson-Forssman-Lehman syndrome: Mental retardation, seizures, nystagmus, stunted growth, microcephaly, hypogonadism, obesity, large ears, and epilepsy; both autosomal recessive and x-linked recessive forms exist.

Boettcher cells: Cells located on basilar membrane of cochlear duct; provide mechanical structure for organ of Corti sensory cells.

Bogaert disease (Bogaert-Scherer-Epstein disease, van Bogaert disease): Mental deterioration, multiple xanthomas (esp. on tendons), cataracts, lip and tongue paralysis, and atherosclerosis; onset occurs in young adults. Condition is caused by abnormal cholesterol and bile metabolism, with high levels of 5α-cholestan-3β-ol.

Bogart-Bacall syndrome:
Voice dysfunction in professional voice users, resulting in breaks, variable pitch, and resonance; caused by poor musculoskeletal tension and overuse.

Bogg reagent: Solution of 25 ml concentrated hydrochloric acid in 75 ml H_2O added to solution of 25 g of phosphotungstic acid in 125 ml H_2O.

Bogorad syndrome:
Unilateral tearing produced by chewing food or placing spicy food in mouth; caused by damaged and partially regenerated facial nerve fibers.

Bogros space: Surgically developed fat-filled area in preperitoneum used to visualize hernias (and part of external iliac artery) in laparoscopic repair of groin hernias.

Böhler angle: Measurement of talocalcaneal joint as seen on lateral radiographic view; normally 25° –40° but greatly reduced in crush fractures of calcaneum.

Bohler sign: Used to detect meniscus injuries of knee. Patient lies supine and examiner rotates foot to place valgus stress on knee; positive for lateral injuries if pain is present in lateral knee or pain occurring in medial knee during varus rotation.

Böhler splint: Device used to maintain alignment and provide traction for spiral finger fractures.

Böhler-Braun frame: Adjustable metal frame often used to apply traction in severe ankle fractures.

Bohman procedure: Cervical fusion of bone grafts using triple spinous process wiring via posterior approach.

Bohme reagent: Material used to detect presence of indole in a sample.

Bohn nodule: See Epstein pearls.

Bohomoletz bone: Ulnar fragment found in upper distal limb stump in Freire-Maia disease.

Bohr atom: Depiction of atom in which electrons are able to occupy discrete, fixed orbits due influence of quantum forces.

Bohr effect: Shift in oxygen–hemoglobin dissociation curve with change in blood pH; decrease in pH (increased concentration of carbon dioxide and hydrogen ions) shifts curve to right, making it easier for hemoglobin to unload oxygen.

Bohr equation: Expression used to calculate physiologic dead space for gas and estimate number of alveoli with impaired perfusion contributing to dead space; equation is $V_D = (F_E - F_A) \times V_T(F_I - F_A)$, where V_D is dead space, F_E is fractional concentration of gas in expired gas, F_A is fractional concentration of gas in alveolar gas, F_I is fractional concentration of gas in inspiratory gas, V_T is tidal volume.

Bohr magneton: Unit of magnetic moment; equals $eh/4\pi mc$, where e is electron charge, h is Planck constant, m is electron mass, and c is speed of light.

Boivin antigen: O antigen of any gram-negative bacteria.

Boley retractor: Handheld retractor for displacing small amounts of tissue or delicate vascular structures.

Boley retractor

Boling burner: Component of atomic absorption photometer used for atomizing solution.

Bollinger body: Cellular inclusions found in fowlpox.

Bologna syndrome: Hyperkeratotic streaks running along sides of each finger to palm; autosomal dominant condition.

Bolton point: Top of retrocondylar fossa curvature; lies between condyle and basal surface of occipital bone.

Bolton triangle: Imaginary arc formed by lines running between Bolton point nasion (depression at root of nose just inferior to eyebrows), and sella turcica.

Boltzmann constant: 1.38066×10^{-23} J/K; represents energy per temperature unit of 1 degree of freedom in molecule (x, y, z component of vibration, rotation, or velocity).

Bombay blood phenotype: Patients homozygous for H gene that provides substrate for production of A and B blood antigens. Regardless of their ABO genotype, they are functionally type O (type O_h).

Bonanno catheter: Tube placed percutaneously into peritoneal cavity or bladder.

Bonchardat reagent: Mixture of 1% iodine in dissolved aqueous solution of 1% potassium iodide; acts as alkaloid reagent.

Bonferroni inequality: Expression described mathematically as $\alpha T < K\alpha$, where αT is the true probability of wrongly concluding that a difference exists at least once, K is the number of statistical tests performed, α is the cutoff value for the test statistics, and T is the type of test performed. In experimental design, aim is to minimize αT, which functionally describes chance of obtaining value exceeding an acceptable cutoff level.

Bonferroni method: Multiple comparison method used in ANOVA studies.

Bonferroni *t* test: Statistical technique using Bonferroni inequality to isolate differences between comparisons; describes error rate for all comparisons taken as group. Method is best used when only few comparisons are used [e.g., if 3 comparisons are made while maintaining the

chance of at least 1 mistake to < 5%, chance of error for each test is 1.6% (0.05/3)].

Bongiovanni syndrome: 3-hydroxysteroid dehydrogenase deficiency.

Bonneau syndrome: Congenital syndactyly of fingers, polysyndactyly of toes, and cardiac defects.

Bonner position: Abduction, flexion, and outward rotation of thigh seen in inflammation of hip joint.

Bonnet sign: Positive for sciatica if thigh adduction causes pain.

Bonnet syndrome: Combination of Fothergill and Bernard syndromes.

Bonnet syndrome: Vivid hallucinations experienced by elderly blind or partially blind patients, often at night; no brain lesion usu. discernible.

Bonnier syndrome: Lesion in lateral nucleus of vestibular nerve (Deiter nucleus) or tract, causing ocular disturbances (e.g., paralysis of accommodation, nystagmus, diplopia), limb weakness, trigeminal neuralgia, sleepiness, vertigo, and deafness.

Böök syndrome (PHC syndrome): Premature gray hair, excessive sweating of palms and soles, and hypoplastic teeth prone to cavities.

Borchardt triad: Inability to pass nasogastric tube, pain, and violent retching occurring in gastric volvulus.

Borchgrevink method: Technique used to measure

platelet aggregation at small wound opening.

Border-Sedgwick disease: See Louis-Bar syndrome.

Bordet-Gengou agar: Culture medium using combination of glycerin, potato, and blood.

Bordet-Gengou bacillus: *Bordetella pertussis* .

Bordet-Gengou phenomenon: Complement fixation.

Bordier-Fränkel sign: Bell phenomenon.

Borema gastropexy: Surgical treatment of gastroesophageal reflux disease; establishes intra-abdominal segment of esophagus (in absence of fundal wrap).

Borg scale: Method of scoring perceived exertion on scale of 6–20 (barely perceptible effort to very, very difficult); used in post-MI rehabilitation training phase.

Borg scale: 1982 scale scoring perceived exertion of patient on scale of 0–10 (none to maximal).

Borgorad syndrome (crocodile tear syndrome): Profuse tearing during eating; caused by abnormal connection of autonomic fibers to the lacrimal gland instead of the salivary gland.

Born-Haber cycle: Mathematical relationship between lattice energy of ionic compounds, ionization energy, heats of atomization, and electron affinity.

Bornholm eye disease: Hypoplasia of optic nerve heads causing myopia, astigmatism, and visual deficits; X-linked inheritance.

Borovskii disease: See Aleppo boil.

Borrel blue: Silver oxide stain used to identify spirochetes.

Borrel body: Granules inside of Bollinger bodies in fowlpox.

Borrmann classification: System used to describe gastric adenocarcinoma. Type 1, polypoid masses projecting into lumen in absence of necrosis or ulceration; type 2, ulcerated masses/fungating lesions with sharp margins; type 3, ulcerated with diffuse margin; type 4, diffusely infiltrating through wall (linitis plastica).

Borsch bandage: Temporary bandage covering both abnormal and healthy eye.

Borsieri sign (line): Positive if white line that results when fingernail drawn across skin subsequently turns red; seen in early scarlet fever.

Bose hook: Small, curved sharp-tip retractor used in tracheostomy.

Bosniak classification: System used to categorize renal cysts according to their malignant potential based on CT criteria. Class 1, simple cyst; class 2, cyst with benign calcification or hyperdensity or cyst with septations < 1 mm in width; classes 3 and 4, wall thickening, aggressive calcifications, abnormal density not fulfilling criteria of hyperdense cyst, nodular septations, multiloculated masses.

Bostock catarrh: Hay fever; also used to describe allergic rhinitis from molds, duct, mites, and other pollens.

Boston bivalve cast: Removable "splint in half" with "step cuts."

Boston examination: Test used to evaluate writing, comprehension of written language, speaking ability, and auditory comprehension; responses are scored on ± scales, rating scales, and subjective examiner observation. Exam is useful for classifying patients by different aphasia subtypes.

Boston sign: When gaze is directed downward, upper lid moves partially downward, stops, undergoes spasm, and then continues downward; occurs in Graves disease.

Bosworth fracture: Oblique fracture of distal fibula with proximal fragment pulled posteriorly and medially of tibia.

Bosworth technique: Surgical procedure using bone pegs for treatment of Osgood-Schlatter disease.

Bosworth technique: Surgical repair for neglected rupture of tendo calcaneus. Patient is placed in prone position with tourniquet on thigh. Midline posterior calf incision is made; scar tissue is dissected from ruptured ends; and a strip of gastrocnemius tendon is detached completely, except at anchoring area just proximal to rupture. Strip is then woven in a figure-of-8 manner through each free end.

Botallo duct: Ductus arteriosus.

Botallo ligament: Ligamentum arteriosum; remnant of embryonic ductus arteriosus.

Böttcher cells: Small, polygon-shaped cells in cochlea; lie between basilar membrane and Claudius cells.

Böttcher crystals: Microscopic precipitates that form when a drop of ammonium phosphate is added to prostatic fluid.

Bouchard aneurysm: See Charcot aneurysm.

Bouchard coefficient: Quantity of urine/total mass of solids in urine.

Bouchard index: Measure of amount of adipose tissue in individual; equals weight (kg)/height (dm). Normal index value of male is 4200 g.

Bouchard node: Osteophytic overgrowth at proximal interphalangeal joint; seen in osteoarthritis.

Bouchardat treatment: Diet for control of diabetes that stresses avoidance of carbohydrate-rich food.

Boucher-Neuhauser syndrome: Hypogonadism, chorioretinal dystrophy, and spinocerebellar ataxia; onset in adolescence to early adulthood.

Bouchut respiration: Breathing pattern in pediatric

bronchopneumonia; inspiration is shorter than expiration.

Bouchut tube: Device used to intubate larynx.

Bougard paste: Mixture containing arsenic, starch, flour, zinc chloride, mercuric sulfide, and mercuric chloride.

Bouillaud disease: 1800s term for rheumatic fever (esp. endocarditis, pericarditis, joint inflammation).

Bouillaud sign: Abnormal sound on auscultation over right heart apex; found in cardiomegaly.

Bouillaud sign: Chest wall retraction seen in adherent pericardium.

Bouin fixative (fluid): Histologic fluid; composed formaldehyde, picric acid, and glacial acetic acid solution.

Boulton solution: Phenolated solution of iodine.

Bonnet-Dechaume-Blanc syndrome: Arteriovenous malformation with unilateral multiple shunts and aneurysms in orbit, maxilla, nasal cavity, carotid area, and hypothalamus; rare condition that often manifests as intractable epistaxis. Palliation involves external carotid ligation and repeat intracranial resection.

Bourgery ligament (oblique popliteal ligament): Broad, thin band of fibrous connective tissue running obliquely from medial tibial condyle to lateral femoral condyle; merges with semitendinosis tendon; pierced by popliteal vessels and nerves.

Bourne test: Radiography of centrifuged urine samples taken after barium enema; presence of even minute amount of barium indicates colovesical fistula.

Bourneville disease: Tuberous sclerosis; also associated with pheochromocytoma.

Bouveret syndrome: Rapid onset of persistent nausea and vomiting after eating; cause is gallstone obstructing lumen of duodenum.

Bouveret-Cotton syndrome (Bouveret-Hoffmann syndrome): Paroxysmal atrial tachycardia; may progress to congestive failure in prolonged episodes or with underlying heart disease. Condition is also associated with Wolff-Parkinson-White syndrome and biliary tract pathology. Onset occurs in childhood; boys affected almost exclusively. Treatment is digitalis, phenylephrine, Valsalva and Müller maneuvers, and unilateral carotid sinus stimulation.

Bouvier maneuver: Technique used to determine type of surgical procedure needed to correct claw hand. Examiner prevents hyperextension of metacarpophalangeal joint, and patient then attempts to extend fingers; positive if patient extends fingers at interphalangeal joint. Adequate correction then can be expected with "anticlaw" procedure only.

Bovie cautery: Commonly used type of unipolar cautery

with cutting and coagulation modes; used to control bleeding during surgery.

Bowden cable: Braided steel cable that runs inside tube; used in shoulder harnesses for arm prosthesis for patients who do heavy work.

Bowden control system: Bowden cable attached to arm prosthesis at 2 or more sites.

Bowditch law: "All or none" law; describes contraction of myocardial muscle cells.

Bowditch phenomenon (staircase phenomenon): Incremental increase in muscle contraction upon repeated stimulation.

Bowen disease: Squamous carcinoma in situ appearing anywhere on mucosal or skin surface; reddish, scaly lesion enlarges with itching. Treatment is surgical excision, cauterization, and topical 5-fluorouracil.

Bowen disease: Submucosal nodules on trachea and bronchial walls; associated with cough, wheezing, hoarseness, and dyspnea. Condition is seen mostly in men > 50 years of age.

Bowen pulsator: Hand-powered piston used in external chest compressions. Baseplate is placed behind patient, and mounted vertical arm on piston is attached to lever.

Bowen syndrome: Low weight, respiratory insufficiency, knees fixed in extension, and hips fixed in semiflexion. Condition is rare, congenital, and autosomal

recessive, with death occurring in perinatal period.

Bowers arthroplasty: Hemiresection interposition arthroplasty used in lieu of classic Darrach procedure for treatment of unstable and painful distal radioulnar joint; preserves styloid attachment of triangular fibrocartilage complex and ulnocarpal ligament complex.

Bowie stain: Visualizes basophilic cytoplasm and specific granules found in juxtaglomerular cells.

Bowman capsule: Visceral layer of glomerular capsule that forms beginning of renal tubule; composed of squamous cells that surround the kidney.

Bowman glands: Tubular serous glands that bathe olfactory mucosa and cilia.

Bowman lacrimal probe: Device used to dilate and correct defects of lacrimal ducts; may be double-ended or one-sided with eye.

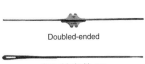

Doubled-ended

One-sided with eye

Bowman lacrimal probes

Bowman layer (membrane): Most anterior layer of corneal stroma, which lies deep to epithelium and superficial to stroma; is composed of uniform, firmly compacted collagen fibrils that do not undergo edema readily.

Bowman space: Space between parietal and visceral layers of glomerular capsule of kidney.

Bowman tube: "Tubes" formed between lamellae of cornea secondary to injections.

Bowman-Birk protease inhibitors: Group of serine protease inhibitors found in some plants.

Boyce sign: Positive for esophageal diverticulum if palpation of lateral neck causes gurgling sound.

Boyd amputation: Foot amputation using talectomy and tibiocalcaneal arthrodesis; performed in children to preserve leg length and bone growth centers.

A. Syme
B. Boyd
C. Chopart
D. Lisfranc
E. Transmetatarsal

Boyd amputation

Boyd approach: Surgical technique for exposure of posterior proximal radius and ulna. Arm of supine patient is pronated and draped over chest. Slightly curved incision is started 2.5 cm proximal to olecranon and extended subcutaneously to 1/4 length of proximal ulna; insertion of anconeus is sharply dissected off olecranon; and anconeus muscle and extensor carpi radius are retracted medially off ulna along with origin of supinator (which requires subperiosteal elevation). Interosseous recurrent artery can be ligated if more exposure is needed.

Boyd graft: Dual-onlay bone graft used to correct congenital pseudoarthrosis of tibia; best performed in patients with type 4 stress fractures with minimal gap between bone ends. Procedure uses two 2 cm × 11 cm cortical tibial bone grafts placed as struts on either side of tibia to bridge open space. The gap between bone is then packed with cancellous bone.

Boyd perforating veins: Vessels that connect greater saphenous vein to deep venous system below knee.

Boyd-Andersen technique: Surgical procedure used to repair distal ruptures of biceps tendon; involves curvilinear incision over anterior elbow and second incision on posterolateral aspect of elbow. Thick suture is placed through retracted tendon edge, passed through radius and ulna, and then positioned into "trap door" made in radial tuberosity.

Boyd-Griffin classification: System used to describe extracapsular fractures of femoral neck region. Type 1, intertrochanteric and easily reduced; type 2, intertrochanteric with comminution; type 3, subtrochanteric with minimum of 1 fracture line running through or distal to lesser trochanter; type 4, trochanteric and subtrochanteric fractures that require 2-plane fixation.

Boyd-Stearns syndrome: Vitamin D–resistant rickets, acidosis, glycosuria, and hypochloremia.

Boyden chamber: Device used to test for chemotaxis of cells, esp. leukocytes. Chemotactic factor is placed in 1 chamber, with a millipore filter placed between it and 2nd chamber that is filled with cells to be tested.

Boyer bursa: Fluid-filled sac beneath hyoid bone.

Boyer cyst: Painless enlargement of Boyer bursa.

Boyes grading: System used to describe function of finger flexor tendons after injury or operation; e.g, grade 5 is salvage only.

Boyes procedure (abduction): Method of tendon transfer to restore thumb abduction.

Boyes procedure (adduction): Method of tendon transfer to restore thumb adduction.

Boyes procedure (finger extension): Method of tendon transfer to restore finger extension.

Boyes procedure (flexion): Method of tendon transfer to restore metacarpophalangeal flexion.

Boyes procedure (wrist extension): Method of transfer of pronator teres to extensor carpi radialis brevis to restore wrist extension.

Boyes test: Used to check for boutonnière deformity; positive if there is less distal interphalangeal flexion with extension of proximal interphalangeal joint than in contralateral finger.

Boyle law (Mariotte law): Volume of known quantity of compressible gas is inversely proportional to pressure applied to it; equation is $V = k/P$, where V is volume, k is constant, P is pressure.

Bozan maneuver: Traction, abduction, and internal rotation applied to leg and pelvis to reduce femoral neck fractures.

Bozeman operation: Procedure used to correct vaginal–uterine fistulas.

Bozeman uterine dressing forceps: Device used in gynecologic surgery.

Bozicevich test: Used to detect trichinosis in serum.

Bozzolo sign: Appearance of pulsatile arteries inside nostrils; sometimes seen in thoracic aortic aneurysm.

Braasch catheter: Ureteral catheter used to dilate and measure inner radius of ureter via bulb tips of different sizes.

Bracht maneuver: Procedure used in breech delivery; after delivery has progressed to umbilicus, newborn's body and extended legs are supported with anterior rotation, and body is then held against mother's symphysis pubis until delivery is complete.

Bracht-Wächter body: Focal inflammatory cell aggregations (neutrophils and lymphocytes) in myocardium; seen in bacterial endocarditis.

Brachet fold (mesolateral fold): Right-sided portion of primitive mesentery running to right side of liver.

Brachmann-de Lange syndrome: Congenital mental retardation, short stature, hypertrichosis of head and face, and limb abnormalities ranging from camptodactyly of 5th fingers to phocomelia.

Brackett-Osgood technique: See Abbott approach.

Bradbury-Eggleston syndrome: Idiopathic orthostatic hypotension with low level of epinephrine that is not responsive to exercise or position change; also marked by anhidrosis, nocturnal polyuria, impotence, dizziness, syncope, bradycardia, and sphincter deterioration. Condition occurs in early morning hours during warmer months in older men; may be progressive. Treatment is volume expansion.

Bradford fusion: Treatment method for kyphoscoliosis by fusion of vertebral bodies through a staged anterior-posterior approach.

Bradford method: Technique used to measure protein concentration using a shift in the absorption maximum of the dye when Coomassie brilliant blue is bound to the protein to be measured.

Bradshaw test: Positive for presence of Bence Jones protein if layering acid–dilute urine mixture over hydrochloric acid produces ring.

Bragard sign (stretch test): Used to discriminate between nerve or muscle etiology of lower back pain; leg is kept straight as it is flexed at hip. If pain is increased when foot is dorsiflexed, nerve etiology is likely at L4, L5, or S1 levels; if no increase occurs, muscle etiology is likely.

Bragg curve: Used to describe increasing intensity of ionization emanating from ionizing particle–losing velocity.

Bragg peak: Slowly increasing initial dose of energy followed by sharply defined maximum close to end of energy range; occurs when negatively charged pions are delivered to tissues. Important in radiation therapy of deep tissues.

Brailsford disease: Shortened bones of feet and hands with lax skin around fingers and growth retardation; frequent infections (respiratory and ear) cause significant morbidity and death.

Brain reflex: Positive when extension of previously flexed hemiplegic arm occurs on placement in quadrupedal position.

Brain syndrome: Exophthalmos associated with pain; however, vision usu. not affected. Condition is also seen with eyelid edema. Treatment is steroids and antibiotics.

Brand procedure
(opponensplasty): Method of tendon transfer to restore thumb opposition.

Brand procedure: Method of tendon transfer to restore metacarpophalangeal flexion.

Brand tendon anastomosis: Use of fascia lata graft to effect palmaris longus tendon.

Brandt syndrome
(acrodermatitis enteropathica, Danbolt-Closs disease): Symmetric rash starting as vesicles and progressing to erythematosquamous type lesions, GI pain and diarrhea, alopecia, paronychia, conjunctivitis, photophobia, schizoid-type personality disorders, and stunted growth; onset in infancy. Condition is possibly related to jejunal malabsorption of zinc as serum zinc levels are decreased. Treatment is long-term daily oral zinc administration.

Brandt-Andrews maneuver
(Andrews maneuver): Method of delivering placenta; uterus is manually elevated by pressure placed between pubis and uterine fundus with gentle traction on cord.

Brandywine imperfection
(Shields syndrome): Easily eroded deciduous and permanent teeth with amber-colored dentin; autosomal dominant condition seen chiefly in southern Maryland (may be variant of Capdemont syndrome).

Branemark implant:
Titanium dental screw (permanently placed) used in both maxillary and mandibular tooth prosthesis.

Branemark technique:
Surgical placement of Branemark implants; most commonly performed with 5 implants into totally edentulous mandible. 3-layered approach to mandible allows visualization of mental nerve and final closure of lingual-based flap away from implants.

Branham reaction: Significant slowing of pulse occurring when main artery to limb with high-flow arteriovenous fistula is occluded.

Brant-Daroff exercises:
Performed for remission of benign paroxysmal positional vertigo. Patient sits on edge of bed and quickly reclines with symptomatic ear down; after vertigo resolves, patient sits up and repeats same procedure. Exercises are performed 3 times/day until no vertigo is experienced for 2 consecutive days (usu. about 2 weeks).

Brauch-Romberg sign: See Romberg test.

Brauer dysplasia: Congenital malformation of face marked by absence of subcutaneous fat ("forceps scar") at temporal regions, causing eyes to slant outward and upward with either absent or multiple eyelashes; autosomal dominant condition associated with visceral organ malignancy.

Brauer-Foerster technique:
Surgical correction of misshapen nostril performed during cleft lip repair. Columellar lengthening is

effected by making 2 sickle-shaped incisions in superior and alar rims, forming flaps that are rotated medially and sutured together. Disadvantage is tip necrosis, affecting repair.

Braun anastomosis:
Procedure performed between afferent and efferent bowel loops in conjunction with gastroenterostomy; prevents recycling of enteric contents. Anastomosis usu. done in setting of Billroth 2 reconstruction after hemigastrectomy.

Braun canal (Kovalevsky canal): Anatomic space in embryo connecting archenteron and posterior neural tube.

Braun episiotomy scissors:
Small, sharp-tipped scissors used for cutting tissue.

Braun-Falco syndrome: See Marghescu syndrome.

Braun-Fernwald sign (Braun-von Fernwald sign): Fullness and softening of fundus at implantation site of fetus; occurring at 7–8 weeks' gestation.

Braunwald sign: Weakening of pulse immediately after premature ventricular contraction.

Brazelton scale: Method for assessment of infant behavior by observing responses to environmental events.

Brazilian blastomycosis:
Paracoccidiomycosis.

Brazilian ophthalmia:
Degeneration of cornea secondary to vitamin A deficiency.

Brazilian pemphigus:
Superficial acantholysis with rare bullae, crusty erosions and erythematous patches; almost identical to pemphigus foliaceus. Likely vector is arthropod.

Brazilian purpuric fever:
Infection with *Haemophilus influenzae* type B in children causing purulent conjunctivitis, abdominal pain, fever, vomiting, purpura, variable disseminated intravascular coagulation, and death. Condition occurs in São Paulo, Brazil, and central Australia. Treatment is ampicillin, cefotaxime, and chloramphenicol; poor prognosis.

Bregeat disease: Congenital angiomas of eye, orbit, contralateral forehead, and thalamus extending to choroid plexus. Treatment is excision if possible.

Bremer disease (Passow syndrome): Congenital spinal cord disorder caused by abnormalities appearing during closure of primary medullary plate and tubulation; marked by spina bifida, mental retardation, facial asymmetry, paralysis of CNs VI and VII, kyphoscoliosis, sacral hair growth, and malformed extremities.

Brendt and Harty classification (modified):
System used to describe bone necrosis after acute injury in talus. Stage 1, normal radiograph with abnormality evident on MRI or bone scan (usu. due to repeat mild trauma); stage 2, partial separation of subchondral fragment (single event); stage

2a, formation of cyst (repeat mild trauma); stage 3, total fragment separation that maintains anatomic position (single event); stage 4, total fragment separation with loss of anatomic position (single event).

Brennemann syndrome: Mesenteric and retroperitoneal adenitis causing abdominal pain, nausea, vomiting, and fever; clinically indistinguishable from appendicitis. Condition usu. follows upper respiratory infection.

Brenner nodules: Nodular masses found in cyst wall in some Brenner tumors.

Brenner tumor: Usu. nonhormone-producing fibroepithelial tumor of ovary with slight malignant and endocrine-active potential; grossly identical to fibroma with histopathology showing "coffee bean" pattern. Tumor originates from surface epithelium, ovarian stroma, rete ovarii, and Walthard rests.

Breschet bones: Variably present small bones found in ligaments joining sternum and clavicle.

Breschet canals: Diploic canals that contain diploic veins.

Breschet hiatus: Opening at cochlear apex connecting scala vestibula and scala tympani.

Breschet sinus: Paired sinuses of dura matter originating at meningeal vein near small wing of apex of sphenous bone; drains into anterior cavernous sinus.

Breschet veins: Occipital, frontal and temporal diploic veins of skull; form sinuses in cancellous skull between laminae.

Brescia-Cimino fistula: Anastomosis of radial artery to cephalic vein in forearm or proximal wrist for hemodialysis access; easy to construct and has longest patency.

Breslow method: System for staging melanoma based on depth of skin penetration, taken from top of granular level to deepest penetration or from base in ulcerated lesions; considered more reliable in predicting biological behavior than Clarke level. Ocular micrometer is used to obtain accurate values. Level 1, ≤ 0.75 mm; level 2, 0.76–1.5 mm; level 3, 1.51–3.0 mm; level 4, > 3.0 mm.

Bretonneau angina: Diphtheria.

Brett syndrome (Janus syndrome): Radiologic finding of unilateral opaqueness in lung field; seen in pulmonary artery atresia of tetralogy of Fallot and truncus arteriosus with solitary pulmonary artery.

Breus mole (hematomole): Tuberous subchorional hematoma found in decidua of ovum. Treatment is surgical excision.

Brewer infarct: Purplish, pie-shaped discolorations of kidney parenchyma seen in pyelonephritis.

Brewer point: Tip of costovertebral angle; tenderness here indicates kidney infection.

Brewerton view: Radiographic patient positioning technique used to reveal fractures of metacarpal; back of hand is placed on table holding film. Metacarpophalangeal joints are flexed 65°, and x-ray tube is tilted 15° to ulnar side of vertical.

Brewster effect: See Broca-Sulzer effect.

Bricker procedure (loop): Diversion of urinary flow through anatomic conduit to skin; uses isolated segment of ileum on vascular pedicle to form end-ureter to side-of-ileum anastomosis.

Briesky disease: Early 1900s term for genital atrophy (clitoris, labia, frenulum) occurring in elderly women.

Bright blindness: Visual loss (in absence of retinal or optic disk lesion) occurring in uremia.

Bright syndrome: Postinfective glomerulonephritis most commonly seen in boys 3–7 years of age but occurring in both sexes at any age; marked by backache, headache, oliguria, hematuria, and vomiting seen 10 days after upper airway infection (usu. streptococcal). 50% of adult patients develop chronic kidney disease.

Brill disease (Brill-Zinsser disease): Recrudescence of previous typhus infection, with milder symptoms than first illness; usu. occurs years after initial, acute episode. Condition is due to persistence of Rickettsiae in lymph nodes; usu. Weil-Felix negative.

Brill-Symmers disease (Brill-Boehr-Rosenthal disease): Splenomegaly with follicular adenopathy with better survival than other lymphomas; now considered category of non-Hodgkin lymphoma.

Brinell number (hardness number): Determination of relative hardness of material; made by measuring diameter of indentation when steel ball is pressed on surface with known load.

Briquet syndrome (conversion reaction): Psychiatric disorder of females (highly unusual in males) with underlying psychic stresses manifested as hemiplegia, ataxia and loss of speech, sight, and hearing in absence of organic lesions; high correlation with borderline/antisocial personality disorder. Condition is associated with significant sexual dysfunction and multiple surgeries.

Brissaud disease: See Peyronie disease.

Brissaud dwarf: Short stature associated with infantile myxedema.

Brissaud infantilism: Infantile myxedema.

Brissaud reflex: Contraction of tensor fasciae femoris muscle upon lightly stroking sole.

Brissaud scoliosis (sciatic scoliosis): Deviation of lower lumbar spine away from leg with sciatica symptoms.

Brissaud-Marie disease (conversion reaction): Psychiatric disorder of females (highly unusual in males) with underlying psychic stresses manifesting as unilateral spasm of tongue and lips.

Brissaud-Sicard syndrome (Brissaud-Lereboullet syndrome): Unilateral facial spasm with contralateral paralysis caused by lesion in pyramidal tract before nucleus 7 in inferior and anterolateral pons.

Bristow symptom (sign): Cervical cord disease with neck flexion, leading to increased pyramidal deficit, (which improves on neck extension). Caused by lesion in descending corticospinal tract.

Bristowe disease: Particularly severe mental status changes occurring in frontal lobe–corpus callosum tumors; begins with personality changes and memory loss and proceeds to hemiplegia, apraxia, confusion, stupor, coma, and death.

British test: Pain with knee extension, quadriceps contraction, and pressure on patella; indicates knee injury.

British thermal unit (BTU): Quantity of energy needed to raise temperature of 1 lb of H_2O from 39° F to 40° F.

Broadbent disease: Intraventricular cerebral hemorrhage preceded by severe headache and vomiting.

Broadbent registration point: Midpoint of imaginary line running from nasion–postcondylar plane to center of sella turcica.

Broadbent sign: Pulsations detectable on left lateral chest wall, which are synchronous with cardiac contractions; seen in aneurysms of left atrium.

Broadbent sign: Retraction of skin and tissue on left posterior chest wall between 11th and 12th ribs; seen in pericardial adhesions.

Broadbent test: Used to determine which cerebral hemisphere is dominant for language. Different words are presented to each ear at same time; right-handed patients report hearing words going into right ear 1st.

Broca angle: Angle formed by imaginary lines drawn from auricular point and glabella to anterior nasal spine.

Broca aphasia (expressive aphasia): Enunciation of slow, nonfluent words with much effort; speech consists of nouns and verbs only with spoken phrases of 4 words or less. Condition is associated with impaired verbal naming and writing. Reading comprehension is usu. preserved. Cause is lesion in left cerebral cortex, near frontal operculum and anterior to precentral gyrus.

Broca convolution: Area of left hemisphere in inferior frontal gyrus containing motor area for speech function.

Broca diagonal band: Posterior lateral part of the anterior perforated substance lying between olfactory triangle and optic chiasm and tract.

Broca fissure: Anterior ascending rami of cerebral lateral sulcus.

Broca motor area: Opercular and triangular parts of inferior frontal gyrus and surrounding prefrontal cortex; transforms neural representations to articulatory sentences. Lesions to area may cause motor aphasia.

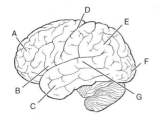

A. Frontal lobe
B. Inferior frontal gyrus
   (Broca area)
C. Temporal lobe
D. Central sulcus (Rolando)
E. Parietal lobe
F. Occipital lobe
G. Transverse gyrus of
   Heschl (auditory area)

Broca motor area

Broca parolfactory area: Small portion of medial cerebral hemispheres, directly in front of subcallosal gyrus.

Broca-Sulzer effect (Brewster effect): With brief flash of light of fixed, small area and duration, enlarging target initially causes increase in brightness. However, beyond critical area, brightness of target dims with further increase in size.

Brock operation: Procedure used to correct pulmonic valve stenosis; part of pulmonic valve is excised using transventricular approach.

Brock syndrome (Graham-Burford-Mayer syndrome): Inflammatory/infectious process resulting in hilar lymphadenopathy and obstruction of left (lingual) bronchus or right middle bronchus; also leads to recurrent hemoptysis and pneumonitis. Treatment is surgical if response to antibiotics is poor.

Brockenbrough catheter: Device using curved metallic needle to pierce intra-arterial septal wall and inject dye into left ventricle when aorta cannot be traversed.

Brockenbrough sign: Weakening of pulse immediately after premature ventricular contraction; sometimes seen in idiopathic hypertrophic subaortic stenosis.

Brocq-Pautrier syndrome: Median rhomboid glossitis associated with candidiasis of mouth, along with dryness of mouth and burning pain when eating spicy foods. Treatment is antifungal agents and cessation of smoking.

Brodel white line: Vertical white line noted on anterior kidney.

Broders classification: System used to describe histologic grades of lip cancer (grades 1–4).

Broders classification: System used to describe histologic grades of gastric cancer; correlates well with prognosis. Grade 1, 5-year survival is 65%; grade 5, 5-year survival is 11%.

Broders index: General description of "malignancy" of tumor based on degree of differentiation. Grade 1, 25% undifferentiated cells; grade 2, 50% undifferentiated cells; grade 3, 75% undifferentiated cells; grade 4, 100% undifferentiated cells.

Brodie abscess: Well-demarcated lytic lesion seen on radiographs of children with osteomyelitis; represents chronic abscess surrounded by sclerotic bone and dense fibrous tissue. Condition usu. occurs with pain but no fever. Cause is *Staphylococcus aureus* or *S. albus*.

Brodie bursa: Fluid-filled sac located between medial tendon of gastrocnemius, femoral condyle, and joint capsule.

Brodie disease: Cystosarcoma phylloides in breast; tumors usu. benign in adolescents. Treatment is simple surgical resection.

Brodie ligament: Transverse humeral ligament.

Brodie sign: Black spot appearing on glans penis caused by urine leaking into spongiosum; seen in gangrene of penis.

Brodin disease: Inflammation of mesenteric lymph nodes,

causing clinical appendicitis-like and duodenal stenosis-like symptoms.

Brodmann area: Numbered areas of cerebral cortex corresponding to different functions and distinguished by differing arrangements of their 6 cell layers.

Brodmann area 4 (primary somatomotor area): Portion of posterior portion of frontal lobe, just anterior to central sulcus; controls motor activity of body.

Brodmann area 19 (peristriate area): Portion of occipital cortex partially encircling striate cortex; functions in processing visual sensations.

Brodmann area 28 (entorhinal area): Posteroinferior piriform area, which includes caudal part of parahippocampal gyrus.

Brodmann areas 41 and 42: Contiguous auditory areas located near anterior transverse gyrus.

Brønsted-Lowry acid: Chemical species that functions as proton donor and forms one-half of conjugate acid–base pairs [e.g., NH_4^+ (acid) and NH_3 (base)].

Brooke ileostomy: Ileal diversion onto anterior abdominal wall; important that ileum is brought 2 cm above skin to make nippled exit.

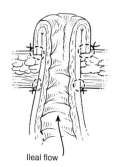

Ileal flow

Brooke ileostomy

Brooke-Fordyce trichoepithelioma: Multiple small facial skin lesions, esp. in nasolabial folds; onset in late childhood. Only rarely are lesions malignant (e.g., basal cell epithelioma).

Brooker classification: System used to describe ectopic ossification in hip area. Class 1, bone formation in soft tissue around hip joint; class 2, bone formation originating from proximal femur or pelvis with minimum of 1 cm between fragments; class 3, same as class 2 but with < 1 cm between bony surfaces; class 4, hip bone ankylosis.

Brookmeyer-Crowley interval: Nonparametric confidence interval for determining median survival time of homogenous population by inverting generalization of sign test for censored data.

Brooks disease: Immunodeficiency syndrome type 6; marked by chronic recurrent nasal, lung, and ear infections, as well as varicella and papilloma virus infections. Condition is associated with normal quantity of natural killer and B cells but decreased IgG production and CD4 and CD8 lymphocytes. Onset occurs in early childhood to early adulthood; X-linked inheritance.

Brooks-Jenkins procedure: C1/C2 spinal fusion using wire to secure bone grafts placed between lamina.

Brophy operation: Technique for repair of cleft palate. Freshened edges of palate are brought together and sutured with reinforcing lead plates.

Broselow tape: Measuring tape used in pediatrics to estimate child's weight; marked in increments in weight categories (50th percentile weights). Method is much more accurate than clinician's visual estimates, esp. for children < 25 kg. Each color-coded length/weight category is labeled with appropriate equipment sizes and drug doses.

Brossard disease: Weakness in small muscles of calves and feet, rectus muscle, and shoulder girdle; fasciculation occurs in absence of degeneration.

Broviac catheter: Device introduced in 1973; uses Silastic catheter inserted into jugular, subclavian, or cephalic vein with distal tip in superior vena cava or right atrium and proximal end tunneled under skin that exits on chest wall. Dacron cuff in subcutaneous tunnel anchors catheter and provides barrier to infection; available in different sizes and lumens. Heparin flushes to prevent clotting of lumen are required.

Browing vein: Superior part of inferior anastomotic vein.

Brown syndrome: Shortening of superior oblique muscle tendon sheath; causes backward head tilt, bilateral ptosis, congenital strabismus, limited eye elevation in adduction, and choroidal coloboma. Condition may be congenital or acquired (e.g., toxins, drugs). Treatment is surgery.

Brown tissue forceps: Instrument used to grasp skin during wound closure.

Brown-Brenn stain: Modification of Gram stain.

Brown-Dodge method: Computer-aided technique for quantitative angiography; uses projection of selected cinematographic frames with 5-fold magnification onto screen. Selected segments of coronary artery are traced by hand from perpendicular views onto computer, which reduces lesion image to true scale and corrects for optical out-of-plane magnification and pincushion distortion.

Brown-Norway rats: Strain of laboratory animal; useful in studying vasculitis syndromes.

Brown-Roberts-Wells apparatus: Globe-shaped frame clamped onto patient's head in stereotactic brain surgery.

Brown-Séquard syndrome (sign): Destruction of lateral half of spinal cord; results in ipsilateral plegia, vibration loss, and contralateral temperature and pain sensation loss.

Brown-Vialetto-van Laere syndrome: 1 of 2 known forms of progressive bulbar paralysis in children; presents with deafness, followed 4–5 years later by palsy of CNs VII, IX, X, XI, and XII, with swallowing and speech problems, shortness of breath, shaking, limb weakness, and sleepiness. Condition is autosomal recessive with variable involvement of CNs III, V, and VI. Death is via respiratory loss.

Browne operation: Method of hypospadias repair; uses epithelialization of lateral wound margins to form urethral floor and intact epithelial strip to form roof.

Bruce effect: Arrest of pregnancy when newly pregnant female mouse is exposed to odor of strange male mouse.

Bruce protocol: Most commonly used exercise tolerance treadmill test.

Bruch membrane (lamina vitrea): 2-mm thick strip of pigment epithelium at choroid–optic cup junction; lies between retinal pigment epithelium and choroid. Deterioration contributes to age-related macular degeneration.

Bruck syndrome: Congenital joint contractures in setting of osteogenesis imperfecta; autosomal recessive condition.

Brücke lens: Double-concave and double-convex lens combination; provides long working distance.

Brücke lines: Broad bands seen in muscle fibrils; alternate with thinner Z bands.

Brücke muscle (meridional fibers): Longitudinal fibers in outer ciliary body of eye; insert into scleral spur.

Brücke reagent: Modification of Mayer reagent; solution of 120 g mercuric iodide and 50 g potassium iodide in 1 L H_2O.

Brücke-De Lange syndrome: Congenital muscular hypertrophy and muscle rigidity with mental retardation; white matter and thalami have multiple cavities. Death occurs within 1 year of onset.

Brudzinski sign: Flexion of knees and hips in response to neck flexion when in supine position; suggests meningeal inflammation.

Brudzinski sign: Elbow flexion with jerky movements in response to pressure on area just below cheekbone; suggests meningeal irritation.

Brudzinski sign: Flexion of 1 hip with passive flexion of opposite hip; suggests meningeal irritation.

Brudzinski sign: Bilateral leg/hip flexion positive with pressure on pubic bone.

Brueghel syndrome (lingual-facial-mandibular spasms, Meige syndrome): Spastic movements of face, including lip retraction, mouth opening, platysma contraction, and tongue protrusion; also variably associated with torso and limb dystonia and torticollis. Facial movements are similar to those caused by chronic neuroleptic use; etiology is unknown.

Condition is usu. seen in women in late middle age. Only treatment with proven efficacy is botulin toxin injections.

Brug filariasis: Disease that occurs in Malaysia and India; vectors are *Anopheles* and *Mansonia* mosquitoes.

Brugsch index: Comparison of body width vs. body length; equals chest circumference (in.) × 100/height (in.).

Brunati sign: Appearance of corneal opacities; indicates impending death due to either typhoid fever or pneumonia.

Brunauer syndrome (Brauer-Brunauer-Fuhs syndrome, Fuhs syndrome): Punctate thickening on palms and soles; occasionally associated with scant hair, crooked teeth, sensorineural hearing deficits, and corneal opacities. Onset occurs in adolescence.

Bruner incisions: "Zigzag" incisions used for volar approach to digit for flexor tendon surgery and repair of neurovascular bundles; useful if extension onto palm is needed.

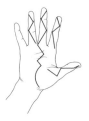

Bruner incisions

Brunhilde virus: Type of poliovirus strain.

Brunn membrane: Nasal epithelium.

Brunner glands: Mucus-secreting submucosal glands found only in duodenum; often extend through muscularis mucosae to the deep mucosa. Glands secrete pepsinogens.

Brunner gland adenoma (gastric adenomyoma): Aberrant location of hamartomatous-type lesion in antrum or pylorus; composed of Brunner glands intermixed with smooth muscle.

Brunnstrom method: System of therapeutic exercise that concentrates on reflex or proprioceptive neuromuscular facilitation to develop voluntary muscle control.

Bruns frontal ataxia: Lesion (e.g., infection, tumor) in frontal lobe causing broad-based gait with short, flat-footed steps; patient tends to lurch backward.

Bruns medium: Glucose, glycerin, camphorated spirit, and distilled H_2O; used to mount fresh tissue specimens.

Bruns sign (syndrome): Episodic vomiting, vertigo, and headache occurring with sudden head movement due to obstruction of CSF flow or destruction of vestibular mechanism. Cause is cysticercus infestation, tumor in cerebellar midline, or colloid cyst in 4th ventricle.

Brunschwig operation: Surgical removal of total pelvic organs and tissues, usu. for locally invasive carcinoma.

Brunschwig operation: Seldomly performed method of pancreatoduodenectomy.

Brunstig syndrome: Recurrent eruptions of vesicles appearing on head and neck resulting in scarring; affects mostly middle-aged men.

Brunton otoscope: Device for looking into ear; light is funneled into ear canal from source located to one side.

Brushfield spots: White spots scattered circumferentially in iris in newborns; may be present in normal infants but is strongly suggestive of Down syndrome.

Brushfield-Wyatt syndrome: Occurrence of port-wine stain in trigeminal nerve distribution in setting of calcified angiomas in cerebral hemispheres; also with hemianopia, hemiplegia, and mental retardation.

Bruton disease (X-linked agammaglobulinemia): Severe immunodeficiency disease with onset at 6 months of age (after disappearance of maternal immunoglobulin) of serious infections. X-linked recessive condition marked by lack of B cells with deficiency in all immunoglobulin classes, Peyer patches, and lymph node germinal centers, along with defective tonsillar and appendiceal crypts. T lymphocytes are normal. Pyogenic infections (e.g., *Giardia lamblia*, rotavirus) recur; 50% of patients have rheumatoid arthritis and scleroderma signs. Death occurs in childhood due to pulmonary infection. Treatment is antibiotics and immunoglobulins.

Bruyn-Went syndrome: Infantile spastic paraplegia and

progressive athetosis in setting of Leber disease (optic atrophy).

Bryan-Morrey approach (Mayo approach): Surgical approach to elbow. Arm of supine patient is placed on sandbag on chest, 15-cm longitudinal incision is made lateral to medial epicondyle and medial to olecranon tip, and ulnar nerve is located at medial border of triceps.

Bryant ampulla: Portion of artery that contains clot; usu. proximal to slight constriction of artery.

Bryant line: Vertical border of iliofemoral triangle.

Bryant sign: Lowering of axillary skin folds; seen in dislocation of shoulder.

Bryant traction: Method of overhead traction in infants to keep thighs flexed to 90° and knees extended.

Bryant triangle: Imaginary area formed by line from anterior superior spine directed vertically to table (with patient supine), line from superior greater trochanter in long axis of thigh to intersection of 1st line with table, and line from anterior superior spine to top of greater trochanter.

Bryce-Teacher ovum: Human ovum noted historically and incorrectly as youngest existing specimen during its study in 1908.

Bryson sign: Decreased thoracic expansion occasionally seen in Graves disease.

Buchanan syndrome: Truncus arteriosus, with cyanosis, dyspnea, respiratory infections, polycythemia, and cardiomegaly. Treatment is surgery; 25% mortality.

Buchman disease: Aseptic necrosis of medial cuneiform.

Buck fascia: Deep penile fascia that binds 3 cavernous bodies together.

Buck operation: Resection of proximal tibia and fibula and patella.

Buck traction (extension): Skin traction of leg used for knee injuries and temporary fixation of hip fractures.

Buck-Gramcko method: Classification system based on functional end-result after primary repair of finger flexor tendons.

Buckey syndrome (hyperimmunoglobulinemia E syndrome; Immunodeficient state with IgE > 5000 IU/ml, increased neutrophils and eosinophils, pustular skin lesions, lung abscesses, and lymphadenopathy; infections tend to be mycotic or staphylococcal.

Buckler syndrome: See Biber-Haab-Dimmer dystrophy.

Buckley syndrome: Increased levels of IgE.

Budd cirrhosis: Hepatomegaly caused by intestinal intoxication.

Budd-Chiari syndrome (Rokitansky syndrome): Hepatic vein obstruction; usu. caused by thrombosis in IVC secondary to hypercoagulable states, vena caval webs (esp. in China), tumors, trauma, and bone marrow transplantation, and most commonly polycythemia vera. Condition can also be idiopathic. Disorder leads to hepatomegaly and ascites (most reproducible finding). Diagnostic test is hepatic venography or increasingly spiral CT scan. Standard treatment has been anticoagulation, venous bypass, or if failure occurs liver transplantation. Recent developments in nonoperative care include angiographic approach with local thrombolytic therapy to open vena cava, angioplasty, and intravascular stenting.

Budge center (genital center): Area of sacral spinal cord responsible for mediating reflexes controlling genital erection.

Buerger disease (Billroth-von Winiwarter disease, endaortitis obliterans, Winiwarter-Manteuffel-Buerger disease): Pain in extremities similar to intermittent claudication caused by medial arterial sclerosis; also affects small veins and lymphatics. Disease occurs almost exclusively in men and is related to tobacco use, cold, malnutrition, and collagen vascular disorders. Condition manifests initially at rest and in absence of significant physical findings; often accompanied by migratory phlebitis. As disease progresses, exacerbations may cause trophic changes, ulcers, and gangrene. Only effective treatment is complete cessation of tobacco.

Buerger sign: Pallor in extremity on elevation and rubor on dependency; indicates

advanced ischemia. Condition is caused by significantly restricted arterial inflow and chronic dilatation of peripheral vascular bed, esp. postcapillary venules.

Buerger-Gruetz disease (essential hyperlipidemia): Absent or defective lipoprotein lipase that removes chylomicrons from plasma; onset at 1st fat intake in childhood. Symptoms and signs include diffuse eruptive xanthomas, abdominal pain and fever, hepatosplenomegaly, failure to thrive, and repeat bouts of pancreatitis. Treatment is reduction of all types of dietary fat to 20% of total caloric intake, elimination of alcohol, and avoidance of certain drugs (e.g., estrogen, diuretics, β -blockers).

Buford complex: Normal anatomic variants consisting of cord-like middle glenohumeral ligament, loosely attached superior labrum, and large sublabral hole.

Bugbee electrode: Electrocautery device used in cystoscopy.

Buhot cells: Phagocytes that contain engulfed leukocytes with Alder-Reilly granulations in leukocyte cytoplasm; stain strongly metachromatic with toluidine blue.

Buie pile clamp: Curved, ring-handle, locking clamp used to occlude hemorrhoids.

Bumke pupil: Dilation of pupil under psychological stress or stimulation.

Bunge amputation: Method involving total stripping of

periosteum from distal bone stump.

Bünger bands: Coalescence of sheath cells to form bands of syncytium during regeneration of peripheral nerves.

Bunnell classification: System used to describe injuries of finger flexor tendons.

Bunnell incision: Midlateral volar incision used to surgically approach digit.

Bunnell procedure: Tendon loop reconstruction to restore stability to distal radioulnar joint.

Bunnell procedure: Tendon transfer to restore metacarpophalangeal flexion.

Bunnell procedure: Tendon transfer to restore thumb adduction.

Bunnell reconstruction: Flexor tendon pulley reconstruction; optimizes tendon excursion into finger flexion.

Bunsen burner: Commonly used bench-top device in which gas is mixed with air before ignition; provides complete oxidation.

Bunsen-Roscoe law: Product intensity and duration of illumination determine quantity of photochemical effect.

Bunyan bag: Sac used to cover wet dressings to prevent skin maceration; made of waterproof material.

Burch procedure: Method using modified Lloyd-Davies position and retropubic approach through Pfannenstiel incision to effect urethropexy. Bladder is swept off superior pubic rami, vagina is tented by fingers placed intravaginally, and sutures are used to secure both sides of bladder neck to Cooper ligament on symphysis pubis.

Burdach column (fasciculus cuneatus): Ascending sensory spinocerebral nerve fibers.

Burdach fissure: Groove formed by lateral insula surface and inner operculum surface.

Bureau-Barriere disease: Bullous lesions on soles of feet progressing to chronic perforating ulcers; usu. seen in adult male alcoholics with poor nutrition. Cause is radicular sensory neuropathy.

Buren disease: See Peyronie disease.

Burford-Finochietto self-retaining rib retractor: Instrument used in chest surgery.

Burger sign: See Heryng sign.

Bürger-Grütz syndrome: Type 1 familial hyperlipoproteinemia.

Burka syndrome: Variant of Dubin-Johnson syndrome that lacks development of jaundice.

Burke syndrome (De Martini-Balestra syndrome, vanishing lung syndrome): Progressive bleb/bullae formation in lungs; marked by cough, dyspnea, and wheezing in absence of inhaled chemical irritants.

Burkhalter procedure (opponensplasty): Tendon transfer to restore thumb opposition.

Burkitt lymphoma (tumor): B-cell lymphoma associated with Epstein-Barr virus; endemic to parts of Africa. Tumor mass usu. presents in jaw, cervical lymph nodes, and salivary glands; very good response to cyclophosphamide.

Burmese pyramid: See tower of Hanoi.

Burnett syndrome: End-stage milk-alkali syndrome marked by severe hypercalcemia, renal failure, and phosphate retention; leads to conjunctivitis, mental confusion, headache, and dizziness.

Burns disease: Aseptic necrosis of pediatric humeral trochlea.

Burns ligament: Lateral border of saphenous hiatus.

Burns space (suprasternal space): Anatomic area formed by division of superficial neck fascia as it attaches to front and back of manubrium; contains fat, sternal heads of sternomastoids, small veins, and communicating branch between anterior jugular veins.

Burow operation: Technique used in plastic surgery in which triangular sections of skin adjacent to flap are resected to allow removal of standing cones ("dog ears").

Burow solution: Aluminum acetate topical solution added to glacial acetic acid and H_2O; contains approximately 5% aluminum acetate. Uses include mouthwash or wet dressing (diluted form).

Burow vein: Vessel formed by confluence of inferior epigastric veins and vein originating from bladder; drains into portal vein.

Burr cells: Acanthocyte cells seen in liver disease.

bursa of Achilles tendon: Fluid-filled sac between posterior surface of calcaneus and calcaneal tendon.

Burton disease: Congenital small mouth, dislocated lenses, pursed lips, stunted growth, and malformed limbs.

Burton line (sign): Bluish discoloration at tooth line seen in chronic lead poisoning.

Buruli ulcer (Bairnsdale ulcer): Gigantic, painless ulcers, usu. occurring on legs (at trauma sites); seen in tropical Africa and Australia. Lesions caused by *Mycobacterium ulcerans* infection.

Bury syndrome (Crocker-Williams syndrome): Symmetric, bilateral papular nodules on dorsum of hands and occasionally knees, elbows, wrists, and ankles; associated with polyarthritis. Condition is considered a cutaneous vasculitis. Onset occurs in middle-age adults. Treatment is topical steroids and dapsone.

Busch umbilical scissors: Instrument used in obstetrics.

Busbi syndrome: See Rowley-Rosenberg syndrome.

Buscacca nodule: Large granuloma of iris; associated with anterior uveitis.

Buschke disease: Localized scleredema, usu. sharply demarcated from normal skin and appearing 1st on face or neck, which may spread to arms and chest; associated with arthralgia, myalgia, malaise, and preceding infection. Condition may also involve parotid, eyes, and pericardial effusions; usu. remits spontaneously or responds to treatment with hyaluronidase or steroids. Etiology is unknown.

Buschke-Ollendorff disorder (Albers-Schönberg syndrome type 2, Curth syndrome): Bone lesions of Albers-Schönberg disease in combination with skin lesions of Schreus disease; marked by firm, yellowish nodules on buttocks and posterior thighs that occur in streaks. Course is usu. benign.

Buschke-Fisher-Braver syndrome: Development of keratosis on palms; may herald presence of internal malignancy. Onset at 15–30 years of age.

Buschke-Löwenstein tumor (Buschke-Löwenstein condyloma, verrucous carcinoma): Low-grade squamous carcinoma found on penis, vulva, and perineum; resembles a giant condyloma.

Buselmeier shunt: U-shaped external arteriovenous dialysis shunts placed in wrist.

Busquet disease: Foot pain worsened by walking; metatarsal bones show osteoperiostitis. Etiology is unknown.

Bussiere-Escobar syndrome: Stunted growth; eyelid ptosis; micrognathia; "winged" skin around knees, elbows, and neck; cryptorchidism; and vertebral anomalies; autosomal recessive condition.

Butcher saw: Instrument used in amputations; blade can be adjusted to different angles.

Byar-Jurkiewicz syndrome: Congenital hypertrichosis and enlarged gums. Kyphosis and large breast fibroadenoma may occur later in life.

Byers dysplasia: Variant of corneal spondyloepiphyseal dystrophy with punctate lesions, which does not affect vision; arises in infancy.

Byler disease: Defective excretion of conjugated bile salts causing recurrent jaundice, infections, cirrhosis, and hepatosplenomegaly; autosomal recessive condition. Treatment is liver transplantation for inevitable liver failure.

Bywaters lesion: Small, painless brown spots on nails and painful maculopapular lesion on finger pads; due to necrotizing angiitis often seen in rheumatoid disease.

Bywaters syndrome (crush syndrome): Sequelae of renal failure (e.g., edema, oliguria) seen after crush/ischemic injury to large muscle mass or body part.

Cabot ring body: Lines in "figure-of-8" pattern seen in RBCs in severe anemias; stain blue with eosinate methylthionine chlorides.

Cabrol operation: Surgical method of aortic root replacement; used in patients with Marfan disease.

Cacchi-Ricci disease: Medullary sponge kidney with cystic areas interspersed with normal tissue; marked by inguinal pain, colic, nocturnal polyuria (usu. with proteinuria,) and recurrent UTIs, with relatively benign course. Onset occurs at any age.

Caffey disease (Caffey-Silverman disease, infantile cortical hyperostosis): Bone disorder in infants with fever and inflammatory swelling; mandible, ribs, and sometimes skull and orbits show soft tissue masses with underlying hypertrophy. Condition occurs in both sporadic and autosomally dominant forms, with onset usu. before 6 months of age. Corticosteroids relieve symptoms until usu. spontaneous recovery.

Cagot ear: See Aztec ear.

Cairns operation: (goniospasis): Seldomly performed surgical treatment of glaucoma using a thin filament passed through the ivis to apply traction on the angle of the anterior chamber of the eye.

Cairns syndrome (akinetic mutism): Marked by one of several states of altered consciousness (e.g., persistent vegetative state, "locked-in" syndrome). Multiple etiologies include large bilateral lesions in cerebral frontal lobes or basal ganglia, global demyelinization, and severe hydrocephalus.

Cairns syndrome: Residual neurologic deficits/lesions occurring in children who have recovered from meningitis; marked by hydrocephalus, impaired vision, and focal neurologic deficits. Condition due to thickened arachnoid with chronic inflammatory reaction.

Cajal cell: Astrocyte.

Cajal cell: Horizontally positioned neuroglia cell found in molecular layer of cerebral cortex.

Cajal nucleus (interstitial nucleus): Collection of nerve cells lying at rostral end of medial longitudinal fasciculus; has reciprocal projections to vestibular nuclei and also connects to spinal cord.

Cajal stain: Silver impregnation technique used to visualize gray matter neurofibrils.

Cajal trichrome stain:
Technique used to visualize and distinguish connective tissue from muscle; uses basic fuchsin, indigo carmine, and picric acid to stain nuclei bright red, cytoplasm orange, and collagen fibers blue.

Caldani ligament: Fibrous tissue connecting inferior surface of clavicle, 1st rib, and subclavius tendon to inner edge of coracoid process.

Caldwell-Luc operation:
Surgical approach to maxillary antrum; incision is made high in gum area above premolar teeth.

Caldwell-Moloy classification: System used to categorize shape of female pelvis as android, gynecoid, anthropoid, or platypelloid.

California encephalitis:
Severe frontal bilateral headaches, fever, vomiting; and convulsions; abrupt onset. Cause is 1 of 14 related strains of bunyavirus. Disease is associated with long convalescence but has excellent prognosis.

California mastitis test
(Schalm test): Used to detect subclinical mastitis in cows. Bromcresol purple, milk, and anionic substance are mixed together and rapidly rotated; gel formation is positive finding.

Callahan procedure: Cervical fusion using wires to secure bone grafts to facets.

Callander amputation: Leg amputation at knee joint; patella is removed and soft tissue is formed into long posterior and anterior flaps.

Callaway test: Positive for humeral dislocation if circumference of shoulder is greater than contralateral shoulder.

Call-Exner vacuole (bodies): Microscopic, rounded intercellular vacuoles filled with acidophilic and eosinophilic fluid; found in ovarian granulosa cells.

Callison fluid: Diluting medium used for counting RBCs; composed of formaldehyde, Löffler aniline methylene blue, sodium chloride, glycerin ammonium oxalate, and distilled H_2O.

Calmette-Guérin bacillus (BCG): *Mycobacterium bovis* strain made avirulent by hundreds of culture cycles on unfavorable bile–glycerine medium. BCG is used as human immunization against TB; given via a single intradermal injection to newborns in developing and some Western countries and patients at risk for developing resistant TB. Maximum of 1 skin tuberculosis test should be performed in BCG-inoculated patient (this test is usu. negative) due to development of systemic reaction. BCG is also used as intravesical chemotherapy for superficial transitional cell carcinoma of bladder.

Calori bursa: Fluid-filled sac between aortic arch and trachea.

Calot triangle: Anatomic space in porta hepatis formed by cystic artery anteriorly and superiorly, hepatic duct medially, and cystic duct inferiorly.

Calvert formula: Expression used to calculate dose of chemotherapy; equation is dose (mg) = AUC × (GFR + 25), where AUC is under the curve and GFR is glomerular filtration rate.

Calvin cycle: Step in photosynthesis in which carbon dioxide is attached to 5-carbon sugar and then reduced to other sugars.

Camera syndrome: Intermittent and progressive diffuse bone pain; typically worse at night. Condition is associated with overlying trigger point but absence of swelling and erythema; onset in middle age.

Camerer law: Children of equal weight have equal caloric requirements regardless of age.

Cameron suture method: Continuous horizontal mattress suture; runs distally and then proximally in an over-and-over method to secure cut end of large vein.

Cameroon haplotype: 1 of 4 major sickle cell gene clusters on arising on chromosome 11; marked by gene abnormalities.

Camitz procedure: Transfer of palmaris longus under thenar tissues and attachment to radial side of proximal thumb phalanx; used to correct carpal tunnel syndrome.

Camp stockings: Graduated compression stockings.

Campailla-Martinelli dwarfism: Variant of Hunter-Thompson type dwarfism. Congenitally normal-appearing infant with growth deformities evident in 1st year; marked by short distal extremities, abnormal epiphyses, "frozen" elbow, thoracic kyphosis, and enlarged 1st toe. Condition is autosomal recessive, with normal mental development.

Campbell approach: Surgical approach to posterior elbow that allows for wide exposure in open reduction of "T" fractures of humeral condyles. Triceps muscle is split longitudinally, ulnar nerve is identified and retracted medially and then tissue is removed from lower humerus by subperiosteal dissection.

Campbell De Morgan spots (cherry angioma): Benign hemangiomas appearing usu. on trunk in adults and face and ears in elderly; common condition caused by dilated venules. Treatment is laser coagulation or excision.

Campbell ligament: Fibrous connective tissue that suspends axillary tissues.

Campbell technique: Method for viewing lacrimal duct system after injection of radiopaque contrast material. Microfocusing tube is used to immediately image the duct system, and film plane is removed to moderate distance from patient.

Camper fascia: Superficial globular fatty layer of fascia on ventral abdominal wall;

continuous with Camper fascia of thigh.

Camurati-Engelmann syndrome (progressive diaphyseal dysplasia): Thickening of diaphysis of long bones; marked by bone pain, fatigue, waddling gait, anemia, and elevated sedrate. Onset usu. occurs in childhood, often with waddling type of gait. Treatment is glucocorticoids.

Canada balsam: Substance used to mount histology specimens after staining and rinsing and before cover slip is applied.

Canadian classification: System for description of angina pectoris developed by Canadian Cardiovascular Society. I, angina only with strenuous or prolonged exertion; II, slight limitation of ordinary activity (e.g., walking or climbing stairs rapidly or walking more than two blocks brings on symptoms); III, marked limitation of ordinary physical activity; IV, angina with any physical activity and variable angina at rest.

canal of Arantius: Ductus venosus.

canal of Corti: Spiral canal in organ of Corti.

canal of Cotunnius: Single passageway connecting canaliculus cochlea and aqueductus vestibuli.

canal of Guidi (pterygoid canal, vidian canal): Horizontal space running through bottom of medial pterygoid plate of sphenoid bone to just inferomedial to foramen rotundum; carries pterygoid vessels and nerves.

canal of Hering: Bile ductule; located on periphery of hepatic lobule. Walls are formed by hepatocytes on 1 side and ductule cells on other.

Canale-Kelly classification: System used to describe fractures of talus. Type 1, minimal displacement with maximum of 1 blood supply possibly compromised; type 2, subtalar displacement with 2–3 blood supplies possibly compromised; type 3, dislocation of talar body from subtalar joint and ankle; type 4, talar neck fracture with displacement of body fragment away from ankle or displacement of talar head away from talonavicular joint.

Canavan disease (sclerosis): Spongy degeneration of white matter in brain with relative axonal preservation and Alzheimer type II astrocytes in gray matter; also with spasticity, seizures, psychomotor degeneration and macrocephaly. Lesions are located in central white matter and occasionally in cerebellum and basal ganglia; associated with aspartoacyclase deficiency. Autosomal recessive condition that usu. presents in mid- to late infancy; occurs more commonly in Jews and tends to be associated with lighter complexion and hair. Disease may progress to death in several months to years.

Cannon disease: Benign, white, spongy lesions developing in both sexes at any age in oral and labial mucosa and occ. in vaginal and anal mucosa; autosomal dominant condition.

Cannon-De La Paz syndrome: Early 1900s term for symptoms of increased epinephrine secretion (sweating, tachycardia, flushing) caused by emotional stress.

Cantelli sign (doll's eyes sign): Dissociation between movements of eyes and head; for example, eyes moving to left when head is turned to right or eyes moving down when head is tilted up.

Cantlie line: Imaginary line running from gallbladder to just left of inferior vena cava; delineates right and left lobes of liver.

Cantor tube: Single-lumen, long intestinal tube inserted through nose and allowed to travel to small intestine; uses balloon filled with mercury at tip to aid in passage through bowel. Tip is weighted and carried distally via peristalsis (thus not indicated in ileus). Device is useful in recurrent partial small bowel obstruction due to adhesions (esp. caused by radiation enteritis); also sometimes used in small bowel obstructions due to malignancy. FDA has recently banned tube secondary to risk of mercury poisoning.

Cantrell line: Imaginary line running between gallbladder fossa and inferior vena cava; separates right and left lobes of liver.

Cantrell pentalogy: Congenital abnormality of lower sternum; with supraumbilical abdominal wall defect and defects of anterior diaphragm, heart (usu. VSD), and pericardium.

Cantu disease: Large skull, mental retardation, wide-set eyes, hyperextensible joints, cardiac defects, wrinkled skin on soles and palms, and small vertebral bodies; associated with advanced paternal age.

Cantu disease: Hyperkeratotic soles and palms and brownish macular lesions on feet, face, and forearms; autosomal dominant condition developing during adolescence.

Cantwell-Ransley technique: Penile elongation and urethroplasty used to improve cosmetic appearance in epispadias and bladder extrophy in children. Corpora are mobilized proximally and rotated, urethra is positioned ventrally, and neurovascular structures are placed in dorsal midline; distal vertical incision and horizontal closure allows neomeatus to reach glans tip.

Capdepont disease (Stainton disease): Defective dentinogenesis with abnormal deciduous and permanent teeth; marked by translucent, small, and orange-tinted teeth that wear to gum level with normal chewing. Condition is autosomal dominant.

Capgras syndrome (phantom double): Psychiatric condition occurring in absence of psychosis in which patient is convinced that significant person (usu. spouse) has been replaced by another person, despite all persuasion to contrary; conditon more common in women.

Caplan syndrome (Colinet-Caplan syndrome): Rheumatoid arthritis, pulmonary fibrosis, and nodular infiltrates in lung; seen typically in miners' pneumoconiosis.

Capner procedure: Incision and drainage of thoracic spinal abscess; uses anterolateral exposure.

Capute-Rimoin-Konigsmark syndrome: Congenital deafness, brown spots on face (onset in 2nd year), and occasional syndactyly; autosomal dominant condition.

Carcassone ligament (puboprostatic ligament): Thickened portion of pelvic diaphragm; runs laterally from prostate to pelvic fascia tendinous arch and medially to pubic bone.

Carcassone perineal ligament (transverse perineal ligament): Thickened anterior border of perineal membrane; runs across subpubic angle posterior to deep dorsal vein of penis.

Cardarelli sign (Castellino sign): Indication of aortic arch aneurysm if laryngotracheal tube shows transverse pulsations.

Carden amputation: Above-knee amputation at distal femur; uses 1 large soft tissue flap to close wound.

Carducci test: Evidence of boutonnière deformity if proximal interphalangeal extension is restricted 20° with full metacarpophalangeal and wrist flexion.

Carey-Coombs murmur: Mid-diastolic murmur heard in acute rheumatic fever; best detected at apex of heart.

Carey-Fineman-Ziter syndrome: Rare ophthalmoplegia, weakness, and hypotonia in setting of Möbius-like disease.

Carini disease (Seeligman disease, alligator baby): Diffuse bright red skin developing into large peeling flakes in neonates or infants; condition may recur depending on underlying etiology.

Carl Smith lymphocytosis: Acute onset of fever, diarrhea, abdominal pain and distention, neck or generalized adenopathy, and sometimes meningeal signs; several infectious etiologies likely. Condition is most typical in young adults; 2–3 week incubation period.

Carleton spots: Areas of sclerosed bone seen in gonorrhea.

Carlson syndrome (fish eye disease): High serum levels of triglycerides, VLDL, and LDL, with severe corneal opacities (resembling fish eyes) causing vision loss; associated with defect in cholesterol acyltransferase gene. Treatment is corneal transplantation.

Carman sign (Carman-Kirklin sign, meniscus sign): Crescent-shaped radiologic shadow caused by gastric ulcer crater; if convexity points downward, ulcer is distal to incisura; if convexity points upward, ulcer is on lesser angle.

Carmi syndrome: Aplastic skin on scalp and GI atresia; associated with high α-protein content of amniotic fluid. Autosomal recessive condition also seen with winged axillary skin and lid ectropion.

Carmody-Batson operation: Procedure used to repair fractures of zygoma or zygomatic arch (cheekbone) by making incision in gums above molar teeth.

Carnett sign: Method used to determine etiology of abdominal pain in which patient tenses abdominal muscles. If palpation causes tenderness, etiology is parietal. If palpation does not cause tenderness (and tenderness occurs with relaxed muscles), cause is intra-abdominal.

Carnevale syndrome: Mental retardation, drooping eyelids, strabismus, hip dysplasia, cryptorchidism; and elbow contractures; rare condition.

Carney complex (NAME syndrome, Russell-Rees syndrome): Pigmented lesions over entire body surface (worse in summer), subcutaneous myxoid neurofibromas, and atrial myxomas; onset occurs in early infancy. Cushingoid symptoms due to adrenal cortex adenoma/hyperplasia occur in 2nd decade. Condition is also occ. associated with adenomas of thyroid, pituitary, and testes.

Carney triad: Occurrence of symptoms and signs of 2 of the following tumors: gastric lymyosarcoma; lung chondroma; or extra-adrenal paraganglioma. Condition usu. affects young women.

Carnoy solution: Combination of 1 part glacial acetic acid, 5 parts saturated picric acid, 5 parts 40% formalin, and 3 parts absolute ethanol; used as acid fixative for viewing cell nucleus and chromosomes.

Caroli disease: Progressive cystic degeneration of intrahepatic bile ducts; usu. requires liver transplantation. Two forms exist; less severe form (15% of cases) are associated with recurrent cholangitis and medullary sponge kidney, and more severe form has periportal fibrosis and a lower incidence of sponge kidney.

Carpenter syndrome (acrocephalopolysyndactyly type 2): Presence of skull malformations (e.g., acrocephaly), premature closure of skull sutures, odd facies, brachysyndactyly of fingers, polysyndactyly of toes, obesity, hypoplastic genitalia, congenital heart defects, abdominal hernias, and mental retardation; rare autosomal recessive condition.

Carpentier-Edwards prosthesis: Artificial heart

valve (mitral or aortic) made of xenograft material (usu. porcine); does not require anticoagulation but does have shorter life span than synthetic valves.

Carpentier-Edwards prosthesis

Carpue operation: Late 1800s technique for surgical reconstruction of obliterated nose; developed by military surgeon to treat battlefield casualties.

Carr-Barr-Plunkett syndrome: 48XXXX genotype with congenital mental retardation, wide-set eyes, small mouth, clinodactyly, and webbed neck.

Carr-Purcell-Meiboom-Gill technique: Method of measuring intensity of signal in MRI of heart at different echo times to allow calculation of T2 (transverse) relaxation time.

Carr-Purcell pulse sequence: Variant of basic spin-echo model of multipulse nuclear MRI; creates additional spin-echoes by repeated isochromatic refocusing.

Carraro syndrome: Rare hypoplastic or absent fibula and deafness.

Carrel patch: Elliptical segment cut from wall of donor artery encompassing the opening of arteries leading to a graft organ; allows end-to-side anastomosis without impinging on lumen. Patch is fixed at superior and inferior ends with 5–0 or 6–0 prolene.

Carrel-Dakin fluid: Dilute solution of sodium hypochlorite.

Carrington-Liebow variant: Form of Wegener granulomatosis with pulmonary pathology and some extrapulmonary pathology but with absence of kidney disease.

Carrión disease: See Bartonellosis.

Carson-Neill disease: Homocystinuria; after normal perinatal period, onset of seizures occurs at 6 months of age, with development of mental deficiency, dislocation of lenses, speech deficiency, clumsiness, and deficiency of cystathionine β-synthetase. Also with buildup of homocystine and methionine in preschool years. Screening test is positive cyanide nitroprusside reaction in urine. Treatment is low-methionine diet with anticoagulant and antiplatelet drugs.

Carter-Horsely-Hughes syndrome: Diffuse familial intestinal polyposis in both large and small bowel; rare autosomal dominant condition.

Carter-Sukavajana syndrome: Atrophy of cerebello-olivary tract with gait ataxia and Parkinson-like symptoms; X-linked condition that occurs in males, with onset from childhood to middle age.

Cartwright blood group: Yt blood group, containing erythrocyte antigens Yt^a and Yt^b.

Carvallo sign: Early, soft systolic murmur that accentuates with inspiration. Occurs in tricuspid regurgitation; usu. best heard at lower left sternal border.

Casoni test: Evidence of hydatid infection if injection of hydatid fluid into skin causes wheal-and-flare reaction; now largely supplanted by more sophisticated serum tests.

Caspersson cells (type B): Cells containing small amount of nuclear DNA and large amounts of nucleolar RNA.

Casser ligament: Triangular-shaped fibrous connective tissue running from posterior surface of incisura tympanica to malleolar neck or head.

Cassidy syndrome: See Bjoerck disease.

Cassirer syndrome: Sensory disturbances in limbs (e.g., paresthesias, sweating, coldness) caused by emotional stress or cold exposure; skin appears dusky and mottled with elevation of extremities improving cyanosis. Onset occurs in childhood; more prevalent in girls. Condition often improves after 1st pregnancy or in 3rd decade.

Castaneda bottle: Container that holds both solid agar and broth; used to culture fastidious organisms from blood specimens.

Castellani bronchitis: Bronchial inflammation caused by spirochete invasion.

Castellani dermatosis: Papules and pilosebaceous follicles located on bilateral facial cheeks; condition considered benign. Onset occurs at puberty; affects black persons in Mediterranean region and Central America.

Castellino sign: See Cardarelli sign.

Castillo catheter: Thin, J-shaped device inserted into brachial vessel to inject dye for coronary angiography.

Castle factor: Intrinsic factor.

Castleman disease: Lymph node hyperplasia secondary to reactive proliferation of B-cell lymphocytes, with 2 distinct subtypes: mediastinal and diffuse multicentric adenopathy. Associated with collagen vascular disease, myasthenia gravis, amyloidosis, and nephrosis; in 25% of cases B-cell lymphoma or Kaposi sarcoma develops. Treatment is radiation.

Castroviejo needle holder: Fine-tipped needle holder with cross-action locking mechanism; used in sewing vascular anastomosis requiring fine suture sizes.

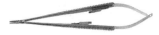

Castroviejo needle holder

Catel-Manzke syndrome: Signs of Pierre Robin disease with additional anomalies of both index fingers and variable presence of dislocatable knees.

Catel-Schwartz-Jampel syndrome: Myotonic chondrodysplasia marked by abnormal growth by 1 year of age, as well as facial and limb myotonia; autosomal recessive condition.

Cattaneo sign: Indication of tracheobronchial lymph node enlargement if reddish spots appear over spinous processes of thoracic vertebrae when palpated.

Cattell maneuver: Reflection of right colon and small bowel anteriorly and medially to expose inferior vena cava, right renal vessels, 4th part of duodenum, aorta, and uncinate of pancreas; performed by dividing along white line of Toldt lateral to cecum and ascending colon. Procedure should be performed in all zone 1 (centromedial), traumatic injuries.

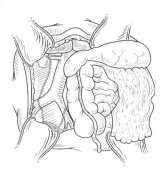

Cattell maneuver

Cattell personality inventory: Self-report inventory used to assess presence of personality traits; based on scores of 16 different scales.

Catterall hip score: System used to describe pediatric avascular necrosis of femoral head (Legg-Calvé-Perthes disease). Grade 1, femoral head compression seen only on frog-leg lateral film; grade 2, central compression on frog-leg lateral and AP views; grade 3, majority of femoral head involved; grade 4, entire femoral head involved.

Cauchois-Eppinger-Frugoni syndrome (Opitz syndrome): Thrombophlebitis of splenic vein causing left upper quadrant abdominal pain, fever, and splenomegaly.

Cauhepe-Fieux syndrome: Lateral deviation of jaw while chewing.

Cayenne pepper spots: Red punctate angiomatous lesions found in margins of Schaumberg disease lesions.

Cayler syndrome: Congenital asymmetric crying facies; also associated with kidney, limb, and vertebral body abnormalities. Condition is more common on right side. Up to 10% of patients have cardiac abnormalities (usu. VSD).

Cazenave vitiligo: See Jonston alopecia.

Cecil operation: Method of hypospadias repair; new urethral segment is constructed and buried in scrotum and then separated from scrotum in a 2nd operation.

Cecil operation: 3-stage repair of urethral stricture; uses excision of strictured segment via a ventral approach, followed by construction of a new urethral segment buried in scrotum and then separated from scrotum in a 2nd procedure.

Cedell fracture: Fracture line running through posterior talus bone of foot.

Ceelen-Gellerstedt syndrome (idiopathic pulmonary hemosiderosis): Recurrent cough, dyspnea, and hemoptysis; due to focal fibrosiderosis and hemorrhages of lungs. Onset (usu. sudden) occurs in childhood; more prevalent in boys. Chest radiograph shows changing pattern of ill-defined opacities. Condition is considered to be autoimmune derangement and associated with Goodpasture, Wegener, and Churg-Strauss syndromes.

Cegka sign: Lack of variation in cardiac dullness during respiration; seen in pericardial adhesions and fibrosis.

Celand-Arnold-Chiari malformation: See Arnold-Chiari malformation (type I).

Celani stain: Method that uses peroxidase reaction to visualize blood smears; stains nuclei pale red, peroxidase-containing granules blue, cytoplasm of leukocytes pale pink, and RBCs yellow.

Celestin tube: Plastic tube used as esophageal stent in obstructing esophageal cancer; allows patient to handle secretions and avoid cervical esophagostomy.

Cellano allele: Homozygous K allele of Kell blood group.

cells of Cajal: Horizontally arranged cells occurring only in layer 1 of cerebral cortex; processes run laterally.

cells of Corti: All cell types in organ of Corti.

cells of Hensen: Outer border of cells in organ of Corti; provide structural support for hair cells.

cells of Martinotti: 1 of 5 cell types in cerebral cortex; axons point toward surface.

cells of van Gehuchten: See Golgi cell (type 2).

Celsius thermometer: Instrument that measures temperature using Celsius scale.

Celsus alopecia (vitiligo, area): See Jonston alopecia.

Cenani-Lenz syndactyly: Disorder similar to Apert disease with addition of short and fused ulna and radius, fused metacarpals, and abnormal phalanges; autosomal recessive condition.

central canal of Stilling: See Cloquet canal.

central cloudy dystrophy of Francois: Small, grayish patches with surrounding whitish zones developing in deep, axial parts of corneal stroma; vision generally not affected. This autosomal dominant condition is often confused with Fuchs dystrophy.

Cervenka disease: See David-Stickler disease.

Cervòs-Navarro syndrome: Inflammatory reticuloendotheliosis causing chronic or acute encephalitis;

histologically marked by perivascular infiltration with lymphocytes, histiocytes, and plasma cells.

Céstan-Chenais syndrome: Marked by lesions of nucleus ambiguus, restiform body, and descending sympathetic tracts; also with hemiplegia and loss of proprioception and tactile sense on contralateral side. Condition is due to occlusion of vertebral artery below origin of posterior inferior cerebellar artery; results in paralysis of soft palate, pharynx, and larynx, as well as Horner syndrome on ipsilateral side.

Ceylon sore mouth: Tropical sprue.

Chaddock sign: Irritation of skin in external malleolus area, leading to extension of big toe on same side; seen in corticospinal pathway lesions.

Chaddock sign (reflex): Pressure or scratching at ulnar side of palmaris longus or flexor carpi radialis, leading to flexion of wrist and extension and spreading of fingers; seen in corticospinal tract lesions (upper motor neuron).

Chadwick sign: Dusky, bluish mucosa found in vagina and cervix at 8–12 weeks of pregnancy.

Chadwick-Bentley classification: System used to describe distal tibial fracture through epiphysis in children. Group 1, no involvement of epiphysis; group 1a, fracture and lateral separation of distal fibula (abduction mechanism); group 1b, fracture and posterior separation of metaphysis fragment (hyperplantar flexion/supination mechanism); group 1c, fracture of anteromedial tibial metaphysis with posterior displacement (external rotation/supination mechanism); group 1d, fracture of tibial metaphysis posteromedially and distal fibular shaft fracture with medial displacement (adduction mechanism); group 2, epiphyseal fracture with displacement of vertical lateral fragment; group 3, combinatiion of Salter type 4 fracture with Salter type 1 or 2 (adduction mechanism).

Chagas disease (American trypanosomiasis): Systemic disease caused by infection via direct bite by reduviid or "kissing" bug, *Trypanosoma cruzi;* endemic to South America. Disease is associated with megacolon, achalasia due to destruction of ganglion cells in Auerbach plexus and, sudden cardiac death (in young adults). There is no effective antibiotic treatment.

Chagasia: Subgenus of *Anopheles* mosquitoes found in South America.

Chamberlain filter: Porcelain-based bacterial filter available in several different porosities.

Chamberlain line: Imaginary line at base of skull running between dorsal tip of foramen magnum and dorsal margin of hard palate; normally lies above tip of odontoid process of axis.

Chamberlain method:
Radiographic positioning
technique using AP projection
of pelvis, hip joints, and lumbar
vertebrae to determine
differences in leg lengths.

Chamberlain procedure:
Transverse parasternal incision
with dissection of deep tissues;
allows for excisional lymph
node biopsy of paratracheal and
aortopulmonary nodes.

Chambers-Pratt syndrome:
Absence of fructose-1-
phoshpate liver aldolase in
kidney, liver, and small bowel;
marked by vomiting,
convulsions, cachexia,
hepatomegaly, jaundice, edema,
and ascites. Autosomal
recessive condition manifests in
infancy when fructose or
sucrose is 1st ingested.
Treatment is fructose-free diet
and liver transplantation (if liver
failure occurs).

Champey plate: Monocortical
plate for fixation of craniofacial
fractures and osteotomies.

**Chanarin-Dorfman
syndrome:**
Hepatosplenomegaly and scaly
skin developing in infancy;
delayed onset of nystagmus,
cataracts, and gait problems.
Etiology is intracellular buildup
of triglyceride due to impaired
long-chain fatty acid oxidation.
Leukocytes show vacuolation
(Jordan anomaly). Treatment is
medium-chain triglyceride diet.

Chance fracture: Unstable
fracture of vertebral body
separating spinous processes
from bony arch, leading to
horizontal fracture line through
vertebral body; mechanism is
severe, acute flexion.

Chandler disease: Aseptic
necrosis of femoral head; usu.
seen in middle-aged men.

Chandler syndrome: Corneal
edema, glaucoma, endothelial
dystrophy, and stromal atrophy
of iris; glaucoma usu. results.

**Chandra-Khetarpal
syndrome:** Levocardia,
bronchiectasis, and sinus
abnormalities; possible variant
of Kartagener syndrome.
Congenital condition usu.
manifests in infancy with
repeated fever episodes with
sequelae of bronchiectasis.
Treatment is antibiotic therapy
and surgery to remove abnormal
lung.

Chang algorithm: Technique
for correction of attenuation in
SPECT computers; uses map of
attenuation coefficients in
thorax to determine average
attenuation at each pixel
throughout image. Algorithm
overcorrects at center of image
(esp. if iterative calculations are
not performed) and may
introduce artifacts in cardiac
imaging.

Channing solution:
Potassium iodide and mercury
solution.

Chaoul tube: Low-voltage x-
ray tube positioned 2 cm from
skin surface; produces
significant but superficial
ionizing radiation to tissues.

Chapman mixture: Opium
and copaiba mixture.

Chaput fracture: Break running through Chaput tubercle; due to tension applied by anterior tibiofibular ligament.

Chaput tubercle: Anterior lateral tubercle of distal tibia; attachment site of anterior tibiofibular ligament.

Charcot angina: Global insufficiency of blood flow to supply metabolic tissue demand during exertion; marked by cold extremities, weakness, cramps, and pain. Condition improves with rest.

Charcot arteries (lenticulostriate arteries): Several arteries branching off anterior choroidal and middle cerebral arteries; supply internal capsule, globus pallidus, and striatum of brain. Vessels usu. enter base of brain anteriorly through substantia perforator.

Charcot cirrhosis: Primary biliary cirrhosis.

Charcot foot: Deformity resulting from arthropathy; occurs in tabes dorsalis and end-stage diabetes mellitus.

Charcot gait: Ataxic gait occurring in Friedreich ataxia.

Charcot joint: Pain and swelling in joint; followed by development of deformity, loss of mobility, and "bag of nuts" on palpation; seen as sequela of diabetes, leprosy, tabes dorsalis, and syringomyelia.

Charcot sign: Raised eyebrow seen in lateral facial paralysis; if attempt is made to contract facial muscles, eyebrow is lowered.

Charcot spine (neuropathic joint disease): Articular cartilage destruction in spine with formation of osteophytes and subchondral bone in disorganized pattern. Causes include syphilis, diabetes, tumors, trauma, syringomyelia, and transverse myelitis.

Charcot syncope (carotid sinus syncope): Sudden onset of dizziness, fainting, headache, slurred speech, convulsions and systemic vagal signs (e.g., bradycardia, hypotension), and peripheral dilation. Caused by pressure on carotid sinus (e.g., tight neck clothing, sudden head turning). Treatment during attacks is atropine (if vagal signs present) or amphetamines.

Charcot triad: Jaundice, fever, and right upper quadrant pain; diagnostic for cholangitis. Occurs in 50%–70% of cases; fever is most common sign.

Charcot triad: Scanning speech, nystagmus, and intention tremor occurring in multiple sclerosis.

Charcot vertigo: Acute onset of coughing followed by syncope, diaphoresis, and occ. seizures; most common in obese middle-aged men with high intake of alcohol and tobacco.

Charcot walker: Restraint orthotic walker used to provide prolonged support and protection in diabetic neuropathic arthropathy of foot; usu. custom-built, with rigid boot that encloses ankle and foot completely. Walker is typically used after initial cast immobilization.

Charcot-Böttcher crystalloids: Slender, thread-like structures 10–25 μm long; unique to Sertoli cells of human testes. Occur in both benign and malignant cells.

Charcot-Bouchard aneurysm: Miliary aneurysms in small arteries exposed to hypertension; probably not associated with increased risk of bleeding.

Charcot-Leyden crystals: Lance-shaped crystals representing destroyed leukocytes; seen as eosinophilic structures under hematoxylin–eosin stain. Crystals are typically found in chronic mucous bronchitis of asthma, helminthiasis, or intestinal amebiasis.

Charcot-Marie-Tooth-Hoffman disease: Slowly progressive motor and sensory neural muscular atrophy, with peripheral nerve demyelination and anterior horn cell degeneration; begins with distal extremities (esp. peroneal nerve, causing foot drop) and moves proximally. Condition has dominant, recessive, and X-linked forms.

Charcot-Willbrand syndrome: Agraphia and visual agnosia caused by arterial lesion in angular gyrus of dominant side; patients unable to describe common objects not in immediate view.

Charles law (Gay-Lussac law): Pressure exerted by a fixed volume of gas is directly proportional to its temperature. Equation: $V = kT$, where V is volume, k is constant, and T is temperature.

Charles procedure: Classical, 1-stage excisional procedure for surgical treatment of lymphedema of leg; uses radical excision of subcutaneous tissue and skin from ankle to knee. Past results were usu. poor, and procedure is rarely performed today.

Charles Ruppe syndrome: Fibrous dysplasia of skull and facial bones.

Charleston-Bending brace: Orthotic back brace used in nonoperative treatment for juvenile idiopathic scoliosis.

Charlevoix syndrome: See Andermann syndrome.

Charlin syndrome (Charlin-Sluder syndrome, Harris syndrome): Cluster headache in setting of severe inflammation of eye.

Charmat syndrome: Clinical occurrence of splenomegaly and macroglobulinemia; seen in Africa.

Charnley arthroplasty: Hip replacement surgery using Charnley prosthesis.

Charnley prosthesis: Low-friction hip joint.

Charnley scale: Evaluates preop and postop hip surgery patients; scores pain, function, and range of motion.

Chassaignac syndrome (Chassaignac-Laehmung

syndrome, nursemaid elbow):
Pain and subluxation of arm
starting in infancy; caused by
excessive muscle stretching.
Treatment involves reposition
supination of forearm.

Chassaignac tubercle
(carotid tubercle): Anterior
bony prominence of transverse
process of C6 vertebrae, which
is sometimes palpable; occurs
lateral and slightly cephalad to
C6 posterior tubercle. Carotid
artery lies just anterior.

Chassard-Lapiné position:
X-ray film technique used to
obtain superior-inferior view of
pelvic outlet, opacified bladder,
or rectum. Patient sits on film,
spreads legs wide, and leans
forward.

Chattel syndrome: Unilateral
weakness and palsy of facial
muscles or vocal cords; onset in
infancy. Treatment is B-complex
vitamins.

Chauffard point: Anatomic
area just below clavicle and
equidistant from each end; site
of tenderness in gallbladder
disease.

Chaussier sign: Pain in
epigastric area; seen in
eclampsia.

Chavany-Brunhes syndrome
(Fitzsche syndrome):
Headaches occurring after
fatigue, stress or immobilization
of head and neck; associated
with calcification of falx.

**Cheadle-Moeller-Barlow
syndrome:** See Barlow
syndrome.

Cheattle hernia repair:
Procedure using preperitoneal
approach.

Chédiak-Higashi disease
(anomaly, syndrome): Albinism,
photophobia, recurrent
infections (esp. periodontal),
lymphomas, and neurologic
deficits, with abnormal
lysosomes, which appear as
giant cytoplasmic granules; rare
autosomal recessive condition.
Disorder is associated with
deficiency in natural killer cell
activity and antibody-dependent
cellular cytotoxicity.
Accelerated phase of disease
(occurs only in positive Epstein-
Barr virus patients) is marked
by fever, pancytopenia,
jaundice, hepatosplenomegaly,
lymphadenopathy, and
neurologic deterioration.

Cherney incision:
Suprapubic, transverse incision
of rectus muscles off pubic
bone; used to gain access to
reproductive organs in women.
Technique originally described
as using bilateral ligation of
inferior epigastric vessels to
allow greater incision width;
provides excellent access to
Retzius space and pelvic
sidewall.

Chester porphyria: Variant
with absence of
photosensitivity; reduced
activity of porphobilinogen
deaminase and
protoporphobilinogen oxidase.

Chester-Erdheim disease:
Diffuse lipogranulomatosis of
internal organs and bones.

Cheyne nystagmus (Cheyne-Stokes nystagmus): Rhythmic movements of eyes in synchrony with crescendo–decrescendo breathing.

Cheyne-Stokes respiration (sign): Alternating periods of deep breathing and apnea; may occur normally during sleep in children and elderly. Pathologic causes are bilateral brain damage, drug-induced respiratory failure, uremia, and heart failure.

Chiari net: Group of fibers representing remnants of septum spurium and sinus venosus; occ. seen on right atrial wall.

Chiari-Frommel syndrome: Amenorrhea, prolonged lactation, uterine hypoplasia, and atrophic endometrium due to abnormal prolactin secretion; most commonly seen in 1st-time mothers.

Chick-Martin tests: Used to determine disinfectant properties.

Chiclero ulcer: See Aleppo boil.

Chiene test: Indicator of femoral neck fracture if positive.

Chievitz layer: Transiently present layer of fibers between inner and outer neuroblastic lamina of optic cup.

Chievitz organ: Embryonic epithelial growth that develops behind parotid gland; may disappear entirely or merge with parotid gland.

Chievitz organ (paraorgan): Epithelial nests on intraoral sensory nerve endings; easily confused with perineural involvement of epidermoid cancer.

Chilaiditi syndrome (wanderleber syndrome): Intermittent entrapment of colon between liver and diaphragm; pain, vomiting and distention seen mostly in children at end of day. Treatment is dietary and reclining position.

Child classification: System originally conceived to predict mortality from surgical shunting operations for variceal bleeds; now used as measure of liver disease and reserve. Basis is clinical ascites, encephalopathy, nutritional status, serum albumin, and bilirubin: mortality for A, B, and C is < 2%, 10%, and 50%, respectively.

Childs-Phillips procedure: Mostly abandoned technique of external plication of small bowel and mesentery to prevent episodic obstruction in multiply recurrent bowel obstruction.

Chimani-Moos test: Used to detect malingering in deafness.

Chinese anise (Indian anise): Dried fruit of *Illicium verum;* oil used as carminative and stimulant.

Chinese ginseng: See Korean ginseng.

Chinese hamster ovary cells: Well-established experimental strain of fibroblasts used in biomedical research.

Chiray disease: Abnormal motility of biliary system; most commonly presents as nausea, right upper quadrant pain, anorexia, avoidance of fatty foods, and variable headache. Condition may be due to atonic state and flaccid gallbladder or hyperkinetic state and spasmodic sphincter of Oddi.

Choix fever: Disease occurring in Northern Mexico that is identical to Rocky Mountain spotted fever.

Chopart amputation (mediotarsal amputation): Early surgical procedure for foot amputation. Incision passes dorsally between talus and navicular medially and calcaneus and cuboid laterally. Plantar flap should extend to 2 cm from metatarsal heads; anterior tibialis and extensor tendons must be sutured to plantar flap.

Chopart joint (transverse tarsal joints): Junction between hindfoot (talus and calcaneus)

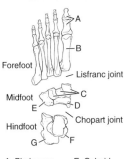

A. Phalanges
B. Metatarsals
C. Cuneiforms
D. Navicular
E. Cuboid
F. Talus
G. Calcaneus

Chopart joint

and midfoot (navicular, cuboid, and cuneiforms).

Chopart dislocation: Disarticulation of cuboid and navicular bone across calcaneus and talus.

Chotzen syndrome: Type 3 acrocephalosyndactyly; autosomal dominant condition marked by mild asymmetry of head and fusion of 2nd and 3rd fingers and toes.

Christ-Siemens-Touraine syndrome: Derangement in temperature regulation, reduced or absent perspiration, hypotrichosis, partial or total anodontia, sunken cheeks, thickened lips, abnormal nails, saddle-shaped nose, dysphagia, increased respiratory infections, and stunted development. Congenital condition has X-linked inheritance, with occasional presentation of mild clinical syndrome in female carriers.

Christensen agar: Medium used to detect urease production by *Proteus*.

Christensen-Krabbe disease: See Alpers disease.

Christian disease: Short thumbs with shortened distal phalanges, metatarsals, and metacarpals; congenital autosomal dominant condition occurring equally in both sexes.

Christian disease (Christian-Andrews-Conneally syndrome): Mental retardation, dysphagia, hypotonia, seizures, craniosynostosis, microcephaly, wide-set eyes, cleft palate, torticollis, ear abnormalities, abducted thumbs, and hirsutism; congenital autosomal recessive condition.

Christmas disease (hemophilia B, factor IX deficiency): Congenital deficiency of factor IX; clinical syndrome very similar to classic hemophilia but with milder symptoms.

Christopher spots: See Maurer dots.

Chudley syndrome: Severe mental retardation, obesity, hypogonadism, stunted growth, odd facies with almond-shaped palpebral fissures, anteverted nostrils, and macrostomia; X-linked inheritance with onset in infancy.

Chung classification: System used to describe invasiveness of vulvar melanoma invasion. Stage 1, intraepithelial; stage 2, < 1 mm; stage 3, 1–2 mm; stage 4, > 2 mm; stage 5, into subcutaneous fat.

Churchill caustic: Solution of iodine and potassium iodide.

Churg-Strauss syndrome: Allergic vasculitis marked by involvement of small and medium-sized arteries (esp. in lungs), fever, weight loss, myalgia, headache, and respiratory distress. Cutaneous biopsy shows eosinophilic vasculitis.

Churukian-Schenk modification: Histologic staining technique used to produce argyrophilic reaction.

Chvostek sign (tremor, reflex, Chvostek-Weiss sign, Weiss sign, Schultze sign): Contraction of facial muscles elicited by tapping over facial nerve anterior to ear; occurs in hypocalcemia, tetany, and 5% of normal patients.

Ciarrocchi disease: Maculopapular rash between 3rd and 4th finger.

Cierny-Mader classification: Description of osteomyelitis based on anatomy of bone infection and physiology of the host; originally developed to describe long bone osteomyelitis.

Cincinnati incision: Incision used for exposure of lateral, medial, and posterior hindfoot, as well as medial and lateral midfoot, esp. in surgical soft tissue release in correction of clubfoot. Patient is placed in prone position. Incision through skin and subcutaneous tissue is started at 1st metatarsal joint and runs parallel to sole, around heel (cephalad to heel skin crease), extending onto lateral foot to calcaneocuboid joint. Achilles tendon is then severed with Z-shaped incision to expose deeper structures.

Cinderella syndrome (Ramirez syndrome, erythema dyschromicum persistens): Disseminated grayish, macular lesions appearing on limbs and trunk but sparing scalp, soles, and palms; may enlarge and coalesce. Condition is histologically marked by vacuolization of cells in Malpighian layer, perivasculitis in upper 1/3 of cutis, and edema of dermal papillae. Onset is from childhood onward.

circle of Willis: Series of arterial collaterals found (with much anatomic variation) in brain; provide connection between vertebral–carotid and hemisphere–hemisphere circulations. Ring of arteries circles optic chiasm, infundibulum, tuber cinereum, and posterior perforated space.

circles of Haller: Arterial and venous arcades in eye.

circles of Weber: Skin area in which patient is able to sense two different tactile stimuli.

circular muscle of Santorini: Smooth muscle fibers surrounding urethra.

circumscribed melanosis of Dubreuilh: Lentigo maligna melanoma.

Citelli syndrome: Mental deficiency and insomnia associated with tonsillar or sinus infection.

Ciuffo syndrome: Pulmonic stenosis, atrial septal defect causing a widely split 2nd heart sound, and absence of anterior ECG readings in precordial leads; rare condition.

Civatte poikiloderma: See poikiloderma of Civatte.

Civinini canal: Small opening off facial canal traversed by chorda tympani nerve as it enters tympanic cavity.

Civinini ligament: Fibrous connective tissue band running from superior edge of lateral pterygoid plate to spine of sphenoid bone.

Civinini process (pterygospinous process): Small, spiny ridge on posterior edge of lateral pterygoid plate of sphenoid; acts as attachment site for pterygospinous ligament.

Clado anastomosis: Joining of appendicular and ovarian arteries in appendicular-ovarian ligament.

Clado ligament: Variably present peritoneal fold running from mesoappendix to infundibulopelvic ligament.

Clanton-DeLee algorithm: Method for determining treatment for symptomatic osteochondritis dissecans in adults. Conditions are described as: no cartilage separation; early separation with no displacement; late separation with displacement, loose body in nonweight-bearing area; and loose body in weight-bearing area.

Clapton line: Appearance of greenish line on gum; seen in copper poisoning.

Clara cell: Nonciliated, cuboidal, secretory-appearing cell lining bronchioles at junction of alveolar branches.

Clark levels: Staging system of melanoma based on depth of skin penetration. 1, above basement membrane; 2, into papillary dermis; 3, at papillary/reticular dermal junction; 4, into reticular dermis; 5, into subcutaneous fat.

Clark nevus: Dysplastic melanotic nevi with notched, irregular borders on lesions; considered premalignant and marker for increased risk for melanoma. Lesions occur in 5% of white population.

Clark procedure: Separation of distal part of pectoralis major muscle from proximal part and insertion of distal part into biceps tendon.

Clark rule: Early 1900s calculation to determine pediatric drug doses; weight of child (lb)/150 × adult dose.

Clark sign: Inability to detect liver edge with percussion of abdominal wall when abdomen is distended due to peritonitis.

Clarke body: Intranuclear inclusions seen in alveolar breast sarcoma.

Clarke column (anterior pyramidal tract): Nucleus dorsalis of spinal column; runs in dorsal horn from C7–L3.

Clarke sign: Evidence of chondromalacia in patella if pain occurs behind bone when quadriceps is contracted and pressure is applied to patella.

Clarke-Hadfield syndrome: Congenital pancreatic atrophy with infantilism, obesity, and hepatomegaly.

Clarkson syndrome: Idiopathic systemic leaky capillaries (lung parenchyma spared), leading to acute shock-like collapse; fluid and proteins < 900,000 d infiltrate organs. Condition is rare, with unknown etiology. Treatment is aggressive replacement of fluid and crystalloids.

Clatworthy shunt (mesocaval shunt): Treatment of portal hypertension; inferior vena cava is ligated at junction of both common femoral veins and anastomosed to superior mesenteric vein.

Clauberg unit: Measure of progestin activity.

Claude sign (hyperkinesia reflex): Rapid extension or retraction of extremity (even in condition of total paralysis) following painful stimuli; seen in patients with motor disturbances, most commonly corticospinal tract abnormalities or hemiparesis.

Claude syndrome: CN III palsy with contralateral ataxia; often due to occlusion of proximal posterior cerebellar artery.

Claudius cell: Large cube-shaped cells found near organ of Corti (along with Böttcher cells) in external spiral sulcus.

Claybrook sign: Transmission of heart sounds and respiratory sounds to abdominal area; occurs in perforation/rupture of intra-abdominal organs. Detection of sounds is due to their transmission through intra-abdominal fluid, exudate, and blood.

Cleaves position: X-ray film technique using rolled film axial projection to visualize shoulder joint of patients who cannot abduct arm; provides image of glenohumeral joint, greater and lesser tuberosities, bicipital groove, and coracoid process.

Cleeman sign: Creasing of skin just above the patella; seen in femur fracture with "bayonet-like" displacement of fragments.

Cleland ligaments: Fibrous tissue on dorsolateral finger that stabilizes skin when bending finger; runs adjacent to neurovascular bundle.

Clemens solution: Potassium arsenate and bromide solution.

Clevenger fissure: Inferior occipital fissure.

Clifford disease: See Ballantyne disease.

Cloquet canal (hyaloid canal): Opening running from eye lens to optic disk in fetus and posteriorly through vitreous in serpentine manner but not extending to optic disk in adults; traversed by hyaloid artery and continuous with Berger space.

Cloquet ganglion: Enlarged portion of nasopalatine nerve as it traverses anterior palatine canal.

Cloquet hernia: Femoral hernia.

Cloquet ligament: Connective tissue band in spermatic cord representing remnant of processus vaginalis.

Cloquet node (Rosenmüller node): Deep femoral node located in femoral canal; may be mistaken for femoral hernia when enlarged.

Cloquet septum: Thin fascial layer continuing from transversalis fascia that partially closes femoral annulus, which is surrounded by adipose tissue; traversed by lymphatic channels.

Cloquet sign: Placement of clean needle into biceps muscle that exhibits oxidation on surface if patient is still alive; early technique used to determine if death has occurred.

Cloudman melanoma: Black, easily detectable melanoma originally described in female DBA mice; now used as a metastatic melanoma inducer when transplanted into other DBA mice and BALB/C mice.

Clough-Richter disease: 1920s term for erythrocyte autoagglutination.

Clouston syndrome (ectodermal dysplasia): Discolored, thickened nails, chronic paronychia, thickened skin over joints, hyperkeratosis of palms and soles, and variable mental retardation; onset in infancy.

Cloward technique: Method of anterior diskectomy with placement of bone graft (usu. harvested from ilium) into empty disk space. Depth of interspace is measured and a drill is positioned with aid of drill guide, hole is made overlying empty disk space with preservation of posterior cervical rim of adjacent vertebral bodies, and Cloward bone dowel is passed transversely through ilium avoiding iliac crest (after skin incision is made just below iliac crest and anterior muscles are stripped off). Procedure requires use of cervical collar for 8–12 weeks postop.

Clutton joint: Late manifestation of congenital syphilis; marked by painless synovitis and effusions of large joints, esp. knees and elbows. Onset is 8–15 years of age. Treatment is conservative management.

Coats disease: Formation of yellowish exudate under retina. Clinical variations include elevation and detachment of retina with no vascular changes; retinal findings with fresh arteriole retinal hemorrhages; and retinal findings with deafness, mental retardation, and muscle weakness. Treatment is diathermy.

Coats disease: Idiopathic retinal telangiectasia very similar to Leber aneurysm, except usu. thought of as occurring in children (male predominance); marked by accumulation of exudative subretinal fluid and retinal detachment. Vascular lesions appear as "red light bulbs" in retinal periphery. Condition usu. occurs unilaterally.

Cobb angle: Angle of curvature of spine in scoliosis as determined on full-length radiographic views.

Cobb brace: Orthopedic brace used to correct curvature of spine in growing children; typically used when curvature is < 40%.

Cobb method: Assesses scoliosis; angle of curvature defined by lines running from inferior edge of lower vertebrae with greatest tilt and superior edge of upper vertebrae.

Cobb syndrome (Cushing-Bailey-Cobb syndrome): Posterior vertebral destruction due to encroachment of a bone or cord angioma.

Cochin China diarrhea: Tropical sprue.

Cochrane syndrome: Leucine-sensitive hypoglycemia.

Cockayne syndrome (Neill-Dingwall syndrome): Ataxia, dwarfism, mental retardation, blindness, deafness, flexion contractures, cataracts, retinal atrophy, microcephaly, and paralysis; autosomal recessive condition leading to death in 2nd–3rd decade.

Cockayne-Touraine syndrome: Variant of epidermolysis bullosa; bullae develop on head and extremities (usu. after trauma). Condition may be severe, leading to mutilation; associated with hypertrichosis, hyperhidrosis, scaly skin, and dystrophic nails. Inheritance may be autosomal dominant or autosomal recessive (Kallin syndrome). Treatment is corticosteroids, antibiotics, and avoidance of trauma.

Cockett perforating veins: Vessels connecting posterior

communicating vein to deep venous system in leg.

Cockroft-Gault method: Method for calculation of creatinine clearance value is reduced by 15% for women. Equation: Creatine clearance = $(140—age) \times$ Weight (kg)/27 $\times$ serum creatinine (g/100 ml).

Codivilla extension: Device using nail placed through bone distal to fracture with weights attached to provide traction.

Codman Castaneda kit: Instruments specifically designed for infant cardiovascular surgery.

Codman Diethrich kit: Instruments for coronary artery bypass surgery.

Codman exercises: Maneuvers used to increase range of motion in shoulder capsulitis (frozen shoulder). Patient keeps knees extended and bends torso at 90°; examiner gently swings affected arm like pendulum.

Codman IMA kit: Instruments for handling internal mammary artery and small-vessel anastomoses.

Codman sign: Indication of supraspinatus tendon rupture if arm can be passively abducted without pain and if contraction of deltoid muscle causes pain.

Codman triangle: Area seen on radiographs outlined by periosteum being lifted off cortex by tumor (usu. osteosarcoma) and then readhering to normal bone.

Codman tumor: Benign chondroblastoma with pain, tenderness, and swelling at long bone epiphyses. Condition is more prevalent in males, with onset in adolescence to early adulthood. Treatment is excision.

Codman-Mentor cautery: Bipolar cautery with coagulation of tissues placed between tips; minimizes damage to adjacent tissues.

Coffin-Lowry syndrome: Mental deterioration, muscle weakness, clubbing, joint hypermobility, scoliosis, abnormal facies, genitourinary tract abnormalities, and bone deformities. Onset occurs in early infancy; gene defect is in ribosomal S6 kinase2 *(Xp22.3-p22.1)*.

Coffin-Siris syndrome: Stunted growth, absent or hypoplastic distal 5th finger, hirsutism in lumbosacral region, elbow dislocation, and sparse skull hair; congenital condition with female-to-male ratio of 4:1.

Cogan microcysts: Milky, pinpoint cysts developing in epithelium and basement membrane in setting of anterior corneal dystrophy; usu. centrally located and filled with nuclear and cytoplasmic debris. Cysts have surrounding "fingerprint" or "map-like" lines that surround cysts; can cause blurred vision and corneal erosions.

Cogan oculomotor apraxia: Inability to move eyes in 1 or both horizontal directions;

patient must turn head to view object in periphery. Condition is more prevalent in males and esp. noticeable in children.

Cogan syndrome (Cogan-Guerry syndrome): Onset of vertigo and endolymphatic hydrops of cochlea in young adults; condition marked by interstitial keratitis, eye pain, vision loss, vertigo, tinnitus, hearing loss, and variable periarteritis nodosa and aortic valve disease. Treatment is early, large doses of corticosteroids and cylcophosphamide and cyclosporin; poor prognosis for hearing and vestibular function.

Cogan-Reese syndrome: Unilateral glaucoma, development of iris nodules and ectopic pupil, and Descemet membrane.

Coghillian sequence: Successive stages in development of the tadpole; basis of early theory that specific behavior patterns develop from process of individuation (head-to-tail, central-to-peripheral axes) and behavior is not an accumulative, additive process.

Cohen syndrome (Pepper syndrome): High-arched palate, microcephaly, antimongoloid eyelid slant, tapered extremities, simian palmar crease, lax joints, syndactyly, scoliosis, cubitus valgus, hypotonic muscles, obesity in childhood, and mental retardation; rare congenital condition.

Cohen technique (advancement technique):

Procedure for ureteral reimplantation or correction of ureteral reflux; uses a tunnel through bladder wall across trigone (not toward bladder neck). Technique is good for use in small bladders and avoids risk of neohiatus formation but does not allow easy access to ureteral orifices.

Coindet disease: Acute enlargement and pain in thyroid gland caused by iodide administration; occurs both in thyroid disease and normal thyroid states. Condition is more common in females. Agents associated with immediate or delayed onset (years later) are amiodarone, contrast dyes, and seaweed.

Cohn solution: Aqueous solution containing ammonium tartrate, magnesium sulfate, calcium phosphate, and monopotassium acid phosphate; used to culture yeasts and molds.

Cohn test: Used to measure visual perception using different-colored embroidery figures.

Cohnheim artery (terminal artery): Artery that diminishes directly into capillaries without branching.

Cohnheim field (area): Loosely grouped fibrils separated from each other by narrow sarcoplasmic regions seen in cross-section of muscle.

Cohnheim theory: Early 1900s hypothesis that tumors occur due to abnormal embryonic development.

Colcott-Fox disease:
Impetigo; caused by
Staphylococcus or
Streptococcus infection of sweat
glands.

Cole hematoxylin: Variation
of hematoxylin stain; uses
mixture of warm distilled H_2O,
1% iodine in 95% distilled
ethanol, hematoxylin, and
aqueous ammonium alum.

Cole method: Technique for
anchoring tendon to bone; uses
wire suture passed on straight
needle through hole in bone.

Cole sign: Deformed duodenal
contour on radiography, which
indicates presence of duodenal
ulcer.

Cole-Jessner syndrome: See
Goltz syndrome.

Cole-Liebermann syndrome:
See Goltz syndrome.

Coleman test: Evidence for
flexibility of cavovarus foot
deformity if loss of varus
deformity occurs when lateral
foot and heel are placed on 2 cm
step.

**Coleman-Meredith
syndrome:** Fracture or
dislocation of spine with
associated spinal cord injury.

Coley toxin: Heat-killed
combination of *Serratia
marcescens* and *Streptococcus
pyogenes*; used in combination
with radiotherapy and surgery
to improve results when treating
osteogenic sarcoma or non-
Hodgkin lymphoma of bone.
Mechanism involves stimulating
host immune system against
tumor.

Coller hemostatic forceps:
Fine, curve-tipped, ring-handle,
locking forceps placed on small
vessels to control bleeding.

Colles fascia: Superficial
perineal fascia covering
external genitalia; attaches on
each side to lower margin of
ischiopubic ramus and to ischial
tuberosity.

Colles fixator (Ace-Colles
fixator): External fixation device
used in treatment of
comminuted distal radial
fractures; manipulation and
traction of ligaments and
capsules pull bone pieces into
place.

Colles fracture ("dinner fork"
deformity: Buckle-type fracture,
usu. resulting from fall on
outstretched hand; occurs at
distal radius with dorsal
displacement and angulation.

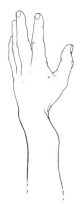

Colles fracture

Colles ligament (reflex
inguinal ligament): Triangular-
shaped fibrous connective

tissue band running from pubic bone and lacunar ligament medially and upward to linea alba; lies superficial to inguinal aponeurosis and deep to superficial abdominal ring.

Colles space: Space under perineal fascia containing labial (or posterior scrotal) neurovascular bundle, bulbous urethra, bulbocavernosus muscle, ischiocavernosus muscle, and transversus perineal muscle.

Collet-Bonnet syndrome: Facial palsy occurring in setting of Villaret syndrome.

Collet-Sicard syndrome (Vernet-Sarganon syndrome): Variant of Villaret syndrome without accompanying Horner syndrome; due to lesion (e.g., infection, tumor, trauma, adenopathies) in retropharyngeal space, resulting in ipsilateral paralysis of CN IX–XII. Condition also leads to inability to swallow, anesthesia of posterior tongue, trapezius and sternocleidomastoid paralysis, and hemiatrophy of tongue.

Collier sign: Eyelid retraction due to lesions in posterior commissure of brain; usu. bilateral (e.g., retraction due to thyroid disease) and symmetrical (unlike thyroid disease).

Collings knife: Device used in urologic surgery to cut tissue via electrocautery. For example, cutting current is used to make incision of ureteral meatus to allow passage of stone impacted at cystoureteral junction.

Collip unit: Amount of parathyroid extract needed to increase amount of serum calcium by 5 mg in 15 hours in 20-kg dog.

Collis gastroplasty: Antireflux procedure using 280° gastric fundoplication.

Colombian tick fever: Term for disease occurring in Colombia that is identical to Rocky Mountain spotted fever.

Colombo syndrome: Congenital inability to metabolize lysine; marked by vomiting, diarrhea, seizures, coma, spasticity, and impaired mental functioning. Condition affects urea synthesis and causes high levels of ammonia; cause is defect in L-lysine nicotinamide adenine dinucleotide oxidoreductase activity. Treatment is strict dietary restriction of protein.

Colonna classification (Delbet classification): System used to describe pediatric hip fractures. Type 1, fracture through epiphysis; type 2, fracture through femoral neck; type 3, fracture through neck/trochanter; type 4, intertrochanteric fracture.

Colonna operation: Method of reconstructing intracapsular femoral neck fractures.

Colonna-Ralston approach: Technique for access to posteromedial distal tibia; involves C-shaped incision anterior to medial malleolus; anterior retraction of tibialis posterior and flexor digitorum longus tendons; and posterolateral retraction of flexor hallucis longus, posterior tibial vessels, and tibial nerve.

Colorado tick fever: Mild fever without rash caused by arbovirus infection; rarely fatal. Disease occurs in Pacific and Rocky Mountain states of U.S. Tick vector is *Dermacentor andersoni.*

Colton blood group (Co blood group): Presence of antigens on chromosome band 7p14; antigenic polymorphisms at this locus have allowed DNA analyses of homozygous patients for nonsense mutations that prevent formation of channel-forming integral protein in RBCs.

column of Bertin: Normal variant in which remnant of polar parenchyma of embryonic subkidneys that fuse to form normal kidney persists; usu. found at junction of middle and upper third of kidney. Condition is diagnosed on ultrasound by appearance of lateral notching of renal sinus and junctional parenchymal line.

column of Clarke: Nucleus dorsalis of spinal cord; contains many prominent neuron cell bodies.

Combette syndrome: Congenital aplasia of cerebellum.

Comby sign: Appearance of whitish plaques on mucosa of the mouth and gums; early indication of measles infection.

Comfort-Steinberg syndrome: Familial relapsing pancreatitis with incomplete recovery between attacks; marked by diffuse abdominal pain and eventual development of diabetes mellitus. Onset usu. occurs by 15 years of age. Treatment is steroids and surgery with mixed results.

Comly syndrome: Chronic methemoglobinemia marked by cyanosis of mucosa and skin and variable metabolic and respiratory symptoms; due to high level of nitrates in well water. Treatment is avoidance of contaminated water and IV methylene blue (1 mg/kg) [in severe cases].

Comolli sign: Triangular swelling over fracture area; seen in scapular fractures.

Compton effect (scattering): Change in wavelength of x-rays or gamma rays due to interaction of electron orbiting nucleus and incidental photon, resulting in scattered photon of lower energy and recoil electron; most commonly seen in gamma rays 0.5–1.0 mEv and in medium-to-low atomic number absorbers.

Concato disease (Bamberg syndrome): Progressive, malignant accumulation of effusions in peritoneum, pleural cavity, and pericardium; may be idiopathic or tubercular.

Condon procedure: Technique using anterior iliopubic tract repair for correction of inguinal hernias. For indirect hernias, transversus abdominis arch is sutured to iliopubic tract from internal inguinal ring to pubic tubercle; sutures can be placed lateral to cord to reconstruct internal ring if needed. For direct hernias, sutures are placed between transversus abdominis superiorly to Cooper ligament and pubic tubercle below.

Condorelli syndrome: Fatty infiltration of mediastinum in obese patients; leads to irregular breathing when supine, impaired sleep, and mild facial cyanosis.

Condy fluid: Potassium and sodium permanganate solution; used as disinfectant.

Cone scalp retractor: Ring-handled, self-retaining retractor.

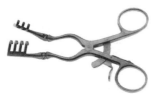

Cone scalp retractor

Congo blue (trypan blue, Niagara blue): Sodium salt of toluidin-diazo-diamino-naphthol-disulfonic acid; used to stain and identify protozoa.

Congo floor maggot: *Auchmeromyia luteola.*

Congo red: Staining method that uses hematoxylin to stain nuclei blue and congo red to stain amyloid red; also very efficient technique for detecting amyloid in histologic specimens (makes use of both polarized and unpolarized light).

Congo red test: Indicator of amyloidosis if 60% of IV injection of Congo red disappears after 1 hour.

Congolian red fever: Typhus that occurs in mice.

Conley incision: Incision used for exposure on anterior neck and lower mandible.

Conn syndrome (Conn-Louis syndrome): Primary hyperaldosteronism due to increased secretion of aldosterone from unilateral benign (glomerulosa layer) adenoma (85%), bilateral adenomas (5%) or bilateral adrenal hyperplasia (10%); marked by decreased renin secretion, hypervolemia, alkalosis, hypokalemia, hypernatremia, hyperchlorhydria, headaches, hypertension (esp. diastolic), polydipsia, and polyuria. Hypertension is surgically correctable in this condition.

Connell suture: Suturing technique used to "turn the corner" to complete deep, anterior layer when hand-sewing bowel anastomosis; allows inversion of structures as suture is tightened. Suture is placed outside-to-inside, then inside-to-outside on 1 side of bowel, is crossed to other side of anastomosis using an outside-to-outside suture, and is then repeated.

Connell-Ohio face mask: Anesthesia face mask designed to conform to Caucasian facial features.

Conrad-Bugg trapping:
Condition that occurs in ankle
fractures when soft tissue (usu.
posterior tibial tendon) is
caught between bony fragments.
Treatment is open reduction.

**Conradi syndrome
(Huenermann syndrome):**
Congenital bone and skin
disorder marked by scoliosis,
club foot, short proximal long
bones, macro- or microcephaly,
and syndactyly; also with mental
retardation and pulmonary
arterial stenosis. 25% of patients
have whorl-like yellow plaques
over total skin area. Death is
common within 1st year of life.

Conradi-Drigalski agar:
Culture medium containing dye
crystal violet; allows growth of
gram-negative organisms while
inhibiting growth of gram-
positive organisms. Agar is used
to isolate organsims from feces
such as *Salmonella typhi* and
other intestinal flora.

**Conradi-Hünermann
syndrome:** Large skin pores,
shortened and asymmetric
extremities, ventricular septal
defect, patent ductus arteriosus,
and early punctate mineralization.

Contarini syndrome: Ovarian
cancer associated with serous
and chylous effusions.

Convisart disease:
Dextroposed aorta associated
with tetralogy of Fallot.

Conway disease: Congenital
bowing of long bones seen in
hypophosphatasic dysplasia and
osteogenesis imperfecta.

Conway mammoplasty:
Method of reduction
mammoplasty using subtotal
breast amputation with free
transplantation of areolar
complex.

Cooley anemia: Thalassemia
major (homozygous β-
thalassemia); marked by striking
skull manifestations of widening
of diploë and atrophy of outer
table, severe anemia, debilitation,
and early death. Condition
occurs as 4 genetic variants.

Cooley aorta clamp: Ring-
handled, locking clamp with
curved tips; used to occlude
vascular structures.

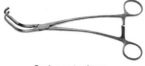

Cooley aorta clamp

Coolidge tube: Device that
generates x-ray radiation using
massive tungsten anode and
spiral filament of incandescent
tungsten as cathode.

Coombs direct test: Lab test
using RBCs to detect antibody
to RBCs or complement;
positive (abnormal) in leukemia,
lymphoma, systemic lupus
erythematosus, collagen
vascular diseases, and
erythroblastosis fetalis, as well
as with methyldopa, levodopa,
and cephalothin.

Coombs indirect test: Lab
test using serum that contains
antibody, which may be used for
RBC typing; positive (abnormal)
in isoimmunization from

previous transfusions or improper cross-matching.

Coonrad-Morrey device: Total elbow prosthesis with semiconstrained device manufactured from a titanium-based alloy; uses basic hinge articulation with pin that runs through polyethylene bushings to secure ulna.

Cooper breast: Pain of neurologic origin in breast tissue.

Cooper disease: 1800s term for benign fibrosis of breast tissue, usu. occurring unilaterally in upper outer quadrant; palpation indicates firm, indurated mass. Treatment is excision.

Cooper disease: Recurrent, chronic pain in testis; may have organic or psychiatric etiology.

Cooper fascia (fascia propria): Combined layer of femoral sheath and septum crurale partially ensheathing femoral hernia at ring.

Cooper hernia: Retroperitoneal hernia.

Cooper hernia: Femoral hernia with additional component bulging into scrotum, toward obturator foramen and labium majus.

Cooper laser: Device used at settings of 25 W in rapid intermittent superpulse mode for radial incisions in fimbriae in correction of hydrosalpinx.

Cooper ligament (pectineal ligament): Thickened fascia in transversalis fascia attached to linea terminalis, which fuses to periosteum of superior pubic ramus; forms floor of femoral ring and inferior border of femoral canal orifice and acts as insertion site of iliopubic tract.

Cooper ligament hernia repair: Procedure used to repair femoral hernia through groin approach. Cooper ligament is approximated to transversus abdominis aponeurosis medially; transition suture is placed between iliopubic tract, Cooper ligament, and transversus aponeurosis; and then lateral sutures are placed between iliopubic tract and transversus aponeurosis. A relaxing incision should always be used.

Cooper suspensory ligament: Connective tissue bands suspending mammary gland.

Cooper testis: Pain in testis caused by neuralgia.

Cooperman-Miura syndrome: Malposition of uvula of tongue causing irritation of tongue and uvula, with headaches, temporomandibular joint pain, and respiratory disorder. Treatment is mechanical intervention to prevent malposition.

Coopernail sign: Ecchymotic splotches sometimes seen on labia, scrotum, and perineum in pelvic fractures.

Cope disease: Bullous lesions developing on legs in absence of sun exposure, trauma, or inflammatory changes; usu. resolve after fluid aspiration without scar formation.

Cope introducing system: Cope needle, obturator, and accessory equipment; used for percutaneous placement of wire into kidney calyx through posterior approach to effect ureter dilation.

Cope law: Highly differentiated genera have only few organisms, whereas relatively undifferentiated genera have many types of organisms.

Cope needle: Cutting needle used for percutaneous needle biopsy.

Cope sign (psoas sign): Indication of appendicitis if flexion of hip causes pain.

Corbin technique: Wide-angle frontal projection of ribs.

Cordis stent: Flexible, balloon-expandable, single tantalum wire forming zigzag intravascular stent; originally developed as coronary stent and now being investigated for peripheral vascular application.

Cords disease: Visual loss with creamy exudates found in detached retina; defect is usu. unilateral and in temporal fields. Condition is typical in young boys; most common cause is toxocariasis. Treatment is antibiotics and anticoagulation.

Cori cycle: Lactate produced by muscles is transported to liver and converted to glucose, from which it is transported to muscles for reuse.

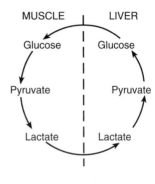

Cori cycle

Cori disease: See Forbes disease.

Cornell protocol: Exercise tolerance test procedure.

Corner-Allen test: Onset of endometrial changes seen in rabbit ovaries after injection of progesterone assay (18 hours after mating).

Corning filter: Bacteria filter using sintered glass.

corpus luysii (subthalamic nucleus): Small, lens-shaped structure located in ventral thalamus just dorsal to cerebral peduncle; carries motor fibers.

corpus of Oken: Fetal excretory organ; long vertical tubule in lower pole joined by horizontal, twisting tubules.

Correra line: Outline of lung fields seen on plain film radiograph of thorax.

Corridor procedure: Surgical treatment for atrial fibrillation.

Corrigan disease: Benign form of rheumatoid arthritis with abrupt onset in elderly; usu. resolves after several months. Serum rheumatoid factor is typically negative.

Corrigan disease: Aortic regurgitation, usu. due to bicuspid aortic valve and frequently asymptomatic until adulthood; congenital condition much more prevalent in males. Condition manifests with subtle weakness, lethargy, and sensation of neck pulsation, or less commonly with acute onset of cardiac failure; often associated with other cardiac malformations. Required treatment for correction is surgery.

Corrigan pulse: Carotid pulse marked by "water hammer" upstrokes (high-amplitude pulse with rapid upstroke); positive sign of large diastolic runoff seen in advanced, chronic aortic regurgitation.

Corrigan respiration: Shallow, blowing inspiration occurring in febrile states.

Corrigan sign (line): Indication of chronic copper poisoning if purple line occurs at tooth/gum line.

Corrigan sign: Expanding pulsatile mass seen in abdominal aortic aneurysm.

Corson bipolar scissors: Used in gynecologic surgery.

Corti ganglion: Collections of neurons found within spiral canal of modiolus; bipolar cells send processes centrally to cochlear nuclei in brainstem and peripherally through foramina nervosa to spiral organ.

Corti membrane: Sensory membrane of organ of Corti made of soft protein substance; adjacent to spiral organ and connected to hair cells.

Corti organ: Specialized hair cells that receive sound vibrations and transmit them as nerve impulses to brain; located on basilar membrane of inner ear in 2 rows sloping against one other. Cells are widest at helicotrema, where low-frequency sounds are received, and narrowest at base, where high-frequency sounds are heard.

Corti tunnel: Anatomic space running between 2 rows of hair cells in organ of Corti; triangular in cross-section.

Coschwitz duct: Arch-like structure on dorsum of tongue; believed to be vein.

Cosman-Roberts-Wells frame: Stereotactic frame used in brain surgery.

Cossio-Berconsky disease: Atrial septal defect occurring in association with Pick disease.

Costa disease (acrokeratoelastoidosis): Disorder of keratinization; marked by nodular, yellowish lesions on soles and palms that sometimes extend to dorsum of hands and feet. Treatment is topical or systemic vitamin A.

Costello-Dent disease: Tetany due to

hypoparathyroidism in association with osteitis fibrosa cystica generalisata.

Costen syndrome (temporomandibular joint syndrome): "Loose" temporomandibular joint due to resorption or degeneration of joint tissues; marked by earache, tinnitus, decreased hearing, dizziness, and nystagmus. Condition is sometimes associated with herpes appearing in external ear canal. Some controversy exists regarding diagnosis; many oral and head and neck surgeons are unconvinced of the temporomandibular joint etiology. Treatment is dental/oral surgery or injection of corticosteroids.

Costenbader accommodator: Handheld device used to determine "near point" accommodation.

Cote-Katsantoni syndrome: Mental retardation, otosclerosis, atrial septal defect, stunted growth, neutropenia, and ectodermal dysplasia.

Cotswolds classification: 1989 modification of Ann Arbor staging classification for Hodgkin disease.

Cotte operation: Presacral neurectomy.

Cotting operation: Method of repairing ingrown toenail; side of the affected toe is resected down to and including ingrown nail.

Cottle disease (wide nose disease): Onset of lacrimation and crusting of nose mucosa when walking from warm environment to cold environment; most common in elderly women. Cause is obstruction of Hasner valve due to inferior turbinate hypertrophy. Treatment is placing small cotton ball in vestibule.

Cotton fracture: Posterio-inferior fracture and forward dislocation of tibia.

Cotton-Berg syndrome (tender fracture): Fracture in lateral head of tibia; caused by impact against lateral femoral condyle, resulting from violent abduction.

Cotrel traction: Pelvic and cervical traction using sling in initial treatment of scoliosis.

Cotrel-Dubousset instrumentation: Posterior spinal fixation device used to treat trauma, tumors, and degenerative conditions.

Cotugno disease: Sciatica.

Cotunnius nerve (nasopalatine nerve): Nerve passing through sphenopalatine foramen and running downward and forward in vomer groove between periosteum and mucosa to incisive (anterior palatine) canal; communicates with nasal branch of anterior superior alveolar nerve.

Cotunnius space: Space within membranous labyrinth.

Coudé catheter: Urinary catheter similar to Foley catheter but with curved, stiff tip. Useful in male patients with enlarged prostate.

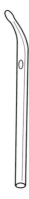

Coudé catheter

Couinaud nomenclature

(French nomenclature): System used to describe liver anatomy; divides parenchyma into 8 segments based on hepatic vein drainage and portal pedicle branches, with counterclockwise numbering. Scheme allows preop planning for less-than-lobar resections. Segment 1, caudate lobe; segments 2–4, left lobe; segments 5–8, right lobe.

coulomb (C): Unit of electrical charge (SI nomenclature) equal to charge carried across surface by 1 ampere of current in 1 second; alternately described as 6.25×10^{18} electrons.

Coulomb law: Attractive or
repulsive force between 2 charged bodies is inversely proportional to square of distance between them and directly proportional to amount of charge on each body.

Coulter technique (counter
technique): Sensitive, automated method for determining sizes of RBCs in serum sample; produces histogram that can be used when attempting to determine if fetal blood is contaminated by maternal blood.

Councilman bodies: Hyaline
bodies that stain eosinophilic on light microscopy; represent necrotic, shrunken cells phagocytosed by Kupffer cells and hepatocytes. Structures are typically seen in acute, viral hepatitis and yellow fever.

Cournand catheter: Thin
device with opening at tip that is inserted into heart chambers to measure pressure.

Courvoisier law: Obstruction
of common bile duct by stone rarely causes ductal dilation; other causes of ductal obstruction commonly cause dilation.

Courvoisier sign (Bard-Pic
disease): Enlarged, palpable, nontender gallbladder sometimes seen in cancer of pancreatic head.

Courvoisier-Terrier
syndrome: See Courvoisier sign.

Coutard law: Last site to
repair itself after radiation of mucous membrane tumors is site of origin of tumor.

Couvelaire uterus
(uteroplacental apoplexy): Widespread extravasation of blood into uterine musculature

and occ. beneath tubal serosa and connective tissue of broad ligaments; seen in severe cases of placental abruption.

Cova point: Tip of costolumbar angle; tenderness during pregnancy may occur here due to kidney infection.

Cowden disease (multiple hamartoma syndrome): Hamartomas and polyps (e.g., juvenile, inflammatory, lipomatous) occurring in GI tract, most commonly in stomach and colon; also with lesions and papillomas in mouth, keratoses on limbs, and tricholemmomas. Condition is associated with increased benign and malignant thyroid and breast disease.

Cowdry type 1 inclusion bodies: Nuclear inclusions made of protein and nucleic acid, which stain eosinophilic; seen in cells infected with varicella-zoster or herpes simplex viruses.

Cowen sign: Contralateral pupil constriction when light is shown into 1 eye; seen in Graves disease.

Cowper fascia (cremasteric fascia): Thin membranous connective tissue covering cremaster muscle.

Cowper glands (bulbourethral glands): Two small tubuloalveolar structures in urogenital diaphragm near bulb of urethra; secrete mucus-like substances into urethra during erotic stimulation.

Cowper ligament: Pectineal segment of fascia lata.

Cowtown hemoglobin: High-oxygen affinity hemoglobin with histidine replaced by leucine close to c-terminal; causes hemoglobin levels of 18–19 g/dl.

Cox proportional hazards method: Technique allowing multivariate analysis of time-related events; assumes hazard functions of all potential risk factors are proportional. Method identifies risk factors, parametrically computes their coefficients and P values, from which odds ratios or relative risks can be exponentiated.

Coxe syrup: Syrup of Squill; used to treat hives.

Cozen test: Indicator of "tennis elbow" if pain occurs in lateral epicondyle region when examiner attempts to forcibly flex patient's extended wrist (with clenched fist).

Cozen-Brockway plasty: Z-plasty used for release of congenital constriction rings; requires minimum of 3 operative stages. Constriction is excised with undermining of skin edges, which are reapproximated with interrupted sutures (except in area where incisions representing top and bottom portion of Z have been made).

Crabtree effect: Inhibition of oxygen consumption on addition of glucose; seen in tissues with a significant aerobic glycolysis.

Crafts test: Positive result is great toe extension after blunt tip stroking upward over dorsal ankle; occurs in pyramidal tract lesions.

Craig needle: Percutaneous biopsy needle; provides long, thin tissue core.

Craig test: Technique used to assess forward torsion of femur or femoral anteversion. Patient lies prone with knees bent at 90°. Examiner rotates leg laterally until limit of movement is reached or greater trochanter is parallel with floor; angle formed by lower leg with vertical estimates degree of anteversion.

Craigie tube: Apparatus used to separate motile from nonmotile bacteria; slanted, hollow glass tube is inserted into semisolid medium and inoculated with bacteria, and motile organisms group on outside of tube.

Crain syndrome: Recurrent, indolent, erosive osteoarthritis in distal interphalangeal joints with eventual involvement of proximal joints; associated with mucous cysts over involved joints. Condition mainly affects middle-aged women.

Cramer 2.5 reagent: 100-ml aqueous solution of 6 g potassium iodide and 0.4 g mercuric oxide; provides correct formulation so that 2.5 ml of 10 N acid will neutralize 10 ml of reagent to phenolphthalein end point.

Crampton test: Used to measure overall physical condition based on pulse and blood pressure lying down and standing. Score of 75 is good condition; score of 65 indicates poor physical condition.

Crandall syndrome: Condition marked by segmental twists in hair shafts (pili torti).

Crane-Heise syndrome: Cleft lip and palate, short neck, micropenis, cryptorchidism, talipes equinovarus, and hypertelorism; rare autosomal recessive condition.

Crawford classification: System used to describe thoracoabdominal aneurysms based on diameter. Low risk, < 5 cm; moderate risk, 5–6 cm; high risk, > 10 cm.

Crawford hook: Thin, malleable metallic device; used to retrieve Crawford probes from nasal lacrimal duct system.

Crawford probe: Thin, malleable metallic device with bulb tip on 1 end; used to intubate nasolacrimal duct system.

Crawford tube: Thin, hollow, Silastic tube with bulb tip; used to intubate nasolacrimal duct system, esp. in laceration repair. Device is very flexible and can be difficult to pass but is easily removed with Crawford hook.

Credé prophylaxis: Application of 1% silver nitrate eye drops in neonate; prophylactic treatment of gonococcal ophthalmia.

Creteil hemoglobin: High-oxygen affinity hemoglobin with serine replaced by asparagine; results in hemoglobin levels of 21 g/dl.

crescent sign of Caffey:
Subchondral lucency in femoral head seen in Legg-Calvé-Perthes disease; caused by avascular necrosis.

Creyx-Levy syndrome
(reversed Sjögren syndrome): Gastric, nasal, oral, and lacrimal hypersecretions in setting of cervical spine arthritis; also with calcification of cervical lymph nodes and tendons and increased sedimentation rate.

Crichton-Browne sign:
Tremor in outer angles of mouth and eyes seen in early paresis.

Crigler-Najjar syndrome (type I):
Persistent, severe (> 20 mg/dl) unconjugated bilirubinemia presenting in 1st few days of life; kernicterus occurs without aggressive treatment by continuous phototherapy or liver transplantation. Cause is defect in glucuronyl transferase; absence of bilirubin diglucuronide is pathognomonic. No decrease in serum bilirubin is seen after phenobarbital administration.

Crigler-Najjar syndrome (type II)
(Arias syndrome): Milder condition of unconjugated bilirubinemia (6–20 mg/*dl*); neurologic deficits occur but are less severe than in type I. Onset is usu. in infancy but as late as 2–10 years of age. Cause is defect in glucuronyl transferase; absence of bilirubin diglucuronide is pathognomic.

Decrease in serum bilirubin after phenobarbital administration differentiates this condition from type I.

Crile hemostatic forceps:
Fine, curved or straight-tipped, ring-handle, locking forceps placed on small vessels to control bleeding.

Crile retractor:
Handheld, doubled-ended retractor.

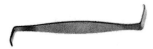

Crile retractor

Crile-Wood needle holder:
Locking needle driver with relatively fine tip.

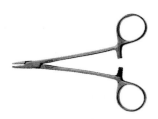

Crile-Wood needle holder

Crimean-Congo hemorrhagic fever:
Viral fever; humans become infected via body fluid contact with infected humans or animals. Vector is *Hyalomma* ticks.

criminal nerve of Grassi:
Branch of right posterior vagus that courses behind pylorus.

Crocker-Williams syndrome: See Bury syndrome.

Crocq disease: See Cassirer syndrome.

Crohn's disease: Inflammatory bowel disease with chronic transmural inflammation of alimentary track marked by noncaseating granulomas and "skip areas"; most common sites of inflammation are terminal ileum and colon, with additional involvement of skin, eyes, and joints (25% of cases affect small bowel only, and 25% affect colon only). Fistulas between bowel loops are common; also found are abdominal cramps, nonbloody diarrhea, perforation, and perianal abscesses. Transmural inflammation and granulomas are pathognomonic; on contrast studies, mucosa shows cobblestone appearance due to deep linear ulcers; most common complication is obstruction. Condition is most common surgically treated disease of small bowel. Medical treatment is optimized (bowel rest, antibiotics, steroids) before surgery is considered. Bowel resection margins are to grossly normal bowel; 50% recurrence rate of significant disease after resection. Crohn's patients have 75 times greater risk of adenocarcinoma of small bowel with poorer prognosis (and increased risk of bladder cancer) than non-Crohn's patients. Primary drug treatment uses corticosteroids for active disease, with response rates of 75%–90%.

Crome syndrome: Congenital cataracts, mental retardation, renal tubular necrosis, and death within 1st year of life; rare, autosomal recessive condition.

Cronkhite-Canada syndrome: Hamartomatous polyps of GI tract causing loss of protein, calcium, magnesium, and potassium; also marked by nail atrophy, alopecia, and hyperpigmentation of skin.

Crooke cell adenoma: Rare lesion of anterior pituitary; sequelae range from mild to severe Cushing disease.

Crooke cell hyalinization: Morphologic indicator of functional suppression of corticotropes; now known to occur both in nontumorous pathology and adenomas. Condition results from accumulation of keratin-type intermediate filaments, which are easily visualized on electron microscopy.

Crooke cells: Basophilic cells in pituitary found in Crooke hyalin degeneration.

Crookes lens: Allows passage of visual light but opaqueness blocks both IR and UV rays.

Crookes space: Area near x-ray tube cathode through which current is passed.

Crosby capsule: Spring-activated biopsy instrument; uses small knife seated inside capsule for collection of intestinal wall specimens.

Crosby syndrome: Hereditary nonspherocytic hemolytic anemia.

Cross syndrome: Congenital gingival fibromatosis, pink skin with freckles and nevi, cataracts, nystagmus, blindness, athetosis, and oligophrenia; rare, congenital, autosomal recessive condition.

Cross-Bevan reagent: Sustance that dissolves cellulose; 2 parts concentrated hydrochloric acid and 1 part zinc chloride.

Crosti reticulosis (Winkelmann disease): High-grade β-cell lymphoma, with 1 or occ. multiple nodular masses appearing on back, neck, or torso; usu. occurring in women in 5th–6th decades. Treatment is chemotherapy, radiation, and steroids, with favorable prognosis.

Crouzon disease (Apert-Crouzon disease, Vogt malformation, Virchow oxycephaly, Franceschetti disease): Craniofacial synostosis with hypoplasia of maxilla, dental malocclusion, prognathism, and exophthalmus. Skull abnormalities include enlarged transverse diameter, short frontal floor fossa, and hypertelorism. Autosomal dominant condition may result in papilledema, blindness, hydrocephalus, epilepsy, and mental retardation.

Crow-Fukase syndrome (POEMS, Takatsuki disease, Shinpo disease): Plasma cell dyscrasia with severe, progressive motor polyneuropathy; *p*olyneuropathy, *o*rganomegaly, *e*ndocrinopathy, *M*-proteins, and *s*kin changes. Condition is marked by anasarca of legs, diffuse hyperpigmentation, hypertrichosis, ascites, pleural effusion, fever, finger clubbing, lymphadenopathy, hepatomegaly, hyperhidrosis, and gynecomastia. Treatment is prednisone, radiation, and cyclophosphamide. Death occurs 2–3 years after onset.

Crozat appliance (Walker appliance): Removable orthodontic device usu. made of precious metal.

Cruetzfeldt-Jakob disease: Spongiform encephalopathy with dementia and myoclonus; highly contagious condition caused by gene mutation in prion. Positive brain biopsy is needed for definitive diagnosis.

Crutchfield clamp: Adjustable occluding device used to reduce carotid artery aneurysms over several days.

Crutchfield tongs: Instrument that provides skull traction by immobilizing cervical spine.

Cruveilhier ligament: Thick, tough fibrous connective tissue bands on palmar surface of hand; runs between collateral ligaments from interphalangeal articulations and metacarpophalangeal articulations.

Cruveilhier ligaments: Adipose-containing synovial membrane in knee joint; runs from infrapatellar adipose body posterosuperiorly to intercondylar femoral fossa.

Cruveilhier plexus (posterior cervical plexus): Nerve tissue in neck; formed from medial branches of posterior primary divisions of CN I and III. Tissue extends from medial branch (great occipital nerve) of CN II.

Cruveilhier sign: Tremor felt when groin area is palpated while patient coughs (similar to jet of H_2O filling a pouch); seen in varices of saphenous vein.

Cruveilhier ulcer: Gastric ulcer.

Cruveilhier-Baumgarten disease: Baumgarten disease with portal hypertension.

Cruveilhier-Baumgarten sign: Easily detectable (with stethoscope) bruit in caput medusa caused by portal hypertension.

Cruveilhier-Baumgarten syndrome: Congenital liver cirrhosis.

Cruveilier disease: See Aran-Duchenne disease.

crypts of Fuchs: Pits found in region of circulus arteriosus minor in the iris.

crypts of Haller (Littre glands): Small glands that secrete smegma; located on inner surface of foreskin of penis.

Csendes procedure: Method used to excise type 4 gastric ulcers near gastroesophageal junction; uses removal of distal stomach along lesser curvature, small part of esophageal wall, and the ulcer with Roux-en-Y esophagogastrojejunostomy.

Csendes ulcer: Type 4 gastric ulcer; occurs high on lesser curvature of stomach. Not associated with acid hypersecretion; condition is believed to be related to defect in mucosal defense.

Cuignet test: Uses series of bars to detect malingering in unilateral visual impairment.

Cullen sign: Ecchymosis in periumbilical area from blood dissecting up falciform ligament; seen in ruptured ectopic pregnancy or acute pancreatitis.

Curie unit: Unit of radioactivity; equals quantity of radionuclide undergoing 3.7×10^{10} disintegrations/sec.

Curling factor: Griseofulvin.

Curling ulcer: GI ulcer occurring in burn patients; causes significant bleeding usu. 4–10 days postburn. Lesions tend to be multiple but nonconfluent; may occur anywhere from esophagus to terminal ileum, most commonly in posterior duodenal wall. Treatment is aggressive prophylaxis against ulcer formation (e.g., antacids, H_2-blockers, omeprazole), adequate nutrition, and control of sepsis. If severe hemorrhage occurs, ulcer is initially oversewed to control bleeding followed by hemigastrectomy and vagotomy.

Currarino syndrome
(Kennedy syndrome): Sacral
bone defects, anorectal defects
(atresia, stenosis, impaired
function) and presacral defects
of the neurocanal and rectum
(hamartomas, cysts, lipomas,
meningitis, meningoceles);
congenital condition more
common in females. Treatment
is surgical correction of
defects.

**Currarino-Silverman
syndrome**: (pectus carinatum):
Growth abnormality of sternum;
marked by premature
obliteration of bone sutures
causing outward projection of
sternum (pigeon breast), with
variable dyspnea. Onset occurs
in infancy. Treatment is surgery
with good results.

Curreri formula: Expression
used to calculate number of
calories required in burn
patients; usu. overestimates
necessary calories. Equation:
Calories = 25 kcal × weight
(kg) + 40 kcal x total body
surface area burned (%).

Curry-Jones syndrome:
Congenital asymmetric facies,
corpus callosum agenesis,
craniosynostosis, atrophic skin
patches, polysyndactyly, and
abnormal gut and mucous
membranes.

Curschmann spiral: Filling of
lumen by mucus, which causes
"whirling spiral" with dark
center on hematoxylin–eosin;
seen on microscopic
examination of bronchus.
Condition is typically found in
asthma.

Curtis-Fisher technique:
Method for correction of
congenital dislocation of knee.

Curtius syndrome: See
Cassirer syndrome.

Curtius syndrome:
Considered variant of
Goldenhar syndrome; marked
by telangiectasia, sparse
eyebrows and eyelashes,
congenital cataracts,
hemihypertrophy of tongue,
unilateral enlargement of teeth,
unilateral polydactyly, and
clubfoot. Condition occurs in
autosomal dominant and
recessive forms.

curve of Carus: Axis of
normal pelvis.

curve of Ellis and Garland:
See Ellis line.

Cushing disease: Condition
leading to bilateral adrenal
hyperplasia and Cushing
syndrome symptoms; clinical
features (incidence) include
obesity (94%), facial plethora
(84%), hirsutism (82%),
menstrual disorders (76%),
hypertension (72%), muscle
weakness (58%), back pain
(58%), and striae (52%). Cause is
hypersecretion of ACTH from
pituitary source (usu. adenoma
identified in 60%–70% of cases).
Treatment is transsphenoidal
resection of tumor with
adjunctive radiation and
medical therapy.

Cushing neuroma: Acoustic
neuroma; female-to-male ratio,
3:1. Treatment is surgical
removal.

Cushing syndrome:
Hyperadrenocorticalism caused by ectopic ACTH source (extra-adrenal or extrapituitary neoplasm) or adrenal hyperplasia. Manifestations include moon facies, buffalo hump, truncal obesity, peripheral muscle wasting and weakness, striae, hypertension, diabetes, osteoporosis, hypokalemic alkalosis, bruising, acne, hirsutism, emotional lability, and menstrual abnormalities. Dexamethasone test is used to determine source of ACTH; 2 g dexamethasone is given PO q6hr with 24-hour urine collection for free cortisol on 2nd day. Pituitary source of ACTH usu. shows suppression of free cortisol, and ectopic source usu. does not.

Cushing syndrome (chiasmal syndrome): Space-occupying lesion (usu. suprasellar meningioma) in area of optic chiasm; marked by progressive bitemporal field defects and primary optic atrophy.

Cushing triad: Bradycardia, hypertension, and irregular breathing seen in increased intracranial pressure.

Cushing ulcer: Gastric or peptic ulcer due to acid hypersecretion after brain surgery. Ulcers tend to be multiple but nonconfluent; more likely to perforate than cause significant bleeding.

Cushing vein retractor: Handheld device used to retract small vascular structures.

Custer cell: Cell with protoplasmic tendrils that

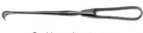

Cushing vein retractor

replace normal lymph cell; seen in disease of reticuloendothelial system.

Cutter vaccine (incident): Inactive polio vaccine that was contaminated with live polio virus; caused 260 cases of poliomyelitis after inoculation.

Cuvier ducts: Embryologic short venous channels emptying into left atrium; right channel forms superior vena cava.

Cyon nerve: Branch of vagus nerve in rabbits; stimulation lowers blood pressure.

Cyriax syndrome (Davies-Colley syndrome): Pain in chest wall sometimes accompanied by shock that occurs after arm movement, sneezing, or deep inhalation. Cause is injury to synovial membrane of ribs 8–10 with slippage of rib, causing compression of intercostal nerve.

Czapek solution: Aqueous solution of magnesium and iron sulfate, glucose, potassium chloride, sodium nitrate, and monopotassium phosphate.

Czapek solution agar (Czapek-Dox medium): Medium used to culture and identify yeasts and molds, esp. *Aspergillus* species.

Czermak space (spaces of Owen): Minute spaces in outer dentin of tooth root.

Dabska syndrome:
Endovascular angioendothelioma occurring in children; causes diffuse swelling. Any area can be affected; metastasis possible. Etiology is unknown. Treatment is wide surgical excision.

D'acosta syndrome: Onset of nausea, vomiting, headache, mood changes, and insomnia occurring several hours to days after ascent to high altitude, with pulmonary and cerebral edema; death ensues in severe cases. Cause is hypoxia with increased ventilation rate and resulting respiratory alkalosis. Treatment is acetazolamide and descent (if severe).

Da Costa syndrome: Orthostasis in setting of panic attacks.

Dagnini reflex (Aschner-Dagnini reflex): Percussion on radial side of back of hand, causing extension and adduction of wrist; seen in corticospinal tract lesions.

Dahl rat: Sodium-sensitive and sodium-resistant strains that are animal models for human hypertension as it relates to dietary content of salt.

Dahl S rat: Sodium-sensitive hypertensive rat; animal's blood is also sensitive to dietary levels of potassium.

Dahlberg syndrome: Congenital lymphedema, nephropathy, hypoparathyroidism, mitral valve prolapse, and shortened digits.

Dakin-Carrel fluid: Dilute sodium hypochlorite solution.

Dalby mixture: Tincture of opium.

Dalen-Fuchs nodules: Enlarged and proliferated pigment cells found in eye in "sympathetic ophthalmia."

Dalmatian insect powder (Persial insect powder): Pyrethrum flowers.

Dalrymple sign: Variably present retraction of upper eyelid that contributes to exophthalmos of Graves disease.

Dalton law (law of partial pressures): Pressure exerted by each gas in mixture of gases is proportional to its percentage in mixture. Alternate description: total pressure of gas mixture is sum of partial pressures of each individual gas.

dalton unit [atomic mass unit (amu)]: Unit of mass that is 1/2 atomic mass of carbon-12 isotope; equals 1.66041×10^{-24} g.

Dalton-Henry law: When gases are dissolved in fluid (i.e., blood), amount of gas dissolved is same as if it were pure gas; important when giving anesthesia.

D'Amato sign: Movement of location of dullness on percussion from ipsilateral vertebral area when sitting to contralateral heart region when recumbent; seen in pleural effusion.

Damoiseau line: See Ellis sign.

Damus-Kay-Stansel technique: Portion of 1st stage of Norwood procedure for treatment of hypoplastic left heart.

Dana disease: Hereditary benign essential tremor that chiefly affects head, neck, and arms; worsened by stress, fatigue, and cold. Onset occurs in 6th decade for men and later for women. Progressive for some years and then appears to stabilize. Condition is autosomal dominant

Dana operation: Posterior rhizotomy.

Danbolt-Closs disease: See Brandt syndrome.

Dance sign: Sensation of "empty abdomen" when palpating right lower quadrant; suggests diagnosis of intussusception in children.

Dandy aneurysm: Arterial dilation of internal carotid artery in anterior cavernosus sinus area.

Dandy operation: Severing of trigeminal nerve; approach is from posterior cranial fossa.

Dandy scalp hemostatic forceps: Curve-tipped (and curved to 1 side), ring-handle, locking forceps placed on small vessels to control bleeding before suture ligation or cautery.

Dandy ventriculostomy: Operation on 3rd ventricle of brain.

Dandy-Walker malformation: Hydrocephalus due to atresia of foramens of Magendie and Luschka; results in an intracerebellar cyst connected to an enlarged 4th ventricle with hypoplasia of cerebellar vermis. Condition is most commonly found in childhood but occurs in adults with syringomyelia; associated with maternal use of coumadin during pregnancy.

Dane method: Mayer hematoxylin, tap H_2O, phloxine, Alcian blue, and orange G solution; used to stain nuclei brown, mucopolysaccharides blue, and keratin and prekeratin red-orange.

Danielson method: Repair of incompetent tricuspid valve in Ebstein malformation; uses interrupted mattress sutures to obliterate atrialized right ventricle.

Danubian nephropathy: See Balkan nephropathy.

Danysz phenomenon:
Generally applies to
antigen–antibody reactions,
specifically to toxin–antitoxin
reactions; if toxin is added to
antitoxin in several increments,
more antitoxin is needed to
neutralize it than if same
amount of toxin is added all at
once. Cause is ability of toxin to
bind antitoxin in multiple
proportions.

Dar es Salaam bacterium:
Salmonella salamae.

Darcy equation: Expression
that describes energy loss of
fluid moving through tube as
function of flow velocity (under
both laminar and turbulent flow
conditions). In laminar flow, f is
64/Re, and Darcy equation is
identical to Poiseuille law. P1—
P2 =f (L/4r)ρv2, where f is
friction factor, r is radius, ρ is
density, L is length, and v is
velocity.

Darier disease (variant): See
Hailey and Hailey disease.

Darier sign: Worsening of
itching, redness, and swelling of
urticaria pigmentosa lesions
when rubbed.

Darier-Ferrand syndrome
(dermatofibroma protuberans):
Well-differentiated sarcoma
with small, hard nodules in skin
that coalesce to become
pedunculated and mobile
plaque-like lesions. Rare
condition that occurs in areas of
flexion and can progress to
painful ulcerations. Treatment is
excision with generous margins;
recurrence rate is 20%.

Darier-Roussy syndrome
(subcutaneous sarcoidosis):
Slow-growing, subcutaneous
nonulcerative nodules on trunk
and thighs; usu. flesh-colored or
bluish.

Darier-White syndrome:
Foul-smelling, crusty lesions on
head, neck, trunk, and groin,
and punctate keratosis on soles
and palms; lesions can form in
zosteriform pattern on chest.
Autosomal dominant condition
is seen with a variable degree of
mental retardation and defects
in tonofilament–desmosome
complex. Onset is 10–20 years
of age. Treatment is avoidance
of sun exposure (mild cases),
etretinate or isotretinoin
(moderate cases), or
dermabrasion (severe cases).

Darkschewitsch fibers:
Nerve tracts running from optic
tract to habenular ganglion.

Darling disease
(histoplasmosis): Systemic
mycosis due to *Histoplasma
capsulatum* infection; fungus is
inhaled from bird droppings.

Darrach procedure:
Transverse resection of distal
end of ulna for unstable wrist
joint; usu. provides good pain
relief but may decrease grip
strength and joint stability if not
performed meticulously.

Darrow red: Stain used to
visualize cytoplasm and nuclei
of goblet cells, striated bordered
cells, and nuclei of fibroplasts.

Darrow-Gamble syndrome
(hypochloremic congenital
alkalosis): Profuse, watery

diarrhea in absence of vomiting; seen mostly in infants born prematurely. Abdominal distention with obstructive radiographic findings incorrectly suggests diagnosis of mechanical obstruction. Condition is due to defective jejunal brush-border Na^+/H^+ exchange. Treatment is IV NaCl and KCl initially, followed by 4 g KCl daily.

Darwin tubercle (darwinian tubercle ear): Small elevation in upper rim of ear; congenital condition commonly mistaken for deposition of uric acid crystals in gout.

Daubenton angle (occipital angle): Angle formed by extension of opisthionasial and opisthiobasial lines.

David disease: Intermittant gingival and other mucosal hemorrhages usu. occurring during menstrual periods. Etiology is unknown; possible psychogenic component.

David-Stickler disease (Stickler disease, Wagner-Stickler disease, Cervenka disease): Progressive visual defects (e.g., myopia, astigmatism, vitreous degeneration) leading to blindness, progressive sensorineural deafness, and hypermobility of joints leading to arthritis; congenital autosomal dominant condition. 50% of patients develop mitral valve prolapse.

Davidoff cells: See Paneth cells.

Davidsohn sign: Decreased pupil illumination when light is placed into mouth; caused by tumor or fluid in maxillary antrum.

Daviel operation: Method of cataract extraction; approach is from corneal incision with iris left intact.

Davies disease: Peripheral edema, cyanosis, jaundice, and constrictive cardiomyopathy; seen in Uganda, Sri Lanka, and some South American countries. Treatment is corticosteroids and (in cardiac failure) heart transplantation.

Davis disease (Swiss-type agammaglobulinemia): Congenital achondroplasia and agammaglobulinemia; marked by frequent infections, absence of hair and eyebrows, short limbs, and scaly lesions on skin. Condition is possibly autosomal recessive. Etiology is unknown; poor prognosis with death likely before 1 year of age. Treatment is banked blood (> 21 days), antibiotics, and immunoglobulins.

Davis disease: Uveitis, rheumatoid arthritis-type symptoms, and (variably) hepatosplenomegaly. Treatment is systemic and (to eye) topical steroids.

Davis line (vertical fissure line): Curved strip of translucency arising laterally from right part of diaphragm seen on plain film chest radiograph, which represents caudal end of right major lung fissure; indication of likely cardiomegaly if line seen on right side or loss of lower lung volumes if seen bilaterally.

Davis loop: Mechanical device inserted via urethra and bladder into ureter to effect stone removal; now largely replaced by Seguira, Gemini, or Nitinol baskets.

Davis muscle pedicle graft: Used in hip arthrodesis.

Davison syndrome: Occlusion of anterior spinal artery of medulla oblongata; results in flaccid paralysis and loss of sense discrimination.

Davson-Danielli model: Phospholipid bilayer model of cell membrane with lipids sandwiched between 2 protein layers; 1st proposed in 1935.

Dawbarn sign: Evidence of subacromial bursitis if pain occurs when palpating bursa when arm is at side; pain disappears when arm is abducted.

Dawidenkow syndrome: Muscular atrophy in scapular and peroneal areas, fasciculations, glove-and-stocking distribution of sensory disturbances, and variably present pes equinus.

Dawson fingers: Hyperintense lesions radiating from ventricles representing perivenous demyelination; seen on T2-weighted brain MRIs of some patients with MS.

De Barsy syndrome: Rare degeneration of elastic tissue in skin and retina; marked by mental retardation, progeria-like facial features, cutix laxa, dwarfism, dislocation of 1st toe and thumb, and hip dysplasia.

De Clerambault syndrome: Sudden onset (usu. in women) of delusion that a particular man is in love with patient; object of attention is usu. public or prominent figure. Patient believes inevitable rejection by person is a form of love; condition may eventually lead to assaults or violent behavior toward pursued male.

De Crecchio syndrome (Apert-Gallais syndrome, female congenital adrenal hyperplasia): Rapid onset of virilization in XX female newborn; pubic and axillary hair appears by 3 years of age, with subsequent deepened voice, lack of breast development and menses, and hypertrophic clitoris. Varying degrees of external genitalia may be present. No sodium-wasting occurs. Etiology is excessive adrenal androgen secretion, deficiency of 21-hydroxylase, and decreased cortisol production. Increased ACTH and 17-OHP. Treatment is cortisone/hydrocortisone 25–100 mg IM for 7–10 days and frequent dosing thereafter.

D'Espine sign: Indicator of bronchial lymph node enlargement if pectoriloquy over spinous processes is heard below C7 in infants and level of tracheal bifurcation in adults.

de Galantha stain: Stain used to demonstrate sodium urate monohydrate crystals in gout.

De Haas-Houtsmuller syndrome: Fuchs heterochromia occurring in association with von Recklinghausen disease.

De Jeans syndrome: Pain in floor of orbit, double vision, and eye bulging caused by tumor or infection.

de la Camp sign: Dullness over 5th and 6th vertebrae in bronchial lymph node TB.

De la Chapelle syndrome (neonatal osseous dysplasia type 1): Cleft palate, laryngeal stenosis, tracheobronchomalacia, short limbs, triangular ulna and fibula, and genitourinary abnormalities; cartilage forms "ring" around chondrocytes. Condition is autosomal recessive, with death occurring shortly after birth.

De Martel-Wolfson intestinal anastomosis clamp: Metal "alligator" jaws with hinge at 1 end and fastener at other end; usu. placed transversely across outer bowel wall. No ring handle is used.

De Meyer syndrome: Congenital cleft face with varying degrees of severity; 20% of patients have mental retardation. Treatment is facial reconstructive surgery.

de Morsier syndrome: Childhood onset of seizures, precocious sexual development, mental deterioration, and possible acromegaly.

de Musset sign: See Musset sign.

de Mussy point: Tip of 10th rib; very tender with palpation in diaphragmatic pleurisy.

de Quervain disease: Thickened bulbous tendon sheath, causing "snapping" in distal interphalangeal joint when tendon passes through sheath on flexion and extension. In children, condition occurs in thumbs with equal sexual prevalence, and in adults it affects all fingers and is more prevalent in women.

de Quervain disease: Thyroiditis with enlargement and tenderness of thyroid, pain in neck area radiating to ear, headache, and hyperthyroid symptoms; usu. abrupt onset after upper respiratory infection. Treatment is analgesics, anti-inflammatory agents, and steroids; severe cases may require radiation.

de Quervain fracture: Fracture of scaphoid bone of wrist with volar subluxation of fragments and lunate.

De Sanctis-Cacchione syndrome: Xeroderma pigmentosum; marked by skin tumors, microcephaly, mental retardation, paralysis, convulsions, speech disorders, photophobia, gonadal hypoplasia, pneumonia, and hepatomegaly. Cause is inability to repair DNA damaged by UV light (280–310 nm). Subtypes A–H have variable expression of signs and symptoms.

De Souza disease: Rare form of amyloidosis with formation of bulbous lesions around joints only; autosomal recessive condition.

De Vaal syndrome (congenital aleukia): Congenital absence of leukocytes with primitive development of thymus and bone marrow; possibly autosomal recessive. Death from intractable infections occurs in first days of life. Antibiotics and bone marrow transplantation are ineffective.

de Vincentiis operation: Goniotomy for congenital glaucoma.

Dean-Barnes disease: Familial porphyria cutanea tarda. 50% of patients have only skin lesions on exposure to sunlight and skin trauma (e.g., edema, redness, bullae formation, scarring); also with abdominal pain (can mimic surgical abdomen) and neurologic sequelae. Condition has variable penetrance, with females less affected than males. Defect is in uroporphyrinogen decarboxylase; during attacks levels of porphyrins, porphobilinogen, and aminolevulinic acid are increased.

Deaver abdominal retractor: Hand-held retractor used in laparotomy.

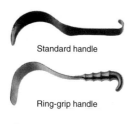

Standard handle

Ring-grip handle

Deaver abdominal retractors

Deaver incision: Incision through right anterior rectus muscle sheath with medial retraction of tissues.

DeBakey classification: System used to describe aortic dissection. Type 1, extends past ascending aorta and arch; type 2, stays proximal to ascending aorta; type 3, begins in descending aorta and extends distally.

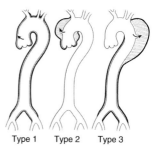

Type 1   Type 2   Type 3

DeBakey classification

Debove membrane: Thin layer of tissue between epithelium and tunica propria in lung, trachea, and GI mucosa.

Debré disease: See Petzetakis disease.

Debré phenomenon: Absence of measles rash at site of injection of immune serum; seen in patients with measles.

Debré-Fibiger syndrome (Debré-Fibiger-von Gierke syndrome; Pirie syndrome): Sodium-losing congenital adrenal hyperplasia with virilizing characteristics similar to those found in simple virilizing congenital adrenal hyperplasia for both male and female (De Crecchio syndrome); marked by acute addisonian crises and enlargement of zona reticularis and fasciculata and atrophy of zona glomerulosa. Onset is 1st week of life or later if induced by infection. Treatment is NaCl 3–6 g in 1st 24 hours and desoxycorticosterone 2 mg IM with pellets implanted on long-term basis.

Debre-Fittke syndrome: Congenital form of cutis laxa marked by persistent fontanelles, hip dislocation, pigeon breast, scoliosis, and flat feet; autosomal recessive condition.

Debré-Sémélaigne syndrome (Kocher-Debré-Sémélaigne syndrome): Cretinism associated with muscular pseudohypertrophy and myotonia; autosomal recessive condition.

Deelman effect: Carcinoma tends to localize when lab animals are inoculated through multiple scratches or puncture sites (scarification).

Deetjen body: Platelet.

Degos acanthoma: Superficial, scaly, brownish plaque usually found as singular lesion on leg or arm.

Degos disease (malignant atrophic papulosis): Rare thrombotic disease that manifests as 2–5-mm pinkish cutaneous lesions eventually becoming umbilicated and developing depressed, whitish centers that represent infarcts. Condition may also occur in small intestine with multiple bowel perforations, with variable infarcts in nervous tissue. Treatment is aspirin and dipyridamole, which has limited success.

Dehne cast: Spica cast covering thumb, index, and middle fingers; for treatment of navicular fractures.

Deiters cells: Outer supporting phalangeal cells in organ of Corti.

Deiters nucleus: Lateral nucleus of vestibular nerve; located in midbrain.

Deiters nucleus syndrome: See Barré syndrome.

Dejan syndrome: See Rochon-Duvigneaud syndrome.

Dejean syndrome (orbital floor syndrome): Anesthesia in trigeminal nerve distribution, diplopia; and exophthalmos; caused by lesion in orbital floor.

Déjérine paraplegia: 1800s term for nerve damage caused by prolonged compression in opioid intoxication.

Déjérine radicular: Pain and sensory and motor changes resulting in compression, inflammation, or irritation of nerve root.

Déjérine sign: Indicator of herniated disk etiology of radiating pain in extremities if Valsalva maneuver (e.g., coughing, straining at stool) worsens pain.

Déjérine syndrome (bulbar syndrome): Progressive bulbar palsy due to lesion in medulla or its nuclei with resulting paralysis of cranial nerves.

Déjérine syndrome (diphtheritic polyneuropathy): Polyneuropathy similar to tabes dorsalis caused by lesions of posterior column of spinal cord and peripheral nerves; due to infection by Corynebacterium diphtheriae.

Dejerine-Klumpke syndrome: Injury or lesion of inner cord of brachial plexus; marked by numbness, hyperesthesia, pain on ulnar side of arm, and atrophy of hand muscles (flexor digitorum muscles, interosseous muscles, and thenar, hypothenar and flexor carpi ulnaris) with eventual paralysis. Also associated with vision defects and Horner syndrome.

Dejerine-Lichtheim phenomenon: See Lichtheim sign.

Dejerine-Mouzon syndrome: Unilateral lesion (tumor, infection, hemorrhagic) in parietal lobe causing abnormality of vibration, temperature, tactile, and pain sensation; also associated with tactile agnosia, aphasia, and Gerstmann syndrome if dominant lobe is involved and anagnosia if nondominant lobe is involved.

Dejerine-Roussy syndrome: Hemianesthesia to sensory and stereognostic stimuli with decreased or absent perception of body position and passive movement; also with variable hemiplegia, hemiparesis and dysarthria. Application of cold can cause jerky motor action. Cause is lesion in thalamus (lesion involving nucleus ventralis posterolateralis or thrombosis of thalamogeniculate artery) contralateral to affected side; cause is very rarely white matter lesion in contralateral parietal lobe.

Dejerine-Sottas atrophy (hereditary motor-sensory neuropathy type 3): Lower extremity weakness and atrophy and sensory loss progressing to involvement of arms; also marked by variable kyphoscoliosis, clubfoot, nystagmus, fasciculations, and Romberg sign. Onset occurs in childhood. Histopathology is significant for hypertrophic neuropathy and onion bulb shape of nerves. Death occurs in 3rd–4th decade.

Dejerine-Thomas atrophy (olivopontocerebellar atrophy): Degeneration of olivary nucleus, ventral pons, middle cerebellar peduncles, or cerebellar cortex; causes a variety of clinical presentations resembling Parkinson disease (e.g., tremors, ataxia, speech impairment). Onset is in middle age with progression to total incapacitation within 10 years.

Del Castillo syndrome: Dysgenesis of germinal cells with normal Sertoli and Leydig cells. Men have normal secondary sexual characteristics, libido, and erections but are sterile.

Del Castillo syndrome
(Argonz-Del Castillo syndrome):
Amenorrhea and galactorrhea
due to hyperprolactinemia in
nulliparous women; likely due
to microtumor in pituitary.

Del Rio Hortega method:
Staining method used to
visualize astrocytes of brain.
Cell outlines, processes, and
glial fibers are stained light
brown. Procedure is also used
to modify Golgi method to
visualize oligodendrocytes of
brain.

**Del Rio Hortega modified
stain:** Modification of
ammonium silver carbonate
method used to visualize liver
tissue; stains hepatocytes pale
violet and reticular fibers black.

Delaborde tracheal dilator:
Curved, blunt-tipped, ring-
handled instrument used to
enlarge trachea; opens using
bivalve mechanism.

Delafield fluid: Histologic
fixative; uses alcohol and acetic,
osmic, and chromic acids.

Delbert cast: Short-leg cast
providing lateral stability with
cut-away anterior-posterior heel
portions to allow dorsiflexion
and plantar flexion.

Delbet classification: See
Colonna classification.

Delbet sign: Indicator of
adequate collateral blood flow
in extremity with main arterial
obstructive lesion (e.g.,
aneurysm, atherosclerosis) if
tissue remains viable distally.

DeLee catheter: Tube used
for suctioning meconium and

amniotic remnants from nose
and mouth of neonate.

DeLee operation: Method of
rotating fetal head using
obstetrical forceps.

DeLee suctioning:
Evacuation of oropharynx of
newborn either immediately
after delivery of head (before
1st breath) or immediately after
delivery; intended to reduce risk
of meconium aspiration at birth.

Delhi boil (sore): See Aleppo
boil.

**Delleman-Orthuys
syndrome:** Congenital
periorbital skin tags, scalp tags
with thickened skin rings
around them, small mouth, bony
skull abnormalities, corpus
callosum agenesis, and
poroencephalopathy.

Delmege sign: Flattening of
deltoid muscle seen in early TB.

Delorme operation:
Procedure that uses perineal
(transanal) approach with
removal of mucosa of prolapsed
rectum performed initially and
followed by plication of
prolapsed muscle wall.

Delta nail: Triangular
orthopedic nail with
interlocking screws used in
femoral shaft fractures.

Demarquay sign: Frozen
larynx with speaking and
swallowing seen in tracheal
syphilis.

Demarquay syndrome
(Demarquay-Richet syndrome,
van der Woude syndrome):
Lower lip fistulas with pit-like

openings at vermillion border that may secrete saliva; also marked by "winged" popliteal fossa skin and genitourinary malformations. Condition occurs in about 1.2% of facial cleft patients; associated with gene defect in location 1q32–41.

DeMartini-Balestra syndrome: See Burke syndrome.

DeMeester procedure: Radical esophagectomy with splenectomy, resection of stomach and colon interposition graft; usu. for treatment of esophageal cancer.

DeMeester reflux score: Numeric system used to evaluate 24-hour pH study results; > 19 is abnormal.

Demianoff sign: Evidence of lesion in lumbar erector spinae muscle if patient lying in dorsal decubitus position feels severe pain when lifting extended leg 10°.

Demling formula: Fluid resuscitation treatment plan used in burn patients; uses Dextran 40 in saline administered at 2 ml/kg/hr for 1st 8 hours and then lactated Ringer's solution in sufficient quantity to maintain target urine output (usu. minimum: 30 ml/hr).

Demours membrane: See Descemet membrane.

Denecke spirillum: *Vibrio tyrogenus.*

Denhard mouth gag: Mechanical device used for forcibly opening clenched jaws

that uses ratchet mechanism with processes placed between molars; best suited for mouth that is already opened several degrees.

Denholz appliance: Orthodontic device with vestibular acrylic portion, coil-spring segments, and wire arch.

Denis Browne splint: Device used for correction of talipes equinovarus.

Dennie line: Groove under lower eyelid; seen in some patients with allergic disorders.

Dennie-Marfan syndrome: Weakness leading to paralysis, convulsions, vomiting, and mental deterioration, caused by congenital syphilis; early childhood onset. Treatment is penicillin.

Dennis Browne operation: See Browne operation.

Dennis intestinal clamp: Long (241 mm), straight, locking, ring-handle clamp, with relatively long jaw length (57 mm), nontoothed tips and longitudinal serrations.

Denny-Brown syndrome: Hereditary sensory radicular neuropathy.

Denonvilliers fascia: Extension of endopelvic fascia covering anterior extraperitoneal rectum and lying between prostate and rectum; important landmark in radical prostatectomy.

Denonvilliers ligament (aponeurosis): Rectovesical

septum; splits at base to allow passage to rectoprostatic space of Proust.

Denonvilliers operation: Method of repairing a defective lateral nostril; uses triangular flap taken from ipsilateral side.

Denucé ligament: Fibrous tissue that runs between distal radius and ulna.

Denver shunt: Peritoneovenous shunt for intractable ascites; results in high rate of sepsis and DIC.

Denver test (developmental screening test; DDST): Used to assess gross motor, fine motor, language, and adaptive and social skills; screens large numbers of children quickly (4 weeks–6 years of age) and with little training.

Denys-Drash syndrome (Drash syndrome): Association of Wilms tumor and urogenital abnormalities (usu. causing renal failure in 1st years of life). Cause is mutation in WT1 gene involved in DNA sequencing.

Denys-Leclef phenomenon: Increased capability of leukocytes to carry out phagocytosis when stimulated by immune serum.

Derby nail: Orthopedic nail used for intramedullary repair of femoral shaft fractures; has barbs at distal tip and washer at proximal end to prevent rotation.

Derbyshire neck: Generic term used to describe both bronchocele or goiter.

Dercum disease (Anders disease): Panniculitis with painful, tender subcutaneous nodules; also with headache, hypohidrosis, and amenorrhea. Condition is usu. found in older obese women with significant weight gain.

Derry syndrome: Type 2 gangliosidosis; marked by locomotor ataxia, loss of speech ability, increasing lethargy, startle response, respiratory infections, epilepsy, and visual impairment. Onset of autosomal recessive condition occurs at 1–2 years of age. Cause is acid beta galactosidase deficiency (chromosome 3).

Desault apparatus: A type of bandage.

Desault dislocation: Dislocation of distal radius with volar displacement.

Desault sign: Change in arc of rotation described by greater trochanter from circular (in normal femur) to nonexistent; seen in intracapsular femur fracture.

Desbuquois syndrome: Dwarfism, hypoplastic limbs and hands (micromelia), vertebral bodies with coronal clefts, abnormal ossification centers in hand causing finger deviation, and variable mental retardation and glaucoma; condition manifests in 1st year of life.

Descemet membrane: Thin, elastic, posterior part of basement membrane of cornea; secreted by corneal endothelium. Membrane grows throughout life and thickens in old age and with certain dystrophies.

Descot fracture: Break running through posterior distal tibia.

Desjardins point: Intersection of a imaginary line drawn to right lateral side from umbilicus and the right midaxillary line; marks location of pancreatic head.

Desmond syndrome (Senter syndrome, KID syndrome): Ichthyosiform erythroderma and sensorineural deafness; also with variable vascularized corneas, cryptorchidism, and flexion contractures. Cause is glycogen storage disease with excess glycogen deposition in skin and liver, sometimes progressing to cirrhosis in middle age. Condition may require liver transplantation.

Destot sign: Large scrotal hematoma (also under inguinal ligament) seen in pelvic fractures.

Determan syndrome: Temporary episodes of hypokinesia (disinclination to move body part) caused by focal brain ischemia in carotid system.

Deutschländer disease: Fracture of 2nd–3rd metatarsal caused by prolonged and repeated walking; nodularity forms due to bone callous. Pain responds to rest.

DeVega annuloplasty: Pursestring sutures placed around incompetent tricuspid

valve annulus to reduce size of obturator.

Deventer pelvis: Pelvis with smaller anterior-posterior skeletal dimension than normal.

Devergie syndrome (Hebra syndrome, Kaposi syndrome, Tarral-Besnier syndrome): Erythema over entire body with scaling of face and scalp, thickened palms and soles, and variable lymphadenopathy; papules may crust and ulcerate. Infantile form is more severe with treatment efficacy. Acquired form usu. appears in adolescence or later; treatment is etretinate or isotretinoin.

Devic disease (Devic-Gould disease, Erb-Devic disease): Bilateral acute inflammation and demyelination of optic nerves, often with subsequent demyelination or frank necrosis of spinal cord; considered multiple sclerosis variant. Condition leads to blindness, pain, and loss of sphincter control.

Devonshire colic: Lead poisoning.

Dew sign: Caudal shifting of resonance area in right subdiaphragmatic hydatid abscess when patient moves onto hands and knees.

di Guglielmo syndrome: Variant of acute myelogenous leukemia with leukoblasts as predominant cell type.

Di Saia syndrome: Congenital mental retardation, seizures, blindness, skeletal deformities, and respiratory infection;

caused by maternal coumadin intake during pregnancy. Bone defects are caused with 1st-trimester exposure, and CNS defects are caused with 2nd–3rd trimester exposure.

Diallinas-Amalric syndrome (Amalric syndrome): Deafness occurring with macular dystrophy. In inherited type (autosomal recessive), onset occurs at 5 years of age, with progressive deafness. In acquired type, onset is from birth, with nonprogressing partial deafness.

Diamond-Blackfan syndrome (anemia): Progressive RBC aplasia manifesting in 1st year of life; also with chronic erythroid hypoplasia and mildly abnormal WBC and platelet counts. Clinical features include variable hepatosplenomegaly, short stature, webbed neck, thumb defects, and mental retardation; often incorrectly classifed as type of aplastic anemia. Treatment is corticosteroids and multiple blood transfusions.

Dick test: Intradermal injection of group A streptococcal purified erythrogenic toxin causes small red lesion in 24–48 hours.

Dicker-Opitz syndrome (acrorenal syndrome): Rare autosomal dominant condition with varying malformations of kidneys and extremities.

Dickinson syndrome: See Alport syndrome.

Didiee projection: Radiographic positioning technique for evaluation of unstable or dislocating shoulder joint; patient lies prone and central ray is positioned to enter shoulder from lateral oblique position.

Dieffenbach operation: Method of closing triangular soft tissue defects; uses quadrangular advancement flap.

Diego blood group: Blood group with erythrocyte antigens Di^a and Di^b; Di^a is most commonly seen in Chinese and Japanese peoples and in South American Indians.

Dieterle stain: Method used to demonstrate *Legionella*, *Campylobacter*, *Treponema*, and *Borrelia*.

Diethrich bulldog clamp: Fine-tipped clamp with cross-action opening mechanism; used to control vascular structures.

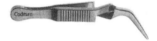

Diethrich bulldog clamp

Dietl syndrome: Episodic acute abdominal pain and hydronephrosis exacerbated in a standing position; typically seen in thin, older women. Cause is intermittent ureteropelvic junction obstruction caused by nephrophthosis.

Dietlen disease: Inflammatory adhesions between diaphragm and pericardial sac, resulting in feeling of epicardial "pulling" and tachycardia during inspiration. Treatment is surgery.

Dietrich syndrome: Pain and decreased range of motion in toe joints, esp. 2nd or 3rd. Both sexes are affected, with onset from infancy to late teens. Cause is fusiform enlargement of proximal interphalangeal joint.

Dieulafoy ulcer: Pinpoint gastric arterial bleeding from artery running from submucosa to mucosa caused by mucosal erosion; usu. occurs in proximal stomach. Diagnosis is made using angiography. Treatment is endoscopic sclerosis, or if needed, simple wedge resection.

DiGeorge syndrome (thymic hypoplasia): T-cell deficiency characterized by severe infections, absent thymus, abnormal parathyroid and heart, abnormal ears, congenital defects of the great vessels, and micrognathia. Male predominance is 2:1. Death occurs within 1st months of life. Cause is defect on chromosome 22q11. When receiving transfusions, patients require irradiated blood.

Dilling rule: Method used to estimate pediatric drug doses; age (years)/20 × adult dose.

Dillon disease: Alcoholic ketoacidosis.

DiMauro-DiMauro syndrome: Defect in carnitine palmitoyl-transferase, which causes muscle cramps and rapid fatigue during exertion; also with myoglobinuria developing after fevers, cold exposure, and high fat intake. Condition is autosomal recessive and very rare in females. Treatment is low fat intake and increased carbohydrates before exertion.

DiMauro-Hartlage disease: Variant of McArdle disease with congenital onset of global muscle weakness. Cause is defect in phosphorylase (chromosome 11q13). Death occurs from respiratory failure in 1st months.

Dimmer keratitis: Eyeball pain, increasing tearing, and photophobia after minor trauma to eyeball. Treatment is topical antibiotics and analgesics.

Dingman technique (nostril rotation): Procedure used to surgically correct misshapen nostril. Reorientation is performed by lengthening shortened nasal columella. Superior flap based on medial crus and lateral flap based on alar base are fashioned, and superior flap is rotated more cephalad with lateral flap repositioned to close just created defect. Disadvantage is narrowing of nostril size.

Diogenes cup: Small, concave anatomic space formed when 4th and 5th metacarpal bones are manipulated radially.

Disse space: Area between hepatocytes and sinusoidal walls, which carries lymphatic fluid of liver; site of amyloid deposition in amyloidosis of liver.

Dittel operation: Rarely performed enucleation of

hypertrophied prostate via an external incision.

Divry-van Bogaert syndrome: Spasticity, seizures, stunted growth and mental retardation; also marked by diffuse angiomatosis of cerebral cortex and meninges, acrocyanosis and cutis marmorata. Condition is autosomal recessive, with onset in infancy.

Dixon Mann sign: See Mann sign.

Dix-Hallpike maneuver: See Bárány maneuver.

Doan-Wiseman syndrome: Splenic dysfunction with trapping and destruction of granulocytes; marked by neutropenia, variably enlarged spleen, pain in left upper quadrant and fever. Condition is more common in women. Treatment is splenectomy.

Doan-Wright syndrome: Clinical and laboratory presentation of splenic pancytopenia; marked by anemia, neutropenia, thrombocytopenia, splenomegaly, and bone marrow hypoplasia. Condition can be congenital, primary, or secondary in etiology. Treatment is splenectomy.

Dobell solution: Compound solution of sodium borate.

Dobie globule: Inclusion in center of transparent disk of muscle fibril.

Dobie line (layer): See Amici disk.

Dobriner syndrome (Berger-Goldberg syndrome, Watson syndrome): Hereditary coproporphyria with onset usu. before puberty; autosomal dominant condition. Clinical expression during attacks ranges from asymptomatic to fatal; marked by recurrent abdominal pain, neurologic deficits, psychiatric disturbances, and hepatic insufficiency. Cause is partial defect in coproporphyrin oxidase with deficient conversion of coproporphyrinogen-9. Treatment is high-carbohydrate diet, heme arginate, and general supportive care.

Dockhorn syndrome: Variant of Alport syndrome with absence of deafness.

Dodd perforating veins: Vessels connecting greater saphenous vein system to deep venous system in leg.

Döderlein bacillus: Normal aerobic (gram-positive rod) lactobacilli found in vagina; appears shortly after birth and flourishes in acid environment, which is variably present throughout life.

Doege-Potter syndrome: Hypoglycemia secondary to production of insulin-mimicking substances from mesenchymal tumors.

Doehle-Heller disease: Syphilitic infiltration of aorta causing aortic aneurysm, aortic insufficiency, and coronary artery ostial stenosis; associated with "bell-like" or "tambour-like" auscultation. Condition is clinically symptomatic in untreated or undertreated cases (more common in men) in 5%–10% of patients, usu. 10–25 years postinfection. Treatment is antibiotics and, if needed, surgery.

Dohi syndrome: Hypopigmented and hyperpigmented lesions on dorsum of hands.

Döhle inclusion body: Ovoid, blue-staining inclusions seen in neutrophil cytoplasm; composed of rough endoplasmic reticulum RNA. Structures found in normal pregnancy, burns, aplastic anemia, infections, and some toxic states.

Dohlman disease: Cataracts with central cornea more affected than periphery; most commonly seen in children of Scandinavian descent. Autosomal dominant condition.

Dolan lines: Outlines of cortical bones in Waters view of midface, which roughly approximates profile on an elephant's head. Line 1, orbital line; line 2, zygomatic line; line 3, maxillary line.

Dolder bar: Device used to stabilize overlay denture with clips; bar is fixed to teeth roots or dental implants.

Dolman test: Used to determine eye dominance by having patient hold card with small hole in center with both hands and align light source on other side.

Dombrock blood group: Erythrocyte antigen; commonly found in Caucasians.

Donath-Landsteiner phenomenon: Occurrence of hemolysis in blood sample if specimen is cooled to 5°C and then rewarmed; seen in patients with paroxysmal hemoglobinuria. (See Dressler syndrome.)

Donders glaucoma: Advanced open-angle glaucoma.

Donders test: Investigates color vision using light source with colored glass walls.

Done nomogram: Used to determine level of salicylate intoxication and need for intervention.

Donné bodies: Colostrum corpuscles.

Donohue syndrome: Acanthosis nigricans, insulin resistance, and dwarfism.

Donohue syndrome (leprechaunism): Growth and osseous growth retardation, wide-set eyes, mental retardation, large ears, scant subcutaneous fat, hypoglycemia, and hirsutism; associated with defect in cell insulin receptor. Male-to-female ratio is 1:2. Life span is greatly shortened.

Donovan body: *Calymmatobacterium granulomatis;* causes granuloma inguinale, a chronic granulomatous, ulcerative, skin disease. Disorder is most commonly found in U.S. amoung homosexual African-American men. Histology specimens appear as bipolar safety pin-shaped inclusions in macrophages.

Donovan solution: Solution of arsenic iodide and mercury iodide.

Doppler effect (phenomenon): Change in pitch or frequency as an object emitting sound moves past relatively stationary listener (or vice versa).

Doppler equation: Expression of Doppler effect as $fd = 2f_0(v\cos\theta/c)$, where f_0 is original frequency of ultrasound beam, v is velocity of blood flow in vessel being studied, θ is incident angle between vessel and ultrasound beam, and c is speed of sound (1540 m/sec in tissue).

Doppler shift: Concept closely related to Doppler effect that can be expressed as change in sound frequency returned from sound at fixed frequency aimed at moving target; based on detecting movement of RBCs in vessels.

Doppler ultrasound: Basic method of ultrasound diagnosis using backscatter frequency-shift mode; determines direction and velocity of blood flow using ultrasound reflections of moving cells within body.

Doppler velocity detector: Method that provides qualitative estimate of direction of pulse contour and flow velocity using analog waveforms; also gives audible flow signal useful in distinguishing arteriovenous fistulas.

Dorendorf canal: Supraclavicular fullness in aortic arch aneurysm.

Dormandy-Porter syndrome: Familial fructose–galactose intolerance.

Dormia basket: Collapsible device threaded into common bile duct through fresh T-tube tract or cystoscopically through urinary bladder into ureter; can be expanded to trap and mechanically remove a stone.

Dornier HM3 lithotripter: Earliest (and still most powerful) model of extracorporeal shock wave ultrasound machine; although introduced in early 1980s, it remains popular because of its high power. Device is most commonly used today for stones in kidney and upper ureter; usu. requires IV sedation.

Dorothy Reed cell: See Reed-Sternberg cell.

Dorph disease (cast syndrome): Chronic vomiting caused by mechanical decompression of 4th portion of duodenum; classically described in patients with spinal curvature treated with full-body cast.

Dorr ratio: Width of femoral canal at midpoint of lesser trochanter/width of femoral canal 10 cm distal.

Dorrance hook (type 5XA): Lightweight metal hand prosthesis; permits desk work.

Dorrance hook (type 7):
Durable metal hand prosthesis;
permits grasping of tools, knife,
or nails. Typically users are
men.

Dortmundt tank: Settling
tank for sludge processing in
water treatment plants.

Doss syndrome: Rare variant
of porphyria caused by
defective ALA dehydratase;
marked by variable clinical
picture, with abdominal pain,
neuropathy, vomiting, limb pain,
muscle hypotonia, and
respiratory insufficiency.
Condition is exacerbated by
alcohol and stress. Urine shows
greatly increased levels of ALA
and porphyrins.

Douglas abscess: Suppuration
in rectouterine pouch.

Douglas ligament: Fibrous
tissue that forms rectouterine
pouch; fold of peritoneum
running from rectum to broad
ligament on either side.

Douglas line (fold; linea
semicircularis): Line marking
lower end of dorsal
ensheathment of rectus muscle
by transversus muscle fascia.

Douglas pouch (space, cul-de-
sac): Rectouterine pouch lined
by parietal peritoneum; mass in
this area is palpable on rectal
exam.

Douglas septum: Embryonic
structure developing into fetal
rectum; derived from fusion of
Rathke folds.

Dover powder: Opium (10%)
and ipecac powder.

**Dow-Van Bogaert
syndrome:** Late onset of
choreiform movements after
resection of cerebellar
hemisphere.

Dowd-Ponka repair: Method
of repair for lumbar (Petit and
Grynfeltt) hernias; uses skin
incision over hernia, ligation of
sac, and removal of lipoma if
present with placement of
Marlex or Prolene patch over
defect. Latissimus dorsi and
external oblique are
approximated as far as possible
(avoiding undue tension) over
patch and sutured to edges, and
gluteal flap is then swung up
over remaining exposed patch
and sutured to patch with skin
closed above this.

Dowling-Degos syndrome:
Onset in early adulthood of
progressive, usu. freckle-like
pigmented lesions on axilla,
groin, buttocks, and
inframammary folds caused by
elongated rete ridges;
associated with mental
retardation, acne-type lesions at
mouth, and trichilemmal cysts.
Condition is autosomal
dominant.

**Dowling-Meara
epidermolysis:** Severe, diffuse
serous and hemorrhagic
blistering originating in basal
cells of skin. Onset occurs in
infancy; condition diminishes
through childhood and usu.
leaves no residual scars.
Treatment is warm saline soaks
and strangely, improves with
onset of fever.

Down syndrome: Trisomy 21
associated with moderate

mental retardation, flattened nasal bridge, small ears, prominent epicanthal folds, duodenal atresia, Brushfield spots, and marbled appearance of skin of newborns.

Downey cell: Atypical lymphocyte always occurring in infectious mononucleosis; 3 types occur. Type 1, foamy, basophilic cytoplasm with kidney-shaped nucleus; type 2, less mature than type 1 cells with relatively less basophilic cytoplasm and plasmacytoid nucleus; type 3, fine chromatin-type cytoplasm and 1–2 nucleoli.

Downs analysis: Radiographic-based measurements of skull used in orthodontic diagnosis and treatment.

Downs Y axis: Angle formed by Frankfort horizontal plane and imaginary line connecting sella turcica and gnathion; assesses forward and downward mandibular growth.

Dox medium: See Czapek solution agar.

Doyen intestinal forceps: Long (235 mm), straight or curved tip, locking, ring-handle forceps; has long jaw length (105 mm), slightly concave and nontoothed tip, and diagonal serrations.

Doyen vascular toothed intestinal clamps: Long (229 mm), straight or curved tip, locking, ring-handle clamp; has slightly concave long jaw length (95 mm), nontoothed tip, and 2 × 3 vascular teeth serrations on jaws.

Doyle operation: Paracervical uterine denervation.

Doyne choroiditis: Honeycomb retinal degeneration. Onset usu. occurs in 3rd decade with white spots forming in peripapillary areas; slow progression to white confluent area with visual loss in 75% of cases.

Drabkin solution: 0.2 g potassium ferricyanide, 0.05 g potassium cyanide, and 1 g of sodium bicarbonate in 1 L H_2O; used to lyse RBCs.

Drake aneurysm clip: Instrument used to occlude brain aneurysms.

Drapanas shunt (interposition mesocaval shunt): Surgical treatment for portal hypertension using short Dacron graft anastomosed between inferior vena cava and superior mesenteric vein.

Drash syndrome: See Denys-Drash syndrome.

Drawer sign: Method for detection of torn anterior or posterior cruciate ligament. Patient lies flat and draws leg up and foot rests flat on floor. Examiner grasps top of calf and pulls toward self for ACL evaluation and pushes away for PCL evaluation. Movement of tibial head > 1 cm is positive result.

Dresbach anemia: Sickle cell anemia.

Dressler syndrome (Harley syndrome): Paroxysmal hemoglobinuria prompted by exposure to cold; marked by shaking chills, back and leg pain, headache, abdominal cramps and fever, jaundice, transient splenomegaly, paresthesias, urticaria; and cyanosis. Condition is associated with syphilis infection, but most cases are idiopathic. Wide range in temperature drop is needed to initiate attacks. Treatment is avoidance of cold exposure and steroids; course is usu. benign.

Dressler syndrome: Pericarditis, pneumonitis, pleurisy, fever, chest pain, and friction rub following MI or open-heart surgery; possible cause is development of autoantibodies. Treatment is aspirin, indomethacin, or steroids with usu. good response.

Dreuw disease: Sudden onset of small, irregular patches of scalp hair loss; unknown etiology. Condition tends to occur in epidemic outbreaks. Hair does not always regrow.

Drew syndrome: Corneal decomposition due to "intermittent touch" after incorrectly placed intraocular lens in cataract surgery.

Drew-Smythe catheter: Tube used to induce labor by iatrogenic rupture of membranes.

Dreyfus syndrome: See Hobaek syndrome.

Drinker respirator: Iron lung.

Dripps classification (ASA classification): System used by anesthesiologists to describe physical status of patient. Class 1, normal patient in good health; class 2, mild to moderate systemic disease; class 3, severe, systemic disease (limited activity but not incapacitated); class 4,severe, life-threatening systemic disease; class 5, mortality likely within 24 hours even with surgery.

Drobin syndrome: Anterior uveitis, lymphadenopathy, and acute interstitial nephritis; likely caused by unknown virus. Treatment is topical steroids to eye and tapering dose of IV prednisone.

Drummond sign: "Whiffing" sound audible with mouth open during respiration; seen in patients with aortic aneurysm.

du Toit modified staple: U-shaped metal staple used to fix tendons/ligaments to bone.

Duane syndrome: Combination of congenital thenar hypoplasia and progressive retraction of eyeball into skull with loss of abduction; usu. left eye is affected but can be bilateral. Hereditary condition is autosomal dominant.

Duane syndrome (Stilling-Türk-Duane syndrome): Congenital eye abnormality, with retraction of eyeball on adduction and impaired or absent abduction; more prevalent in females. Condition also has impaired convergence ability; associated with malformations of ears, face and teeth Klippel-Feil syndrome, and heterochromia iridis. Syndrome occurs bilaterally in 15%–20% of patients.

Duane test: Measurement of ocular heterophoria using prisms and combustion light source.

Duarte disease: Variant of Mason-Turner syndrome.

Dubin-Johnson syndrome (Sprinz-Dubin syndrome, Sprinz-Nelson syndrome): Congenital defect in liver secretion of conjugated bilirubin and other anions; follows benign course with intermittent jaundice and mild right upper quadrant pain. Sometimes 1st presentation is with pregnancy or contraceptive pills.

Dubini chorea (electric chorea): Acute, fatal form of chorea due to involvement of CNS.

Dubois abcesses (disease): Small thymic cysts lined with squamous epithelium and filled with neutrophils; seen in congenital syphilis.

Dubois sign: Shortened 5th finger in congenital syphilis.

Dubois syndrome: Systemic lupus erythematosus.

Dubois-Dubois equation: Expression used to estimate body surface area (m^2); = Weight(kg) $\times$ 0.425 $\times$ Height(m) $\times$ 0.725) $\times$ 71.84.

Dubowitz score: Method for evaluation of gestational age of infants based on presence of neurologic signs and muscle tone.

Dubowitz syndrome: Low-birth-weight dwarfism, eczema, and odd facies; associated with neuroblastoma, aplastic anemia, and lymphoma/leukemia. Autosomal recessive condition is also associated with mental retardation, severe caries, missing lateral eyebrows, coarctation of aorta, occluded right internal carotid artery, and aberrant right subclavian artery.

Dubreuil-Chambardel syndrome: Dental caries of incisors (esp. upper) occurring in adolescence; some dentists question whether this is separate entity.

Duchenne muscular dystrophy: Type of muscle disease with progressive muscular weakness and pseudohypertrophy of muscles; X-linked recessive condition. Defect is absence or derangement of dystrophin.

Duchenne paralysis: See Erb palsy.

Duchenne sign: Convexity of the epigastrium during inspiration; seen in pericardial effusions or paralysis of diaphragm.

Duchenne sign: Indicator of low ulnar nerve paresis and intact extrinsic muscles if fingers 4–5 claw when metacarpophalangeal joint is hyperextended and interphalangeal and distal interphalangeal joints are flexed.

Duchenne-Erb syndrome (paralysis): Limp, medially rotated, pronated arm caused by lesion of upper brachial plexus; affected muscles (supplied by C5–C6) are supraspinatus, infraspinatus, deltoid, biceps, brachialis, brachioradialis, and supinator.

Duckert deficiency: Factor XIII deficiency; see Laki-Lorand factor.

Duckworth phenomenon: Clinical onset of respiratory arrest preceding cardiac arrest in patients with intracranial pathology.

Ducrey bacillus: *Haemophilus ducreyi.*

Ducrey test (Ito-Reenstierna test): Intradermal injection of inactivated *Haemophilus ducreyi* to diagnose chancroid.

duct of His: See His canal.

duct of Vater: See His canal.

ducts of Cuvier: Common cardinal veins of heart.

Dudley-Klingenstein disease: Jejunal tumor (benign or malignant) causing abdominal pain, melena, abdominal distention, and tachycardia.

Duffy antigen: Serum protein (2 allele) receptors for malaria-causing Plasmodium vivax.

Duffy group: See Kell blood group.

Dugas test: Indicator of shoulder dislocation when ipsilateral hand is placed on opposite shoulder and patient cannot bring elbow to chest wall.

Duhamel procedure: Definitive surgical treatment for Hirschsprung disease; uses a rectorectal endoanal pull-through with rectorectal space dissected down to tip of coccyx and preservation of sacral nerves. Submucosal space of rectum is then dissected via perineal incision, side-to-side anastomosis is performed with remaining anterior aganglionic wall, and rectum is left in-situ. Procedure is usu. performed at 6–12 months of age.

Duhot line: Imaginary line running from sacral apex to superior iliac spine.

Duhring disease: Dermatitis multiformis; skin inflammation marked by any combination of papular, vesicular, bullous, or pustule lesions.

Dührssen incisions: Early surgical technique of childbirth consisting of radial cervical incisions made at 2, 6, and 10 o'clock positions in cervix when immediate delivery is necessary before cervix is fully dilated; now performed only with entrapment of fetal head in incompletely dilated (> 7 cm) cervix in breech presentation. Major complication is severe hemorrhage.

Dührssen operation: Vaginofixation of uterus.

Duke inhaler: Hand-held device used to deliver methoxyflurane by self-administration; used in some obstetric patients.

Duke test: Measurement of bleeding time.

Dukes classification: System developed in 1932 to describe colorectal carcinoma. Stage A, lesion confined to bowel wall; stage B, lesion penetrates through bowel wall but does not involve lymph nodes; stage C, regional lymph nodes involved. Technically, there is no Dukes stage D lesion.

Dukes-Filatow disease: Early 1900s term for rubeola.

Dulbecco modification: Variation of Eagle minimum essential medium; used for transport media for 1st 24 hours for recovery of split-thickness skin grafts.

Dumdum fever: Infection of internal organs with *Leishmania*.

Dumon stent: Solid-walled silicone device placed in tracheobronchial tree with rigid bronchoscope to prevent recurrent tumor growth from obstructing airway. It is inserted folded and opened with plunger tube device; the rough outer surface anchors it.

Dumon-Radermecker syndrome: Severe mental retardation, childhood onset of seizures, and middle-age onset of ataxia and dysarthria; rare autosomal dominant condition. Histology is marked by large amount of cytoplasmic material in brain and some cranial nerve cells.

Duncan curette: Scoop-shaped surgical instrument with long handle inserted through vagina to obtain endometrial biopsy specimens.

Duncan folds: Loose, redundant peritoneum adhering to uterus after delivery.

Duncan mechanism: Placental extrusion after childbirth associated with free vaginal bleeding before delivery. Separation of placenta from uterine wall occurs first at periphery and descends sideways to vagina. Maternal surface appears first at introitus.

Duncan syndrome: Acute, usu. rapidly fatal (80%) fulminant liver failure or aplastic anemia on infection with EBV; X-linked inheritance. Patients appear immunologically and clinically normal before infection, with exaggerated antibody response and cytotoxic reaction after infection. Patients surviving 1st week usu. develop rapidly growing, high-grade B-cell lymphoma.

Duncan-Bird sign: See Bird sign.

Dunfermline scale: Used to categorize nutritional condition for children. 1, excellent; 2, acceptable; 3, requires supervision; 4, medical intervention required.

Dunlop traction: Type of skin and skeletal traction using weight placed on lower arm to stabilize elbow or supracondylar fractures.

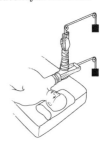

Dunlop traction

Dunn device: Anterior fixation device for thoracic and lumbar spine; no longer used because of unacceptably high rate of vascular complications.

Dunn procedure: Method for posterior stabilization of myelomeningocele deformity via contouring L-rod.

Dunnett test: Statistical measure used for multiple comparisons against 1 control group; best preceded with ANOVA to establish significant differences between groups. Measure is more sensitive than Bonferroni t test.

Dunningham disease (lipoatrophic diabetes): Loss of subcutaneous fat on extremities and (variably) trunk, usu. not in genital region; also associated with thickened nails, premature tooth eruption, and tongue papillae. Both autosomal dominant and sporadic inheritance have been reported.

Dunphy sign: Suggestion of appendicitis when coughing worsens right lower quadrant pain.

Duplay operation: Method of hypospadias repair; uses epithelization of lateral wound margins to form urethral floor and intact epithelial strip to form roof.

Dupré syndrome: Aseptic meningitis usu. occurring in children with acute febrile illness; marked by positive Kernig sign, stiff neck, headaches, seizures, and occ. coma. Lumbar puncture shows increased intracranial pressure and proteins. Treatment is diuretics and control of ICP.

Dupuy syndrome: See Frey syndrome.

Dupuy-Dutemps operation: Procedure to correct stenosis of lacrimal duct using tissue from opposing eyelid.

Dupuytren amputation (Lisfranc amputation): Disarticulation of arm at shoulder joint.

Dupuytren contracture (disease): Fibrosis in palmar fascia causing flexion contracture of 4th and sometimes 5th finger.

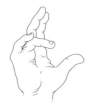

Dupuytren contracture

Dupuytren fracture: Spiral fracture of distal fibula with tear of inferior tibiofibular ligaments.

Dupuytren hydrocele: Loculated hydrocele found in tunica vaginalis testis.

Dupuytren sign: Indication of sarcomatous bone degeneration if pushing on bone causes crackling sound.

Dupuytren sign: Indication of congenital dislocation of femoral head if it moves up and down on palpation.

Duran-Reynals factor: Hyaluronidase.

Durand syndrome: Diffuse angiokeratosis of skin, loss of psychomotor abilities with tremor and spasticity, coarsening of facies, and repeat infections. Autosomal recessive condition seen in patients of southern Italian extraction.

Durand syndrome: Congenital lactose intolerance. Associated with abnormal gastric mucosa and vomiting; autosomal dominant condition. Treatment is lactose-free diet with good response.

Durand-Nicolas-Favre disease: Lymphogranuloma venereum.

Dürck nodes: Aggregation of lymphocyte cells found in perivascular tissue throughout spinal cord and brain; seen in human trypanosomiasis.

Duret lesion: Leakage of blood into tissues surrounding 4th ventricle; seen after slight head trauma.

Durham tube: Jointed tracheostomy tube.

Durham tube: Test tube used to measure bacterial gas production.

Duroziez sign: "Whooshing" murmur auscultated in femoral artery; seen in severe aortic regurgitation.

Dutch-Kentucky syndrome: See Hecht-Beals syndrome.

Dutcher body: Invagination of cytoplasm with immunoglobulin particles into nucleus; seen in normal plasma cells and neoplastic lymphocytes. Structure is periodic acid–Schiff positive.

Dutton disease (relapsing fever): Disease occurring in central Africa caused by *Borrelia duttonii*.

Duval lung grasping forceps: Straight, ring-handle, locking forceps used to retract lung tissue; tips are triangular and open.

Duval procedure: Distal resection of pancreas with pancreaticojejunostomy; used to palliate chronic pancreatitis.

Duvenhage virus: Serotype of Lyssavirus, which causes rabies-like illness in humans in South Africa.

Duverney foramen: See foramen of Winslow.

Duverney fracture: Type of hip fracture with injury to anterior-superior iliac process; mechanism is usu. direct trauma (lateral to medial).

Duverney glands: See Cowper glands.

Dwyer instrumentation (osteotomy): Device that provides internal fixation and correction of anterior thoracic and lumbar spine fusions with compression force only; best for correcting lordosis between T10 and L4. Screw and staple unit is inserted after disks have been removed, and titanium cable is then threaded through keyhole in the screw and screw-heads are pulled together. Best for correcting lordosis.

Dyke-Davidoff-Masson syndrome: Congenital underdevelopment of skull and sinuses, mental retardation, impaired speech development, and seizures.

Dyke-Young syndrome: Mid-1900s term for macrocytic hemolytic anemia.

Dzierszynksy disease: Hyperplastic bone growth of clavicles, sternum, skull, and phalanges.

Eadie-Hofstee equation: Linearized form of Lineweaver-Burk equation. $V = (-V[S])(K_m + V_{max})$, where V is reaction velocity, [S] is substrate concentration, and K_m is Michaelis-Menten constant; allows determination of K_m from experimental data.

Eagle syndrome: Elongated or traumatized styloid process causing ear and throat pain and feeling of foreign body in back of throat.

Eagle-Barrett syndrome (triad syndrome, prune belly syndrome): Thin, weakened abdominal wall; bladder hypertrophy with hydroureter; and undescended testes. Condition is usu. associated with other anomalies (bilateral cryptorchidism, cardiac septum defects, intestinal malrotation, sternal and rib deformities, talipes equinovarus, congenital hip dislocations, scoliosis, and syndactyly). 5% of cases occur in girls; incidence is 1 in 30,000–50,000 live births.

Eales disease: Retinal ischemia and neovascularization of unknown etiology; usu. bilateral. Vitreous bleeding is often presenting sign; condition usu. affects men 20–30 years of age.

Earle sign: Tenderness on rectal exam associated with hematoma; occurs in pelvic fractures.

East African trypanosomiasis: See Rhodesian sleeping sickness.

East coast fever: See African coast fever.

Eastern equine encephalitis: CNS inflammation occurring in north and central America and West Indies. Insect vectors are *Aedes* and *Mansonia* mosquitoes; animal hosts are horses and birds.

Eaton agent: *Mycoplasma pneumoniae.*

Eaton-Lambert syndrome: Paraneoplastic condition (usu. small-cell lung carcinoma) with fatigue and muscle weakness in pelvic and thigh muscles, dry mouth, and decreased deep tendon reflexes at rest; due to autoantibody depletion of voltage-sensitive calcium channels with impaired activity and acetylcholine release. Nonmalignant cases are associated with other autoimmune conditions.

Eaton-Littler reconstruction: Procedure used to alleviate pain in osteoarthritis of wrist; 1/2 of either flexor or extensor tendon is left attached distally, with proximal free end passed through base of metacarpal to simulate atrophied ulnar collateral ligament.

Eberth line: Microscopic jagged lines seen at junction of myocardial cells.

Ebner glands (glands of von Ebner): Serum-secreting glands associated with circumvallate papillae on posterior tongue.

Ebola virus: RNA virus with lipoprotein envelope similar in structure to Marburg virus; initially isolated in Republic of the Congo (formerly Zaire).

Ebola virus disease: Hemorrhagic fever with 1-week incubation period followed by fever, severe diarrhea, limb pain, and coughing; mortality is 50%–70% in 1st 10 days.

Ebstein angle (cardiohepatic angle): Angle formed by imaginary line drawn horizontally through endpoint of hepatic dullness and an upright line drawn to right of sternal edge at end of cardiac dullness.

Ebstein lesion: Epithelial cell necrosis and hyaline deposits seen in renal tubules in diabetes mellitus.

Ebstein malformation (anomaly): Congenital atrialized right ventricle, tricuspid incompetence (fused anterior/posterior leaflet), and functional pulmonary outflow obstruction causing cyanosis; no gender predilection. Accessory pathways usu. found in right free wall or posterior septum. Diagnosis involves cineangiocardiography.

Eck fistula: End-to-side portocaval shunts in dogs performed in late 1800s.

Ecker fissure: Vertical groove on the back of gyrus angularis; sometimes forms part of border of anterior occipital lobe.

Economo disease (lethargic encephalitis): Global epidemic in 1915–1925; marked by headache, apathy, drowsiness, and ophthalmoplegia. No etiology or virus has been discovered; high mortality rate with marked residual deficits.

Edelman syndrome: Atrophic pancreatitis with secondary fatty liver infiltration.

Edelman-Galton whistle: Tests hearing in higher tone (4000–80,000 cycles/sec) range.

Edgarton-Grand procedure: Transfer of tendons to restore thumb adduction.

Edinburgh method: Test used to assess hip dysplasia in newborns; measures space between lateral ischium to most medial edge of femoral metaphysis on radiograph. Normal value is 4 mm; diagnostic if = 6 mm.

Edinger fibers: Visual pathway fibers in amphibians.

Edinger-Westphal nucleus (accessory oculomotor nucleus): Group of cell bodies dorsal to somatic portion of oculomotor nuclear complex; carries parasympathetic nerve fibers of CN III to ciliary ganglion and sphincter pupillae of eye. Lesions at site cause pupil sphincter paralysis and loss of accommodation of pupil.

Edman reaction: Stepwise chemical removal of amino acids from peptide amino terminus. Edman reagent is coupled to protein and then cleaved to protein with 1 less residue; this cleavage product is then extracted, volatized, and identified by gas chromatography.

Edman reagent: Phenylisothiocyanate.

Edna towel clamp: Blunt-tipped, nonperforating, ring-handled surgical instrument used to fasten drapes on sterile field.

Edwards hypothetical system: Schematic embryonic double-arch system for great vessels of mediastinum; anomalous malformations can be better visualized by abnormal regression of right dorsal 4th dorsal arch or left 4th dorsal arch.

Edwards instrumentation: Posterior spinal rod and sleeve used to treat spinal trauma.

Edwards syndrome: Trisomy in group E chromosomes (16–18); 2nd to trisomy 21 (Down syndrome) in frequency. Features include mental retardation, congenital heart disease, spina bifida, and esophageal and biliary atresia; death usu. occurs in 1st–2nd year of life.

Edwards-Collett classification: System used to describe congenital heart malformations. Type 1, truncus arteriosus with 1 arterial trunk giving off aorta and main pulmonary artery; type 2, right pulmonary arteries originating adjacent to each other off dorsal wall of truncus; type 3, right and left pulmonary arteries originating from either side of truncus; type 4, proximal pulmonary arteries missing.

Edwardsiella: Small, motile, gram-negative rods with peritrichous flagella; member of Enterobacteriaceae. *E. tarda* may cause acute gastroenteritis and sepsis.

Edwards-Patau syndrome:
Mental retardation, failure to thrive, abnormal ears, flexion deformities of digits, and congenital heart defects; caused by trisomy 18. Female-to-male ratio is 3:1. Death usu. occurs in 1st year.

Egas Moniz procedure:
Frontal lobotomy. Technique was 1st reported in 1936 for treatment of mental illness; awarded Nobel Prize in Physiology and Medicine in 1949.

Egawa sign: Indicator of ulnar nerve and interosseus muscle paralysis. Ability to flex middle finger but not being able to deviate it radially and ulnarly is positive.

Egger line: Inner aspect of Wiegert ligament of eye lens; partially delineates Berger space.

Egger syndrome (Joubert facial anomalies, Joubert-Boltshauer syndrome): Lobulated tongue, mouth hamartomas, and polydactyly of digits; autosomal recessive condition associated with 4th ventricle posterior fossa cyst and cerebellar vermis hypoplasia.

Eggers plate: Surgical device used to provide opposition of bony fragments.

Egyptian chlorosis: See Griesinger syndrome.

Egyptian conjunctivitis
(trachoma): Infectious condition of cornea and conjunctiva caused by infection with *Chlamydia trachomatis*; marked by pain, tearing, and photophobia.

Egyptian splenomegaly:
Splenic enlargement secondary to portal hypertension being caused by bilharzial fibrosis.

Ehlers-Danlos syndrome type 1 (gravis): Classic form of collagen disease. Marked by severe joint hypermobility; easy bruising; varicose veins; and velvety, fragile, hyperextensible skin. Cause is defect in type 5 collagen. Autosomal dominant.

Ehlers-Danlos syndrome type 2 (mitis): Autosomal dominant condition similar to type 1 but with less severe symptoms; caused by defect in type 1 collagen.

Ehlers-Danlos syndrome type 3 (familial hypermobility): Less severe skin changes than with other types of this syndrome but marked by most severe joint hypermobility.

Ehlers-Danlos syndrome type 4 (acrogeric; ecchymotic; vascular): Translucent skin with visible veins; marked by spontaneous rupture of aorta or intestines and normal joints. Cause is defect in type III procollagen.

Ehlers-Danlos syndrome type 5 (X-linked): Similar to type 2 syndrome but with X-linked recessive inheritance pattern.

Ehlers-Danlos syndrome type 6 (ocular-scoliotic):

Scoliosis, fragility of eye tissues, hyperextended joints, and loose skin; autosomal recessive condition caused by defect in lysyl hydroxylase deficiency.

Ehlers-Danlos syndrome type 7 (arthrochalasis multiplex congenita): Hyperextended joints and soft, velvety skin; caused by defect in conversion of procollagen to collagen.

Ehlers-Danlos syndrome type 8 (periodontal): Periodontitis and soft skin; unknown etiology.

Ehlers-Danlos syndrome type 9 (cutis laxa occipital horn syndrome): Reclassified as disease of copper transport; see Menkes disease.

Ehlers-Danlos syndrome type 10: Symptoms similar to type 2 syndrome; unknown etiology but possibly related to defect in fibronectin.

Ehlers-Danlos syndrome type 11 (familial joint instability): Reclassified as part of familial articular hypermobility syndromes.

Ehlers-Danlos type Beasley-Cohen: Mental retardation, soft/stretchable skin, atrophic muscles, and hearing defects.

Ehlers-Danlos type Friedman-Harrod: Mild joint laxity, periodontal disease, hernias, scoliosis and aortic rupture.

Ehlers-Danlos type Hernandez: Mental retardation, ecchymosis, joint hyperlaxity, stunted growth, winged scapula, and cryptorchidism; caused by abnormal proteodermatan sulfate synthesis.

Ehlers-Danlos type Viljoin: Presence of wormian skull bones and etiology of joint hyperlaxity; similar to type 3 syndrome.

Ehrenfried disease: Congenital cartilage disorder; short stature, deformed hands, excrescences of diaphyseal long bones, scapula and ribs. Sarcomatous degeneration is common; condition is autosomal dominant.

Ehrenritter ganglion: Variably occurring superior or jugular ganglion of CN IX that lies on posterior nerve trunk in upper jugular foramen; no branches arise from it.

Ehret phenomenon: Estimates diastolic blood pressure during blood pressure cuff examination. Sudden throb in brachial artery is palpable during cuff release and pressure drop; corresponds to diastolic blood pressure.

Ehret syndrome: Muscle pain, atrophy, and contracture seen after prolonged immobilization. Treatment is sustained physical therapy.

Ehrlich aldehyde reagent: 80 ml concentrated hydrochloric acid, 380 ml ethyl alcohol, and 4 g paradimethylamino-benzaldehyde; used to detect presence of urobilinogen in urine and feces. Positive reaction is development of red color when reagent is added to test substance.

Ehrlich anemia: Aplastic anemia.

Ehrlich diazo reagent: Mixture of hydrochloric acid, sulfanilic acid, and sodium nitrate used to detect and quantify bilirubin (detected as azobilirubin via spectroscopy), specifically in diagnosis of measles, typhoid fever, and liver disease.

Ehrlich method: Technique for quantification of urobilinogen using *p*-dimethylaminobenzaldehyde as coloring agent.

Ehrlich unit: Equals 1 mg of urobilinogen.

Ehrlich-Biermer disease: See Biermer disease.

ehrlichiosis: Tick-borne disease marked by fever, chills, malaise and rash; occurs in acute form and is generally self-limited. Condition also occurs as coinfection with Lyme disease; although controversial, some experts propound chronic infection state with need for prolonged antibody treatment. Diagnosis is by antibody tests for human granulocytic ehrlichiosis and human monocytic ehrlichiosis. Treatment in adults is doxycycline.

Eichhorst atrophy: Progressive muscle degeneration of femorotibial compartments; results in toe contraction.

Einhorn regimen: Highly effective chemotherapy regimen for metastatic testicular cancer; uses cisplatin, VP-16, and bleomycin.

Einhorn string test: Early 1900s technique to determine site of bleeding in upper GI tract.

einsteinium: Synthetic, radioactive element; atomic number, 99; most stable isotope, Es-254; half-life, 276 days.

Einthoven law: Electric potential in lead 2 of ECG equals sum of potential differences in leads 1 and 3.

Einthoven triangle: Imaginary triangle drawn between standard limb lead placement in ECG; apices are at left hip and shoulder and right shoulder.

Eisenlohr syndrome: Early 1900s term for paralysis resulting from bulbar lesion.

Eisenmenger disease (complex): Development of increased pulmonary vascular resistance and right-to-left shunting in patient with preexisting left-to-right shunt; most common causes are large ventricular septal defect and patent ductus arteriosus. Death results from endocarditis, thrombosis, or heart failure. Optimal treatment is closure of communication of connection at earliest possible date; once pulmonary hypertension develops, treatment is heart and/or lung transplantation.

Eklund modification for mammography: Technique using compression of breast implant and displacement of breast tissue with modification of radiographic views.

Ekman-Lobstein syndrome (osteogenesis imperfecta type 4): Variant of Beighton disease with normal hearing and sclera; autosomal dominant condition caused by defect in collagen metabolism.

El-Naggar electrode: See Nashold electrode.

El Tor vibrio: Strain of *Vibrio cholerae* causing hemolytic cholera; develops partial resistance to chemotherapy regimens.

Elejalde syndrome (acrocephalopolydactylous dysplasia): Large birth weight, cystic kidneys, extra digits, acrocephaly, and craniosynostosis; rare autosomal recessive condition.

Elek test: Immunodiffusion test for toxigenic strains of *Corynebacterium diphtheriae.*

Elgin table: Apparatus used in physical therapy; uses a pulley–weight system at 1 end that allows for strength and endurance exercises of lower extremity. Patient lies prone, supine, or in lateral decubitus position.

Eliakim disease: Development of liver granulomas and dysfunction; causes include many microbial infections, sarcoid, Wegener granulomatosis, Hodgkin disease, melanoma, and drugs.

Elliot B solution: Artificial CSF solution used in infusion

manometrics of spinal subarachnoid space.

Elliot procedure: Trephination of eyeball with scleral flap for treatment of glaucoma.

Elliot sign: Indurated edge of skin lesion in syphilis.

Elliot sign: Small, scattered point-like scotoma extending from blind spot.

Elliot-Maher guidelines: Criteria used to diagnose Beckwith-Wiedemann syndrome; presence of 3 major features or 2 major and 3 minor features required.

Ellis sign (line, Ellis-Garland line): Curved line of dullness of chest wall detectable in reabsorbing pleural exudate.

Ellis-Jones technique: Procedure used to correct displacement of peroneal tendons; involves longitudinal incision posterior to lateral malleolus with creation of flap of tendo calcaneus inserted into hole drilled into lateral malleolus; effect is to "bind" tendons in place.

Ellis-van Creveld syndrome: Dwarfism, polydactyly (esp. hands), atrial septal defect, "knock knees," urogenital defects, and mental retardation (30%); autosomal recessive condition most commonly seen in Pennsylvania Amish.

Elmslie-Trillat transplant: Relocation of tibial tuberosity to reinforce anteromedial capsule after release of lateral retinaculum; transferred bone should be in line of axis of femur when knee is flexed to 45°.

Eloesser flap: Procedure used for long-term drainage of empyema cavity. Modern variations involve removal of 2 ribs with skin sutured to pleura and packing of cavity with wet-to-dry dressings. Granulation obliterates cavity over months, and thoracoplasty or muscle flaps may hasten healing.

Elpenor disease: Intoxication hallucinosis; classically described after alcohol abuse. After partially awakening from sedative state, patient acts bizarrely or abnormally, esp. if in unknown surroundings.

Elsahy-Waters syndrome (bronchoskeletogenital syndrome): Rare association of hypospadias, cleft palate, jaw cysts, wide-set eyes, nystagmus, pectus excavatum, seizures, and mental retardation.

Elsberg syndrome: Acute urinary retention due to neurologic dysfunction in genital herpes.

Elsberg test: Used to distinguish location (intracerebral vs. extracerebral) of lesions affecting sense of smell; based on fatigability to odor detection and other functional variations.

Elschnig disease (pearls): Chronic conjunctivitis seen after lens trauma or cataract removal; usu. mild visual loss, pain, and itching. Foamy, large globules (Elschnig pearls) form on conjunctiva. Treatment is antibiotics and topical anti-inflammatory drugs.

Elschnig disease: Congenital lower eyelid ectropion, wide-set eyes, laterally lengthened palpebral fissures, and frequent cleft palate.

Elschnig spots (acute): Localized yellow areas visible in retinal pigment epithelium on ophthalmoscopic exam, which represent hypertensive choroidopathy; caused by fibrinoid necrosis within choriocapillaris.

Elschnig spots (chronic): Darkened pigment areas developing over several weeks in areas of acute yellow Elschnig spots.

Elsner asthma: Angina pectoris.

Elson middle slip test: Evidence of ruptured central extensor tendon slip of proximal interphalangeal joint. When finger is flexed 90°, central slip is intact; if proximal interphalangeal joint can extend and distal interphalangeal joint is flail, central slip is not intact.

Ely sign: Indicator of femoral nerve irritation, lateral thigh contracture, or tightness of rectus femoris if prone patient flexes calf onto thigh and gluteus muscles retract and hip abducts.

Embden-Meyerhof-Parnas pathway (glycolysis): Common pathway for fermentation of glucose seen in microbial metabolism. Aldolase and kinase transform G6P to 2 triose phosphates with net gain of 2 ATPs and either lactate or ethanol, depending on microbial species.

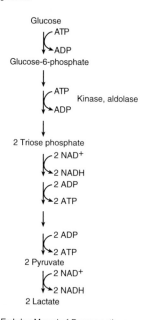

Embden-Meyerhof-Parnas pathway

Emerson effect: Increase in photosynthesis efficiency in plant cells if long exposure to long-wavelength energy is supplemented by simultaneous exposure to short-wavelength energy.

Emery-Dreifuss syndrome (muscular dystrophy): Onset in early childhood of slowly progressive muscle weakness starting in legs (children walk on tip-toe) followed by weakness in shoulder muscles; atrial conduction abnormalities, chest pain, and recurrent syncope occur in young adulthood. Condition may be associated with mental retardation. Disease severity varies widely. Inheritance is X-linked, and syndrome occurs almost exclusively in males; female carriers may develop heart block. Type 2 muscle fibers predominate. Gene defect is in Xq28 region.

Emery-Nelson syndrome: Mental retardation, stunted growth, claw toes, flat facies, and deformities of hands; congenital condition with variable penetrance.

Emmert-Gellhorn pessary: Hollow-stemmed instrument placed into vagina to support uterus or rectum mechanically; variation of Gellhorn pessary.

Emmet operation: Surgical repair of laceration in perineum.

Emmet operation: Suture repair of lacerated uterine cervix.

Emmet operation: Creation of vaginal-urinary bladder fistula to allow drainage of urine in cystitis; largely abandoned technique.

Emmon modification: See Sabouraud agar.

Emmonsia: Now classified as *Chrysosporium*.

Emmonsiella (*Ajellomyces*): Heterothallic fungi similar to Ascomycetes; contains *E. capsulata*, which is form of *Histoplasma capsulatum capsulatum* and *H. capsulatum duboisii*.

Ender nails: Long, flexible metallic strips usually placed multiply in humeral medullary to fix humeral fractures.

Endo agar (medium): Medium used to culture and identify *Salmonella typhi*; contains lactose, fuchsin, sodium sulfite, and soda solution.

Engebretsen technique: Procedure for repair of torn anterior cruciate ligament; uses anteromedial incision to form small tunnel in tibia. 8-mm Kennedy LAD is passed into joint through tunnel, intercondylar notch, and posterior capsule. Tension is then applied to proximal LAD to tighten attached anterior collateral ligament stump and pull it towards femoral stump.

Engel alkalimetry: Method for determining blood alkalinity; uses titration of litmus paper with known amounts of tartaric acid, which turn litmus paper red.

Engel disease: Congenital myasthenia gravis.

Engel syndrome: Rare deficiency in skeletal muscle carnitine; marked by childhood onset of progressive weakness with variable cardiomyopathy. Treatment is daily carnitine; steroids, and a high-carbohydrate, low-fat diet.

Engel-Aring syndrome (transient Cushing disease): Intermittent hypothalamic discharge occurring every 2 weeks to months. Episodes last 3–5 days and are marked by tachycardia, hypertension, depression, nausea, vomiting, and weight fluctuation; also with abdominal striae and obesity but absence of buffalo hump. Treatment is dexamethasone.

Engel-von Recklinghausen disease (von Recklinghausen disease type 2): Renal osteodystrophy marked by end-stage kidney disease and hyperparathyroidism.

Engelmann disease (progressive diaphyseal dysplasia): Cortical bone disease with increased bone density (less severe than Albers-Schonberg disease) and abnormal tubulation in long bones; variable occurrence in flat bones. Cortical thickening occurs in midshaft area and progresses toward epiphyses.

Engels catarrh: See Bostock catarrh.

English sweating fever: Pestilence and death occurring during Middle Ages in Great Britain; occurred in several epidemic-like episodes.

Engstrom respirator: Device that provides sine wave airflow via a piston-driven, volume-controlled device.

Enroth sign: Eyelid fullness seen in Graves disease.

Entner-Doudoroff pathway: Alternate pathway of glucose fermentation in microbial metabolism. Unique step is dehydration with G-phospho-gluconate with production of pyruvate and triose phosphate.

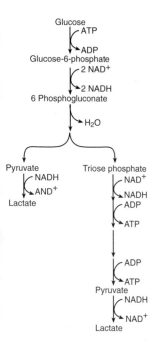

Glucose

ATP

ADP

Glucose-6-phosphate

2 NAD⁺

2 NADH

6 Phosphogluconate

H_2O

Pyruvate

NADH

AND⁺

Lactate

Triose phosphate

NAD⁺

NADH

ADP

ATP

ADP

ATP

Pyruvate

NADH

NAD⁺

Lactate

Entner-Doudoroff pathway

Epley maneuver: Canal repositioning maneuver used to treat benign paroxysmal positional vertigo; can be performed in office by otolaryngologist. Treatment has long-term effectiveness.

Epstein disease: Deafness, glomerulonephritis, and variable aortic cystic medial necrosis in association with megathrombocytopenia.

Epstein nephrosis: Chronic tubular kidney inflammation; associated with hypothyroidism and other endocrine disorders.

Condition is most common in young women.

Epstein pearls: Small, whitish, gingival cysts found in midline of hard palate in newborns, which disappear several weeks after birth; due to retained secretions.

Epstein-Barr virus: DNA virus associated with Burkitt lymphoma, nasopharyngeal cancer and lymphoma in transplant recipients, and mononucleosis. 80%–90% of healthy adults have EBV antibodies.

Erb atrophy: See Duchenne muscular dystrophy.

Erb disease: Juvenile muscular dystrophy; onset usu. at 20–39 years of age, with proximal arm muscle most commonly involved first (Erb-type) or, rarely, lumbosacral region muscles involved first. Facial muscles are involved late in disease. Condition is usu. slowly progressive with somewhat shortened life span.

Erb palsy (Erb-Duchenne palsy): Arm on affected side shows adducted shoulder, extended elbow, pronated forearm, and flexed wrist—"porter's tip" position; caused by disruption of upper roots (C5–C7) of brachial plexus due to acute, severe flexion of spine in opposite direction from side of injury. Condition can occur in motorcyclists who skid on crash helmet, in birth injuries, or in gun shots to shoulder.

Erb point: Anatomic point located at angle formed by

clavicle and posterolateral edge of sternocleidomastoid (2–3 cm above clavicle at C6 level). Electrodes testing motor conduction of brachial plexus are best placed here.

Erb-Charcot disease: Rare involvement of spinal cord in syphilis; manifests several years after primary infection with gradual progression to paraplegia. Condition does not respond well to antibiotics.

Erb-Goldflam disease: Myasthenia gravis.

Erben reflex: Slowing of pulse when head and torso are quickly tilted forward to 90°; caused by vagal stimulation.

Erdheim disease (Gsell-Erdheim disease): Cystic necrosis of aorta, often with acute rupture; usu. seen as part of Marfan disease but may occur alone.

Erdheim disease (Scaglietti-Dagnini disease): Variant of acromegaly, with hypertrophy of vertebrae, disks, and clavicles; leads to pain and kyphosis.

Erdheim necrosis (cystic medial necrosis): Degeneration of medial layer of aorta with necrosis of elastic fibers, cyst formation, and mucoid infiltration; usu. results in aortic dissection.

Erdheim-Chester disease: Systemic xanthogranulomatosis with infiltration of kidney, heart, lungs, retroperitoneum, and (rarely) eyeball with yellow eyelid nodules. Treatment is systemic corticosteroids.

Erhard test: Used to detect malingering in deafness.

Erich arch bar: Intermaxillary fixation device; made of malleable alloy.

Erichsen sign: Indication of sacroiliac etiology of back pain if forcefully compressing iliac bones together worsens discomfort.

Erlenmeyer flask: Glass container with flat base and funnel-shaped body.

Ermengen bacillus (van Ermengen bacillus): *Clostridium botulinum;* gram-positive rod that causes botulism.

Erni sign: Cavernous tympany heard over previously filled apical cavity.

Ernster-Luft syndrome: Hypermetabolic state with normal thyroid function and tests, with sweating, intense thirst, weakness, increased body temperature and tachycardia; caused by defect in oxidative phosphorylation with mitochondrial respiration not coordinated with phosphorylation.

Erwinia: Facultatively anaerobic, gram-negative, motile rod. Bacterium is primarily pathogenic in plants; can cause human septicemia if contamination occurs in IV solutions.

erythroplasia of Queyrat: Squamous carcinoma-in-situ of

vulva or penis. Treatment is complete excision with frozen section evaluation of margins.

Escamilla-Lisser syndrome: 1930s term for presentation of visceral manifestations of hypothyroid disease in absence of significant external signs; marked by ascites; atony of heart, bowel, and bladder; and menorrhagia and anemia.

Escat procedure: Surgical ligation of internal maxillary artery via transmaxillary sinus approach.

Escheler disease: Congenital lateral deviation in muscle movements.

Escherich bacillus: *Escherichia coli.*

Escherich sign: Contraction of lip, tongue, and jaw muscles after inner lip or tongue is tapped; seen in tetany.

Escherichia: Gram-negative rod found normally in GI tract; only species is *E. coli.* Bacterium is occ. pathogenic in gut (traveler's diarrhea) and causes serious CNS, urinary, and peritoneal infections. Some strains produce exotoxins and mimic shigellosis.

Espildora-Luque syndrome: Ophthalmic artery embolus with reflex spasm of middle cerebral artery; causes unilateral blindness and transient contralateral hemiplegia.

Esser operation (epithelial inlay operation): Technique to reepithelialize deep and chronically nonhealing wound; uses placement of epithelialized graft of epidermis in wound for 10 days with subsequent removal of this mold.

Essex-Lopresti fracture: Comminuted radial head injury with dislocation of distal radioulnar joint; results from forearm injury.

Essig splint: Method for stabilizing fractured tooth; uses thin stainless steel filament wrapped around (lingually and labially) part of dental arch and secured using individual ligature wires around teeth.

Estes operation: Surgical technique to improve fertility in absence or pathology of Fallopian tubes; ovary is moved from normal anatomic position and reimplanted into uterine cornu.

Estlander flap: "Lip switch" flap similar to Abbe flap but used in reconstructing lateral defects involving lateral commissure; uses triangular tissue flap, most commonly from lower lip.

Estlander operation: Largely abandoned surgical procedure using resection of ribs in empyema to allow collapse of chest wall to close empyema cavity.

Estren-Dameshek syndrome: Congenital aplastic anemia in absence of developmental abnormalities.

Eternod sinus: Plexus connecting vessels of chorion and inferior yolk sac.

Euro-Collins solution: Organ preservation solution used for cold storage of organs since 1970s.

European blastomycosis (torulosis): Systemic cryptococcosis via respiratory infection due to cryptococcus neoformans serotypes A, B, C and D; seen most commonly in HIV. Condition causes meningitis, organomegaly, and skin nodules. Prophylaxis is fluconazole. Treatment is amphotericin.

European hookworm: *Ancyclostoma duodenale;* parasitic intestinal nematode found in humans and other mammals.

European tarantula (wolf spider): *Lycosa tarentula;* bite is poisonous.

Eustace Smith sign: See Smith sign.

Eustachian tube: Canal connecting nasopharynx and inner ear extending from anterior wall of tympanic cavity and running inferiorly, medially, and anteriorly; has bone and cartilage components.

Evans blue (T-1824): Bluish powder injected intravenously to act as dye in measuring blood volume.

Evans syndrome: Idiopathic thrombocytopenia with variable purpura and hemolytic anemia; associated with dermatomyositis and pregnancy.

Eversbusch operation: Surgical correction of upper eyelid ptosis; uses resection of levator muscle through external skin incision.

Ewald node (sentinel node): Enlarged supraclavicular node; may herald intra-abdominal tumor.

Ewald tube: Large-bore plastic tube used to aspirate stomach contents.

Ewald-Hudson dressing forceps: Short, straight, thin-tipped device with tweezer-type handle and horizontal tip serrations.

Ewart sign: Dullness to percussion at lower left scapular angle seen in pericardial effusion.

Ewing sarcoma: Aggressive malignant small cell tumor of bone forming histologic pseudorosettes; usu. occurs in males before 25 years of age. Condition can occur in any bone, but long bones (esp. around knee) are most commonly affected; causes pain and swelling and often complaints of mild trauma preceding presentation. "Onion-skinning" is apparent on radiography.

Ewing sign: Indication of frontal sinus outlet obstruction if tenderness occurs at upper inner orbital angle.

Ewingella: Bacterium belonging to Enterobacteriaceae; occ. seen in human infections.

Faber anemia (Hayem-Faber anemia, Kasnelson anemia, Kilud-Faber anemia, Witt anemia): Currently used to describe hypochromic anemia and achlorhydria; clinical features similar to pernicious anemia.

Faber test: See Patrick test.

Fabricius bursa: Origin of B lymphocytes in birds; forms as epithelial outpouching of gut.

Fabry disease (Anderson-Fabry disease, Ruiter-Pompen disease, Sweeley-Klionsky disease): Inborn error of glycosphingolipid metabolism; marked by tiny red punctate lesions of skin, corneal and lens opacities, hypohidrosis, acroparesthesias, and vascular disease of internal organs. X-linked recessive condition is caused by deficiency in α-galactosidase A with accumulation of ceramide trihexoside in endothelial cells, fibrocytes, and pericytes.

Faget first sign: Tachycardia with high fever and subsequent bradycardia (50 beats/min) with continuing high fever in 24–48-hour period; occurs in 1st stage of classical presentation of yellow fever.

Faget second sign: Development of shock with increased pulse rate secondary to bleeding; occurs in late stage of classical presentation of yellow fever.

Fahr disease: Symmetric cerebral calcification with clinical presentation ranging from mild rigidity, athetosis, and dystonia to Parkinson's disease; also with mental retardation. Calcific deposits occur in basal ganglia and capillary walls. Inheritance patterns are variable.

Fahr-Volhard disease: Acute onset of chronic or episodic headache, abdominal pain, weight and visual loss, dyspnea, diastolic pressure > 130 mm Hg, cardiomegaly, and neurologic deterioration. Treatment is aggressive antihypertensive medications, dialysis, and kidney and/or heart transplantation.

Fahraeus-Lindqvist effect: Occurrence of lower blood viscosity in small-diameter vessels (< 1.5 mm) vs. large-diameter vessels; due to movement of blood cells in single file in smaller vessels.

Fahrenheit scale: Widely used temperature scale; H_2O boils at 212° F and freezes at 32° F.

Fahrenheit thermometer: Instrument that uses Fahrenheit scale to measure temperature.

Fairbank disease: Abnormally soft, mucinous hyaline cartilage in epiphyses. Condition manifests before puberty with pain on walking and coxa vara, genu valgum, shortened stature, stubby hands, and thickened nails.

Fairbanks changes: System now used to describe degenerative changes in knee seen on anterior-posterior radiographs. Grade 0, normal; grade 1, osteoarthritic changes from margin of femoral condyles; grade 2, joint space narrowing; grade 3, flattening of femoral condyle.

Fairbanks test (apprehension test): Used to detect dislocation of patella. Supine patient flexes knee to be tested to 30° while examiner slowly pushes patella laterally with thumbs. If patella is dislocated, patient reflexively tightens quadriceps muscle.

Fajans-Conn standards: Criteria used in scoring glucose tolerance test.

Fajersztajn sign: Indicator of sciatica, pain is caused by hip flexion of affected side when leg is straight; no pain is caused if hip flexion is performed when leg is flexed. Alternative description: pain occurring on affected side when leg is straight and contralateral hip is flexed.

fallopian aqueduct (facial canal): Superior foramina in fundus of internal auditory meatus; transmits facial nerve.

fallopian ligament: See Poupart ligament.

fallopian tube: Anatomic structure that carries ova from ovaries to uterus; 2 trumpet-shaped tubes emanating from superior uterus running in superior border of broad ligament. Segments are isthmus, ampulla, infundibulum, and fimbriae.

Falls-Kertesz syndrome: Double-row eyelids, leg lymphedema with hypoplastic or absent thoracic duct, photophobia, and variable webbed neck; autosomal dominant condition.

Falret disease (cyclothymia): Bipolar disorder.

Falta coefficient: Percentage of ingested sugar eliminated from body.

familial Mediterranean fever: Episodic fever, abdominal pain, chest pain and erysipelas; sometimes associated with amyloidosis. Condition occurs in Armenian and Sephardic Jews.

Fananas cell: Specialized glial cell in molecular layer in cerebral cortex.

Fanconi anemia: Aplastic anemia usu. appearing in childhood with renal failure, cardiac malformations, hyperpigmentation of skin, and hypoplastic radii or thumbs; carries 10% risk for acute myelogenous leukemia. Chromosomes show excessive fragility. Disease is associated with positive diepoxybutane test results. Condition is autosomal recessive.

Fanconi renotubular disease (adult-type) [Luder-Sheldon disease]: Same features as Fanconi-DeToni syndrome, with addition of fractures, pain, and later onset. Condition may occasionally result from delayed onset of congenital form but is usu. due to heavy metal poisoning or malignancy (esp. myeloma).

Fanconi-Bickel disease: Onset of glycogen accumulation in liver and kidney cells by 1 year of age with vitamin D–nonresponsive rickets; marked by increased serum alkaline phosphatase, hypophosphatemia, and hypoglycemia. Condition is autosomal recessive.

Fanconi-DeToni syndrome: Renal rickets with dwarfism; usu. resistant to vitamin D administration.

Fanconi-Hegglin disease: Positive serology for syphilis occurring in some viral pneumonias.

Fanconi-like syndrome: Chronic lung infections, recurrent pneumothorax, pancytopenia, osteomyelitis, and skin malignancy; rare autosomal recessive condition.

Fanconi-Tuerler syndrome: Congenital cerebellar ataxia, nystagmus, dysmetria, and mental retardation; unknown etiology.

Fansler proctoscope: Instrument inserted into rectum with inner trocar in place; trocar is removed to inspect lumen.

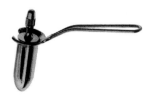

Fansler proctoscope

Far Eastern hemorrhagic fever: See Korean hemorrhagic fever.

Farabee syndrome: Fused middle phalanges, short proximal phalanges, thumb ankylosis (brachydactyly type A1), and variable mental retardation.

Farabeuf amputation: Leg amputation using large flap to close wound.

Farabeuf triangle: Anatomic area with borders formed by facial vein, hypoglossal nerve, and internal jugular vein.

farad unit: SI unit for electrical capacitance equal to 1 coulomb/volt.

Faraday effect: Result of planar rotation of polarized light seen when solutions are placed in magnetic field.

Faraday law (of electrolysis): Oxidization or reduction of 1 equivalent of chemical moiety requires 1 faraday of electrical charge.

Faraday law (of electromagnetic induction): Relationship between rate of change of magnetic field and resulting current.

faraday unit: Amount of electrical charge in 1 mole of electrons (96,487 coulombs).

faradic effect: Muscle contraction occurring when electrical frequency is $< 10,000$ cycles/sec.

Farber disease (lipogranulomatosis): Deficiency in ceramide trihexosidase with accumulation of ceramide and resultant disorder in sphingolipid metabolism. Manifests shortly after birth with mental retardation, hepatomegaly, joint swelling, and fatty infiltration of viscera. Autosomal recessive condition.

Farmer-Mustian syndrome: Episodic attacks of ataxia, vertigo, and diplopia with onset in childhood to early adulthood; associated with progressive cerebellar disease. Condition is autosomal dominant.

Farnsworth test (panel D-15 test): Used to detect abnormalities in color vision by testing ability to detect hue differentiation.

Farnsworth-Munsell test (100-hue test): Used to test color vision, esp. ability to detect differences in chromaticity. Macular pathology usu. has < 400 errors, whereas cone dystrophies usu. have > 500 errors.

Farr test: Measures capacity of radiolabeled antigen to bind with antibody (which is precipitated using ammonium sulfate); can be used for all immunoglobulin classes.

Farrant fluid: Acacia dissolved in glycerol and warm saline; used to form mounting medium with index of refraction of 1.43.

Farre tubercles: Palpable masses beneath capsule occurring in liver cancer.

Farre white line: Area where mesovarium inserts into hilus of ovary.

Fasanella-Servat procedure: Surgical procedure used to correct mild ptosis of eyelid secondary to congenital or acquired involutional conditions or to correct Horner syndrome; does not affect final positioning or prominence of lid crease. Small stab wound in skin in lateral border of lid crease is made with eversion of upper lid; 2 small hemostats are clamped across superior tarsus, inferior Müller muscle, and conjunctiva (avoiding imbrication of skin and levator aponeurosis); 6–0 mattress suture is run 1 mm above hemostats, which are then removed; and tissue is resected at crush line. Suture is then run from medial to lateral to rejoin superior tarsal edge to inferior Müller muscle.

Faulk-Epstein Jones syndrome: Drooping of eyelids with posterior fusion of lumbosacral vertebrae.

Favre syndrome (Favre-Chaix syndrome): Venous stasis skin changes and ulcers occurring in legs; more common in males.

Favre-Racouchot syndrome: Chronic skin changes caused by prolonged and excessive exposure to sun; marked by thickened skin, comedones, and cysts caused by degeneration of collagen.

Fazekas criteria: Standards used on MRI to distinguish small vessel disease from multiple sclerosis lesions.

Fazio-Londe disease (atrophy): Progressive bulbar paralysis with onset in childhood; marked by loss of motor neurons in trigeminal, hypoglossal, facial, and ambiguous nuclei, as well as bilateral ptosis, facial weakness, dysarthria, and swallowing difficulty. Death occurs within 1–2 years of onset.

Feagin test: Used to detect inferior shoulder instability. Patient stands with arm extended out to side and parallel to floor with hand resting on examiner's shoulder, and examiner clasps hands on arm just distal to deltoid and pushes down. If patient grimaces or looks apprehensive, anterior-inferior instability is present.

Fechtner syndrome: Variant of Alport syndrome with macrothrombocythemia and cytoplasmic inclusions in eosinophils and neutrophils; also with sensorineural deafness, nephritis, and congenital cataracts.

Federici sign: Indicator of ruptured viscus and free air if cardiac sounds are auscultated over abdomen.

Feer disease: See Bilderbeck disease.

Fegeler disease: Nevus flammeus occurring in trigeminal nerve distribution with limb weakness and hyperesthesia.

Fehling solution: Sodium hydroxide, copper sulfate, and potassium tartrate solution used to detect solutes with reducing ability (e.g., sugars). Positive result is formation of yellow-red copper oxide precipitate.

Feingold diet: Diet postulated to reduce hyperkinetic behavior in attention deficit disorder; eliminates salicylates, preservatives [sodium benzoate, monosodium glutamate, butylated hydroxyanisole (BHA), butylated hydroxytoluene (BHT)] and artificial colors (esp. FD and C yellow no. 5) and flavors.

Feingold theory: Food additive and colors may cause hyperactivity in children; recent studies have suggested these substances may play role in 5% of cases of attention deficit disorder.

Feiss line: Imaginary line running between plantar surface of 1st metatarsal joint and medial malleolus.

Feldaker disease: Pain and edema in legs with purplish lesions, which may ulcerate; occurs most commonly in obese, middle-aged women in warm weather.

Feldenkrais method: Series of gentle, low-impact exercises to retard loss of muscle mass and movement; intended for elderly or recovering patients.

Felson silhouette sign:
Obscuring of lung interstitial
process by alveolar consol-
idation on chest radiograph.

Felton phenomenon:
Injection of pneumococcal
polysaccharide into mice,
causing immune unrespon-
siveness.

Felton unit: Amount of
antibody needed to protect
white Swiss mouse after being
injected with 1 million fatal
doses of pneumococcus culture;
considered equivalent to NIH
control serum P-11.

Felty neutrophils: Leukocytes
that bind antibodies in
idiopathic thrombocytopenic
purpura.

Felty syndrome:
Hypersplenism with splenomegaly, fever, recurrent
infections, rheumatoid arthritis,
pancytopenia, neuropathy,
recurrent infections, and leg
ulcers; associated with splenic
antibody production. Splenectomy may lessen symptoms.

Ferguson operation: Surgical
resection of internal hemorrhoids. Patient is placed in left
lateral decubitus position with
knees flexed.

Ferguson reflex:
Enhancement of uterine
contractions by mechanical
stretching of cervix.

Ferguson-Critchley ataxia:
Rare familial ataxia with onset
in middle adulthood; clinically
resembles multiple sclerosis.

**Ferguson-Smith epitheli-
oma:** Onset in middle-age of

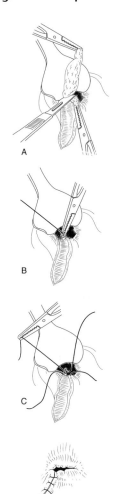

Ferguson operation

multiple, round, reddish skin
lesions with horny, crusty plug in
center; usu. heal over 2–3 months
but repeat attacks are norm.

Fergusson operation:
Resection of maxilla; uses incision running along border of nose and cheek and around ala to midline and bisects upper lip.

fermi (femtometer): Unit equal to 10^{-15} m.

fermium: Synthetic, radioactive element; atomic number, 100; most stable isotope, Fm-257; half-life, 100.5 days.

Fernandez reaction (lepromin test): Test using intradermal injection of suspension of heat-killed *Mycobacterium leprae*. Development of raised papule at 48–72 hours is positive result. Test is not diagnostic for leprosy; many people have cross-reactivity with this antigen.

Ferraro syndrome: 1920s term for adult-form leukodystrophy.

Ferrata cell: Hemohistioblast.

Ferrein ligament: External bands of temporomandibular joint capsule.

Ferrein process (medullary ray): Radiating portion of cortical lobule of kidney arranged axially; these tubules extend from cortex to base of medullary pyramid.

Ferrein tube: Spiral-shaped uriniferous tubules.

Ferriman-Gallwey scale: System for rating hair growth in 11 androgen-sensitive areas (lip, chin, chest, upper back, lower back, upper abdomen, arm, forearm, thigh, leg, and axilla): 0, no growth; 4, frankly virile; > 15, hirsutism.

Feulgen stain (Feulgen-Schiff reaction): Histochemical test for presence of DNA; uses acid hydrolysis to remove purine bases and open furanose ring of 2-deoxyribose, which exposes aldehyde groups. Development of red-purple color with addition of Schiff reagent is positive finding. Glucose, xylose, ribose, and RNA are Feulgen-negative.

fibers of Winslow: Fibrous tissue joining 2 crura of superficial inguinal ring.

Fick angle: Angle between gait direction and foot axis; provides more stable gait and better balance. Normal "angling out" is 5°–10°.

Fick law: Rate of diffusion of material or substance is proportional to its concentration gradient.

Fick phenomenon: Clouding of vision experienced by wearer of contact lenses. Some report seeing halos around light sources.

Fick principle: Blood flow rate equals organ uptake of indicator substance/(inflow indicator concentration—outflow indicator concentration); allows indirect measurement of blood flow through an organ using artificially introduced indicator substance.

Fick principle: Derivation of equation for oxygen saturation of blood; used in obstetrics to allow calculation of oxygen uptake of fetus and uterus by measuring oxygen content of blood from umbilical artery and vein, uterine vein, and maternal artery and the uterine and umbilical blood flow at any 1 time.

Fickler-Winkler syndrome: Atrophy of olivopontocerebellar tracts; clinical symptoms are identical to Menzel syndrome except for absence of involuntary movement and sensory disturbances.

Filipovitch sign: Yellowish coloration of soles and palms seen in typhoid fever.

Filippi syndrome: Mental retardation, syndactyly of toes and fingers, small head, and stunted growth.

Filatov disease (Filatow disease): Infectious mononucleosis.

Filatov-Dukes disease (fourth disease, rose rash): Fever and pink macular rash occurring on torso and neck and moving peripherally. Condition is seen in young children; caused by infection with human herpes virus 6.

Fincher syndrome: Rare combination of sudden onset of subarachnoid bleed accompanied by acute, severe sciatica; most common scenario is bleeding from cauda equina ependymoma precipitated by pregnancy.

Finkel-Biskis-Jinkins virus (FBJ virus): Antigen closely related to this virus may be cause of some animal osteogenic sarcomas.

Finkelstein test: Used to diagnose de Quervain tenosynovitis; also positive in basal joint arthrosis. Patient grasps thumb in palm; pain in radial area on

abrupt movement of hand toward ulnar side is positive finding.

Finn chamber test: Device for testing skin sensitivity; patch with small aluminum cups holding material to be tested for allergic reaction is taped against skin for 24–48 hours.

Finney pyloroplasty (U-shaped pyloroplasty): Incision of pylorus and 1st part of duodenum with reapproximation of anterior duodenal and pyloric margins; used to aid drainage of gastric antrum after selective or truncal vagotomy or vagal nerve interruption with esophagogastrectomy. Procedure is not indicated in duodenal scarring or inflammation or if duodenotomy is made to locate gastrinomas. Full Kocher maneuver should be performed in conjunction with this procedure. Inverted U-shaped incision is made with double-layer closure; 7–10-day gastric decompression is required postop.

Finnish nephrosis: Congenital nephrotic syndrome occurring in people of Finnish descent; marked by missing heparin sulfate sites in glomerular basement membrane. Death usu. occurs in 1st year of life. Condition is autosomal recessive.

Finochietto rib retractor: Large self-retaining retractor with crank handle to "wind open" retracting blades.

Fischer frame (Ace-Fischer frame): Partial ring monolateral bar external fixator for knee; sometimes used to stabilize tibial pilon fractures.

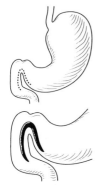

A. Schematic of incision

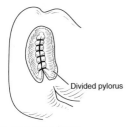

Divided pylorus

B. Closure of back wall

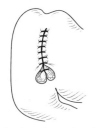

C. 2-layer closure of anterior wall

Finney pyloroplasty

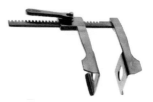

Finochietto rib retractor

Fischer projection: 2-D model of spatial ordering of organic compound; groups to right and left of each carbon are in front of page, and groups above and below are in plane behind page.

Fischer rat thyroid cell line (FRTL-5): Commonly used animal cell model for study of thyroid pathology in vitro; manifests majority of known in vivo responses to thyroid-stimulating hormone.

Fischer-Sargent-Drachman syndrome: Choreoathetosis of lower extremities; autosomal dominant condition with onset in infancy. Condition is not associated with seizures or mental deterioration.

Fischgold line (bimastoid line): Imaginary line at base of skull running from lower tip of one mastoid bone to lower tip of other.

Fish procedure: Cone-shaped wedge resection of femoral head to correct for chronic slipped capital femoral epiphysis.

Fishberg concentration test: Measures urine specific gravity of 3 urine specimens (morning void and after 1 and 2 hours) 12 hours after meal with < 200 ml of fluid in patient at bed rest; specific gravity < 1.024 indicates kidney impairment.

Fisher disease (one-and-a-half syndrome): Lesion in unilateral lower area of dorsal pontine tegmentum, which affects internuclear fibers of ipsilateral medial longitudinal fasciculus, abducens nucleus, and paramedian pontine reticular formation. Condition manifests as palsy of lateral gaze in 1 direction with internuclear ophthalmoplegia in other direction; also associated with slurred speech, vertigo, gait problems, and diplopia.

Fisher exact test: Statistical hypothesis test for homogeneity of 2×2 contingency tables; uses exact significance level (unlike chi-square test) and is useful in replacing this test when expected frequencies are small.

Fisher syndrome (Bickerstaff encephalitis, Miller-Fisher syndrome): Variant of Guillain-Barré syndrome marked by ophthalmoplegia, ataxia, and areflexia secondary to brainstem encephalitis.

Fisher-Adams syndrome: Transient global amnesia lasting 12–24 hours in absence of seizures, aphasia, or loss of consciousness. Triggers include sexual intercourse, pain, stress, or fatigue; possibly related to arterial hypertension and ischemia in inferomedial temporal lobes.

Fisher-Race hypothesis: Rh antigens (pairs Dd, Cc, and Ee) are inherited by each person in 2 sets of 3 antigens, with 1 set contributed by each parent.

Fisher-Race system: Notational description of Rh antigen blood group.

Fisher-Volavsek syndrome: Congenital sparse hair on eyebrows and eyelashes, thickened ends of fingers and toes, onychogryphosis, and later onset of syringomyelia-like symptoms.

Fishman-Doubilet test (rapid serum amylase test): Qualitative test used to determine amylase concentration. Small quantity of starch is mixed with serum and iodine for 5 minutes. Blue means normal level of amylase; yellow means high level of amylase.

Fisk position: Radiographic film technique using superior-inferior projection to image bicipital groove.

Fitch syndrome (Andre syndrome): Low-set ears, hypoplastic mandible, flattened nasal bridge, wide-set eyes, stunted growth, small thoracic cavity, and variable mental retardation; X-linked inheritance with full symptomatology in males. Respiratory infections usu. cause death in 1st 2 years of life.

Fite method: Xylene–peanut oil solution (preserves acid-fastness), Ziehl-Neelsen carbol fuchsin, and methylene blue used to stain lepra bacilli and other acid-fast microbes.

Fitz-Hugh-Curtis syndrome: Diffuse abdominal pain in women; also with fibrotic strands surrounding liver. Cause is classically described as intra-abdominal gonorrhea but also may be due to *Chlamydia*.

Fitzgerald factor (Fitzgerald-Williams-Flaujeac factor, high-molecular-weight kininogen factor): Blood coagulation cofactor; serves as plasma substrate for kallikrein and bradykinin precursors.

Fitzgerald-Williams-Flaujeac trait: Deficiency in high-molecular-weight kininogen; causes prolonged clotting time and PTT.

Flack node: See Keith node.

Flack test: Used to measure physical fitness by having patient take full breath and then blow as long as possible into 40–mm Hg manometer.

Flajani disease: See Graves disease.

Flatau law: Peripheral fibers in spinal cord are longer than more centrally located fibers.

Flechsig tract (direct cerebellar tract, dorsal spinocerebellar fasciculus): Ascending pathway traveling through medulla and inferior cerebellar peduncle.

Fleck syndrome: Diabetes insipidus associated with hypohidrosis, hypotrichosis, coloboma, and syndactyly.

Flegel disease (hyperkeratosis lenticularis perstans): Onset in 4th decade of reddish scaly papules on dorsal foot with progression to legs and dorsal hands; may be associated with higher risk of developing basal and squamous cell carcinoma of skin (in uninvolved areas).

Fleischmann bursa: Fluid-filled sac located beneath tongue.

Fleischner atelectasis: Linear disc-like shadow seen in lower 1/3 of lung field on chest radiograph; represents collapsed alveoli.

Fleischner sign: Radiographic finding highly suggestive of intestinal TB; patulous appearance of ileocecal valve (on both sides) secondary to ulcerations and fibrosis.

Fleming-Mayer flap: Multistage surgical technique for hair transplantation; modification of Juri procedure. Full-thickness scalp flaps from posterior parietal and temporal areas are swung anteriorly and superiorly to partially cover bald area with scalp resection to remove remaining bare skin. Procedure may require initial use of tissue expanders placed under scalp.

Flemming center (germinal center): Spherical collection of actively proliferating lymphocytes in center of lymph nodes, with surrounding capsule of elongated cells.

Fletcher factor (prekallikrein): Blood coagulation factor; active form (kallikrein) enhances Hageman factor. Deficiency is associated with prolonged activated PTT and impaired fibrinolysis and chemotactic activity but no bleeding diathesis; inheritance is autosomal recessive.

Fletcher-Suit system of radiotherapy: Variation of Manchester technique for applying intracavitary (intra-uterine) brachytherapy for cervical cancer; uses flexible "afterloading" system for radium or cesium.

Flexal virus: Arenavirus in Tacaribe complex; rodent is host animal.

Flexner bacillus: *Shigella flexneri*.

Flexner-Wintersteiner rosettes: Groups of tumor cells found in retinoblastoma, with clusters of low columnar cells around central lumen, basally located nuclei, and external limiting membrane-like structure. Morphology is specific for retinoblastoma.

Flier syndrome: Rare combination of acanthosis nigricans, muscle cramps, limb hypertrophy, and insulin resistance.

Flieringa ring: Circular ring placed on eyeball during eye surgery to prevent scleral collapse. Ring is usu. attached using 8 equally spaced 7–0 Vicryl sutures through conjunctiva and episclera and secured with 2 4–0 silk traction sutures at 6 and 12 o'clock positions.

Flint arcade: Arterial-venous anastomosis occurring at base of renal pyramids.

Flint syndrome (hepatorenal syndrome, Heyd syndrome): Progressive kidney failure (in absence of intrinsic kidney parenchyma pathology) due to severe renal arteriolar constriction caused by severe liver disease.

Floegel layer: Granular lamina found in lateral disk of muscle fiber.

Flood ligament: Superior ligament of shoulder joint.

Florence flask: Laboratory glassware with cylindrical neck and spherical body.

Flourens law: Stimulation of semicircular canal produces nystagmus corresponding to the plane of that canal.

Flower index (dental index): Used to describe head size; equals dental length × 100/ basinasal length.

Fluckiger syndrome: Familial hepatic disease, clubbing of digits, and cyanosis; eventually progresses to liver cirrhosis.

Flynn-Aird syndrome: Congenital cataracts, myopia, atypical retinitis pigmentosa, progressive sensorineural deafness, chronic ulcer, ataxia, epilepsy, and dementia.

Foerster syndrome (atonic-astatic syndrome): Congenital mental retardation, seizures, incontinence developing in childhood, and hypotonic muscles; unknown etiology but positive serology for syphilis in some cases.

Foerster-Fuchs spots: Discrete areas of epithelial pigment proliferation, usu. in association with myopic macular degeneration.

Foix syndrome: Lesion in anterior part of red nucleus causing cerebellar ataxia with hyperkinesis.

Foix-Alajouanine syndrome: Spastic paraplegia followed by flaccid amyotrophia; due to vasculitis or pathology of arteries supplying spinal column.

Foix-Chavany-Marie syndrome (bilateral perisylvan syndrome): Bilateral paralysis of movements controlled by CNs V, VII, IX, X and XII; usu. develops after 2nd or later cerebral infarct. Congenital cases due to failure of opercula to form completely have been reported.

Foix-Jefferson syndrome (clivus edge syndrome): Myosis followed by mydriasis, slow pupil response, and paralysis of extraocular muscles; due to increased intracranial pressure affecting oculomotor nerve. Causes include subdural hematoma, aneurysm, or tumor of temporal bone.

Foix-Thevenard syndrome: Tonic postural reflexes due to impairment of basal ganglia; sometimes occurs in Wilson disease, Parkinson's disease, and athetosis.

fold of Marshall: Tissue ridge on medial border of recess formed by left pulmonary artery passing inferior to aortic arch.

folds of Hoboken: Transverse intimal folds protruding into lumen of umbilical artery.

Folin-Ciocalteau reagent: Phosphorus–molybdic acid; used to qualitatively and quantitatively measure phenols, indole, imidazole, and compounds containing certain proteins and tyrosine. Reduced agent (blue color) is measured at 670 nm.

Folius muscle: Lateral ligament of malleus; triangular fibrous tissue running from posterior surface of incisura tympanica to neck or head of malleus.

Folling disease: Phenylketonuria.

Foltz valve: Membranous tissue at lacrimal canal.

Fontaine-Dake stent: Flexible, balloon-expandable, single tantalum wire intravascular stent under investigation for peripheral vascular applications. When expanded, stent has zigzag shape.

Fontan procedure: Surgical palliation of congenital cyanotic heart malformations (hypoplastic left heart, single ventricle, and tricuspid atresia); most commonly performed steps include closure of atrial septal defect and fashioning of valveless conduit between right atrium and pulmonary artery. Complications include low cardiac output, atrial arrhythmias, and obstruction of valveless conduit.

Fontan procedure (fenestrated): Technique of Fontan procedure with creation of 4-mm fenestration that allows right-to-left interatrial shunting and subsequent decompression of right atrium. Trial balloon closure is used before permanent closure is undertaken.

Fontan procedure (modified): Technique used for palliation of tricuspid atresia. Subpulmonic obstruction is relieved and right ventricle is enlarged with valved conduit or aortic homograft placed between right ventricular outflow tract and right atrium.

Fontana-Masson stain:
Method involving fixation in Bouin fluid or paraffin, ammoniacal silver nitrate solution, gold chloride solution, and sodium thiosulfate solution. Counterstain is then used to detect carcinoid tumors, melanoma, and pheochromocytoma. Carcinoid tissue stains brown, and argentaffin and melanin stain black.

Fontana-Masson technique:
Useful method for demonstrating presence of melanin. Sample to be tested is embedded in paraffin; substance that reduces metallic (esp. silver) salts gives positive result.

Fontana methamine–silver stain: Method used to visualize argyrophilic fibers that lie near nucleus in some cells and also argyrophilic fibers in connective tissue in lamina propria.

Fontana space: Space in iridocorneal angle of eye lying between pectinate ligament and trabeculae of sinus venosus; allows aqueous humor to move from anterior eye chamber to sinus lumen.

Foot-Hortega stain: Silver carbonate method that stains reticular lung fibers black.

foramen of Bochdalek: Site of most common diaphragmatic hernia in children; due to failure of fusion of posterolateral pleural-peritoneal folds.

foramen of Bochdalek hernia: Congenital diaphragmatic hernia; intra-abdominal contents herniate into chest, causing hypoplastic lung. Condition is more common on left side. Optimal treatment is stabilization of respiratory condition [including extracorporeal membrane oxygenation (ECMO)] and urgent (but not emergent) reduction.

foramen of Magendie:
Medial aperture of 4th ventricle; connects ventricle with subarachnoid space.

foramen of Monro
(interventricular foramen): Small round channel 2–4 mm wide, which connects lateral ventricle with 3rd ventricle; bounded anteriorly by anterior pillars of fornix and posteriorly by anterior tubercle of thalamus.

foramen of Morgagni hernia: Passage of intra-abdominal contents through small triangular area of diaphragm on either side of xiphoid; 90% of these hernias occur to right of xiphoid and are usu. asymptomatic, even in adults.

foramen of Pacchionius
(foramen ovale): Opening connecting posterior cranial fossa with cerebral cavity; anterior border is clivus (basilar groove), and posterolateral border is free edge of tentorium.

foramen of Rivini: Opening found in Shrapnell membrane in middle ear.

foramen of Vesalius:
Connection occasionally found between foramen rotundum and foramen ovale; carries a small vein from cavernous sinus.

foramen of Winslow (epiploic foramen): Opening connecting greater and lesser sac; bounded by caudate lobe of liver superiorly, duodenum inferiorly, interior vena cava posteriorly, and right margin of lesser omentum (containing common bile duct, hepatic artery, and portal vein) anteriorly.

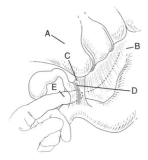

A. Liver
B. Lesser omentum
C. Hepatoduodenal ligament
D. Portal vein
E. Finger through foramen of Winslow

Foramen of Winslow

Forbes disease (Cori disease type 3, glycogenosis type 3): Most commonly occurring glycogenoses, with onset in infancy of weakness, hypotonia, fasting hypoglycemia, and hepatomegaly; associated with mild mental retardation and craving of sweets and carbohydrates. Condition often resolves later in childhood; disease frequently occurs in Israel. Cause is deficiency in debrancher enzyme (amylo-1, 6-glucosidase). Some patients progress to cirrhosis, cardiac failure, and progressive distal muscle wasting.

Forbes-Albright syndrome (Albright syndrome): Amenorrhea and galactorrhea in women with obvious pituitary or suprasellar tumor.

Forchheimer spots: Transient appearance of pinkish spots on soft palate that may coalesce; sometimes seen in rubella and heralds onset of skin rash.

Fordyce angiokeratoma: Multiply occurring dark red dilated venules (4 mm) found on scrotum and vulva; usu. associated with history of venous obstruction.

Fordyce disease (spots): Submucosal hyperplasia of sebaceous glands in buccal and labial areas.

Forel fields (Haubenfelder fields): Three separate areas of ventral thalamus designated as H, H1, and H2. Field H, which is considered to be the area where H1 and H2 merge, lies rostral to red nucleus and medial to subthalamic nucleus and contains fibers from rubrothalamic, pallidofugal, and dentatothalamic tracts. Field H1 roughly comprises thalamic fasciculus, and field H2 is lenticular fasciculus and area where it merges with ventral zona incerta and dorsal subthalamic nucleus.

Forestier-Rotes-Querol spondylosis: Ossification of anterior spinal ligaments with degeneration of intervertebral disks and growth of osteophytes, resulting in eventual ankylosis; occurs in elderly.

Formad kidney: Enlarged, misshapen kidney seen in chronic alcoholism.

formol-Müller fixative: Addition of formaldehyde to Müller fixative.

Forney syndrome: Congenital deafness, bony malformations, and heart defects.

Forsius-Eriksson syndrome (Aland disease): Mental retardation, seizures, retinal degeneration, partial deafness, myopia, nystagmus, and lack of pigmentation in macular area; occurs only in males, with females as carriers.

Forssel nomenclature: System used to describe stomach as containing four areas; fornix, corpus, sinus, and canalis egestorius.

Forssel sinus: Area of stomach with absence of mucosal folds; seen on radiography.

Forssell disease: Increase in RBC mass in setting of renal pathology, most commonly hypernephroma.

Forssman antibody: Immunoglobulin directed against Forssman antigen.

Forssman antigen: Loosely applied term for any substance that causes production of sheep hemolysin with resulting formation of different antibodies.

Förster choroiditis: Rare retinal manifestation of late syphilis; marked by diffuse pigmentation occurring along

major vessels and slowly progressive mixed hyperpigmentation and atrophic retinopathy.

Fort Bragg fever (pretibial fever): Onset of fever with patchy rash on lower legs or variably generalized rash; due to *Leptospira interrogans autumnalis* infection. Condition occurs primarily in U.S. and Japan; source of infection is unknown.

Foshay test: Positive for *Pasteurella tularensis* if tuberculin-like skin test reaction occurs when suspension is injected into skin.

Foshay-Mollaret fever: See Petzetakis disease.

fossa of Rosenmueller (pharyngeal recess): Invagination of lateral wall of nasal pharynx.

Foster Kennedy syndrome: Rare ipsilateral optic atrophy and contralateral papilledema occurring in about 1% of mass lesions (tumor, abscess) in frontal brain lobe.

Fothergill disease: Trigeminal neuralgia; marked by sharp shooting pain distributed over nerve pathways of trigeminal nerve, usu. starting at constant trigger point. Manual stimulation of point causes attack.

Fothergill operation: See Manchester operation.

Fothergill pill: Mercury (calomel), squill, and digitalis.

Fothergill sign: Used to differentiate palpable abdominal wall mass from intra-abdominal mass. Mass is located in abdominal wall if palpation is heightened when patient partially rises from supine position.

Fouchet reagent: 25 g trichloroacetic acid, 10 ml 10% ferric chloride solution, and 100 ml H_2O.

Fouchet stain: Indicator of bilirubin in urine if green color develops when Fouchet reagent is added.

Fountain syndrome: Sensorineural deafness, mental retardation, short stubby hands, full lips, and facial edema.

Fourier analysis (Fourier transform, harmonic analysis, spectrum analysis): Representation of waveform or mathematical function as sum of average direct current level and sine and cosine waves of various frequencies; used in electronics to describe effects of filters and amplifiers that boost each frequency component by amount independent of other frequency components.

Fourmentin index: Used to describe size of thoracic cage; equal to transverse diameter of thorax × 100/anteroposterior diameter of thorax.

Fournier gangrene: Severe infection and necrosis of scrotum and perineum in males; 50% mortality even with aggressive treatment. Most likely cause is *Clostridia* infection. Diabetes is risk factor; marked by subcutaneous crepitance and skin necrosis with foul-smelling, watery, grayish fluid. Necrosis of testicles implies thrombosis of testicular artery and intra- or retroperitoneal infection. Treatment is prompt extensive debridement to several-centimeter margin of healthy tissue and broad-spectrum antibiotics. Diverting colostomy may be beneficial.

Fournier test: Used to assess gait ataxia; performed by having sitting patient rise and walk and stop and turn around quickly at a signal.

Fournier tibia: Thickening and anterior bowing seen in congenital syphilis.

Foville fasciculus: Pontine longitudinal fasciculus.

Foville syndrome (type 1) [Foville-Bruechen syndrome, Foville-Laehmung syndrome]: Hemiplegia with ipsilateral facial paralysis and contralateral eye movement abnormalities (impaired lateral gaze or deviation to ipsilateral side).

Foville syndrome (type 2): Foville syndrome (type 1) with absence of facial nerve (CN VII) abnormality.

Foville-Wilson syndrome: Differing degrees of lateral convergence in the eyes; occurs in multiple sclerosis.

Fowler maneuver: Indicator of rheumatoid arthritis when taut ulnar band and ulnarly deviated intrinsic muscles are seen when digit is placed in normal axial position.

Fowler procedure: Transfer of tendon to restore metacarpophalangeal flexion.

Fowler procedure: Transfer of tendon to restore thumb opposition.

Fowler solution: Potassium arsenite solution.

Fowler test: Indicator of anterior shoulder instability when supine patient's shoulder is abducted and externally rotated and posterior force is applied to humerus. If movement is detected, then instability is present.

Fowler-Stephens procedure (orchiopexy): Surgical correction of undescended testes; can be performed either open or laparoscopically. Optimum age is 1 year in absence of hernia.

Fox sign: Ecchymosis of groin area/inguinal ligament; seen with retroperitoneal hemorrhage.

Fox-Fordyce disease (hidradenitis): Onset in adolescence of severe pruritus in axilla and groin caused by obstruction of sweat glands. Treatment is topical steroids and excisions.

Fraccaro syndrome: Type 1A Parenti-Fraccaro syndrome; hypervascular condition but otherwise with normal cartilage matrix and hypercellular bone. Male-to-female ratio is 2:1.

Fraenkel nodule: Development of growths on cutaneous blood vessels in typhus.

Fraga disease: Addisonian state caused by malaria infection.

Fraley syndrome: Congenital malformation of pelvocaliceal system marked by dilation of affected calices with corresponding atrophy of renal cortex; associated with variable pain, bleeding, and urinary infection.

Frame disease: Osteomalacia occurring in the axial skeleton; usu. with benign clinical course.

Franceschetti disease: See Crouzon disease.

Franceschetti disease (fundus flavimaculatus): Development of yellowish deposits surrounding macula lutea in adolescence or early adulthood; causes loss of central vision with intact peripheral vision.

Franceschetti-Kaufman disease: Damage to corneal epithelium caused by trauma (often herpes infection or previous foreign body); causes pain in eye on 1st opening and variable photophobia.

Franceschetti-Klein syndrome: Treacher Collins syndrome in setting of deafness, external ear abnormalities, and mandibular abnormalities.

Franceschetti-Their syndrome: Spinocerebellar degeneration, corneal atrophy, mental retardation, and multiple lipomas; autosomal recessive condition.

Francis test: Skin test for antibody bound to pneumococci; performed by injecting pneumococcal polysaccharide material into skin. Appearance of wheal with surrounding inflammation is positive.

Francis test: Indication of bile acid in urine if purple color develops when 2 g glucose, 15 g sulfuric acid, and specimen are layered sequentially in test tube.

Francisella: Small, aerobic, gram-negative coccobacillus. *F. tularensis* is virulent organism, causing tularemia in humans; it is transmitted by infected rabbits, fleas, and ticks.

Franco operation: Placement of suprapubic tube in bladder.

François syndrome (chondro-dermal corneal dystrophy): Hand and foot deformities, variable contractures and sub-luxations, and subcutaneous xanthomas; related to lipid storage dysfunction. Onset occurs at 1–2 years of age.

François-Evens syndrome: Development of ring-shaped opacity in corneal epithelium, usu. with benign and nonprogressive course.

François-Haustrate syndrome: Variant of hemifacial microsomia with coloboma in optic disk and microphthalmia.

François-Neetens syndrome (speckled corneal dystrophy): Flat, partially opaque lesions in corneal stoma; usu. does not affect vision. Condition is autosomal dominant, with onset in early childhood or later.

Frank lead system: Com-monly used lead placements in vector cardiography; 7 elec-trodes are used to describe transverse (X), vertical (Y), and sagittal (Z) planes.

Frank operation: See Ssabanejew-Frank operation.

Frank procedure: Nonsurgical pressure technique for creation of vagina in congenital absence. Patient presses successfully larger dilators onto perineum while in lithotomy position; firm pressure for 2 hours/day for several months is required for effectiveness.

Frank-Starling reaction: End-diastolic length of a cardiac muscle fiber (within certain limits) determines pumping force of contraction. Longer length corresponds to increased ventricular end-diastolic volume, causing more forceful contraction.

Fränkel apparatus: Orthodontic device used to provide correct oral function.

Frankel assessment: System used to describe severity of spinal cord injury below level of lesion. A (complete), no motor or sensory reflexes; B (sensory), some sensory reflexes intact but no motor; C, motor reflexes use-less; D (motor useful), sensory and functional motor reflexes, with ability to walk; E (recov-ery), normal sensory, motor, and sphincter reflexes but may retain abnormal reflexes on testing.

Frankel line: White line tracing outer margins of bony epiphysis on plain film; seen in scurvy.

Fränkel sign: Loss of tonicity in hip joint muscles; seen in tabes dorsalis.

Fränkel sign: Excessive laxity of hip joint on passive flexion; seen in tabes dorsalis.

Fränkel test: Evidence of anterior accessory sinus infection if pus is seen in middle meatus after sitting patient bends close to knees and turns head to one side.

Frankenhäuser block: Injection of regional anesthesia into Frankenhäuser ganglion during childbirth.

Frankenhäuser ganglion: Nerve ganglion of visceral sensory fibers from the uterus, cervix, and upper vagina; lies just lateral to cervix.

Frankl-Hochwart syndrome: Neurologic condition marked by Bell palsy, vertigo, and peripheral-type nystagmus.

Franklin disease (γ heavy chain disease): Rare form of plasma cell dysfunction, marked by hepatosplenomegaly, lymphadenopathy, and predisposition to lymphoma; usu. with hypoalbuminemia and normal total serum protein. Cause is overproduction of Fc fragments of γ heavy chains.

Franz sign: Disappearance of palpable thrill after ligation of venous limb of arteriovenous fistula.

Fraser syndrome (Meyers-Schwickerath syndrome, Ullrich-Feichtiger syndrome): Congenital cryptophthalmos (hidden eye), gross abnormality of eyelids, deafness, cleft palate, separated symphysis pubis, abnormal digits, renal hypoplasia, and cardiac abnormalities; autosomal recessive condition with unknown etiology.

Fraser syndrome (infantile hypophosphatasia): Onset of rickets at 6 months of age; also with hypercalcemia, bulging anterior fontanelle, papilledema, proptosis, brachiocephaly, and variably, blue sclera. Predisposition to pneumonia occurs; 50% of fatalities due to this disease result from respiratory infections.

Frauenhofer zone (far field): Area located away from ultrasound transducer where sound waves diverge and pressure wave amplitude decreases at fairly uniform rate. Distance is determined by frequency of sound waves and radius of transducer.

Frazier-Spiller operation: Retrogasserian neurotomy for treatment of idiopathic trigeminal neuralgia; uses approach through middle cranial fossa.

Fredet-Ramstedt operation: Type of pyloromyotomy.

Freeman-Sheldon syndrome (whistling face): Small mouth, dimpling of chin, small nose, equinovarus H -shaped feet, growth retardation, scoliosis, and kyphosis; normal intelligence. Condition is congenital; may be sporadic or autosomal dominant inheritance. Treatment is multiple surgeries on bone/soft tissue.

Freer septum elevator: Delicate, handheld device with

rounded, thin ends; used to loosen atherosclerotic plaque from arterial wall or to separate nasal mucosa and cartilage.

Freer septum elevator

Freese syndrome: Condition that is clinically similar to Costen disease with initiating event through stimulation of myofascial trigger zone (cold, heat, needle stimulation).

Fregoli illusion: Psychiatric disturbance in which patient thinks stranger, a persecutor, is changing appearances to resemble familiar people (e.g., physician, nurse, bus driver); considered variant of Capgras syndrome.

Frei antigen: Antigenic material made from lymphogranuloma venereum organisms cultured in chick embryos.

Frei test: Skin test used for diagnosis of lymphogranuloma venereum; performed by injecting partially purified suspension of chlamydiae into skin. Positive finding is appearance of red indurated lesion > 6 mm within 48 hours.

Freiberg disease: Aseptic necrosis of 2nd metatarsal head ("crushing" type osteochondritis); seen mostly in adolescence.

Freiberg infraction (osteochondrosis of metatarsal head): Overgrowth of bone usually seen in 2nd metatarsal head and occasionally in 3rd,

4th, and 5th metatarsals with anterior foot pain on walking. Also with swelling and erythema. Treatment is surgery performed after resolution of acute episodes and in more severe cases.

Freire-Maia syndrome: Rare congenital absence of the hands and forearms and foot, fibula, and distal 1/3 of tibia; possible retention of Bohomoletz bone. Condition is autosomal recessive.

Frejka splint (pillow): Placement of pillow between thighs of infant to hold legs in flexion and abduction; early technique to correct congenital hip dislocation.

French chalk: Talc.

French-American-British classification: System used to describe categories of acute leukemia. *Acute myelocytic leukemia*—M_1, acute myelocytic leukemia without differentiation; M_2, acute myelocytic leukemia with differentiation (predominantly myeloblasts and promyelocytes); M_3, acute promyelocytic leukemia; M_4, acute myelomonocytic leukemia; M_5, erythroleukemia. *Acute lymphocytic leukemia*—L_1, predominantly "small" cells (twice size of normal lymphocyte), homogeneous population; L_2, larger than L_1, more heterogeneous population; L_3, "burkitt-like" large cells, vacuolated abundant cytoplasm.

Frenkel syndrome: Sequelae of trauma to anterior eye; marked by iris dehiscence, lens opacity, and subluxation and pigment particles behind lens. Condition may arise months to years after injury.

frenum of Morgagni: Fold closely associated with ileocecal valve that partially encircles lumen of colon; is made of joined extremities of valve.

Frenzel lenses: Specialized, 10-diopter lenses that distort vision and make fixation impossible; useful when trying to provoke or screen for nystagmus.

Fresnel fringe: Technique of overfocusing to correct astigmatism in transmission electron microscopy.

Fresnel lens (prism): Soft plastic lens used in eyeglasses to relieve diplopia with prismatic correction.

Fresnel lens: Lens formed by concentric steps cut onto lens surface; acts like much thicker lens.

Fresnel plate: Aperture made of concentric rings that allows entry of gamma rays into gamma camera. Plates form bulls-eye pattern when combined with alternating lead rings.

Fresnel zone (near field): Area near ultrasound transducer where pulses have highly variable pressure amplitude. Area is function of acoustic lenses that shape sound beam, curvature of transducer, and constructive and destructive interferences of 3-D waves.

Freund anomaly: Shortened 1st rib causing decreased expansion of ipsilateral lung apex.

Freund complete adjuvant: Oil- or lipid-based emulsion of an antigen and killed myco-bacteria; elicits much stronger antibody response and cell-mediated reaction than antigen alone.

Freund incomplete adjuvant: Oil-based emulsion of antigen without addition of mycobacteria.

Freund operation: Largely abandoned technique of resecting chest wall cartilage in attempt to improve chest wall mechanics and respiration.

Frey hairs: Handle-mounted stiff bristles used for testing skin sensitivity at pressure points.

Frey procedure: Longitudinal pancreaticojejunostomy (Puestow procedure) with addition of local resection of pancreas overlying ducts of Santorini and Wirsung. This cavity is connected to main pancreatic duct, which is drained by jejunostomy.

Frey syndrome (Baillarger syndrome, Dupuy syndrome, gustatory sweating, von Frey syndrome): Unilateral flushing of face, sweating of cheek and ear lobe and decreased heat sensation; due to injury to parotid gland. When present, condition can be elicited by eating chocolate or hot, spicy food. Previous treatment was procaine injection into auriculotemporal nerve at tragus. One current treatment involves botulinum injection.

Freyer method: Transvesical prostatectomy.

Freyer operation: Largely abandoned technique of suprapubic enucleation of prostate for benign prostatic hypertrophy.

Friderichsen test: Indicator of vitamin A deficiency if stronger or weaker than normal light stimulus causes oculomotor reflex.

Frieburg personality inventory: Self-report inventory used to evaluate presence of personality traits; similar to Minnesota Multiphasic Personality Inventory.

Fried syndrome: Complex of dystrophic nails (thin and brittle); thin, short hair; and few, peg-shaped teeth; autosomal recessive condition.

Fried-Emery syndrome (spinomuscular atrophy type 2): Infantile muscular dystrophy with onset at 3–12 months of age; marked by symmetric proximal muscle wasting and weakness and decreased tendon reflexes. Cause is defect in chromosome 5; condition is autosomal recessive.

Friedländer bacillus: *Klebsiella pneumoniae.*

Friedman test: Early (1950s), reliable test for pregnancy based on detection of gonadal stimulation in experimental animals by human chorionic gonadotropin.

Friedman-Roy syndrome: Mental retardation, slow speech, strabismus, and choroid plexus calcification; congenital autosomal recessive condition.

Friedreich ataxia: Autosomal recessive condition marked by ataxia, speech impairment, cardiomyopathy, diabetes mellitus, absent reflexes, lateral curvature of spine, and sclerosis of dorsal and lateral spinal cord columns; usu. onset during puberty.

Friedreich disease: Onset in adulthood of brief, clinical muscle contractions affecting single motor compartment that worsen with stimulation and disappear with sleep; associated with other neurologic diseases. Condition can occur in familial pattern with autosomal dominant inheritance. Treatment is valproic acid, clonazepam, and 5-hydroxytryptophan.

Friedreich phenomenon: Increased pitch in skodaic resonance of inspiration in pleuritis.

Friedreich symptom (paramyoclonus multiplex): Paroxysmal contractions of trunk and extremity muscles every 1–2 seconds following severe stressor such as trauma, infection, fright, or exhaustion. Spasms disappear with intentional movements and during sleep and are aggravated with emotional stimulation.

Friedreich-Auerbach syndrome (hypertrophic myopathy): Slow, painful enlargement of muscles with variable hyperhidrosis; X-linked recessive condition seen in males 10–20 years of age. Condition may affect any muscle (except heart), including tongue; limbs most often involved. EMG is normal.

Friedrich sign: Emptying of cardiac veins during diastole; caused by constrictive pericarditis.

Frisch bacillus: *Klebsiella pneumoniae rhinoscleromatis*.

Fritzsche syndrome: See Chavany-Brunhes syndrome.

Froehlich syndrome: Obesity, hypogonadism, diabetes mellitus, headache, and mental retardation due to hypothalamic dysfunction (usually midhypothalamic tumor); more common in males.

Fröhlich dystrophy: See Babinski-Fröhlich syndrome.

Froimson-Oh technique: Method used for repair of tendon rupture of biceps brachii. Proximal end of tendon is detached from glenoid and then inserted through keyhole opening made in humerus at floor of bicipital groove.

Froin syndrome: Presence of > 500 mg protein/100 ml in CSF in absence of frank purulence; also seen in chronic meningitis (especially syphilitic), tumor obstruction of the spinal subarachnoid space, and polyneuritis.

Froment sign: Clawing of 4th and 5th fingers and loss of normal extension of interphalangeal joint of the thumb when pinching together tips of thumb and index finger. Cause is ulnar nerve palsy leading to loss of adductor pollicus and deep head of flexor pollicis brevis. Sign is best elicited by having patient pinch piece of paper with thumb and index finger and having examiner try to withdraw it forcibly.

Frommann lines: Transverse lines on nerve axon visible after staining with silver nitrate.

Froriep ganglion: Collection of nerve cells found in embryo in lowest occipital segment.

Frost-Lang operation: Insertion of gold ball into empty eye socket after enucleation; largely of historical interest.

Fruchard orifice (myopectineal orifice): Anatomic area in groin with borders of transverse abdominal and internal oblique superiorly, iliopsoas laterally, pubic pecten inferiorly, and rectus abdominal medially.

Frund sign: Indicator of chondromalacia patella; positive finding is occurrence of pain on percussion when patient maintains sitting position and moves knee to different degrees of flexion while examiner percusses patella.

Frykman-Goldberg procedure: Surgical correction of rectal prolapse. Abdominal incision is made and rectum is completely mobilized (leaving lateral stalks intact). Rectum is sutured posteriorly to endopelvic fascia, and sigmoid resection is then performed to eliminate redundant colon.

Fryns syndrome: Cystic–adenomatoid malformation of viscera, cleft palate, broad and flat nasal bridge, redundant neck skin, and brachytelephalangy; congenital autosomal recessive with death in infancy.

Fuchs coloboma: Small, benign tumor of ciliary body epithelium.

Fuchs disease (blepharochalasis, Fuchs syndrome): Onset in young adulthood of recurrent edema in eyelid (upper more commonly affected than lower) with eventual herniation of periorbital fat and "baggy" eye pouches. Treatment is plastic surgery.

Fuchs dystrophy: Stromal corneal swelling with endothelial guttata; usu. manifests as epithelial edema on wakening and progresses to painless, blurred vision. Temporizing treatments are hypertonic eye drops and ointment, β-blockers, and warm air blown over cornea; when progression occurs, corneal transplant is required.

Fuchs method (modified): Radiographic positioning technique to view styloid processes of temporal bone; head is tilted 13° from horizontal with anterior-posterior direction of central x-ray.

Fuchs syndrome: Nonfebrile variant of Stevens-Johnson syndrome.

Fuchs syndrome (heterochromic uveitis): Color differences in irises, whitish keratic precipitates in cornea, and variable cataracts; onset usu. occurs from puberty to 4th decade. Patients may be predisposed to glaucoma and secondary open-angle glaucoma.

Fuchs syndrome (Fuchs-Kraupa syndrome, Groenouw-Fuchs syndrome): Corneal bullae, erosions and scarring, pain, photophobia, and vision abnormalities; most common in elderly women. Treatment is hypertonic solution and (in advanced cases) irradiation of lacrimal glands and corneal transplant.

Fuhs disease: See Brunauer syndrome.

Fukula operation: Removal of eye lens for treatment of severe myopia; largely of historical interest.

Fukuyama syndrome: Infantile muscular dystrophy with global weakness, mental retardation, large tongue, abnormal teeth, short fingers; and variable seizure disorders; seen primarily in Japan. Death occurs by 12 years of age, usu. because of respiratory infection.

Fuller operation: Rarely performed incision of perineum for drainage of seminal vesicles.

Fulton syndrome: See Adie-Critchley syndrome.

Fürbringer sign: Used to distinguish supraphrenic from subphrenic abscesses. Needle inserted into the abscess cavity shows respiratory movement if abscess is below diaphragm.

Gaenslen sign (test): Positive for sacroiliac cause of back pain if symptoms worsen when pressure is placed on hyperextended thigh with opposite thigh flexed.

Gaffkya: Gram-positive, anaerobic peptococcus.

Gage sign: Translucent "V" on lateral femoral head epiphysis; seen on anterior-posterior plain radiograph in Legg-Calvé-Perthes disease.

Gainsville simulator: Mannequin anesthesia simulator; capable of simulating noninvasive blood pressure measurements and palpable pulses.

Gaisböck syndrome: Mild polycythemia without leukocytosis and splenomegaly; occurs in obese, hypertensive, white, middle-aged men who usu. smoke. Condition may be related to social stressors (e.g. anxiety, overwork).

Galant reflex: Movement of pelvis and shoulders of newborn toward side of stimulation when paravertebral space is palpated when infant is in prone position; disappears at 8 weeks.

Galassi phenomenon: See Westphal pupillary reflex.

Galeati glands: See Brunner glands.

Galeazzi fracture: Fracture of radius with dislocation of ulnar head distally; usu. caused by blow to forearm. Injury most frequently occurs in children. Treatment requires surgical reduction.

Galeazzi sign: Indication of congenital hip dysplasia and functional shortening of femur if knees are at different levels when patient lies supine and flexes knees and hips at right angles.

Galen loop: Variably occurring sensory branch off recurrent laryngeal nerve that joins internal branch of superior laryngeal nerve.

Galen nerve (anastomosis): Small nerve connecting inferior and (usu. internal branch of) superior laryngeal nerve; runs within or posterior to posterior cricoarytenoid muscle.

Galen veins: Vessels formed at interventricular foramen by confluence of choroid and thalamostriate veins; veins run backward, drain basal nuclei, and join at corpus callosum splenium to create cerebral vein.

Gall body: Lipid-containing lymphocyte vacuole; best seen using phase microscopy.

Gallaudet fascia: Deep investing perineal fascia; runs next to bulbospongiosus muscle.

Gallavardin disease (blockypnea): Inhibition of breathing on exertion, with resolution during rest periods; occurs in patients with angina.

Gallavardin effect (phenomenon): "Softening" and slight increase in pitch of midsystolic murmur heard in older patients with aortic stenosis.

galenic system: See vein of Galen.

Gallie spinal fusion: Cervical spinal fusion using wire around C1 lamina and C2 spinous process.

Galloway-Mowat syndrome: Congenital hiatal hernia, microcephaly, vomiting with 1st feeding, glomerulosclerosis, and large ears; autosomal recessive with unknown etiology. Death occurs by 3 years of age.

Galveston Orientation and Amnesia test (GOAT): Test for posttraumatic amnesia.

Gambian sleeping sickness (trypanosomiasis): More chronic and less fatal variant of African sleeping sickness; caused by *Trypanosoma brucei gambiense* via bite of infected tsetse fly (*Glossina*). Early stages are intermittent rash, fever, and edema, followed by lethargy, seizures, coma, and death.

Gambian trypanosomiasis: See Gambian sleeping sickness.

Gamna-Favre bodies: Cytoplasmic inclusion bodies found in lymphogranuloma venereum.

Gamna-Gandy bodies (siderotic nodules): Yellow-brown nodules seen in enlarged spleens due to splenic congestion; represent hemosiderin deposits in perifollicular locations.

Gamstorp disease (adynamia, Westphal hyperkalemia): Familial episodic paralysis with presence of hyperkalemia and recurrent flaccid paralysis with areflexia; attacks last hours to days. Condition occurs suddenly during periods of rest after activity and can be provoked with potassium administration.

ganglion of Valentine: Nerve fibers located at junction of posterior and middle branches of superior dental plexus.

ganglion of Wrisberg (cardiac ganglion): Sympathetic and parasympathetic nerve fibers usu. found in association with superficial cardiac plexus on right side of ligamentum arteriosum.

Ganser syndrome: Psychiatric disturbance of consciousness, with memory lapses, hallucinations, and nonsensical responses to questions; usu. appears suddenly in adolescents and young adults. Condition is transient with complete recovery but can recur.

Gänsslen disease: 1920s term for bone abnormalities seen in setting of hemolytic syndromes.

Gänsslen disease (familial neutropenia): Chronic neutropenia with infections varying from asymptomatic to severe and recurrent. Disorder is usu. associated with periodontal infection and clubbing.

Gantzer muscle: Anomalous head of flexor profundus or pollicis longus muscle; originates from ulnar coronoid process or medial epicondyle. Muscle is associated with anterior interosseous nerve compression.

Ganzfield stimulation (full-field stimulation): Method used to study electrophysiology of eye; uses uniform illumination of entire retinal surface. Technique ensures simultaneous activation of complete retina to allow accurate recordings of voltage drop across extracellular resistance, from which area of retinal functioning can be derived.

Garceau catheter: Thin, cone-tipped device used to dilate ureter.

Garcia disease (cyclic thrombocythemia): Fluctuating (over 2–3 weeks) platelet counts, petechiae, epistaxis, and bruising; rare autosomal dominant condition. Treatment is platelet transfusion and prednisone.

Garcia-Lurie syndrome: Congenitally fused radius and ulna and oligodactyly; probably autosomal recessive.

Garcia-Rock endometrial biopsy curette: Thin metal device (9.5 in. long) positioned in vagina to obtain uterine tissue; has angled tip and suction-and-stopcock mechanism to trap specimen.

Garcin syndrome: Paralysis of CNs III–X (usu. unilateral) due to metastatic disease; may also be result of direct extension of nasopharyngeal or retropharyngeal tumor, infection, or granuloma.

Gardener-Diamond syndrome (erythrocyte sensitization syndrome): Tingling or burning sensation followed by appearance of purpura on face, limbs, and scalp; occurs only in women, most commonly after surgery on reproductive system. Emotional factors impact severity.

Gardner syndrome (multiple familial polyposis): Multiple intestinal polyps (75% malignant transformation), desmoid tumors, epidermal cysts, fibromas, tooth impactions, jaw osteomas, retinal hypertrophy, periampullary cancers, thyroid cancer, and benign bone tumors; autosomal dominant condition. Onset of symptoms usu. occurs by 20 years of age. Treatment is total or subtotal colectomy with fulguration of remaining rectal polyps and surveillance upper endoscopy at 3–5-year intervals.

Gardner-Silengo-Wachtel syndrome (Smith-Lemli-Opitz syndrome): Congenital heart malformation (esp. tetralogy of Fallot), clubfoot, cleft palate, digit malformations, and low-set pinnae; patient is phenotypic female with XY genotype. Condition is autosomal recessive. Death usu. occurs shortly after birth.

Gardner-Wells tongs:
Cervical spine traction using sharp metal pins screwed into skull and attached to hanging weights.

Gardnerella: Gram-negative bacterium. *G. vaginalis*, which is found in 40% of women with no history of prior sexual contact, is common cause of vaginitis.

Garel sign: See Heryng sign.

Gariel pessary: Hollow, rubber instrument inserted into vagina and inflated to support vagina.

Garin-Bujadoux-Bannwarth disease: See Bannwarth syndrome.

Garré disease (osteomyelitis sicca): Bone condition with low-grade infection, enlargement, pain (esp. at night), and sub-periosteal calcification; affects young adults. Causes may include trauma, Hodgkin disease, sickle cell anemia, lupus, or renal failure.

Garrison disease (battle fatigue): Emotional and physical collapse experienced by soldiers who see combat and then are moved to "safe" environment.

Garrod disease (alkapto-nuria): Deficiency of acid oxidase in liver and kidneys; in 1st few days of life, patient's urine becomes black on standing. Features also include blue-black sclerae and ear cartilage developing in 2nd decade, back pain, joint stiffness, and calcification of intervertebral disks.

Garrod pads: Fibrous swelling over dorsum of proximal interphalangeal joints; familial tendency.

Garth view: Radiographic positioning technique for viewing acromioclavicular joint; uses apical oblique view with 45° caudal tilt.

Gärtner bacillus: *Salmonella enteritidis.*

Gartner cyst: Cystic degenera-tion of Gartner duct that may protrude into vaginal lumen and through introitus; often con-fused with cystocele. Cyst may also develop from remnants of Gartner duct, wolffian ducts, or embryonic mesonephros.

Gartner duct: Canal made of narrow vertical tubules lined by ciliated epithelium that extends laterally down vagina to hymen; variably present. Lumen is remnant of wolffian duct.

Gärtner phenomenon:
Anatomic distention of veins in upper extremity when held below level of heart, with ensuing collapse of veins as extremity is elevated above heart.

Gass classification: System used to describe macular degeneration. Stage 1A, discrete area of foveolar detachment and depression with development of yellow macular spot; stage 1B, same as stage 1A with macular ring rather than spot; stage 2, beginning of macular hole; stage 3, macular hole completely formed with halo of subretinal fluid.

Gass disease: Loss of central visual acuity following viral-type illness or in patients with erythema nodosum; usu. resolves spontaneously.

Gasser disease: Hemolytic uremia.

Gasser inclusion: Alder-Reilly–type anomaly in which inclusions involve lymphocytes in mucopolysaccharidoses (except Morquio syndrome); structures stain red-purple with Wright-Giemsa and metachromatically with toluidine blue.

Gasser-Karrer syndrome: Onset in 1st few days of life of acute loss of RBCs caused by administration of RBC toxins (frequently vitamin K analogs). Patients usu. present with transient jaundice with anemia developing in 2nd–3rd week. Treatment is RBC transfusion.

Gasserian ganglion (semilunar ganglion): Collection of nerve cell bodies of trigeminal nerve that lies in floor of middle cranial fossa in anterior surface of petrous part of temporal bone; forms part of sensory system of trigeminal nerve and contributes to maxillary, ophthalmic, and mandibular nerves.

Gatellier-Chastang approach: Posterolateral incision used to gain access to ankle; involves curved longitudinal incision posterior to lateral malleolus. Peroneal tendons are retracted anteriorly with division of fibula and anterior-posterior tibiofibular ligaments.

Gaucher cell: Enlarged macrophage with accumulation of intracellular glucocerebroside; appears as roundish cell 20–80 μm in diameter with characteristic lipid inclusions separated by blue layers that make cytoplasm look like wrinkled tissue paper.

Gaucher disease: Abnormal retention of glycolipidcerebroside in reticuloendothelial system; causes liver, spleen, and lymph node enlargement. Condition is autosomal recessive and due to deficiency of glucocerebrosidase and α-galactosidase in lysosomes. Symptoms of hypersplenism respond to splenectomy, but this does not alter overall course of disease; partial splenectomy can be performed in children to decrease hypersplenism and reduce risk of overwhelming sepsis.

Gaul pits: Indentations in corneal epithelium occurring in some forms of keratitis.

Gault test: Positive for malingering in deafness if "good" ear is closed, noise is made near "bad" ear, and winking occurs on side of "bad" ear.

gauss (abtesla): Unit of magnetic induction; equals 1 maxwell/cm^2 and 10^{-4} tesla.

Gauss points: Area through which principal planes pass on optical axis of lens.

Gaustad encephalopathy: Mental confusion and deterioration arising after portocaval shunt procedure; sometimes does not become clinically important until precipitating event (e.g., infection, trauma, pregnancy, or transfusion) occurs.

Gavard muscle: Muscle fibers in stomach wall that run obliquely.

Gay glands (anal gland): Sebaceous and sweat glands located circumferentially around anus.

Gay-Lussac law: See Charles law.

Gee disease (Gee-Hertener-Heubner disease): Celiac (nontropical) sprue.

Gegenbaur cell: Osteoblast.

Gehrung pessary: Mechanical device inserted into vagina for treatment of cystocele; shaped as ring bent over on itself to form double horseshoe, with one of lever arms being slightly longer than other.

Geiger-Müller counter: Radiation detector used as beta-particle detector and survey meter; cannot distinguish different types or energies of particles.

Gelfard-Hyman disease (familial histicytic dermatoarthritis, Zayid-Farraj disease): Onset in childhood of joint pain, widespread subcutaneous nodules, plaque-like skin lichenification, glaucoma, cataracts, variable hearing loss, and hydronephrosis; autosomal dominant condition.

Gélineau syndrome: Narcolepsy.

Gell and Coombs classification: System used to describe types of allergic (hypersensitivity) reactions. Type 1, anaphylactic type—IgE binds mast cells and basophils via Fc fragment; type 2, cytotoxic type—antigens on cell surface bind antibodies causing opsonization, phagocytosis and variably complement binding and activation; type 3, complex-mediated type—antigen binds antibody to form complexes that activate Hageman factor and complement pathway and cause platelet aggregation; type 4, cell-mediated (delayed) type—antigen activates T cells, which proliferate and turn on macrophages and lymphocytes.

Gellé syndrome: Injury to CN VIII due to infarction or injury to pons; marked by acute onset of deafness, tinnitus, vertigo, and ear pain.

Gély suture (Appolito suture): Method of anastomosing bowel using long, continuous, running suture with needle at both ends. Individual tissue bites are taken in "baseball stitch" pattern.

Gemini hemostatic forceps: Fine, curved-tipped, ring-handle, locking forceps placed on small vessels to control bleeding before suture ligation or cautery.

Gendre fluid (picric acid fixative): Picric acid, 95% ethanol, formalin, and glacial acetic acid; used for detecting glycogen.

Genee-Wiedemann syndrome (acrofacial postaxial dysostosis, Miller syndrome): Congenital agenesis of digits, hypoplastic malar bones, coloboma, cleft facial anomalies, malformed ear cartilage, ectropia of lower eyelids, and variable heart and urogenital defects; autosomal recessive condition.

Gensini catheter: Coronary angiography catheter with side ports for dye injection and end port for passage of pressure monitor into heart chamber.

Gepfert procedure: Surgical procedure using eversion of distal end of fimbria or tubal mucosa in treatment of ectopic pregnancy.

Gerbasi disease: Megaloblastic anemia in infants; caused by breastfeeding from folate-deficient mothers. Treatment is addition of folic acid to diet.

Gerdy fibers (superficial transverse metacarpal ligament:) Thickening of superficial fascia of palm close to fingers.

Gerdy ligament: Fibrous connective tissue providing support to axilla.

Gerdy loop (interatricular loop): Small, distinct collection of muscle fibers located in septum between right and left atria.

Gerdy tubercle: Lateral tibial tubercle; distal insertion site of iliotibial band.

Gerhardt disease: See Weir Mitchell disease.

Gerhardt sign: Loss of laryngeal motion occurring in dyspnea secondary to aortic aneurysm.

Gerhardt syndrome: Paralysis of vocal cords; either congenital (autosomal dominant) or acquired (CN X injury, infection, hemorrhage, or tumor in pons or medulla). Severe cases can lead to suffocation.

Gerhardt test: Used to detect acetoacetic acid in urine. After urine is filtered to remove phosphates, ferric acid is added to produce red color. Positive result is disappearance of red color when sulfuric acid is added.

Gerhardt test: Used to detect urobilin in urine. Positive result is development of yellow-brown color when chloroform, tincture of iodine, and potassium hydroxide is added.

Gerhardt triangle: Triangular area of dullness to percussion above left 3rd rib; occurs occasionally in patent ductus arteriosus.

Gerlier disease: Sudden onset of temporary diffuse muscle palsy and hyperemia of sclera; most typically occurs in warm summer months in young males who come into contact with cows (Switzerland) or horses (Japan). Etiologic agent is unknown. Recovery is usu. spontaneous.

German syndrome: Congenital heart abnormalities (e.g., tetralogy of Fallot, hypoplastic left heart, transposition of great vessels), ear abnormalities, cleft palate, mental retardation, up-slanted eyebrows, and genital abnormalities (e.g., hypospadias, hypertrophic clitoris). Cause is maternal ingestion of trimethadione or paramethadione during pregnancy; 2/3 newborns exposed in utero develop defects.

germinal epithelium of Waldeyer: Single layer of cuboidal epithelium on surface of cortex of ovary.

Gerota fascia: Visceral peritoneum encapsulating kidney; represents natural boundary limiting spread of infection, abscess, or kidney cancer.

Gerota method: Injection of nonsoluble dye into lymphatic system; Prussian blue commonly used.

Gerrard test: Used to detect glucose in urine; positive when potassium cyanide is added to Fehling solution (until blue color begins to disappear) and color change occurs with subsequent heating.

Gerstenbrand syndrome: Mental deterioration following head trauma, with impaired concentration, euphoria, loss of inhibition, social adjustment problems, and seizures.

Gerstmann syndrome (finger agnosia, Gerstmann-Badal syndrome): Rare symptom complex of aphasia with inability to name objects and right–left disorientation; due to focal lesion at junction of parietal and occipital lobes of dominant cerebral hemisphere.

Gerstmann-Straussler-Scheinker syndrome: Rare hereditary (not infectious) prion disease caused by point mutation in gene coding for prions on chromosome 20; marked by ataxia and cerebellar dysfunction in mid-life. Dementia is absent or mild.

Gesell stages (development scales): System used to describe stages of development in normal children from infancy to 5 years of age; includes milestones in motor, visual, reflex, social, adaptive, and language skills.

Getty decompression: Laminectomy and partial facetectomy for decompression of lumbar spinal stenosis.

Ghon tubercle: Bean-shaped shadow seen on chest radiograph of children with lung TB.

Ghon-Sachs bacillus (von Hibler bacillus): *Clostridium septicum;* infects humans only via wounds.

Gianelli sign: See Tournay sign.

Gianotti-Crosti syndrome: Infantile acrodermatitis.

Gianturco-Rosch Z-stent: Device placed by invasive radiologists that is used to open arteries; stent is inserted in collapsed position and then opened when correct position is confirmed using fluoroscopy.

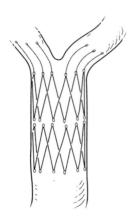

Gianturco–Rosch Z-stent

Gibbon and Landis test:
Used to indicate normal
circulation if temperature in
patient's unimmersed extremities rises when both hands or
both feet are placed in 43°–45°C
bath.

Gibbon hernia (hydrocele):
Large inguinal hernia with
hydrocele.

Gibbs free energy (G): Ther-
modynamic function described
by G = H—TS, where H is
enthalpy, S is entropy, and T is
absolute temperature. ΔG
determines direction in which
chemical reaction proceeds. ΔG
is negative for spontaneous
(exergonic) reactions and
positive for nonspontaneous
(endergonic) reactions.

Gibbs-Donnan effect (equilibrium): Describes movement
of 2 solutions separated by
semipermeable membrane as
function of distribution of ions,
osmotic pressure, and resulting
electrical potential.

Gibney bandage: Tape
applied in several directions to
stabilize ankle ligament strains.

Gibson murmur: Machinery-
like murmur audible throughout
most of systole and diastole
with crescendo thrill in systolic
pulse over site of highest
loudness; occurs in patent
ductus arteriosus.

Giemsa stain: Stain containing
glycerin, methanol, azure II, and
azure II–eosin; used to visualize
blood smears, viral inclusion
bodies, *Chlamydia*, and protozoa (e.g., *Plasmodium*,
Trypanosoma).

Gierke cell: Small Golgi type 2
neurons found in Rolando
substance.

Gierke corpuscle: See Hassall
corpuscle.

Gies reagent: 975 ml 10%
potassium hydroxide solution
and 25 ml 3% cupric sulfate
solution; used for detecting
proteins.

Gifford operation: Type of
keratotomy.

Gifford sign: Upper eyelid
cannot be everted; occurs in
Graves disease.

Gigli operation: Rarely
performed sectioning of pubic
bone laterally to effect rapid
delivery of newborn in arrested
labor.

Gigli saw: Commonly used
bone saw, with thick wire that
attaches to 2 handles after saw

is placed next to bone. Sawing motion is achieved by gripping handles (1 in each hand) and moving arms back and forth, which draws wire across bone surface.

Gil Vernet incision: Posterior, vertical incision made from 12th rib to superior edge of iliac crest and 2.5 cm from erector spinae muscles; used to approach kidney. Method is associated with minimal postop pain but provides limited exposure to upper pole and ureter.

Gila monster: *Heloderma suspectum;* injects venom via bite. Lizard is most common in Arizona and New Mexico.

Gilbert repair: "Sutureless" mesh plug repair used for closing indirect inguinal hernias. Once indirect hernia has been reduced into abdomen, inverted cone-shaped mesh plug is placed into anatomic defect, and another layer of flat mesh is placed on floor of inguinal canal with slit cut into it for spermatic cord. Most surgeons use 2–3 sutures to secure plug and overlaid flat piece.

Gilbert sign: Increased urine excretion in fasting state (vs. digestive state) occurring in cirrhosis.

Gilbert syndrome: See Behçet syndrome.

Gilbert syndrome: Abnormal bile pigment metabolism caused by defect of bilirubin transport into hepatocyte; presents as mild hyperbilirubinemia in absence of other abnormalities.

Gilbert-Dreyfus syndrome: Incomplete male pseudo-hermaphroditism; most common phenotype is man with perineoscrotal hypospadias.

Gilchrest sign: Test for bicipital tendinitis; standing patient lifts 2-lb weight overhead, and arm is then lowered in coronal plane in full external rotation. Positive result is pain or discomfort in the bicipital groove, esp. in 90°–100° of abduction.

Gillepsie syndrome: Rare complex marked by ataxia, aniridia, and mental retardation; autosomal recessive condition with onset at birth to 6 months of age.

Gilles de la Tourette syndrome: Symptom complex with chronic, relapsing-remitting motor and vocal tics, including repetitive sniffing, winking, grunting, sighing, coughing, coprolalia (speaking obscene or scatological terms), echolalia (repeating another person's words) and palilalia (repeating speaker's own phrases). Onset is usu. between 5–15 years of age, and disorder may change in character as patient ages. U.S. prevalence is 0.05%. Cause is unknown. Treatment is clonidine and haloperidol (Haldol).

Gilles technique: Surgical treatment of rounded commissure resulting from reconstructive lip surgery; uses incision of small equilateral triangle of skin with apex at point of desired commissure.

Mucosa of medial lower lip is freed and rotated superiorly, and previous "elbow" of vermilion is rotated to form upper lip.

Gillet test (sacral fixation test): Used to test for pathology in sacroiliac joint. Standing patient pulls up 1 knee and stands on 1 leg while examiner palpates posterior superior spine; test is then repeated on other side. Positive result is minimal movement of spine on side that knee is brought to chest, indicating "blocked" or hypomobile joint.

Gilliam suspension (modified): Uterine suspension technique to prevent adhesions from forming on denuded peritoneal surfaces; has unknown efficacy on increasing fertility. After peritoneal cavity is entered through small incision, 2–0 chromic suture is looped around round ligament 3–4 cm from uterus, and Kelly clamp is placed through internal ring. Chromic suture and round ligament are then brought through internal ring, outside peritoneal cavity, and are sutured to rectus sheath (without encircling it); same technique is performed on other side.

Gillies operation (reduction): Technique of surgical reduction of zygomatic arch fractures; uses incision above hairline in temporal area.

Gillingham modification: Variation of Guiot stereotactic frame used in brain surgery.

Gilmer wiring: Intermaxillary fixation using wires placed around opposing single teeth and then having ends twisted around each other.

Gimbernat ligament (lacunar ligament): Triangular medial attachment of Poupart ligament; apex is attached to pubic tubercle, upper edge is continuous with Poupart ligament, and lower edge is attached to iliopectineal line.

Gimenez stain: Carbol–basic fuchsin and malachite green used to stain *Legionella*, *Chlamydia*, and several other rickettsial bacteria red against green background.

Giordano-Giovannetti diet: Low-protein diet used in chronic renal failure to lessen gut symptoms.

Giraldes organ: Paradidymis.

Girdlestone resection (operation): Removal of head and neck of femur as treatment for severe and refractory hip infections.

Gittes bladder neck suspension (Gittes-Loughlin no-incision urethropexy): Modification of Peyrera needle bladder suspension used in correction of stress incontinence in absence of cystocele; uses 2 suprapubic stab wounds and placement of polypropylene suture via Stamey needle into vaginal canal. (Monofilament suture will pull through vaginal wall, causing fibrosis and tethering of urethra.)

Gitzelman syndrome
(galactose diabetes): GI
disturbances, jaundice,
cataracts, and visual loss
(possibly leading to blindness);
due to deficiency of galactose
kinase activity with onset from
infancy to adulthood. Treatment
is elimination of milk products.

Givens method: Technique
used to assess peptic activity.
Sample of dilute gastric juice is
added to several tubes containing globulin from pea plant. At
specified intervals, tubes are
checked for amount of globulin
that has been broken down.

glands of Wolfring: Minute
tubuloalveolar glands located
above upper edge of tarsal plate
with ducts opening onto
subconjunctival surface.

gland of Zeis: Meibomian
gland at edge of eyelid; blockage
can cause localized abscess
(stye).

Glanzmann disease
(thromboasthenia): Rare
deficiency of platelets caused by
abnormal fibrinogen receptor;
defect is in GPIIb-IIIa. Condition
is autosomal recessive and
marked by prolonged bleeding
time, failure of platelet
aggregation, and defective clot
retraction. Clinical features are
chronic mucocutaneous
hemorrhages, gingival bleeding,
GI bleeding, and menorrhagia.
Total platelet counts are normal.

glaserian fissure: Petrotympanic fissure.

Glasgow coma scale: System
used to assess severity of head

Eyes open	Never	1
	To pain	2
	To verbal stimuli	3
	Spontaneously	4
Best verbal response	No response	1
	Incomprehensible sounds	2
	Inappropriate words	3
	Disoriented and converses	4
	Oriented and converses	5
Best motor response	No response	1
	Extension (decerebrate rigidity)	2
	Flexion abnormal (decorticate rigidity)	3
	Flexion withdrawal	4
	Localizes pain	5
	Obeys	6
Total		3–15

Glasgow coma scale

trauma; reactions are given
numerical value in 3 categories:
eye opening, verbal responsiveness, and motor responsiveness.
Score < 10 is indicative of
severe trauma.

Glasgow sign: Distinctive
sound synchronous with systole
in the brachial artery; indicates
aortic aneurysm.

Glasgow-type dysplasia: See
Holmgren-Connor syndrome.

Glass-Gorlin syndrome:
Absence of teeth and
sensorineural deafness.

Glatzel mirror: Mirrow used
to detect functional patency of
nostrils. Highly polished metal
mirror is held horizontally just
under nose, and size of
condensed moisture on each
side is compared.

Glauber salt: Sodium sulfate; used as oral purgative.

Gleason grade: Pathologic grading of prostate based on histology; ranges from 1 (well-differentiated) to 5 (anaplastic).

Gleason score: Rating of prostate tumors calculated by adding grades for primary and secondary aspects of tumor; ranges from 2 (well-differentiated) to 10 (anaplastic).

Glénard disease: Abdominal muscle weakness causing abdominal pain, nausea, vomiting, constipation, sagging transverse colon; and tachycardia; usu. seen in females. Condition can be congenital or caused by significant weight loss or pregnancy.

Glenn shunt: Cardiopulmonary anastomosis performed bilaterally in correction of hypoplastic heart; uses connection of superior vena cava to right pulmonary artery to correct systemic cyanosis.

Glenn technique: Procedure used to restore symmetry to corner of mouth and lower lip in paralytic distortion of mouth or injury to marginal branch of facial nerve; involves 2–2.5-cm wedge resection of skin lateral to commissure with intentional mismatch of vermilion border of 3 mm and flap of adjoining tissue slid into place.

Glenn-Anderson repair: Technique for reimplantation of ureter to treat vesicoureteral reflux; ureter is mobilized and advanced beneath new submucosal tunnel toward bladder neck.

glenoid ligament of Cruveilhier: Thick, tough fibrous connective tissue on plantar surface of metatarsophalangeal articulations on plantar surface of foot; runs between collateral ligaments of foot.

glenoid ligament of Macalister: Fibrocartilage lip of glenoid cavity rim; deepens glenoid cavity and provides shoulder joint stability.

Gley cell: Large cell in glandular interstitium of testes.

Gley gland: Parathyroid.

Gley gland: Accessory thyroid glands; located along course of thyroglossal duct or occasionally in chest.

Glisson capsule: Fibrous tissue surrounding hepatic artery, common bile duct, nerve fibers, and lymph tissue.

Glisson disease: Rickets.

Glouston syndrome (hidrotic ectodermal dysplasia): Rare complex of abnormal nails (striated, brittle, and thin), chronic paronychial infections, and hyperkeratosis of soles and palms; also associated with abnormal hair development at puberty and mental retardation. Condition is autosomal dominant.

Gluge corpuscle: Granular inclusions found in diseased nerve tissue.

Gmelin test: Used to detect presence of bile pigments in urine. Nitric acid added to normal urine (without bile) results in formation of green, blue, violet-red, and yellow-red rings. Bile pigment is present if green and violet-red rings do not form.

Godfrey cordial: Mixture of sassafras and opium.

Godfrey test: Test of posterior knee instability. Patient lies supine and flexes hips and knees to 90°; positive result is posterior sagging of tibia, which is usu. accentuated if manual posterior pressure is applied.

Godfried-Prick-Carol-Prakken syndrome: Mental retardation, von Recklinghausen (type 1) disease, mongoloid facies, skin defects, and congenital heart block.

Godin syndrome: Localized headache resulting from mechanical pressure to area carrying arteries to site of headache.

Godwin tumor: Benign lymphoepithelial tumor of parotid gland, usu. encapsulated, with slowly progressive lymphoid infiltration; seen most commonly in middle-aged or older women. Previous treatment with small doses of radiation is no longer used because of risk of lymphomatous change.

Goebel disease: Slowly progressive muscle deterioration starting in adolescence, with muscle cells characterized by spheroid-type inclusions; autosomal dominant condition.

Goekay-Tuekel syndrome: Slowly progressive cerebellar ataxia and loss of mental functioning, with onset in childhood; also associated with heart and liver disease.

Goelet retractor: Handheld, double-ended retractor.

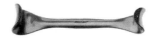

Goelet retractor

Goeminne syndrome: Congenital renal dysplasia, cryptorchidism, multiple keloids, varicose veins appearing at puberty, and torticollis; more severe in males. Location of gene defect is mapped to Xq28.

Goeminne-Dujardin syndrome: Rare congenital synostosis, patella aplasia, and coxa vara.

Goggia sign: Brachial biceps muscle is slapped and then immediately pinched. In normal health, entire muscle shows fibrillary contraction. In disease states (e.g., typhoid fever), only localized response occurs.

Golabi-Rosen syndrome: See Simpson dysmorphia.

Goldberg-Maxwell-Morris syndrome: Sertoli cell tumor.

Goldberg-Shprintzen syndrome: Hirschsprung disease, cleft palate, small head, wide-set eyes, ptosis, learning deficits, and small stature; autosomal recessive condition.

Goldberg-Wenger syndrome: Deficiency of neuroaminidase-β-galac-tosidase; results in gargoyle face, cherry-red macular spot, corneal defects, and dwarfism. Condition is autosomal recessive; may be congenital, or onset may occur in late adolescence. Diagnosis is by leukocyte enzyme test.

Goldblatt kidney: Kidney exposed to obstructed blood flow, causing hypertension; used as experimental model of renin-mediated hypertension.

Goldflam-Erb disease (Goldflam disease): Myasthenia gravis.

Goldie-Coldman hypothesis: Spontaneous mutation contributes to drug resistance in tumors.

Goldman scale: System used to describe cardiac risks in patients undergoing surgery, with total possible score of 53 points; ranges from class 1, < 5 points ($< 1\%$ chance of serious cardiac event) to class 4, > 26 points (highest risk).

Goldman tonometer: Device that is fixed to slit-lamp microscope; used for measuring intraocular pressure.

Goldman-Favre disease: Degeneration of vitreous and retina, causing severe night blindness; onset in childhood. Bone corpuscle pigmentation may occur. Disorder is autosomal recessive.

Goldner procedure (opponensplasty): Technique using transfer of tendons to restore thumb opposition.

Goldner stain: Method used to visualize kidney.

Goldstein procedure: Technique used in treatment of scoliosis.

Goldstein sign: Medially deviated 1st toe seen in trisomy 21 and cretinism.

Goldstein-Reichmann syndrome: 1920s term for acquired cerebellar ataxia.

Goldthwait brace: Back brace used to support thoraco-lumbar spine; runs from above nipple line to pelvis. Device uses 3 leather-covered, metal circular strips positioned around torso.

Goldthwait sign: Used to differentiate sacroiliac and lumbosacral causes of back pain. Patient lies supine and raises one leg, and examiner places hand under lower back and presses pelvis. If pain occurs before pressure is applied, probable cause is sacroiliac sprain. If pain occurs after pressure, probable cause is lumbosacral sprain.

Golgi complex (apparatus, reticulum): Cellular structure that appears on microscopy as "stack of pancakes"; serves as condensation and packaging structure for high-carbohydrate macromolecules and synthesis of lysosomes and membrane glycoproteins. "Forming" face is close to endoplasmic reticulum, and "mature" face points toward cell surface. Best marker enzyme for this structure is glycosyl transferase.

Golgi mixed method: Technique for staining neurons and their cellular processes.

Golgi method: Method of silver impregnation that stains protoplasmic astrocytes and gray matter nerve cell bodies and their processes dark brown.

Golgi neuron type I (cell): Pyramidal neuron with long axons that leave gray matter, pass through white matter, and terminate in periphery of brain.

Golgi neuron type II (cell, cell of Gehuchten): Stellate neuron with short axons that do not leave gray matter; found mostly in cerebral and cerebellar cortex and retina.

Golgi theory: Scientific tenet that interconnections between axons of Deiter cells and Golgi cells play important role in neurotransmission.

Golgi-Mazzoni corpuscles: Specialized nerve endings in subcutaneous tissue of finger-tips; mediates tactile sensation. Morphology is similar to that of Pacinian corpuscles but with larger cone and less branching.

Goll column (fasciculus gracilis): Ascending spino-cerebellar tract.

Goll fasciculus (column of Goll): Ascending fibers running in medial posterior funiculus of spinal cord; terminate in nucleus gracilis of medulla oblongata.

Goll fibers: Fibers originating in vermis of cerebellum and running to Goll nucleus.

Goll tract: Nucleus lying at rostral end of fasciculus of cord in medulla oblongata; cell bodies send processes to thalamus via medial lemniscus.

Gollop-Wolfgang complex: Bifid femur with absent tibia; represents defect in developmental field in fetus. Condition occurs equally in both sexes.

Goltz syndrome (Goltz-Gorlin syndrome, Jessner-Cole syndrome, Liebermann-Cole syndrome): Focal dermal hypoplasia.

Gomez-Lopez-Hernandez syndrome: Abnormal fusion of pons and vermis; associated with microcephaly, short stature, craniostenosis, and variable mental retardation. Condition is also marked by ataxia, trigeminal anesthesia, alopecia, low-set ears, and corneal opacities.

Gomori chrome stain: Method used to visualize and differentiate alpha and beta cells in islet of Langerhans; alpha cells stain red, and beta cells stain blue.

Gomori methenamine stain: Silver solution mixed with sodium thiosulfate and gold chloride and the counter-stain safranin O; stains mast cells and argentaffin granules black.

Gomori stain (Gomori-Takamatsu stain): Means of

identification of connective tissue fibers, secretion granules, phosphatases, and lipases; useful in differentiating epithelial from nonepithelial tumors.

Gomori-Wheatley stain (trichrome stain): Distilled H_2O, acetic acid, chromotrope 2R, light green SF, and phospho-tungstic acid; identifies structure of intestinal protozoa.

Gompertzian growth: Description of reduction in growth rate of tumor as it increases in size.

Gonda sign (Allen sign of foot): Corticospinal tract response with dorsiflexion of toes after downward movement of distal 2nd or 4th toe.

Gonin operation: Technique for reattaching detached retina using thermocautery to involved area; approach is via scleral incision.

Good syndrome: Rare combination of thymoma, red cell aphasia, and hypogamma-globulinemia that causes immunodeficiency state.

Goodall-Power modification: Variation of LeFort colpoceles for complete uterine prolapse, which fashions vagina long enough for vaginal inter-course but much shorter than normal.

Goodell sign: Softening of vagina, cervix, and uterus that occurs in pregnancy secondary to hormonal stimulation effected by fetus at 4–6 weeks' gestation.

Goodenough draw-a-person test: Used to assess general intelligence level of child by having child draw picture of person.

Goodenough-Harris drawing test: Refinement of Goodenough draw-a-person test that evaluates inclusion of body details and clothing.

Goodman syndrome (acrocephalopolysyndactyly type 4): Normal intelligence, congenital heart defect, clinodactyly, and ulnar devia-tion; autosomal recessive condition.

Goodpasture disease: Autoimmune disease affecting glomerular and lung basement membrane; caused by antiglomerular basement membrane antibodies. Presenting features are usu. hematuria and/or hemoptysis.

Goodpasture stain: Identifier of peroxidase reaction.

Goodpasture syndrome: Occurrence of signs and symptoms of Goodpasture disease in setting of other systemic disease (e.g., systemic lupus erythematosus, poly-arteritis nodosa, Wegener granulomatosis, Henoch-Schönlein purpura).

Goodsall rule: States that posterior anal fistulae curve before entering anal lumen; anterior anal fistulae course in straight line to anal lumen.

Goormaghtigh cells (juxtaglomerular cells): Renin-releasing cells in tunica media of afferent glomerular arteriole.

Gordon disease: GI polyposis occurring with protein-losing gastroenteropathy of Ménétrier disease.

Gordon reflex: Positive for brain damage when percussion on lateral thigh causes toes to go up rather than down.

Gordon sign (reflex): Positive when pressure on radial side of pisiform bone causes extension and spreading of fingers; seen in patients with corticospinal tract lesions.

Gordon sign (reflex): Direction of plantar response can be determined by applying pressure to calf; seen in patients with corticospinal tract lesions. Reflex can be used in place of Babinski test when patient voluntarily withdraws from plantar stroking.

Gordon syndrome: Rare disease with normal GFR, metabolic acidosis, hyperkalemia, volume expansion, and low renin and aldosterone levels; associated with enhanced chloride reabsorption. Mineralocorticoids do not produce potassium diuresis as expected.

Gordon test: Used to test for Hodgkin disease; lymph tissue to be tested is injected into rabbit's brain. Positive result occurs if lesions develop in animal's nervous tissue with subsequent paralysis, spasm, and ataxia.

Gordon test: Used to detect globulin or albumin; positive if mixture of spinal fluid to be tested and dilute mercuric chloride forms precipitate after 60 minutes.

Gordon-Cooke syndrome: Condition associated with mental and growth retardation and microcephaly; caused by terminal deletion in chromosome 1, resulting in ring conformation.

Gordon-Overstreet syndrome: 1950s term for mild virilization occurring in cases of ovarian agenesis.

Gordon-Sweet stain: Reticulin stain useful in differentiating epithelial from nonepithelial tumors.

Gorham disease (Jackson-Gorham disease): Massive lysis and resorption of bony skeleton with replacement by vascular fibrous tissue; usu. occurs before 40 years of age.

Gorlin formula: Method for calculation of cross-sectional area of heart valve orifices. $A = \text{flow}/k(P_1 - P_2)$, where A is orifice area (cm^2), flow is blood flow through the valve (ml/sec), $P_1 - P_2$ is mean pressure gradient across the valve, and k is constant (44.3 for aortic valve and 37.7 for mitral valve).

Gorlin sign: Ability of tongue to touch tip of nose; often an indication of Ehlers-Danlos syndrome.

Gorlin syndrome: Basal cell nevus syndrome.

Gosselin fracture: Shearing fracture of both condyles of distal tibia with involvement of tibiotalar articulation; forms V-shape at distal tibia.

Göthlin test: Used to evaluate capillary fragility in diagnosis of scurvy.

Gotthard disease: See Griesinger syndrome.

Gottinger line: Imaginary line running along superior edge of zygomatic arch.

Gottron disease (familial acrogeria): Senile changes occurring in infancy that affect skin and subcutaneous fat on distal limbs; also with short stature and distinctive vascular pattern on chest. Condition is autosomal recessive; more common in females.

Gottron disease: Symmetrical erythematous lesions on hands and feet and variably on face, neck, and thighs; margins of lesion frequently appear orangish.

Gottron sign (papules): Violet, flat papules found on dorsal interphalangeal joints in 30% of patients with dermatomyositis; presence is considered pathognomonic.

Gottstein fibers: External hair cells and nerve fibers forming part of auditory nerve of cochlea.

Gougerot disease: See Hailey and Hailey disease.

Gougerot-Blum disease: Pruritic purplish lesions usu. developing on legs in middle-age persons; most commonly seen in Japanese. Treatment is dapsone and topical and systemic steroids.

Gougerot-Carteaud syndrome: Development of midline warty, papillomatous-type lesions on both anterior and posterior chest; often extends to confluent lesion on neck and pubis. Condition is usu. seen in young women. Treatment is topical and systemic retinoids with good response; tends to recur.

Gougerot-Duperrat-Werther syndrome: Dermatitis nodularis necroticans.

Gougerot-Ruiter syndrome: Cutaneous allergic vasculitis marked by antibody–antigen reaction at vessel wall; causes include microbes, drugs, toxic materials, and neoplasms. Acute form is marked by purpuric, hemorrhagic skin lesions on arms, legs, and buttocks; sub-acute form is marked by papules, urticaria, and necrotic lesions coalescing into plaques; and chronic form is marked by urticaria, petechiae, and maculopapular lesions.

Goulard extract: Lead subacetate solution.

Goulard water: Dilute lead subacetate solution.

Gouley catheter: Solid metal device used to dilate urethral strictures; inserted proximal to blockage by passing over guide-wire via groove on 1 side of catheter.

Gowers sign: Characteristic manner of rising from supine to standing position in tabes dorsalis and some muscular dystrophies with pelvic girdle weakness. Patient first rolls onto side and then rises to hands and knees before using arms to propel torso to upright position.

Gowers sign: Episodic oscillating movement of iris when stimulated by light; occurs in tabes dorsalis.

Gowers tract: Superficial ventrolateral spinocerebellar fasciculus; acts as ascending conduction pathway.

graafian follicle: Fluid-filled cavity in ovary lined with follicular cells and that contains ova. Ripening follicles enlarge in size, move toward surface, and release eggs on bursting; they are transformed into corpus luteum and eventually scattered as corpus albicans.

Graber-Duvernay procedure: Uses technique of drilling channels into femoral head to promote bone circulation.

Grabstald staging: System used to describe invasiveness of urethral cancer in women. Stage 0, carcinoma in situ; stage A, confined to mucosa; stage B, penetration into muscularis; stage C1, penetration into vaginal muscle; stage C2, involvement of vaginal mucosa; stage C3, involvement of clitoris, bladder, or labia; stage D1, involvement of inguinal lymph nodes; stage D2, involvement of pelvic lymph nodes;

stage D3, metastasis to lymph basin cephalad to aortic bifurcation; stage D4, metastatic spread to distant sites.

Gradenigo syndrome: Presence of pus in middle ear, pain in CN V distribution, paralysis of lateral rectus eye muscle (CN VI), eye pain, diplopia, variable pain in temporal or parietal regions on affected side (gasserian ganglion involvement), and CN II–IV paralysis and meningitis; caused by abscess involving petrous bone.

Graefe operation: Technique for removing cataract and lens by laceration of capsule and iridectomy; approach via incision in sclera.

Graefe sign: Slow, jerky downward movement of upper eyelid when patient looks down; occurs in Graves disease.

Graefe test: Used to detect heterophoria by having patient hold prism (base either up or down) at 10° oblique angle from one eye; positive if one of two images is laterally displaced.

Graham law: Relative rates of diffusion of gases is inversely proportional to square root of their densities.

Graham patch: Segment of omentum sutured to oversew repair of perforated peptic ulcer disease (modern variation).

Graham test: Used in radiologic exam of gallbladder; oral or IV tetraiodophthalein sodium is given.

Graham-Burford-Mayer syndrome: See Brock syndrome.

Graham-Kendall test (memory for designs test): Measure of short-term memory for geometric configurations in different spatial arrangements.

Graham-Steell murmur: Diastolic murmur best heard in pulmonic area with radiation along left sternal edge, which is characterized by loud, high-pitched pulmonic valve closure sound (P2) with decrescendo quality; due to pulmonic valve regurgitation and pulmonary artery hypertension.

Grahmann disease: Lesion in diencephalon causing mental status changes, obesity, hypo-gonadism, and stunted growth.

Gram-negative bacteria: Bacteria that become decolorized by alcohol and require counterstaining with fuchsin or safranin.

Gram-positive bacteria: Bacteria that retain crystal violet–iodine complex.

Gram syndrome: Postmeno-pausal hypertension, rheumatoid arthritis in knee, and pain in fatty tissue.

Grancher sign: Indication of expiratory obstruction if pitch of inspiration and expiration is identical.

Grandy corpuscle (Grandy-Merkel corpuscle): See Merkel tactile cell.

Granger sign: Indication of destruction of mastoid if anterior wall of lateral sinus is visible on plain films in child ≤ 2 years of age.

Granit loop (gamma loop): Reflex arc that involves impulse travel along gamma fibers to intrafusal fibers, causing individual muscle spindles to contract. This contraction causes stimulation of afferent signals, which travel to alpha motoneurons in anterior horn of spinal cord (via posterior route), eliciting stretch reflex.

Grant disease: Onset in adolescents or young adults of diffuse urticaria in response to cholinergic stimulation (exercise, intense emotion); attacks last minutes to hours followed by period in which repeat stimulus does not provoke further urticaria. Treatment is antihistamines or anticholinergic drugs.

Grant syndrome: Variant of osteogenesis imperfecta with blue sclerae, wormian bones, hypoplastic mandible, shoulder dislocations, and bent extremities.

Grashey position: Radiographic positioning technique using anterior-posterior view to image glenoid fossa.

Grashey view: Radiographic positioning technique using lateral view with 10° caudal tilt to image shoulder impingement by acromion.

Grasset-Gaussel phenomenon: Inability of recumbent patient with corticospinal tract lesion to raise both legs simultaneously despite ability to raise each one separately.

Grasset-Gaussel-Hoover sign: Greater downward pressure (as compared to normal) on examiner's hand from unaffected limb when hemiparetic patient attempts to lift contralateral impaired limb.

Graves disease: Autoimmune disease of thyroid marked by thyroid-stimulating hormone receptor antibodies and variable thyrotoxicosis.

Grayson ligament: Fibrous connective tissue running from palmar distal interphalangeal and proximal finger phalangeal joints to lateral finger skin and adjacent to neurovascular bundle.

Grayson-Wilbrandt syndrome: Degeneration of cornea with lesions ranging from mottling to small grayish raised spots, with variable affect on vision; autosomal dominant condition.

Grebe syndrome (nonlethal achondrogenesis, Quelce-Salgado syndrome): Dwarfism, hypoplastic limbs, obesity, and delayed mental development; autosomal recessive condition.

Grebe-Myle-Loewenthal syndrome (transition form lipomatosis): Systemic lipomatosis; associated with mental retardation, spina bifida, and café-au-lait spots.

Grecian foot: See Morton foot.

Greefe-Prowazek body: See Halberstaedter-Prowazek body.

Greene sign: Lateral displacement as detected on percussion of free cardiac border in expiration; seen in pleural effusions.

Greene thyroid retractor: Handheld retractor with fenestrated blade.

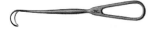

Greene thyroid retractor

Greenfield disease: Metachromatic leukodystrophy.

Greenfield filter (birdcage): Mechanical device resembling badminton birdie placed in inferior vena cava below level of renal veins; used to block passage of large emboli to heart and lungs; also indicated as prophylaxis against development of pulmonary emboli in patients who cannot be anticoagulated or who have had pulmonary emboli while being anticoagulated. Patients should always be asked about presence of this device before central line is placed using Seldinger technique with wire (to avoid catching wire on device).

Greenough microscope: Type of stereomicroscope for focusing on 1 object but with separate compound microscope for each eye.

Gregerson and Boas test: Modification of benzidine test; uses barium peroxide and more dilute benzidine solution to detect blood in feces.

Gregg syndrome: Birth defects and congenital pathology occurring in newborns whose mothers were exposed to rubella in 1st trimester; marked by patent ductus arteriosus, pulmonary trunk stenosis, mental retardation, cataracts, ataxia, hepatosplenomegaly, inguinal hernia, hearing loss, and pneumonia.

Gregory powder: Rhubarb, ginger, and magnesium oxide powder.

Gregory stay suture clamp: Instrument used to pinch together Gregory stay sutures fastening devices.

Greig syndrome: 1920s term for wide-set eyes (hypertelorism).

Greig syndrome (Hootnick-Holmes syndrome, Marshall-Smith syndrome): Dysplasia of frontal and nasal bones and polysyndactyly of feet and hands; also associated with bilateral hip dislocation, ichthyosis, and retinal defects.

Greissinger foot: Multiaxis foot and ankle prosthesis with U-shaped joint to allow movement in all directions; has bumpers to limit dorsi- and plantar flexion.

Greissinger prosthesis: Foot and ankle prosthesis; best results when used in above-the-knee amputations in active patients.

Greither syndrome: Progressive keratosis of palms and soles, sometimes extending to patches on arms and legs; tends to spontaneously regress after many years. Treatment is topical steroids and keratolytic agents and high-dose vitamin A.

Grenet syndrome: Ipsilateral facial anesthesia for pain and temperature changes and contralateral truncal anesthesia for pain and temperature; due to lesions in middle 1/3 of pons, causing crossed sensory paralysis. If lesion extends to motor nucleus of CNS and cerebellar peduncle, syndrome may be associated with ipsilateral mastication paralysis, ataxia, and tremor.

Grey Turner sign: Ecchymosis of flanks and anterior abdominal wall; seen in acute hemorrhagic pancreatitis.

Gridley stain for fungi: Technique using glycol–aldehyde reaction (Bauer reaction).

Grieg test: Used to identify *Vibrio cholerae* with mixture of goat or sheep RBCs and broth from culture to be tested. *V. cholerae* does not produce hemolysis, but other *Vibrio* species do.

Grierson-Gopalan syndrome: Burning pain and cramp-like discomfort on soles, tachycardia with exertion, sweating, and amnesia; caused by severe malnutrition. Condition occurs in India. Treatment is restoration of adequate caloric intake, yeast, and calcium.

Grieshaber technique: Method for removing anterior cataracts using handheld trephine; usu. preset at 0.6 mm, depending on corneal thickness. Trephine is placed on cornea and turned back and forth between fingers to effect tissue removal.

Griesinger sign: Swelling behind mastoid process associated with transverse sinus thrombosis.

Griesinger syndrome (Egyptian chlorosis, Gotthard disease): Infestation with *Ancylostoma duodenale* or *Necator americanus;* causes itching of feet and between toes and progresses to perineal itching, weakness, headache, diarrhea, abdominal pain, tinnitus, cough, and duodenal ulcer symptoms. Infection usu. occurs in barefoot workers in damp soil. Treatment is mebendazole and pyrantel.

Griess test: Used to detect nitrates in saliva; positive if yellow color develops when H_2O, dilute sulfuric acid, and metadiamidobenzene are mixed.

Griffith mixture: Compound iron mixture.

Griffith point: Area of splenic flexure at risk for ischemic colitis.

Griffith sign: Lagging movement of lower lid on gazing upward; occurs in Graves disease.

Grigg test: Used to detect protein (except for peptone); positive if precipitate forms when metaphosphoric acid is added to sample.

Grignard reagent: Magnesium compound coupled with halogen and organic radical.

Grimelius method: Method of producing argyrophilic reaction; uses buffered silver nitrate solution, reduced sodium sulfite solution, and hydroquinone to stain cells that contain significant granules.

Griscelli syndrome: Partial albinism and recurrent immunodeficiency states secondary to neutropenia, hypogammaglobulinemia, and thrombocytopenia; autosomal recessive condition.

Grisolle sign: Distinguishes skin lesion of measles and smallpox by stretching skin over lesion and palpating. In small pox, lesion remains detectable, and in measles, lesion disappears.

Gritti amputation: Removal of lower leg performed at knee joint; patella is retained as a flap over end of femur.

Gritti-Stokes amputation (Stokes amputation): Modification of Gritti amputation; performed at knee joint using anterior soft tissue flap, instead of patella.

Grocco sign: Indication of hepatomegaly when dullness is percussed on anterior abdominal wall to left of midspinal line.

Grocco sign (Korányi-Grocco triangle, Rauchfuss triangle): Triangular area of dullness to percussion on posterior chest wall contralateral to pleural effusion.

Grocott-Gomori methenamine–silver nitrate solution: Chromic acid, methenamine-silver nitrite solution, and light green solution counterstain that stains fungi, *Pneumocystis*, and actinomycetes brown on green background.

Groenouw corneal dystrophy (type 1) [granular corneal dystrophy]: Small granular opacities that occur before 10 years of age, which coalesce to form disk in superior cornea; autosomal dominant condition.

Groenouw corneal dystrophy (type 2) [macular corneal dystrophy]: Macular opacities with irregular borders in cornea that present before 20 years of age, surrounded by cloudy stroma; autosomal recessive condition.

Grondahl-Finney operation: Rarely performed enlargement of gastroesophageal junction.

Groshong catheter: Indwelling central venous catheter; similar to Broviac or Hickman catheter but has 3-position slit at distal (indwelling) tip. Slit normally remains closed when catheter is not in use, opens outward when infusing fluids, and moves inward when aspirating blood. Only saline flushes are required, because catheter lumen has no retained blood after blood is drawn.

Gross test: Used to detect trypsin in feces. Specimen, dilute sodium carbonate solution, Grübler pure casein, 1 g sodium carbonate, H_2O, and toluene are mixed together and incubated. Small samples are removed and tested with dilute acetic acid. If casein remains undigested by trypsin, white color will form. If undigested casein remains after 10–15 hours, there is diminution of trypsin. If color appears, carcinoma should be suspected.

Gross-Groh-Weippl syndrome: Congenital hypoplastic or absent radius, which often occurs with hypoplasia of ulna and hand bones, thrombocytopenia with hemorrhagic episodes, cardiac abnormalities, renal abnormalities, and spina bifida; blood disorder tends to improve with age.

Grossman sign: Cardiac enlargement sometimes seen in pulmonary TB.

Grover disease: Transient eruption of pruritic herpes-like vesicles and papules initially on trunk and then extending to limbs; usu. occurs with excessive sun exposure.

Groves procedure (opponensplasty): Transfer of tendon to restore thumb opposition.

Gruber reaction: See Widal test.

Gruber syndrome (cloverleaf skull, hydrocephalus chondrodystrophics congenitum, trefoil skull): Symptom complex of grossly deformed, trilobed skull, achondroplasia, exophthalmos, and beaked nose; usu. seen only in stillborn fetuses.

Gruentzig catheter: Low-compliance balloon catheter with flexible guidewire attached to tip; used to open arterial blockages (e.g., dilating medial fibroplastic lesions in renal artery).

Grund disease: Distal motor neuropathy marked by muscle stiffness and accompanied by fine muscular twitches and variable cramps and sweating; occurs in localized area or occasionally systemically. Condition appears to regress after several years. Symptoms are lessened by phenytoin.

Gruner-Bertolotti syndrome: Parinaud and von Monakow syndrome occurring in same person.

Grüning magnet: Series of small steel rods used to remove metal particles from eyeball.

Grynfeltt hernia: Passage of intra-abdominal tissue through superior lumbar triangle at junction of 12th rib and internal oblique muscle.

Gsell-Erdheim disease: See Erdheim disease.

Guarnieri gelatin agar: Culture medium used to identify and culture *Streptococcus pneumoniae.*

Guarnieri bodies: Cytoplasmic inclusions in cells affected with smallpox and vaccinia; likely cell response to viral particles.

Gudden commissure (inferior cerebral commissure): Medial root of optic tract; these fibers connect with medial geniculate bodies.

Guérin fold: Ridge of mucosa variably present in fossa navicularis of urethra.

Guérin fracture: Fracture of maxilla.

Guérin glands: See Skene glands.

Guérin sinus: Inpouching located posterior to Guérin fold.

Guérin valve: Variably present mucous membrane in roof of urethral fossa navicularis.

Guérin-Stern disease (arthrogyrposis multiplex congenita, Rocher-Sheldon disease, Rossi syndrome): Multiple (but nonprogressive) joint contractures at birth; frequently with accompanying muscle weakness. Treatment is intensive physical therapy initially and surgery if needed (esp. on ankles) to allow for weight-bearing and walking.

Guérin-Stern disease (arthrokatadysis, Otto disease, Otto pelvis): Primary idiopathic form of malformed pelvis marked by medial wall of acetabulum being medially displaced to ilio-ischial line. Displacement causes abnormal protrusion of acetabulum.

Guerry-Cogan disease: Fingerprint-like wavy lines developing within corneal epithelium in middle-aged or elderly women; associated with variable pain and corneal erosions. Visual deterioration is common.

Guibaud-Vainsel syndrome:
Marble-brain syndrome.

Guibor chart: Chart containing outlines of pictures; used in orthoptic training.

Guibour tube: Thin, hollow, Silastic tube used to intubate nasal lacrimal duct system, esp. in repair of lacerations; stiffer and easier to pass than Crawford tube.

Guillain-Alajouanine-Garcin syndrome: Unilateral loss of some or all cranial nerves, esp. CNs VII, IX, X, XI, and XII; causes include nasopharyngeal tumors, masses at base of skull, trauma, and Schmincke tumors.

Guillain-Barré syndrome (Glanzmann-Salamud syndrome, Kussmaul-Landry disease, Landry ascending paralysis): Onset of lower extremity paresthesias and weakness and flaccid paralysis with progression (hours to days) to trunk, arms, neck, and cranial nerves; also accompanied by fevers, muscle stiffness, and myalgias. Specific etiology is unknown; 50% of cases follow upper respiratory infections. Condition is also associated with bacterial, parasitic, and other viral infections; surgery; vaccines; insect bites; and leukemia and lymphoma. Degree of resolution is variable; plasmapheresis is indicated in severe cases. Supportive ventilation may be required. Prognosis is better in children than in adults.

Guilland sign: Contralateral hip and knee flexion that occurs when soft tissue in quadriceps femoris area is pinched; suggests meningeal irritation.

Gull syndrome: Adult myxedema seen in untreated hypothyroidism.

Gullner disease: Familial hypokalemia marked by muscle cramps, weakness, nausea, and vomiting.

Gunn dot (Marcus Gunn dot): White specks seen on oblique lighting of macula lutea.

Gunn sign ("jaw winking" sign): Elevation of ptotic eyelid when mouth is opened and jaw is moved to one side.

Gunn sign: Appearance of artery crossing over vein on funduscopic exam; seen in essential hypertension.

Günning test (Gunning-Lieben test): Used to detect acetone in urine. Ammonia and tincture of iodine is added alternately until black cloud develops. As cloud clears, iodoform crystals form if result is positive.

Günther disease (congenital erythropoietic porphyria): Porphyria secondary to defect in uroporphyrinogen synthase III; marked by severe skin photosensitivity causing skin friability and vesicles, hemolytic anemia, and red-brown teeth. Condition is autosomal recessive.

Günz ligament: Segment of obturator membrane.

Günzberg test: Used to detect hydrochloric acid in stomach juice. Hydrochloric acid is present if bright red color develops when phloroglucin and vanillin are dissolved in alcohol, added to gastric juice, and heated. Brown-red color indicates absence of hydrochloric acid.

Guthrie muscle: Muscle fibers comprising urethral sphincter; compresses membranous part of urethra. Origin is at pubic ramus, insertion is at median raphe, and innervation is via perineal nerve.

Guthrie test: Used to detect phenylalanine in blood; positive if β-2-thienylalanine does not stop growth of *Bacillus subtilis*.

Gutierrez disease: Horseshoe kidney usu. fused on inferior pole; has male-to-female ratio of 2:1.

Gutzeit test: Used to detect arsenic if yellow color develops on paper wetted with acid silver nitrate and exposed to fumes from zinc, sulfuric acid, and specimen.

Guy pill: Combination of mercury, digitalis, and squill.

Guyon amputation: Distal below-the-knee amputation; transection is just proximal to malleoli.

Guyon canal: Anatomic space in wrist through which ulnar artery and nerve pass; bordered on medial side by pisiform bone, on lateral side by hook of hamate bone, along deep surface by transverse carpal ligament, and on superficial side by volar carpal ligament.

Guyon sign: Indication of floating kidney when firm pressure into flank or abdominal musculature results in feeling of object hitting fingers (ballottement).

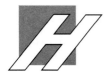

Haab disease (degeneration): Age-related maculopathy, with slow progressive degeneration of retinal cones; usu. bilateral. Onset occurs at advanced age.

Haab stria: Horizontal striations of cornea; usu. due to congenital glaucoma.

Haagensen criteria: System that describes locally advanced breast tumors; uses presence of peau d'orange that causes arm edema or erythema, involvement of supraclavicular nodes, and involvement of internal mammary nodes.

Haagensen test: Change in breast contour noticeable when woman leans forward at waist; may herald breast mass or malignancy.

Haas disease: Avascular necrosis of humeral head in children.

Haas syndrome: Complete bilateral polysyndactyly with finger flexion; autosomal dominant condition.

Haber syndrome: Childhood onset of rosacea-type lesions developing on face with erythema and telangiectasia. In adulthood, lesions become warty and also appear on thighs and torso.

Haber-Weiss reaction: Chemical formula describing combination of superoxide anion and hydrogen peroxide to form hydroxyl radical.

Haboush universal nail: H-shaped plate inserted into neck and head of femur and then bent onto side of femur; used in intracapsular hip fractures.

Haddad-Riordan arthrodesis: Fusion of intra-articular wrist surfaces; uses iliac crest bone graft.

Haden disease: 1940s term for hereditary hemolytic spherocytosis.

Hader dentures: Type of mandibular implant–supported overdentures.

Haeckel law (theory): Development of individual organism mimics successive stages of entire species in its development from primitive to higher form.

Haenel sign: Absence of pain when direct pressure is applied to eyeball; seen in advanced neurosyphilis.

Haff disease: Rhabdomyolysis accompanied by severe myoglobinuria; etiology is consumption of fish containing toxic levels of industrial wastes.

Hagedoom syndrome: Arrested development of anterior vitreous of eye; related to Axenfeld syndrome.

Hageman factor: Coagulation cascade factor XII, which is converted to its activated form (factor XIIa) by contact with either foreign surface or kallikrein; activation initiates intrinsic pathway. Factor XII deficiency, an autosomal recessive condition, results in prolonged activated partial thromboplastin and whole blood clotting times.

Hager reagent: Potassium hydroxide and iron ferrocyanide; used for detecting sugars in urine.

Haggitt system: Classification of GI polyps. Level 1, dysplastic cells above muscularis mucosa of head of polyp; level 2, cell invasion into neck of polyp (junction of normal colonic epithelium in adenomatous epithelium); level 3, polyp stalk involved; level 4, bowel submucosa involved but no involvement of muscularis. All patients with level 4 polyps, and some with level 3 polyps, should undergo segmental colon resection.

Hagie pin: Device used in repair of femoral neck fractures.

Haglund deformity ("pump bump"): Prominent bone formation on posterosuperior calcaneus.

Haglund disease: Fracture of calcaneus at Achilles tendon insertion in children; no damage to periosteum or soft tissue usu. occurs.

Haglund process: Normal posterosuperior calcaneal tuberosity.

Haglund syndrome: Pain on lateral heel; caused by bursitis, callus, or poorly fitting shoes.

Hahn oxine reagent: 5% hydroxyquinoline dissolved in alcohol.

Hahn sign: Repetitive side-to-side head turning in pediatric cerebellar disease.

Haight anastomosis: Technique for repair of esophageal atresia. Mucosa of proximal pouch is anastomosed to distal segment (full-thickness), and proximal segment muscularis is then pulled over anastomosis and sutured to outer layer of distal segment.

Hailey and Hailey disease (Darier variant, Gougerot syndrome): Skin disease marked by chronic eruption of vesicles (leading to erythema and crusting) in neck, groin, and axilla. Condition is autosomal dominant and commonly occurs in hot, humid weather in Jewish people in adolescence or early adulthood.

Haim-Munk syndrome: Recurrent skin infections, gum disease, tapering shape of digits, palmoplantar hyperkeratosis, and claw-like volar curvature; seen in inbred Jewish families in Southeast Asia. Condition is autosomal recessive.

Haines reagent: Solution of 150 parts distilled H_2O, 15 parts glycerin, 2 parts copper sulfate, and 7.5 parts potassium hydroxide.

Hajdu-Cheney syndrome (Cheney syndrome): Short stature, protruding occipital bone, short digits, vertebral body collapse causing height loss, deepened phonation, early tooth loss, and repeated bone fractures, with abnormal bone development and (in distal limbs) bone resorption; autosomal dominant condition.

Hakola syndrome (Nasu-Hakola syndrome): Progressive formation of jelly-filled cysts in brain, bone, and fat starting in 3rd decade; causes dementia, seizures, bone fractures, and GI motility disorders. Condition is seen in Finland and Japan. Death eventually occurs.

Halal syndrome (acrorenal-mandibular syndrome): Rare

association of split hands and feet, hypoplastic mandible, renal abnormalities, and genital malformations; autosomal recessive condition.

Halban culdoplasty: Closure of pelvic cul-de-sac performed in combination with hysterectomy; uses permanent sutures placed in anterior-posterior fashion (usu. incorporating posterior margin of mesh) that obliterates space when tied down.

Halban disease: Benign ovarian tumor causing amenorrhea and persistent corpus luteum function. Treatment is excision.

Halberstaedter-Prowazek body (trachoma body): Cytoplasmic inclusion bodies found in epithelial cells from conjunctiva infected with trachoma.

Haldane apparatus (chamber): Device with valves used to give oxygen, which prevents loss during inspiration and expiration; used to perform metabolic studies on animals.

Haldane effect: Enhancement of carbon dioxide dissociation from hemoglobin by binding of oxygen to hemoglobin (e.g., as occurs in gas exchange in lung).

Hale syndrome: Deficiency of long-chain acyl-CoA dehydrogenase, causing adrenoleukodystrophy-type condition with hypoglycemia, cardiomegaly, hepatomegaly, and hypotonia.

Halifax procedure: Spinal fusion involving lamina of C1 and C2.

Hall antidote: Aqueous solution of quinine hydrochloride and potassium iodide; used to treat mercuric chloride poisoning.

Hall disease: Early term used for pseudohydrocephalus associated with cachexia.

Hall method: Technique that demonstrates bilirubin in tissues by staining specimens with Fouchet reagent and Gieson solution. Biliverdin stains green, muscle stains yellow, and collagen stains red.

Hall sign: Tracheal "shudder" detectable during diastole in aortic aneurysm.

Hall technique (Hall-Pankovich technique): Procedure using multiple flexible medullary nails to fix severe, comminuted fractures of humeral shaft. In distal fracture, distal portholes are placed anteriorly.

Hall-Pankovich procedure: Placement of many small Ender nails to repair midhumeral fractures.

Hall-Riggs syndrome: Congenital mental retardation, chronic vomiting, stunted growth, microcephaly, large lips, and anteverted nostrils; autosomal recessive condition.

Hallauer glasses: Greenish lenses that block out ultraviolet and blue light.

Hallberg effect: Opposite electrical fields exist for crests and troughs of short-standing wave field.

Halle point: Intersection of imaginary lines running horizontally between anterior superior iliac spines and running vertically from center of pubic spine; approximates point where ureter crosses pelvic brim.

Haller aberrant duct: Small spiral tube originating from lower epididymal canal.

Haller arches: Lateral arcuate ligament formed by quadratus lumborum muscle fascia.

Haller arches: Medial arcuate ligament formed by psoas fascia.

Haller duct: Aberrant coiled tube branching off lower part of canal in epididymis.

Haller habenula: See Scarpa habenula.

Haller isthmus: "Pinched in" tissue area between fetal ventricles and atria.

Haller layer: Vascular sheath of choroid.

Haller membrane: Vascular layer of choroid between choriocapillary and suprachoroid layers.

Hallerman-Doering syndrome: Deafness and band keratopathy of eyes; associated with reduction of calcium turnover, but paradoxically patients are usu. normo-calcemic.

Hallerman-Streiff-François syndrome (Audry syndrome, Fremerey-Dohne syndrome, Ullrich syndrome): Congenital hypoplastic mandible, small face, beaked nose, cataracts, alopecia, and delayed psycho-motor development. Treatment is surgical correction of individual deformities; uncorrected conditions can be fatal in infancy or early childhood.

Hallervorden syndrome (Poser syndrome): Onset in childhood of progressive loss of cerebral myelin causing mental and neurologic deterioration followed by visual, speech, and hearing loss; minimal brain inflammation and large number of scattered sudanophilic cells found on autopsy.

Hallervorden-Spatz syndrome: Childhood onset of progressive cerebellar ataxia, dysphagia, loss of mental function, blindness, skin pigment abnormalities, and muscle atrophy; likely disorder of iron storage. Condition is autosomal dominant. Death occurs 10–20 years after onset.

Hallgren syndrome: Congenital deafness, primary pigment degeneration of eyes, ataxia, seizures, and variable mental retardation and psychosis. Condition is most common in Sweden (3/100,000 frequency); autosomal recessive inheritance.

Hallion test: See Tuffier test.

Hallopeau syndrome (Csillag syndrome, Zambusch syndrome): Small, whitish oval macules and papules on trunk, neck, vulva, vagina, and penis; found largely in women at menopause but may occur with spontaneous remission in girls at puberty. In women, condition causes vulvar atrophy and dyspareunia. Syndrome has possible autoimmune etiology. Treatment is palliative with steroids and excision of leukoplakia.

Hallopeau syndrome (Hallopeau-Leredde syndrome): Pustules in mouth and areas of flexure, followed by warts with central erosion; considered benign variant of pemphigus. Etiology is unknown; serum antibodies to interocular substances have been found. Condition occurs equally in men and women of middle age, with spontaneous remissions.

Hallopeau-Siemens syndrome: Large bullae on skin and mucosa, alopecia, and mental retardation. Bullae rupture spontaneously, leaving scars, miliary cysts, webbing between fingers and toes, and strictures of tongue. Condition is autosomal recessive. Prognosis is poor, with carcinoma developing in scars.

Hallpike maneuver: Test for vertigo; positive if rapid rising from sitting to standing position with head tilted to one side causes dizziness and nystagmus.

Hallwachs effect (photo-electric effect): When short-wavelength energy is imported to matter, ejection of electrons results.

Halstead-Reitan battery: Psychometric test used to assess cognitive function that samples wide array of functions and is able to detect subtle deficiencies; administration time is 5–8 hours.

Halsted hemostatic forceps: Long (178 mm) curved or straight-tipped, locking forceps placed on small vessels to control bleeding before suture ligation or cautery; available with nontoothed tips and 1×2 teeth on tips.

Halsted hernia repair: Method identical to Bassini repair except spermatic cord is placed into subcutaneous tissue; rarely performed today.

Halsted maneuver: Procedure used to diagnose thoracic outlet syndrome. Sitting patient turns head to contralateral side and hyperextends neck while examiner first palpates radial artery in limb to be tested and then observes for loss of pulse while applying downward traction on arm.

Halsted mastectomy (operation): Radical mastectomy; no longer performed. Procedure included resection of pectoralis major and minor muscles as well as breast tissue, subcutaneous fat, and skin.

Halsted mosquito hemo-static forceps: Short (90–127 mm), curved or straight-tipped, locking, ring-handle forceps placed on small vessels to control bleeding before suture ligation or cautery.

Halsted theory of breast cancer: Wide, aggressive local control of disease is needed for resection for cure; hematogenous spread is of little importance. Theory is now largely discredited.

Halushi-Behçet syndrome: See Behçet syndrome.

Ham test (acid serum hemolysis test): Used to detect paroxysmal nocturnal hemo-globinuria. 9 parts acidified fresh normal ABO-compatible serum is added to 1 part of 50% washed patient RBCs. Positive result is cell lysis (cells are sensitive to complement at pH of 6.5–7.0). Test is also positive in 15% of cases of aplastic anemia.

Hamas prosthesis: Arm prosthesis using Silastic material at wrist.

Hamblen classification: System used to describe ectopic bone ossification in hip area. Grade 0, no ossification; grade 1, new bone formation occupying < 1/3 femoral head/capsule area; grade 2, new bone formation occupying 1/3–1/2 femoral head/capsule area; grade 3, new bone formation occupying > 1/3 of femoral head/capsule area.

Hamel test: Withdrawal of small amount of blood from earlobe into capillary tube; used to detect occult jaundice. Positive if yellow fluid rises to top after 60–120 minutes.

Hamilton classification: System used to describe androgenetic baldness in men.

Hamilton method: Technique used to tamponade postpartum hemorrhage by placing one fist inside uterus and thrusting superficially, with other hand exerting maximal pressure on lower abdominal wall.

Hamilton test: Used to detect shoulder subluxation; positive if straight rod touches both lateral humeral condyle and acromion.

Hamman sign: "Crunching" crackles best heard in left lateral position; synchronous with heart beat (due to heart beating against air-filled tissue). Causes may be Boerhaave syndrome, pneumothorax, pneumomediastinum, or mediastinitis.

Hamman syndrome: Media-stinal emphysema causing dyspnea and inspiratory pain behind sternum; seen as radiolucent stripes on lateral radiograph. Cause is rupture of alveolus or viscus, with tracking of air into chest.

Hamman-Rich syndrome: Idiopathic pulmonary fibrosis with nonspecific inflammation in interalveolar septa.

Hammar myoid cell: Thymic striated muscle found in birds and reptiles.

Hammarsten test: Used to detect globulin in solution; positive if precipitate forms when saturated with magnesium sulfate.

Hammarsten test: Used to detect bile pigment (biliverdin); positive if green color develops when nitric acid, hydrochloric acid, and alcohol are added.

Hammerschlag method: Rather cumbersome method for determination of specific gravity of blood specimen. 1 drop of blood is placed into chloroform–benzene mixture with a known specific gravity (1.050), and benzene or chloroform is added until blood droplet becomes motionless. Then specific gravity of entire mixture is measured.

Hammon procedure: Bone graft after 1st metatarsal osteotomy to remove dorsal bunion.

Hampson unit: Unit of x-ray exposure; equals 0.25 of erythema dose.

Hampton hump: Rounded densities on chest radiograph near costophrenic sinus above elevated diaphragm; strongly suggests infarction due to pulmonary embolus.

Hampton line: Radiolucent collar seen at base of gastric ulcers on upper GI series; corresponds to ring of granulation tissue.

Hanau law of articulation: Law that governs development of masticatory surface to guarantee balanced articulation; also applies to making dentures.

Hancock amputation: Modification of Pirogoff amputation of foot; talus is divided with retained portion used in flap after it is positioned next to calcaneus.

Hancock valve: Porcine valve used to replace mitral or aortic valves; does not require anticoagulation but has shorter life than artificial valves.

Hand-Schüller-Christian disease: Histiocytosis with skull and bone lesions similar to eosinophilic granuloma.

Hanes plot: Linearized version of Michaelis-Menten equation; $([S]/V) = (1/V_{max})[S] + (K_m/V_{max})$, where $[S]$ is substrate concentration, V is reaction velocity, and K_m is Michaelis-Menten constant. Plot allows K_m values to be calculated from experimental data.

Haney-Falls syndrome: Congenital mental retardation, short stature, misshapen cornea, and brachydactyly.

Hanger-Rose skin test: Used in diagnosis of catscratch fever (Petzetakis disease).

Hanhart syndrome (type 1): Stunted growth and variable mental deterioration, with lack of secondary sex characteristics, low libido, and fat deposits developing on abdomen and breast; associated with multiple pituitary hormone deficiencies. Condition is autosomal recessive, with onset in mid-childhood in closely inbred groups in Switzerland and on small Adriatic islands.

Hanhart syndrome (type 2): Onset from birth of type 1 signs and symptoms with addition of hypoplastic jaws, missing teeth, and limb malformations.

Hanhart syndrome (type 3): Limb malformations, cleft palate, hypoplastic jaws, mental retardation, and variable renal and uterine abnormalities.

Hanhart syndrome (type 4): Diffuse lipomas in subcutaneous tissue, photophobia, excessive tear production, anhidrosis, corneal lesions, small jaws, missing fingers and toes, and mental retardation.

Hank solution: Commercially prepared balanced salt solution; used in reimplantation of avulsed tooth. Tooth should be gently swirled in a shallow dish of solution to remove debris before reinserting.

Hankow fever: Infection with *Schistosoma japonicum.*

Hann filter: Multiplicative attenuation correction used to develop accurate reconstructions in SPECT images.

Hannover canal: Potential separation between anterior and posterior suspensory ligament fibers of lens.

Hannover intermediate membrane: Enamel.

Hanot disease: Autoimmune hepatitis causing bile duct obstruction and cirrhosis leading to liver failure. Treatment is liver transplantation.

Hanot-Roessle syndrome: Early term for intrahepatic cholangitis.

Hansen disease (bacillus): Leprosy caused by *Mycobacterium leprae.*

Hansen disease: Autoimmune neutropenia marked by persistent, recurrent infections. Treatment is antibiotics and steroids.

Hantaan virus: Hantavirus that causes hemorrhagic fever with renal complications.

Happle disease (chondrodysplasia punctata): Skin erythema, striated hyperkeratosis, alopecia, early severe respiratory distress, and stunted growth; X-linked recessive condition, which is possibly related to steroid sulfatase deficiency.

Hapsburg jaw: Severely forward jutting lower jaw.

Hapsburg lip: Thickened, bulbous lower lip; often seen with Hapsburg jaw.

Hardcastle disease: Bone dysplasia associated with medullary fibrosarcoma degeneration and cataracts. Tumor is extremely aggressive. Condition is autosomal dominant.

Harden and Young equation: Expression used to describe chemical reaction of glucose fermentation to form alcohol, hexose diphosphate, and carbon dioxide.

Harder glands (harderian glands): Vestigial accessory lacrimal glands located at inner corner of eye; facilitate movement of 3rd eyelid in less advanced animals.

Harding disease: Disorder marked by CNS demyelination on MRI, multiple sclerosis–like clinical phenotype, optic atrophy, oligoclonal bands in CSF, and mutation of mitochondrial DNA.

Harding-Passey melanoma: Tumor originally found in brown mice; now used as inducer of nonmetastatic melanoma when transplanted into other mice.

Harding-Ruttan test: Used to detect acetoacetic acid in urine; positive if acetic acid, sodium nitroprusside, and concentrated aqueous ammonium hydroxide produces violet color.

Hardy-Rand-Rittler plates: Pseudoisochromatic plates used to evaluate color vision.

Hardy-Weinberg equilibrium (law): Proportions of 3 genotypes resulting from 2 alleles remain constant from 1 generation to next; assumes absence of selection, mutation, genetic drift, migration, and nonrandom mating.

Hare splint: Device used to stabilize long-bone injuries (esp. femoral fractures) in field; has metal frame posteriorly with anterior straps and foot braces.

Hark procedure: Z-tendon elongation of flexors and extensors with bone reposition; treatment for congenital talipes valgus.

Harken procedure: Mitral valve commissurotomy; used to treat mitral valve disease.

Harlem hemoglobin C: Form of hemoglobin with 6 Glu→Val and 73 Asp→Asn substitution on β chain; causes normal packed cell volume, isosthenuria, target cells, and anisocytosis.

Harmon approach (modified) [transfer]: Posterolateral approach to tibia; uses longitudinal skin incision. Dissection takes place between peroneal muscles anteriorly and gastrocnemius, soleus, and flexor hallucis longus posteriorly. Procedural steps are detachment of distal soleus from fibula, medial dissection of interosseous membrane, and detachment of tibialis posterior.

Harrigan resuscitator: Handheld pressure sensor (compression pad with force gauge) used to determine adequacy of manual chest compressions.

Harrington rod (for compression): Device that corrects kyphosis in conjunction with spinal osteotomy in patients with ankylosing spondylitis; has posteriorly threaded rod with hooks and nuts to apply compressive force on spine.

Harrington rod (for distraction): Device that corrects curvature of spine in conjunction with spinal osteotomy; has 2 hooks and ratchet mechanism. Instrument is placed posteriorly on spine, and rod is gradually lengthened to correct curvature. Bone fusion is always required for permanent results.

Harrington splanchnic retractor (sweetheart retractor): Handheld device used to retract tissues deep in wound.

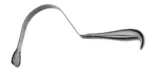

Harrington splanchnic retractor

Harris lines: Radiographic lines that represent growth arrest at long bone epiphyses.

Harris scale: 100-point scale used to describe hip pathology. Function is rated up to 40 points and pain is rated up to 60 points, and the 2 scores are added.

Harris syndrome: See Charlin syndrome.

Harris tube: Mercury-weighted thin plastic tube used to intubate small intestine; currently in disuse because of restrictions on handling mercury.

Harris-Beath footprinting mat: Used to record foot pressure points by having patient ambulate on it.

Harris-Beath procedure: Subtalar and talonavicular arthrodesis for correction of flatfoot.

Harrison disease (Maeda disease): Variant of amyloidosis with deposits isolated to right atrium; marked by bradycardia and/or atrial standstill, cardiomegaly and cardiac failure, and diffuse abdominal pain. Treatment is anticoagulation and pacemaker.

Harrison groove: Horizontal furrow along bottom border of chest corresponding to costal insertion of diaphragm; seen in chronic respiratory diseases and in children with rickets.

Harrison law: 1915 act that legislated regulation of distribution and use of narcotics.

Harrison spot test: Used to detect bilirubin in urine; positive result is production of green-blue color after barium chloride is mixed with sample of urine and filtered and treated with Fouchet reagent.

Hart test: Used to detect oxybutyric acid in urine. Acetic acid is added to dilute urine and boiled, hydrogen peroxide is added to form acetone, and Lange test is then performed.

Hartigan foramen: Opening in lower part of lumbar vertebral transverse process;

variably present and rarely seen in mature skeletons.

Hartley-Krause operation: Excision of gasserian ganglion to relieve trigeminal neuralgia; technique is no longer performed.

Hartmann pouch: Infundibulum of gallbladder; sometimes described as abnormal pouching at gallbladder neck.

Hartmann procedure (pouch): Colon surgery oversewn distal colonic stump; remains intraperitoneal, usu. with marker (nonabsorbable suture). Bowel is decompressed via proximal colostomy, and mucous fistula via anus. Procedure is usu. reversed at later date.

Hartnup disease: Rare genetic abnormal metabolism of alpha amino acids with pellagra-like skin lesions, CNS deficits, cerebellar ataxia, nystagmus, and variable dementia; caused by deficiency in conversion of tryptophan to nicotinic acid. Treatment is nicotinamide and high-protein diet.

Harvard criteria: Early criteria for definition of legal brain death; standards are more stringent, with heavier reliance on EEG, than those now used.

Harvey-Bradshaw index: Numerical system that describes functional activity in Crohn's disease using nonweighted, 1-day scores to assess signs and symptoms. Variables include general well-being, abdominal pain, number of liquid stools per day, abdominal mass, and intestinal and extraintestinal complications.

Hasami fever: Leptospirosis occurring in Japan; cause is *Leptospira interrogans* (serogroup *autumnalis*).

Hashimoto disease (struma, thyroiditis): Chronic autoimmune disease of thyroid due to antibodies to thyroglobulin and microsomes; most common cause of hypothyroidism in U.S. Thyroid is firm and rubbery but nontender. Condition usu. develops in women in 5th–6th decade. Treatment is T_4 replacement when symptomatic; surgery is appropriate in refractory cases.

Hashimoto-Pritzker disease: Congenital, self-healing variant of histiocytosis X.

Hasner valve (lacrimal fold): Ridge of mucous membrane at lower orifice of nasolacrimal duct.

Hassall corpuscle (Gierke corpuscle, Leber corpuscle): Cluster of flattened, spherical cells found in medulla of thymus; arises from 4th pharyngeal pouch. Formation occurs by concentric arrays of epithelial cells containing cytoplasmic filaments and keratohyalin.

Hasson technique: Placement of laparoscopic instruments via cutdown and direct visualization.

Hatchcock sign: Indication of mumps infection if tenderness results from running finger toward angle of jaw.

Haubenfelder fields: See Forel fields.

Haudek niche (sign): Indicator of penetrating gastric ulcer if projecting shadow is evident on radiograph; due to trapped particles of bismuth in ulcer wall.

Haultain operation: Surgical treatment for inverted uterus using posterior approach to uterus via incision in cervical ring; considered modification of Huntington operation.

Hauser index: Description of categories of ambulation in multiple sclerosis.

Hauser procedure: Two partial incisions of Achilles tendon (proximal posterior and distal medial two-thirds) with casting and passive stretching to alleviate tight heel cord.

Hauser procedure: Correction of bunion using removal of medial exostosis and adductor tendon transfer from proximal phalanx to distal metatarsal.

Hauser procedure: Correction of chronic patellar subluxation; involves infero-medial displacement of bone segment with attached infrapatellar tendon.

Haverhill fever: Condition marked by fever, blotchy rashes, and polyarthritis; caused by *Streptobacillus moniliformis* ingested in contaminated milk. Diagnosis is made by culture of organism or serum agglutination test. Penicillin is effective treatment.

Haversian canals: Central canals running longitudinally in long bone that transport blood-borne nutrients to bone cells.

Haversian system (spaces): Anatomic passageway that allows movement of nutrients in bone Osteons Haversian canals and lacunae branch radially to individual bone cells.

Hawaii agent: Virus that causes acute infectious gastroenteritis in both children and adults.

Hawkins classification: System used to describe talar neck fractures. Type 1, minimal displacement with 1 blood supply disrupted; type 2, subtalar dislocation with 2–3 blood supplies disrupted; type 3, complete separation of talus from subtalar joint and ankle.

Hawkins impingement sign: Indication of rotator cuff problem if pain results when humerus is flexed to 90°, horizontally adducted, and internally rotated.

Hawkins keloid: See Alibert disease.

Hawkins sign: Translucent area under subchondral plate of dome of talus seen in avascular necrosis.

Haworth formula: Convention used to represent 3-D cyclic configuration of sugars in 2 dimensions; anomeric carbon is always to right. For α-d or β-L configurations, hydroxyl group is below ring.

Hay test: Used to detect bile salt in urine; positive if small amount of sulfur added to sample to be tested sinks to bottom.

Haycock equation: Expression used to estimate body surface area.

Hayem-Widal-Loutit syndrome: Autoimmune hemolytic anemia.

Hayflick limit: 50 cell divisions or doublings. Cells such as fibroblasts exhibit lipofuchsin and larger size as they approach this limit and old age and death.

Haygarth nodes: Swollen, enlarged joints in arthritis deformans.

Head-Riddoch disease: Sign and symptom complex occurring in patients with quadriplegia. Condition is marked by bradycardia, dilated pupils, hypertension, sweating, flushing, headache, visual disturbances, and variable seizures. Disease results from viscus distention or nerve stimulation below level of spinal lesion.

Heaf test: Test for TB that uses defined pattern of 6 needles fired using set pressure into skin through film of prepared protein derivative (PPD); considered positive if after 3 days, puncture points have coalesced to form circle or more pronounced skin reaction is present.

Heaney hysterectomy retractor: Handheld, double-ended retractor.

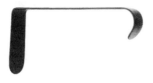

Heaney hysterectomy retractor

Heaney-Simon hysterectomy retractor: Handheld, double-ended retractor.

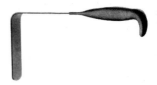

Heaney–Simon hysterectomy retractor

Heath operation: Division of ascending rami of mandible as treatment for ankylosis; largely abandoned procedure.

Heathrow hemoglobin: High-oxygen-affinity hemoglobin with replacement of phenylalanine by leucine in heme pocket; results in hemoglobin values of 16–21 g/dl.

Heberden asthma (disease): Angina pectoris.

Heberden nodes: Osteophytic overgrowth at distal interphalangeal joint seen in osteoarthritis and other conditions.

Hebra disease (prurigo): See Devergie syndrome.

Hecht-Beals syndrome (Dutch-Kennedy syndrome): Congenital inability to open mouth widely, camptodactyly, short stature, talipes equinovarus, and short gastrocnemius; autosomal dominant condition.

Heck syndrome: Benign, multiple, sessile, polyp-type lesions developing on oral mucosa of Native American children and Caucasian adults;

Hedlinger syndrome: See Bjoerck disease.

Heerfordt-Waldenstrom syndrome: Subtype of sarcoidosis with fever, facial nerve palsy, parotid enlargement, and uveitis.

Heffington frame: Device that enables prone patient undergoing lumbar spinal surgery to have hips flexed 90° in operating room by lowering end of table; reverses lumbar lordosis.

Hefke-Turner sign: Enlargement of obturator radiographic shadow caused by pathologic hip lesion.

Hegar sign: Softening of lower segment of uterus; seen in 1st trimester of pregnancy.

Hegenbarth forceps: Small, finger-controlled, cross-action forceps used to apply or remove surgical staples.

Hegesh reaction: Assay for NADH dehydrogenase.

Hehner number: Percentage of nonaqueous fatty acids that can be extracted from total fatty acid content of fats and oils.

Heidelberg analysis: Procedure for diagnosis of gastric hypochlorhydria in which capsule is swallowed with string in place for later removal, with pH recordings of stomach transmitted via radio receiver; bicarbonate challenge is usu. given first.

caused by infection with human papillomavirus.

Heidenhain cells: Parietal and chief cells found in stomach.

Heidenhain law: Glandular secretion is always associated with glandular structure changes.

Heidenhain modification (of Mallory-azan stain): Technique for visualizing tissues of upper esophagus; uses azocarmine to stain nuclei bright red, aniline blue to stain collagen bright blue, and orange G to stain cytoplasm of epithelial cells and muscle orange to red.

Heidenhain pouch: Surgical separation of small stomach pouch from rest of stomach, which drains to exterior; used for study of stomach physiology.

Heidenhain stain: Iron hematoxylin stain.

Heifitz clip: Device used to occlude brain aneurysms.

Heifitz procedure: Excision of ingrown nail and nail bed on affected side.

Heim-Kreysig sign: Retraction of intercostal spaces in synchrony with systole; seen in adherent pericarditis.

Heimlich maneuver: Forcible pressure to epigastrium in setting of suspected acute airway obstruction.

Heine operation: Surgical fashioning of communication between suprachoroidal space and anterior chamber of eye to treat glaucoma.

Heine-Medin disease: Poliovirus (Brunhilde, Lansing, and

Leon strains) affecting children 6 months–15 years of age; causes destruction of anterior horn cells of spinal cord. Mortality rate is 5%–15%. Disease has been largely eradicated in Western countries because of use of effective vaccines.

Heineke-Mikulicz pyloroplasty: Transverse, full-thickness incision in anterior wall of pylorus (1–2 cm on each side of pyloric ring) with double-layer longitudinal closure; requires full Kocher maneuver to avoid undue tension on suture line. Purpose is to aid gastric drainage after truncal or selective vagotomy has been performed or vagus nerve has been severed during esophagogastrectomy. Procedure should not be performed in presence of pyloric scarring or inflammation, and it makes pylorus nonfunctional after truncal vagotomy.

Heiner syndrome (Heiner-Sears syndrome): Condition of infancy marked by failure to thrive, chronic diarrhea, bronchitis, and pallor; cause is likely related to delayed hypersensitivity to cow's milk. Treatment is discontinuation of cow's milk, antibiotics, and (in more severe cases) steroids.

Heinrichsbauer disease: See Herlitz-Pearson disease.

Heintz method: Quantitative method for detection of uric acid in urine. Hydrochloric acid is added to sample, and resulting precipitate and solution are passed through filter, dried, and weighed.

Heinz body: Intracellular inclusion body formed by denatured hemoglobin; removed in splenic cords by pinching-off process known as "pitting."

Heinz body anemia: Any hemolytic anemia characterized by Heinz bodies within erythrocytes.

Heiser mixture: Resorcin, camphor oil, and chaulmoogra oil; used as preantibiotic era treatment of leprosy.

Hektoen agar: Used for isolation and identification of enteric bacteria, esp. *Shigella*, *Salmonella*, and coliforms.

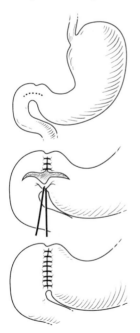

Heineke–Mikulicz pyloroplasty

Hela cell: Phagocytic cell.

Helbings sign: Medial deviation of Achilles tendon from posterior view; seen in flatfoot.

Heller disease: Rare development of groove in nail of thumb; occasionally involves several nails. Condition usu. resolves over several months.

Heller myotomy: Surgical division of circular muscle of lower esophagus; used to treat achalasia. Technique is performed through left chest or (more commonly today) through left chest thorascopic approach. Left vagus nerve is at risk for injury.

Heller test: Used to detect albumin in urine; positive if white substance forms when urine is added to cold nitric acid in test tube.

Heller test: Used to detect blood in urine; positive if red color develops when potassium hydroxide is added and heated.

Heller test: Used to detect glucose in urine; positive if rust-colored precipitate forms when potassium hydroxide is added.

Hellin law (Hellin-Zeleny law): 1 in 89 births results in twins; 1 in 7921 in triplets (89×89); 1 in 704,969 in quadruplets ($89 \times 89 \times 89$); and so on.

Helly fluid: Fixative identical to Zenker fluid, with formalin substituted for glacial acetic acid.

Helmholtz ligament: Segment of anterior malleolar ligament running to greater tympanic spine.

Helmholtz line: Imaginary line running perpendicular to plane of ocular axis of rotation.

Helmholtz theory of accommodation: Convexity of eye lens is determined by degree of relaxation of suspensory ligament.

Helmholtz-Harrington syndrome: Congenital cataracts, abnormalities of hand, mental retardation, and hepatosplenomegaly; unknown etiology.

Helsinki hemoglobin: High-oxygen-affinity hemoglobin with replacement of lysine by methionine in 2,3-diphospho-glycerate binding area; results in hemoglobin levels of 14–16.5 g/dl.

Helvetia blue: See Swiss blue.

Helvetius ligament: Thick-ened longitudinal muscular layer of anterior and posterior surfaces of pyloroantral area.

Helweg bundle (fasciculus): Spino-olivary fasciculus located bilaterally in anterolateral spinal column.

Helweg keratosis (inverted follicular keratosis): Relatively benign, invaginated, cup-shaped tumor developing on skin; formed by squamous cells at center and basal cells at periphery. Treatment is excision.

Helweg-Larssen syndrome (Helweg-Larssen-Ludvigsen syndrome): Congenital anhidrosis or severe hypohidrosis with development of vertigo in 4th–5th decade; autosomal dominant condition.

hemi-Fontan procedure:
Bidirectional superior cardiopulmonary shunt.

Hemming filter:
Bacterial filter that uses centrifugal force to separate organisms; rotating disk forces bacteria-filled fluid through filter.

hemoglobin Alberta:
High-oxygen-affinity hemoglobin with replacement of $\beta101(G3)$ glutamic acid by glycine in $\alpha_1\beta_2$ contact area; results in hemoglobin value of 20 g/dl.

hemoglobin Chesapeake:
High-oxygen-affinity hemoglobin with replacement of $\alpha92(F64)$ arginine by leucine in $\alpha_1\beta_2$ contact area; results in hemoglobin values of 15–20 g/dl.

hemoglobin Constant Spring:
Hemoglobin that causes most common variety of nondeletional α-thalassemia, which is most prevalent in southern China and Southeast Asia, esp. Laos. Gene arises from point mutation (TAA→CAA) in termination codon of α_2 globin gene. Anemia in homozygotes is more severe than in heterozygotes (thalassemia minor). Condition is also marked by reticulocytosis and hepatosplenomegaly.

hemoglobin Gower:
1 of 3 types of primitive embryonic hemoglobin; synthesized in yolk sac erythroid cells. Hemoglobin Gower-1 has globin moiety with 2 ϵ chains and 2 γ chains.

Hemoglobin Gower-2 has globin moiety with 2 α chains and 2 ϵ chains.

hemoglobin Kempsey:
High-affinity-oxygen hemoglobin with replacement of $\beta99$ aspartic acid by asparagine in β chain at contact area; this prevents formation of key hydrogen bonds and results in high-affinity R conformation. Variant results in increased hemoglobin values (17–20 g/dl) but rarely hyperviscosity sequelae.

hemoglobin Malmö:
High-oxygen-affinity hemoglobin, with replacement of $\beta97(F64)$ histidine by glutamine in $\alpha_1\beta_2$ contact area; results in hemoglobin values of 17–21 g/dl.

hemoglobin Portland:
1 of 3 types of primitive embryonic hemoglobin; has 2 γ and 2 β chains.

hemoglobin Wood:
High-oxygen-affinity hemoglobin with replacement of $\beta97$ (F64) histidine by leucine in $\alpha_1\beta_2$ contact area; results in hemoglobin values of 17–22 g/dl.

Hench-Rosenberg syndrome
(palindromic rheumatism): Sudden onset of joint pain and swelling, usu. in late afternoon; most commonly affects fingers, hands, knees, wrists, and ankles. Condition lasts 1–7 days. Moderate elevation in sedimentation rate and WBC count occurs. Treatment is indomethacin and (in severe forms) corticosteroids.

Henck-Assman syndrome:
Benign adult form of Albers-

Schönberg syndrome; autosomal dominant condition.

Henderson arthrodesis: Fusion of intra-articular and extra-articular hip using iliac bone graft.

Henderson fracture: Trimalleolar ankle fracture.

Henderson lag screw: Treatment for hip fractures.

Henderson-Hasselbalch equation: $pH = pK + \log$ [proton acceptor (base)/proton donor (acid)].

Henderson-Jones chondromatosis: Formation of loose bodies with pain and swelling in joints from synovial villi becoming bone and cartilage due to trauma or degeneration; occasional spontaneous resolution.

Hendler test: Used in chronic back pain.

Henke space: Space lying between pharynx and esophagus and vertebral column; contains fibrous connective tissue.

Henle ampule: Twisted, enlarged distal part of ductus deferens.

Henle elastic membrane: Thin fenestrated membrane between middle and outer tunica of arteries.

Henle fenestrated membrane (Bichat membrane): Thin fenestrated membrane in tunica intima of artery.

Henle fiber layer (entoretina): Outer plexiform layer of retina where "flame hemorrhages" can be visualized.

Henle glands: Tubular-shaped glands located in conjunctiva near eyelids.

Henle layer: Outer cell lamina of inner root of hair follicle; lies superficial to Huxley layer and deep to outer root sheath.

Henle ligament (falx inguinalis): Variably present structure representing aponeurotic fibers of internal oblique and transverse muscle tendons running to linea alba and pubic bone attachments.

Henle loop (ansa): Distal segment of nephron; part of renal tubule, with proximal thick, straight segment, thinner loop, and distal thick straight segment.

Henley loop: Esophagojejunostomy; used after complete gastrectomy.

Henle membrane: Posterior border of lamella of Fuchs.

Henle-Coenen test: Assesses back flow from distal segment of transected artery; indicates collateral flow.

Henneberg disease (cataplexy): Sudden onset of muscle weakness and loss of muscle tone; may follow intense emotions (e.g., laughter, fear) and usu. sleep. Partial attacks may involve only dropping of jaw or leg weakness. Condition resolves within minutes of onset. Disorder is chronic in approximately 65% of cases. Treatment is imipramine and clomipramine.

Hennebert syndrome: Spontaneous onset of nystagmus and giddiness in children with congenital syphilis. Treatment is penicillin.

Hennekam syndrome: Congenital mental retardation, mongoloid facies, lower extremity and genital lymphedema, and intestinal lymphangiectasia.

Henning sign: Deformity of stomach angulus in "gothic arch" shape; seen in chronic gastric ulcer.

Henoch syndrome: Henoch-Schönlein syndrome with definite abdominal pathology.

Henoch-Schönlein syndrome: Nonthrombocytopenic purpura, abdominal pain, arthralgias, hematuria, melena, glomerulonephritis, with hypersensitivity vasculitis. With kidney failure, transplantation should be delayed 6–12 months after last episode of purpura.

Henry hernia repair: Technique using preperitoneal approach.

Henry law: Gas solubility in liquid is proportional to partial pressure of gas.

Henschke-Mauch device: Prosthetic knee using hydraulics to control stance and swing phase.

Hensen canal (Hensen duct, Reichert canal): Small passageway connecting cochlear duct and saccule.

Hensen cell: Vertical-shaped supporting cells next to outer phalangeal cells in organ of Corti.

Hensen line (M band): Dark line in center of sarcomere H band.

Hensen node: Cell collection formed at 14 days surrounding the primitive pit on cephalic end of primitive streak of embryo; cells migrate from here to form notochord.

Henshaw test: Used to select specific remedies indicated in homeopathic treatment; flocculation occurs when correct remedy is mixed with blood.

Hensing ligament: Thin peritoneal fold running from proximal descending colon to inner surface of abdominal wall.

hepatic funiculus of Rauber: Proper hepatic artery.

Herbartian psychology (Herbartism): 19th-century school of thought that believed in possible expression of mental processes in mathematical terms; included postulate of the existence of both conscious and unconscious mental processes and the ability to have unconscious thoughts move into conscious level when the emotional state undergoes a force.

Herbert approach: See Russe approach.

Herbert operation: Surgical technique for treating glaucoma; uses displaced wedge-shaped scleral flap. Procedure allows formation of scar tissue with residual opening to facilitate drainage of aqueous humor.

Herbert pits: Conjunctival follicle necrosis with subsequent scarring; most commonly seen after chlamydial infection.

Herbert screw: Short screw (threaded at both ends); used to fix small bone fractures (scaphoid) or osteotomies (bunion treatment).

Herbert screw osteosynthesis: Variably pitched dumbbell-shaped device that provides compression and internal fixation in scaphoid fracture.

Herbert-Fisher classification: System used to describe scaphoid fractures; types B5 and C are now obsolete. Type A1, nondisplaced hairline fracture of tubercle; type A2, nondisplaced hairline fracture of waist; type B1, oblique fracture in distal third; type B2, displaced fracture of middle waist; type B3, proximal pole fracture; type B4, carpal dislocation and fracture; type D1, fibrous union; type D2, pseudoarthrosis; type D3, sclerotic pseudoarthrosis; type D4, avascular necrosis.

Hering law: 1 eye never moves independently of other in normal patients; eyes have bilateral innervation and "yoked" extraocular muscles that receive simultaneous and equal nerve stimulation to effect conjugate gaze.

Hering law: Purity of sensation is function of its intensity and intensity of all simultaneous sensations.

Hering nerve: Branch of glossopharyngeal nerve running to carotid sinus; supplies visceral afferent fibers mediating physiologic status to pressure receptors and chemoreceptors.

Hering test: Used to assess binocular vision. Patient looks through tube with both eyes at vertical string and small sphere suspended at other end of tube either in front of or behind string. Test is positive if patient can tell where sphere is in relation to string.

Herlitz-Pearson disease: Congenital bullous lesions of mucosa and skin and loss of finger- and toenails; marked by significant granulation tissue and severe hypoalbuminemia. Death occurs within 1 year. Condition is autosomal recessive.

Hermodsson fracture: See Hill-Sachs fracture.

Herndon-Heyman procedure: Tendon elongation and lateral and medial foot release for correction of congenital talipes valgus.

Herrick syndrome: Sickle cell anemia; 2 hemoglobin S genes cause full penetrance.

Herring classification: System used to describe Legg-Calvé-Perthes disease. Group A, normal lateral pillar height; group B, pillar height 50%–100% of normal; group C, pillar height < 50% of normal.

Herrmann syndrome: Facial anomalies; pectus carinatum; bilateral malformed digits, wrists, and elbows; and conductive-type deafness. Condition is autosomal dominant.

Hers disease: Cori type-4 glycogenosis and glycogen storage defect with hepatic phosphorylase kinase deficiency, hepatomegaly, and moderately stunted growth. Some variants may also affect muscle and leukocytes. Prognosis is good with administration of glucagon and dietary control of hypoglycemia.

Hersh syndrome: Small mouth, wide-set eyes, scant curly hair, craniosynostosis, and sensorineural hearing deficits; autosomal recessive condition.

Hersman disease: Progressive growth of hands in absence of endocrine abnormality or other gigantism.

Hertel exophthalmometer: Handheld device used to assess prominence or bulging of eyeball; measures distance from lateral orbital bony rim to center of cornea. Normal range is 14–21 mm (average, 16 mm).

Herter infantilism: Infantile celiac sprue.

Herter test: Used to detect indole; positive if blue-green color develops when sample is mixed with 1 drop each of dilute sodium β-naphthoquinone-4-sulfonate and 10% potassium hydroxide solution.

Herter test: Used to detect skatole; positive if purple color develops when acid solution of paradimethylaminobenzaldehyde is added and mixture is heated.

Hertig theory: Etiology of endometriosis is formation of purulent fibrinous exudate with subsequent organization with gland-like structures.

Hertwig-Magendie position (skew deviation): Ocular sign of cerebellar pathology. Subtypes are concomitant deviation (onset of vertical diplopia in all fields), nonconcomitant deviation (vertical diplopia greater in 1 field), and laterally comitant deviation (sudden onset of diplopia with hypertropia in right or left gaze).

Hertwig-Weyers syndrome: Congenital hypoplasia of ulna associated with variable abnormalities of spleen, kidneys, sternum, and jaw.

Herxheimer fibers: Small, spiral fibers in stratum mucosum of skin.

Herxheimer spiral: Minute coil of mucus observed on gynecologic cytology specimens.

Heryng sign: Infraorbital shadow produced by lesion in maxillary sinus when light is placed in mouth.

Herzberg test: Used to detect free hydrochloric acid in stomach juice; positive if moistened paper is treated with Congo red and becomes blue-black on drying.

Heschl gyri (transverse temporal gyri): 2–3 convolutions on brain surface that run transversely on superior temporal lobe and border the lateral (sylvian) fissure.

Hess syndrome (N syndrome): Rare mutation of DNA polymerase α, with mental retardation, overlapping upper eyelids, wide-spaced eyes, spasticity, and elongated head; death occurs in infancy due to leukemia.

Hess test: Used to detect capillary fragility. Previously marked 2.5-cm diameter area (4 cm below elbow) is constricted by manometric cuff for 5 minutes at pressure midway between systolic and diastolic pressure. After cuff is removed, petechiae are counted; value > 10 is marginal to abnormal.

Hessburg-Barron trephine: Instrument used in cataract surgery to enter anterior chamber. After blade is "zeroed" under microscope, 3 quarter-turns are made counterclockwise, and instrument is applied to center of eye under microscope. Under suction, 3 quarter-turns are made in reverse direction (clockwise), and then clockwise quarter-turns are made (either to maximum of 6 turns or until anterior chamber is entered).

Hessel/Nystrom pin: Threaded device used to internally fix fractures of femoral neck.

Hesselbach hernia: Hernia that runs lateral to femoral vessels and under inguinal ligament.

Hesselbach ligament (interfoveolar ligament): Thickened fibers from transversalis muscle that curve medially and downward to internal ring; fibers are attached to lacunar ligament and pectineal fascia.

Hesselbach triangle: Area bordered by lateral rectus sheath, inferior epigastric vessels, Poupart (inguinal) ligament, and floor of inguinal canal; traversed by direct hernia.

Heubner artery (long central artery): Branch of anterior cerebral artery; supplies head of caudate, anterior part of internal capsule, and putamen.

Heuter line: Imaginary horizontal line running horizontal to the medial humeral epicondyle and touches tip of olecranon in elbow extension.

Heuter sign: Test for intact biceps tendon in which arm is pronated and then elbow is flexed under resistance. If tendon is intact, slight degree of supination occurs as biceps is recruited to aid brachialis muscle in flexion (positive finding). If tendon is ruptured, no partial supination occurs (negative finding).

Hey amputation: See Lisfranc amputation.

Hey ligament: Lateral border of saphenous hiatus.

Heyd syndrome: See Flint syndrome.

Heyman procedure: Deltoid ligament and soft tissue release for correction of clubfoot.

Heyman procedure: Soft tissue release and tendon transfers for posterior capsule reinforcement for correction of genu recurvatum.

Hibb-Meary angle: Angle formed by imaginary lines drawn at edge of calcaneal plantar surface and longitudinal of 1st metatarsal.

Hibbs arthrodesis: Extra-articular and intra-articular hip fusion using greater trochanter.

Hibbs procedure: Transfer of extensor digitorum longus to 3rd cuneiform and release of plantar fascia for correction of cavus foot and claw toes.

Hibbs retractor (double-ended)**:** Handheld retractor used to retract tissue in deep surgical fields.

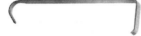

Hibbs retractor

Hibbs spinal fusion (operation)**:** Fusion of lumbar spinous process, facets, and lamina for stabilization. Spinous process of each vertebra to be fused is fractured, and tip is pressed downward to contact vertebra below.

Hibbs test (prone gapping test)**:** Used to compare degree of movement at sacroiliac joints. Prone patient flexes knee to 90°, and examiner rotates hip on side to be tested as far medially as possible and simultaneously palpates sacroiliac joint. Maneu-ver is then performed on other side and findings compared.

Hickey-Hare test: Used to detect diabetes insipidus; positive if IV hypertonic saline does not cause water diuresis.

Hickman catheter: Central venous line with external access; available in various sizes and number of ports. Catheter is anchored subcutaneously with cuff. Heparin flushes are required to prevent clotting of lumen.

Highmore antrum: Maxillary sinus; largest paranasal sinus.

Highmore body (mediastinum testis)**:** Tissue on upper poste-rior border of testis traversed by artery, veins, and lymphatics.

Higouménakis sign: Swelling in inner 1/3 of right clavicle; seen in congenital syphilis.

Hildebrandt test: Used to detect urobilinogen; positive if shaken mixture of 10 parts zinc acetate, 90 parts alcohol, and sample to be tested produces fluorescent green filtrate before or after addition of ammonia.

Hildred formula: Expression for calculation of calories required in burn patients; equals 1800 kcal × total body surface area + 1300 kcal × total surface area of burn.

Hilgenreiner angle (aceta-bular index angle:)**:** Angle formed by line running through both acetabular centers and bordering acetabular slope.

Hilgenreiner line: Imaginary horizontal line on radiograph between femoral head and acetabulum; used in diagnosis of congenital hip dysplasia and hip dislocation.

Hill equation: Expression used to describe fraction of ligand saturation by an enzyme as function of ligand concentration; useful in determining enzyme cooperativity.

Hill gastropexy: Surgical treatment of gastroesophageal reflux disease; establishes intra-abdominal segment of esophagus (in absence of fundal wrap) by fixing stomach posteriorly.

Hill operation: Antireflux procedure performed only through abdominal incision using gastric wrap of 180°; involves posterior approximation of crura followed by anchoring of gastroesophageal junction posteriorly and anteriorly to median arcuate ligament. Intraoperative calibration of plication is absolutely necessary.

Hill sign: Disproportionately higher systolic blood pressure in hypertension of femoral artery compared with systemic value.

Hill-Ferguson rectal retractor: Handheld retractor used to view anal canal.

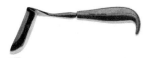

Hill–Ferguson rectal retractor

Hill-Sachs fracture: Compression fracture of head of humerus seen in anterior shoulder dislocation.

Hill-Sachs lesion (hatchet head deformity): Radiographic sign showing indentation of posteromedial humeral head after dislocation.

Hill-Sachs lesion (reversed): Radiographic sign showing indentation of anteromedial humeral head after dislocation.

Hilton law: Motor nerve to muscle sends branches to joint moved by that muscle and to skin overlying that joint.

Hilton muscle: Oblique arytenoid muscle; closes laryngeal inlet. Innervation is via vagus nerve, origin involves dorsal arytenoid cartilage, and insertion is at apex of contralateral arytenoid cartilage.

Hilton white line: Groove between lower edge of internal sphincter and subcutaneous part of external anal sphincter, which forms lower border or pecten; palpable on digital rectal exam.

Hines and Brown test (cold pressor test): Used to evaluate coronary artery disease and vasomotor response in patients unable to undergo exercise stress test. Patient's hand is immersed in ice water, causing vasoconstriction, hypertension, and tachycardia.

Hinman syndrome: Acquired childhood disorder of severe urinary sphincter–detrusor dysfunction; associated with trabeculated bladder, ureteral reflux, hydronephrosis, and frequent urinary tract infections. Condition tends to improve with age; may be learned disorder. Presenting symptoms are daytime and nighttime wetting, recurrent urinary tract infections, and constipation.

Hinshelwood disease: Dyslexia, with reading, spelling, and writing disability; associated with speech defects and occurs with greater frequency in left-handed persons.

Hinze virus: DNA herpesvirus; causes tumors in rabbits.

hippocratic fingers: Clubbing of fingers; Lovibond angle $> 180°$.

hippocratic nails: "Watch-glass nails" found in pulmonary TB and cirrhosis.

Hippocratic oath: Oath demanded of physicians as they begin medical practice: "I swear by Apollo the physician, by Aesculapius, Hygeia, and Panacea, and I take witness all the gods, all the goddesses, to keep according to my ability and my judgment the following Oath: To consider dear to me as my parents him who taught me this art; to live in common with him and if necessary to share my goods with him; to look upon his children as my own brothers, to teach them this art if they so desire without fee or written promise; to impart to my sons and the sons of the master who taught me and the disciples who have enrolled themselves and who have agreed to the rules of the profession, but to these alone, the precepts and the instruction. I will prescribe regimen for the good of my patients according to my ability and my judgment and never do harm to anyone. To please no one will I prescribe a deadly drug, nor give advice which may cause his death. Nor will I give a woman a pessary to procure abortion. But I will preserve the purity of my life and my art. I will not cut for stone, even for patients for whom the disease is manifest; I will leave this operation to be performed by practitioners (specialists in this art). In every house where I come I will enter only for the good of my patients, keeping myself far from all intentional ill-doing and all seduction, especially from the pleasures of love with women or with men, be they free or slaves. All that may come to my knowledge in the exercise of my profession or outside of my profession or in daily commerce with men, which ought not to be spread abroad, I will keep secret and never reveal. If I keep this oath faithfully, may I enjoy my life and practice my art, respected by all men and in all times; but if I swerve from it or violate it, may the reverse be my lot."

Hirano body: Rod-like, actin-containing inclusion body occurring in Alzheimer disease and Guam–parkinsonism dementia complex; usu. arranged in paracrystalline array.

Hiroshima hemoglobin: High-oxygen-affinity hemoglobin with replacement of histidine by aspartic acid in C-terminal area.

Hiroshima procedure: Transfer of long toe flexors anteriorly for correction of equinovarus defect.

Hirschberg sign: Indication of pyramidal tract disease when rubbing inner thigh causes internal rotation and adduction of ipsilateral foot.

Hirschberg sign (adductor reflex of foot): Stroking inner foot from 1st toe to heel causes foot to plantar flex, invert, and adduct.

Hirschberg test: Used to detect muscle weakness causing deviation of eye by noting reflection of light on cornea; less accurate than Krimsky test. Patient's eyes are fixed on midline light source; reflection is noted in cornea as head is turned (7° deviation of eye for each 1-mm displacement of corneal reflex).

Hirschfeld canal (interdental canal): Opening in mandible between lateral and medial incisors; traversed by anastomotic vessels of inferior dental and sublingual arteries.

Hirschmann anoscope: Metal surgical instrument with slightly tapered hollow cylinder, removable inner trocar, and long handle; used to inspect rectum.

Hirschsprung disease: Absence of ganglion cells in rectosigmoid and rectum; usu. presents as complete colonic obstruction in infants (failure to pass meconium in 1st 24 hours) or chronic constipation in children. Male-to-female ratio is 4:1. Definitive diagnosis is rectal biopsy. Dilated segment is proximal to aganglionic area. Surgical treatment is Duhamel, Swenson, Soave, or Boley procedures.

His bundle: AV conducting system of heart; begins in atrial septal wall just in front of coronary sinus and runs beneath medial cusp of tricuspid valve. Left branch pierces interventricular septum and right branch runs beneath supraventricularis.

His bundle ablation: Most common surgical procedure for treatment of atrial fibrillation, which uses catheter to "disconnect" electrical signals of atria and ventricles by ablating conducting tract; corrects unpleasant sensation felt by patient but has no effect on risk of thromboembolism or cardiac hemodynamics.

His bursa: Dilated end of archenteron.

His canal (Bochdalek duct, duct of His, duct of Vater, thyroglossal duct): Structural opening found in fetus between posterior tongue and developing thyroid. Distal part becomes thyroid pyramidal lobe, and proximal part is usu. obliterated.

His perivascular space (Virchow-Robin space): Spaces (or potential spaces) occurring around arteries when entering skull. Inner surface is continuation of arachnoid and outer surface is continuation of pia.

His tubercle: Small prominence on inferior-posterior earlobe.

Hitchcock frame: Stereotactic frame used in brain surgery.

Hitzelberger sign: Ability to feel sensation in external auditory canal; should be included in all medical evaluations of hearing disturbances.

Hitzig test: Used to investigate vestibular apparatus. Normal patient standing with eyes closed and feet together will lean toward positive electrode when galvanic current of 5 mA is applied just in front of ear being tested and negative electrode is held in patient's hand.

Hnevkovski syndrome (vastus intermedius contracture): Adherence of thigh fascia to vastus intermedius with limitation of knee flexion; occurs in girls 1–7 years of age (more common in twins, is usu. unilateral). Treatment is surgical division of fascia and vastus intermedius.

Hobaek syndrome (Dreyfus syndrome, spondylodysplasia): Abnormal ilium and vertebral bodies leading to short trunk and stature; autosomal recessive condition.

Hoboken valve: Ridges protruding from walls into lumen of umbilical cord vessels, esp. arteries.

Hochenegg procedure: Resection of rectum with anal sphincter left intact; procedure is no longer performed.

Hochsinger sign: Hand spasm seen in tetany when inner biceps area is pressed.

Hodges-Lehmann intervals: Nonparametric confidence intervals.

Hodgkin cell: Reed-Sternberg cell.

Hodgkin cycle: Activity of cell membrane characterized by positive feedback mechanism; depolarization causes influx of sodium into cell, which causes further depolarization.

Hodgkin disease (lymphoma): Condition described as having 4 histopathologic types: nodular sclerosis (50% of cases), lymphocyte predominance (best prognosis), mixed cellularity, and lymphocyte depletion; associated with Reed-Sternberg cells. Treatment is radiation (low-stage) and chemotherapy (high-stage) [Ann Arbor classification]; cure rate is 80%.

Hodgkin sarcoma: Lymphocyte depletion form of Hodgkin disease.

Hodgkin staging laparotomy: Procedure involving liver biopsy (performed 1st), lymph node biopsies (splenic, hilar, celiac, para-aortic, iliac, mesenteric, and porta hepatis), splenectomy, iliac bone crest biopsy, and oophorectomy; performed if questions arise concerning low-stage vs. high-stage disease and treatment modalities.

Hodgson procedure: Anterior drainage of C1–C2 TB abscess.

Hoehne sign: Indication of uterine rupture if injection of oxytocic agents do not produce contractions during delivery.

Hoen periosteal elevator: Handheld fork-like metal instrument used to scrape periosteum off bone surface.

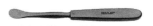

Hoen periosteal elevator

Hoerlein-Weber syndrome: Hereditary methemoglobinemia.

Hoesch test: Qualitative urine screening test used to detect acute episodes of porphyria; urine with twice normal amount of porphobilinogen will turn Ehrlich reagent in acidified solution red.

Hofbauer cells: Large, rounded macrophages found in placenta.

Hoff law (van't Hoff law): Some substances in solution have osmotic pressure identical to gas pressure they would exert if they were in gaseous state and at same temperature and pressure.

Hoffa disease: Hypertrophy of fat pad lying deep to patella, resulting in pain on extension and joint effusions of knee; edges of fat pad become pinched between condyles. Condition is rarely known to affect other joints. Treatment is heel lift (1 cm), quadriceps strengthening, and (in severe cases) excision of fat pad.

Hoffa fracture: Fracture of medial femoral condyle.

Hoffa-Lorenz operation: See Lorenz operation.

Hoffer procedure: Anterior tibial to cuboid tendon transfer for correction of spastic foot inversion.

Hoffman anodyne: Compound spirit of ether.

Hoffman disease: Tenosynovitis in thumb.

Hoffman test: Used to detect tyrosine; positive if mixture of sample and mercuric acid is boiled, nitric acid is added, and red precipitate forms.

Hoffman-Clayton procedure: Excision of proximal phalanges and metatarsal heads to correct toe deformities in rheumatoid arthritis.

Hoffman-Frei test: See Frei test.

Hoffmann duct: See Wirsung duct.

Hoffmann phenomenon: Irritability of sensory nerves under mechanical or electrical stimuli; seen in tetany.

Hoffmann sign (Trömner sign): Positive is flexion of thumb (terminal phalanx) and fingers (2nd and 3rd phalanx) on snapping one of 2nd–4th fingers; seen in corticospinal tract lesions.

Hoffmann syndrome: Congenital everted lower lip;

misshapen and projecting ears; and scant, wooly hair.

Hoffmann syndrome: See Debré-Semelaigne syndrome.

Hoffmann-Zurhelle disease: Growth of unsightly but benign ectopic fat cells in dermis; onset from birth to adolescence. Fat cells most frequent in lower trunk and legs, where they often coalesce to form plaques. Treatment is excision.

Hofmann bacillus: *Corynebacterium pseudodiphtheriticum.*

Hofmeister test: Used to detect peptone in absence of albumin; positive if precipitate forms after sample is mixed with reagent made by combining hydrochloric acid and phosphotungstic acid.

Hofmeister test: Used to detect leucine; positive if metallic mercury precipitates after sample is mixed with mercurous nitrate.

Hogben test: Pregnancy test; positive if female African toad *Xenopus* lays > 5 eggs 4–12 hours after being injected with patient's urine.

Hohl-Moore classification: System used to describe tibial plateau fractures. Type 1, minimal displacement; type 2, local compression; type 3, split compression; type 4, complete unilateral condyle; type 5, bilateral condyles.

Hoige syndrome: Procaine and penicillin G–induced apprehension, fear, hallucinations, tachycardia, systolic hypertension, and rapid-onset seizures; autosomal dominant condition with 6:1 male-to-female ratio.

Hoke procedure: Fusion of the 2 medial cuneiforms and navicular bone for correction of flatfoot.

Hoke procedure: Triple arthrodesis of talar head.

Hoke triple hemisection technique: Method of lengthening Achilles tendon; used in conjunction with split anterior tibial transfer technique in correction of equinovarus foot.

Hoke-Kite procedure: Wedge fusion of talocalcaneal joint and fusion and shortening of talonavicular joint for correction of calcaneocavovarus deformity.

Holden line: Anatomical sulcus running across acetabular capsule; lies below inguinal fold.

Holder angle: See Virchow-Holder angle.

Holländer disease: See Barraquer-Simons syndrome.

Hollenhorst plaques: Atheromatous plaques that act as emboli in retinal vessels.

Holme disease (Alajouanine disease, Foix disease, Marie disease): Progressive atrophy of cerebellar cortex with gait difficulty, hesitant speech, and tremor; most frequently seen in men in 6th and 7th decades. Cerebellar nuclei remain intact with loss of Purkinje cells.

Holmes buffer: Alkaline buffer (pH 7.4–9.0) made of boric acid and borax; used in stains containing silver salts.

Holmes disease: Fused ventricular chamber with great arteries in relatively normal position.

Holmes phenomenon (Gordon Holmes rebound phenomenon, Holmes sign): Attempt to move limb against resistance. On sudden removal of resistance, limb moves in original direction slightly and then jerks back or rebounds. This action is present in normal limbs, absent in limbs affected by cerebellar disease, and exaggerated in limbs with spasticity.

Holmes-Adie syndrome: See Adie syndrome.

Holmes-Rahe scale: Popular point system that measures stress; for example, death of spouse = 100; change in sleeping habits = 16. Total of ≥ 200 points is predictive of development of serious disease.

Holmgren wool test: Used to evaluate color perception by having patient match skein of particular hue to another of same color.

Holmgren-Connor syndrome (Glasgow-type dysplasia): Familial semilethal bone dysplasia with curved, micromelia limbs and severe rib shortening; autosomal recessive condition. Death usu. occurs from respiratory insufficiency in neonatal period.

Holmgrén-Golgi canal: See Golgi complex.

Holstein-Lewis fracture: Oblique humeral shaft fracture in distal 1/3 of bone; may cause radial nerve injury.

Holt-Oram syndrome: Hypoplasia of clavicles, secundum atrial septal defect, 1st-degree heart block, absent or hypoplastic radii, and variable syndactyly; autosomal dominant condition.

Holter monitor: ECG readings recorded over 24-hour period by portable lead–recorder system attached to ambulatory patient; useful in detecting intermittent arrhythmias.

Holth operation: Technique of scleral excision using punched-out sections.

Holthouse hernia: Inguinal hernia that bulges outward into groin.

Holthouse-Batten syndrome: Age-related superficial choroiditis.

Holzbach-Sanders syndrome: Intrahepatic cholestasis, variable jaundice, and pruritus in 3rd trimester of pregnancy; symptoms disappear shortly after delivery. Condition is autosomal dominant.

Holzgreve-Wagner-Rehder syndrome: Variant of Potter sequence with persistent buccopharyngeal membrane, cleft palate, cardiac abnormalities, and stunted growth.

Holzknekt (Holzknecht) sign: Right-sided mediastinal shift during inspiration; seen on chest radiograph in bronchial stenosis.

Holzknekt (Holzknecht) space: Middle lung field seen when chest radiograph is taken in oblique manner (left posterior to right anterior direction).

Homan operation (modified): Staged excision of leg tissue for severe lymphedema. Medial resection is performed 1st, followed by lateral excision.

Homans sign: Pain in calf or popliteal area when examiner dorsiflexes foot; seen in deep venous thrombosis of leg.

Homer-Wright rosettes: Groups of tumor cells seen in retinoblastoma, with no internal limiting membrane; morphologically indistinguishable from rosettes seen in neuroblastoma and medulloblastoma.

Hong Kong ear (Singapore ear): Fungal infection of ear.

Hootnick-Holmes syndrome: See Greig syndrome.

Hoover sign: Patient lying flat is asked to push 1 heel into bed. In normal patients or patients with true paralysis, other leg will lift slightly. In malingering and hysteria states, lifting motion is absent.

Hoover sign: Costal margin movement during inspiration is toward midline; seen in unilateral pneumothorax and pleural effusion and bilaterally in emphysema.

Hope mixture: Acid camphor.

Hope sign: Auscultation of double heartbeat in patients with aortic aneurysm.

Hopkins test: Used to detect lactic acid in gastric juice; positive if red color develops when sulfuric acid and copper sulfate are added to sample, mixture is heated, and thiophene is then added.

Hopkins-Cole test: Used to detect tryptophan; positive if purple color develops when glyoxylic acid and sulfuric acid are mixed with protein sample.

Hopman hump: Saddle deformity seen on lung radiograph in pulmonary embolism.

Hopmann papilloma (polyp): Overgrowth of mucous membranes of nose with papilloma formation.

Hoppe-Seyler test: Used to detect carbon monoxide in blood; positive if red mass develops when sodium hydroxide solution with specific gravity of 1.3 is added to sample. Normal blood forms greenish-brown mass.

Hoppe-Seyler test: Used to detect glucose; positive if green color develops when sample is boiled with potassium chromate and potassium hydroxide.

Horn sign: Pain produced in right lower quadrant and groin by traction on right spermatic cord; occurs in appendicitis.

Horner law: Color blindness is passed between males through asymptomatic females.

Horner muscle (tensor tarsi): Lacrimal portion of orbicularis oculi; originates on posterior lacrimal crest of lacrimal bone and bifurcates to supply fasciculus to each tarsal plate.

Horner sign: See Spalding sign.

Horner syndrome: Classical description is unilateral ptosis (lid droop), miosis (constricted pupil), and anhidrosis (lack of facial sweating); usu. due to interruption of ipsilateral sympathetic nerve supply in neck.

Horsley operation: Ablation of area of motor cortex as treatment for athetoid movement of arms; technique no longer performed.

Horsley sign: Higher temperature sometimes seen in axilla of affected side in hemiplegia.

Hortega cell: Microglial cell.

Horton arteritis: Temporal arteritis.

Horton artery: Temporal artery.

Horton cephalalgia: Cluster headache.

Hosmer device: Arm prosthesis with locking elbow joint and forearm lift assist device.

Hotel Dieu hemoglobin: High-oxygen-affinity hemoglobin with replacement of aspartic acid by glycine in $\alpha_1\beta_2$ contact area, results in hemoglobin values of 20–24 g/dl.

Hotis test: Used to test for bovine mastitis, or garget; positive if yellow flakes develop when fresh milk is incubated for 24 hours with bromcresol purple.

Hounsfield unit (number, CT number): Unit of attenuation in CT imaging; air = -1000 H, water = 0 H, and bone = $+1000$ H.

Houssay animal (phenomenon): Laboratory animal with pancreas and pituitary removed.

Houston loop: Fixation of loop of bowel to underside of abdominal wall. Marking this site and its course running to liver hilum with radiopaque surgical clips allows future percutaneous access to biliary-enteric anastomosis.

Houston muscle: Portion of bulbocavernosus muscle that occludes dorsal vein of penis.

Houston valves: 3 transverse redundant folds of mucosa in rectum; lowest may be palpable (on the left side) on rectal exam.

Houston-Harris syndrome (Parenti-Fraccaro syndrome type 1B): Severely disorganized endochondral ossification with no matrix between cartilage cells; more common in females.

Hovius plexus (Leber plexus): Collection of venous channels near ciliary body that connects to Schlemm canal.

Howard test (split-renal function test): Use of individual ureteral catheterization to measure quantity of urine and values to calculate sodium and creatinine clearance.

Howell test: Measurement of quantity of blood prothrombin via clotting time of sample mixed with oxalate, thromboplastin, and calcium chloride.

Howell-Jolly bodies: Remnants of nuclear material found as inclusion bodies in RBCs, which are eliminated in splenic cords by pinching-off process of "pitting"; structures are more prevalent after splenectomy.

Howship lacuna: Erosions in bone marrow that house osteoclasts.

Howship-Romberg sign: Positive for obturator hernia if pain radiating from inner thigh to knee occurs; due to pressure of hernia mass impinging on obturator nerve.

Hoyeraal-Hreidarsson syndrome: Rare stunted fetal growth, cerebellar hypoplasia, and pancytopenia.

Hoyne sign: When supine patient's shoulders are lifted, head falls backward; seen in poliomyelitis.

Hsieh-Pin syndrome: Trance-like state thought by patient to be due to possession by spirit of deceased relative; not considered pathologic in some cultures.

Huber procedure (opponens-plasty): Transfer of abductor digiti minimi neurovascular bundle to thenar eminence to restore thumb opposition.

Huchard sign: Absence of decreased pulse rate when moving from standing to lying position; seen in hypertension.

Huchard sign: Abnormal percussion sound in pulmonary edema.

Hucker stain: Modification of Gram stain. Smear is fixed by heat, covered with crystal violet, rinsed with Gram iodine, decolorized with acetone in alcohol, and covered with safranin; no blotting is done during staining.

Huddleson test: Brucellosis agglutination test.

Hudson-Stähli line: Horizontal brown pigment at middle/lower third junction of cornea; normal variant seen in 15% of elderly.

Hueck ligament: Network of thin, loose fibers forming 2-part chamber at iridocorneal angle between venous sinus of sclera and anterior eye chamber; aqueous humor filters through network as it passes into bloodstream.

Hueter line: Imaginary line running between humeral medial condyle and top of olecranon when arm is extended.

Hueter sign: Positive for fracture if no bone vibration occurs when auscultating with stethoscope down bone.

Hueter-Mayo procedure: Partial excision of 1st metatarsal for bunion.

Hufner disease: Motor neuropathy causing global weakness ranging to complete paralysis with severe demyelination. Cause is exposure to solvents; weakness progresses even after removal of solvents from environment.

Huggins operation: Orchiectomy performed to remove endocrine stimulation as treatment for prostate cancer.

Hughes classification: System used to describe alkali burns to eye. Grade 1—corneal epithelial injury with no ischemia; grade 2—hazy cornea, iris details intact, ischemia < 1/3 of limbus; grade 3—complete corneal epithelial loss, blurring of iris details, ischemia 1/3–1/2 of limbus; grade 4—opaque cornea with obscured pupil or iris, ischemia > 1/2 limbus.

Hughes syndrome: Gigantism of hands, hyperextensible joints and thickened lips, oral mucosa, and palpebrae.

Hughes-Stovin syndrome: Peripheral vein thrombosis and aneurysm of large and small pulmonary arteries; associated with congenital cardiac defects. Condition almost always affects males 15–35 years of age. Features are fever, hemoptysis (usu. cause of death), optic neuritis, and intracranial hypertension.

Hughston drawer sign (posteromedial and posterolateral drawer sign): Excessive tibial movement; demonstrated when supine patient flexes knee to 80°–90° and hip to 45° and examiner medially rotates foot and pushes on tibia posteriorly. Positive finding indicates possible injury to posterior cruciate ligament, posterior oblique ligament, medial collateral ligament, semimembranosus muscle, posteromedial capsule, or anterior cruciate ligament.

Hughston plica test: Used to indicate anterolateral knee instability; positive if straightening flexed knee with valgus force results in jerky motion 20° from full extension.

Hughston view: Radiographic technique with knee flexed to 60° and imaging performed at 55°; used to detect subluxed patella or femoral condyle fracture.

Huguier canal: Inner portion of petrotympanic fissure; carries chorda tympani nerve.

Huguier sinus: Tympanic groove lying between fenestra rotunda and ovalis.

Huguier-Jersild syndrome (Jersild syndrome): Pelvic lymphatic obstruction caused by ulcer, papula, or herpes lesion; leads to edema and fibrosis. Condition is usu. seen in older women. Treatment is early, aggressive antibiotics.

Huhner test: Aspiration of postcoital vaginal contents to evaluate number and activity of spermatozoa.

Hummelsheim procedure (transposition): Alternative to Jensen procedure for misaligned eyeballs. Split one-half of superior rectus muscle is completely detached and reattached to superior pole of lateral rectus muscle, and split one-half of inferior rectus muscle is completely detached and reattached to inferior pole of lateral rectus muscle.

Humphry ligament: Anterior meniscofemoral ligament of knee; runs from posterior area of lateral meniscus medially and traverses anterior to posterior cruciate ligament.

Hunermann syndrome: See Conradi syndrome.

Hunner ulcer: Interstitial urinary bladder ulcers leading to contracted wall, pain, and fibrosis. Condition occurs much more frequently in women and in middle-age. Treatment is topical silver nitrate, oxychlorosene (Clorpactin), or dimethylsulfoxide.

Hunt atrophy: Degeneration of small muscles of hand due to neurologic process; no occurrence of sensory deficits.

Hunt-Lawrence pouch: Jejunal pouch sometimes used in reconstruction after subtotal gastrectomy to increase gastric reservoir and delay esophageal emptying.

Hunter canal (adductor canal, subsartorial canal): Anatomic space beneath sartorius and between adductor longus and vastus medialis; contains loose alveolar tissue and femoral artery (descending genicular artery branches off within canal) and vein.

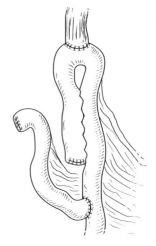

Hunt–Lawrence pouch

Hunter disease: Type 2 mucopolysaccharidosis, with less severe clinical sequelae than with Hurler disease; marked by mental retardation, deafness, chronic diarrhea, dwarfism, and odd facies. Deficiency of lysosomal enzyme sulfoiduronate sulfatase is needed for catabolism of glycosaminoglycan. Inheritance pattern is X-linked recessive.

Hunter ligament: Round ligament of uterus; runs from uterus near fallopian tube through broad ligament and inguinal ring and into labrum major.

Hunter line (linea alba): Median tendinous line between 2 rectus muscles.

Hunter operation: General technique of ligation of artery feeding an aneurysm proximal to area of dilation.

Hunter rod: Arm prosthesis using Silastic rod to build canal for subsequent 2-stage tendon graft procedure.

Hunter-Addison disease: See Biermer disease.

Hunter-Hurler syndrome: See Hurler disease.

Hunterian ligation: Early strategy for ligating parent artery of giant (> 2.5 cm) aneurysms in posterior brain circulation occluding vertebral artery in neck area; now largely superseded by intracranial aneurysm clipping.

Huntingdon sign: Coughing and straining by patient when lying supine with legs over edge of table, causing hip flexion and knee extension; seen in unilateral leg paresis secondary to lesions in pyramidal tract.

Huntington chorea (Mount disease): Gradual onset of choreiform movements, usu. between 30–50 years of age; slow progression to akinesia and demen-tia. Severe coronary disease is common; death occurs within 10–20 years of onset. Condition is autosomal dominant. Treatment is haloperidol (Haldol), chlor-promazine, lecithin, and vitamin E.

Huntington operation: Repair of chronically inverted uterus; rarely performed technique performed through abdominal incision. Invaginated part of uterus is pulled up using forceps, and when uterus is in correct position, packs are placed through vagina to maintain position.

Huppert test: Used to detect bile pigments; positive if yellow and green color develops when sample is mixed with calcium chloride solution and sodium or ammonium carbonate. Washing with H_2O and acetic acid produces green, and mixing with chloroform produces yellow.

Huppert-Cole test: Used to detect bile pigment; positive if greenish-blue color develops when sample is mixed with lime water, sulfuric acid, and dilute potassium chlorate and boiled.

Huriez disease: Onset from birth of scleroderma-like changes to hands with keratoderma of hands; squamous epitheliomas develop in adolescence. Defect occurs on chromosome 2. Condition is autosomal dominant.

Hurler disease (gargoylism, Hunter-Hurler syndrome, Johnie syndrome): Onset in 1st few months of life of physical and mental deterioration; marked by grotesque facial features, hydrocephalus, hirsutism, dwarfism, chest anomalies, retinal degeneration, and hepatosplenomegaly. Cause is deficiency in alpha-l-iduronidase with impaired degradation of heparan and dermatan sulfate. Death usu. occurs by 10 years of age due to cardiac failure and lung infection. Condition is autosomal recessive.

Hurst disease: Acute hemorrhagic encephalitis; usu. preceded by nonspecific respiratory infection 10 days before onset of neurologic symptoms.

Hurst syndrome: Stunted growth, small ears and head, craniosynostosis, dislocated radial heads, and fragile bones.

Hurst-Maloney dilators: Lubricated, tapered bougies placed blindly through mouth (after esophagoscope is withdrawn) to dilate esophageal strictures.

Hürthle cell: Thyroid follicular-type cell with variable enlargement, hyperchromatic nuclei, and granular cytoplasm; described as aggressive variant of follicular cell carcinoma.

Hürthle cell adenoma: Benign tumor of follicular cell origin; treatment is thyroid lobectomy and isthmectomy.

Hürthle cell carcinoma: Malignant tumor with follicular origin; represents 4% of all thyroid cancers. Definitive diagnosis cannot be made on fine needle aspiration. Treatment is total thyroidectomy and (with positive nodes) modified radical neck dissection.

Hurtley test: Used to detect acetoacetic acid; positive if purple color develops when sample is mixed with dilute sodium nitrate and hydrochloric acid, shaken, and then mixed with ferrous sulfate and ammonia hydroxide.

Huschke foramen: Small opening sometimes found in anteroinferior part of temporal plate; represents area of nonossification.

Huschke ligament (gastro-pancreatic fold): Peritoneal fold (containing left gastric artery) running from posterior abdominal wall to lesser curvature of stomach.

Huschke valve: See Hasner valve.

Hutch procedure: Correction of ureteral reflux; commonly performed procedure that can be used with associated congenital diverticulum and does not require ureteral anastomosis.

Hutchinson fracture: Fracture of radial styloid.

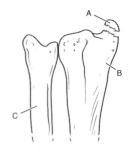

A. Radial styloid
B. Radius
C. Ulna

Hutchinson fracture

Hutchinson freckle: Lentigo maligna form of melanoma; good prognosis when confined to radial growth phase.

Hutchinson notch: Semilunar notch found in lower edge of teeth.

Hutchinson patch (salmon patch): Salmon-colored area seen on cornea in syphilis.

Hutchinson sign: Extension of melanoma lesion into proximal nail fold.

Hutchinson sign: Reddish corneal discoloration and interstitial keratitis seen in congenital syphilis.

Hutchinson sign: Eruption of vesicles on tip of nose due to infection of herpes zoster virus; often heralds onset of ocular involvement.

Hutchinson teeth: Sign of congenital syphilis; permanent upper central incisors most commonly affected are widely spaced, smaller than normal, and notched on biting surfaces.

Hutchinson triad: Deformed teeth, deafness, and keratitis; seen in congenital syphilis.

Hutchinson-Tay syndrome: Age-related guttate choroiditis.

Hutchinson-Weber-Peutz syndrome: See Peutz-Jeghers syndrome.

Huxley layer: One of lamina of inner root sheath of hair follicle.

Huygens eyepiece: Microscope ocular with 2 lenses; introduces lateral color if used with compensating eyepiece and high-power apochromatics or achromats.

Huygens principle: All points on wavefront are sources of production of secondary spherical wavelengths; important in consideration of scatter in ultrasound imaging.

hydatid cysts of Morgagni (paraovarian cysts): Small saclike structures near fimbria or in broad ligament; probably arise on wolffian duct remnants. Structures are clinically benign and found incidentally on ultrasound.

Hyndman sign: See Brudzinski sign.

Hyrtl loop: Variably present arc-like anastomosis of left and right hypoglossal nerves located in geniohyoid muscle.

Iberian cross adder: See Balkan cross adder.

Ideberg classification: Used to describe glenoid fractures of scapula. Type 1, anterior margin avulsion; type 2, horizontal fracture through glenoid fossa with displacement of inferior fragment; type 3, oblique fracture running through glenoid and onto superior scapular border (seen with acromioclavicular fractures); type 4, transverse running through medial border of blade; type 5, type 4 with added separation of inferior glenoid fragment.

Ilizarov technique: Procedure used in corrective osteotomy of tibia.

Illig syndrome: Total growth hormone deficiency leading to small stature at birth, marked dwarfism, and small facies. Treatment is exogenous administration with appearance of growth hormone antibodies after initiation of treatment (synthetic hormone use reduces antibody formation); prognosis is good if disorder is diagnosed and treated early. Condition is autosomal recessive.

Illum syndrome (arthrogryposis multiplex congenita): Fatal disease of infants with abnormal calcium deposits in brain and muscles, mental retardation, contractures of joints, apneic crises, bradycardia, and temp-erature abnormalities; male-to-female ratio of 1:1. Mode of inheritance is unknown but may be autosomal recessive.

India rubber skin: Ehlers-Danlos syndrome.

Indian anise: See Chinese anise.

Indian rhinoplasty (operation): See Carpue operation.

Indiana disease: Variant of Mason-Turner syndrome.

Indiana pouch: Continent urinary reservoir created using colon and terminal ileum; also used as part of pelvic exenteration procedures. Right colon is dissected off retroperitoneal attachments, split longitudinally to 1 side of taenia, and rolled onto itself.

Ingram procedure: Correction of congenital talipes valgus using anterior tendon transfer, Z-lengthening of peroneus brevis tendon, and navicular bone reduction.

Ingram technique: Nonsurgical pressure method to create neovagina in congenital absence using successively larger upright dilators attached to bicycle seat; allows patient to perform tasks while body weight applies pressure in 15–20-minute intervals for 2 hours daily. Full-sized vagina results in 2–12 months.

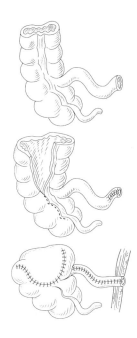

Indiana pouch

Inokucki shunt: Makeshift coronary vein/caval shunt with accompanying splenectomy; used to palliate variceal hemorrhage.

Insall ratio (Insall-Salvati ratio): Length of patella tendon divided by height of patella when knee is flexed 30°; value > 1.3 suggests patella alta.

Iowa scale: Description of preop and postop hip pathology; scored by assessing pain, function, and range of motion.

Irish node: Left axillary metastases due to gastric cancer.

Irvine-Gass syndrome (pseudopathic cystoid macular edema): Development of strand of vitreous material that passes through pupil and becomes attached to cornea 0–3 weeks after intraocular surgery; presents as decreasing vision and sensation of light flashes. Treatment is surgery, with good results.

Irving procedure: Tubal ligation; oviduct is severed, medial end of tube is buried into myometrium posteriorly, and proximal end is buried in mesosalpinx. Technique is least likely method to fail but has highest risk of hemorrhage. Generous surgical exposure is necessary for safe performance.

Isaac-Mertens syndrome: Development of continuous muscle fiber activity (myokymia) in infancy; associated with episodic cyanosis. Increased muscle tone does not remit in sleep. Condition partially resolves as child ages but often results in transient stiffness after movement is initiated. Disorder is autosomal dominant and affects both sexes equally. Treatment is phenytoin, with good results.

Iselin disease (traction epiphysitis): Pain and tenderness over 5th metatarsal bone, esp. on weight-bearing; represents 2nd center of ossification detectable on radiographs in oblique view only. Condition occurs in girls at age of 10 years and boys at 12 years. Playing sports is precipitating factor; disease is often mistaken for fracture with nonunion of epiphyses. Treatment is rest, ice, NSAIDs, and (in severe cases) casting.

Isherwood position:
Radiographic positioning technique of foot to allow imaging of anterior (via oblique lateral view), middle (via medial oblique axial view), and posterior (via lateral oblique axial view) articulations of subtalar joint.

island of Reil (insula): Triangular area lying in floor of sylvan fissure covered by opercula.

Isle of Wight disease:
Disorder caused by tracheal mite of honeybee (*Acarapis woodi*).

islets of Langerhans:
Collection of pancreatic endocrine cells numbering 1 million; contain insulin-secreting beta cells, glucagon-secreting alpha cells (20%–25% total islet cell number), and growth hormone and somatostatin-secreting delta cells.

Isola instrumentation:
Posterior spinal fixation device.

Italian rhinoplasty
(tagliacotian rhinoplasty): Nose reconstruction using flap from arm; flap remains attached to arm until graft forms good union on site on nose.

Itard-Cholewa sign:
Insensate tympanic membrane occurring in otosclerosis.

Ito-Reenstierna test: See Ducrey test.

Ivemark syndrome (type 1):
Congenital hypoplasia or absence of spleen, pulmonary atresia, atrial septal defect, transposition of great vessels, and severe ventricle malformations; death occurs due to heart failure or infection in childhood. Condition is autosomal recessive. Surgery is ineffective.

Ivemark syndrome (type 2):
Ivemark syndrome (type 1) with polycystic kidney disease.

Ivemark syndrome (type 3):
Congenital polysplenia, agenesis of corpus callosum, imperforate anus, short limbs, and malformed external genitalia; autosomal recessive condition is lethal in childhood.

Ives disease: Increased skin photosensitivity ("leopard spots"), swelling, and redness seen in elderly men. Treatment is sun avoidance, systemic steroids, and azathioprine.

Ives-Houston syndrome:
Congenital microcephaly and severe malformations of upper limbs occurring in Cree Indians; usu. results in stillborn fetus or death in infancy from severe apnea. Condition is autosomal recessive.

Ivor Lewis procedure:
Esophagogastrectomy performed through upper midline abdominal incision and right lateral thoracotomy incision; provides good exposure of entire esophagus and azygous vein and protection of left pleural space by aortic arch.

Ivy modification: Variation of Blair procedure for surgical correction of constricted nostril; performed as part of cleft lip repair. Flap is fashioned from lateral ala, moved superiorly and medially, and advanced into defect created after removal of full-thickness tissue wedge below soft tissue facet.

Iwanoff cyst: See Blessig cyst.

Iwashita syndrome (Rosenberg-Chutorian syndrome): Progressive visual and hearing loss and onset of polyneuropathy from birth.

Jaboulay pyloroplasty: Gastroduodenostomy; preferred procedure to bypass severely scarred pylorus.

Jabs-Blaus syndrome: Granulomas developing symmetrically in joints of wrists and hands causing arthritis; uveitis; and skin rashes; autosomal dominant condition with onset in childhood.

Jaccoud sign: Palpable aorta in suprasternal notch.

Jackson bougie: Straight, gum-tipped devices used with rigid esophagoscope for dilating hard esophageal strictures; 26F bougie fits through 45-cm rigid esophagoscope.

Jackson membrane (veil): Variably present thin layer of fibrous tissue running from lateral abdominal wall to (and sometimes covering) cecum; can cause cecal obstruction.

Jackson safety triangle: Anatomic space that delimits area through which trachea can safely be incised to perform tracheostomy; apex is sternal notch, base is bottom border of thyroid cartilage, and sides are inner borders of sternocleidomastoid muscle.

Jackson sign: Lengthened expiration detected over affected lung lobe in TB.

Jackson sign: Wheezing detectable close to mouth in patients with asthma; also occurs in partial occlusion of trachea or bronchus by foreign body.

Jackson syndrome: Paralysis of CNs X, XI, and XII, resulting in unilateral paralysis of soft palate and larynx, sternocleidomastoid and trapezius muscles, and tongue atrophy. Causes include vascular lesions (most common), tumor, infection, and trauma.

Jackson vaginal retractor: Handheld retractor used to view vaginal lumen.

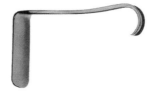

Jackson vaginal retractor

Jackson veil (membrane): Variably present abnormal fibrous bands running across and anterior to colon and deep to peritoneum; may be vascularized. Bands can decrease colonic motility.

Jackson-Barr disorder: Rare conductive deafness due to external auditory canal hypoplasia; also with droopy eyelids, thin nose, misshapen teeth, and skeletal anomalies.

Jackson-Lawler syndrome (Murray disease): Congenital, poorly formed and calcified teeth; thickened, coarse nails; follicular keratosis; epidermoid cysts on chest, neck, and head; and painful, infected cysts on feet in hot weather. Condition is due to defect in keratinization.

Jackson-Pratt drain (JP drain): Surgically placed closed drainage tube with bulb suction (must be released before removal).

Jackson-Rees circuit (Mapleson F circuit): "Noncircle" or "semiopen" anesthesia breathing system.

Jackson-Weiss syndrome: Type of craniosynostosis syndrome associated with defects in FGFR1 or FGFR2 genes.

Jackson-Wisconsin laryngoscope blade: Straight-tipped blade used in tracheal intubation.

jacksonian focal attack: Muscle spasm in synergistic muscles causing clonic-type movements; usu. due to contralateral cerebral lesion.

jacksonian seizures (focal motor seizures, partial motor seizures): Tonic–clonic seizures confined to 1 extremity or side of body, usu. with no loss of consciousness; secondary to lesion in frontal lobe.

Jacob membrane: Rods and cones of retina.

Jacob syndrome: Congenital cleft palate, facial asymmetry, with later onset of recurrent attacks of brachial plexus neuropathy (usu. with cumulative residual deficits).

Jacob ulcer: Rodent ulcer, esp. when located on eyelid.

Jacob-Brenner model: Proposed theory of replication of circular bacterial chromosome. Replication begins at mesosomal site on cell membrane, and chromosome moves past membrane attachment site, unwinding and replicating as it moves.

Jacob-Downey disease: Congenital rheumatoid arthritis, camptodactyly, flexion contractures of fingers, and polyarthritis of large joints in infancy; autosomal recessive condition.

Jacobs disease: Deficiency of riboflavin and vitamin B complex, resulting in conjunctivitis, scrotal pruritus, and fissures in nostrils.

Jacobs instrumentation: Spinal fixation device that uses threaded rods and locking hooks.

Jacobsen syndrome (spondyloepiphyseal dysplasia tarda): Pain in hip and back and stunted growth of torso; posterior superior vertebral plate has characteristic "hump" shape. Onset occurs at 5–10 years of age. Condition is associated with defects at chromosome locations Xq28 and Xp22.

Jacobsen-Brodwell syndrome: Rare renal dysplasia with anemia, neurogenic hearing deficits, visual loss, and diseased gums and teeth.

Jacobson canal: Tympanic canal with small mass of fusiform vascular tissue that Jacobson nerve runs through on way to forming tympanic plexus.

Jacobson cartilage: Narrow strips of cartilage running longitudinally on both sides of lower septal cartilage.

Jacobson nerve: Tympanic branch of CN IX originating from petrosal ganglion (Andersch ganglion).

Jacod disease: Unilateral damage to CNs II through VI; caused by neoplasm located at medial part of medial cranial fossa extending to foramen rotundum, foramen ovale, and superior orbital fissure.

Jacquart angle: See Broca angle.

Jacquemier sign: See Chadwick sign.

Jacquemin test: Used to detect phenol; positive if blue color develops when sodium hypochlorite and aniline are added to sample.

Jacquet dermatitis: Diaper rash.

Jacquet disease: Congenital focal areas of alopecia; may also develop in 1st year of life. Condition is associated with other ectodermal dysplasias or epidermal nevi.

Jadassohn nevus (nevus sebaceous): Nevoid lesion of scalp, which causes alopecia; difficult to diagnose, esp. in children, because scalp discoloration is only slightly yellowish.

Jaeger chart: See Rosenbaum screen.

Jaffe reaction (modified): Quantitative technique to determine serum creatinine; uses centrifugal analyzer and standard reagents.

Jaffe-Campanacci syndrome: Association of von Recklinghausen–type syndrome with nonosteogenic fibromas; marked by pathologic fractures before puberty. Condition also associated with congenital heart abnormalities, mental retardation, eye defects, precocious puberty, and alopecia.

Jahss procedure: Bone resection to release plantar fascia and dorsal wedge resection and excision of metatarsotarsal joint; used for correction of cavus foot and clawtoe.

Jalili-Smith syndrome: Association of abnormally shaped and discolored teeth and progressive dystrophy of rods and cones; photophobia and nystagmus present in 1st years of life.

Jamar dynamometer: Instrument for measuring isometric grasp (kg or lb) in 5 different hand positions.

James fibers (atriohisian connection): Myocardial electrical conduction tract connecting atrium and proximal His bundle; represent continuation of posterior internodal tract.

Jamshidi biopsy needle: 11-gauge needle commonly used for bone marrow biopsy in older children and adolescents; procures minimum biopsy specimen of 1.5 cm^3.

Janeway gastrostomy: Procedure used to gain permanent access to stomach. Full-thickness stomach flap is taken from greater curvature and then closed around catheter and brought out to skin, and mucosal nipple is formed at skin edge.

Janeway lesions: Small nodular hemorrhages on soles and palms; most commonly seen in acute endocarditis.

Jansen test: Used to detect hip osteoarthritis deformans; positive if patient is unable to cross legs (ipsilateral ankle-to-knee).

Jansey procedure: Wedge skin excision for ingrown toenail.

Janus stain: Substance that stains mitochondria in leukocytes bluish green.

Janus syndrome: See Brett syndrome.

Janz syndrome: Juvenile onset of myoclonic epilepsy, with symptoms esp. noticeable in morning; usu. well-controlled with medication.

Japanese B encephalitis: Vector is *Culex* mosquito; animal hosts are birds and domestic animals. Disease occurs in Far East.

Japanese blood fluke (*Schistosoma japonicum*): Trematode that penetrates skin in snail-infested water and migrates to liver and small veins of small intestine; found in Far East. Treatment is praziquantel.

Japanese river fever: Scrub typhus.

Japas procedure: Dorsal tarsal wedge resection and plantar fascia release; correction of high-arched foot.

Jaquet erythema: Diaper rash.

Jarcho syndrome: Thrombocytopenic purpura and hemorrhage in setting of disseminated carcinoma.

Jarcho-Levin syndrome: Congenital odd facies (mongoloid eyes, prominent occiput), short neck, winged scapulae, kyphoscoliosis, protuberant abdomen, and genitourinary malformations; usu. associated with respiratory insufficiency and infections. Thoracic skeleton shows characteristic "crablike" appearance. Condition most commonly occurs in Spanish individuals.

Jarisch-Herxheimer reaction: Abrupt deterioration (e.g., myalgia, chills, fever, headache) seen after onset of treatment with spirochete diseases (e.g., syphilis, Lyme disease); probably due to release of treponemal antigen. Treatment is largely supportive.

Jarjavay muscle: Tissue that arises from ischial ramus and inserts in vaginal constrictor muscle; depresses urethra.

Jatene procedure (arterial switch): Arterial reconstruction in transposition of great vessels in absence of pulmonary outflow tract obstruction. Aorta and pulmonary arteries are severed above valves, great valves are switched, and coronary arteries are transplanted into neoaorta.

Javid shunt: Coiled tubing used to shunt blood around operative field in carotid endarterectomy; has smooth finish on ends and different proximal and distal

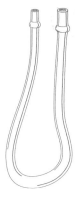

Javid shunt

diameters with flanges to prevent displacement. Shunt is anchored in place using Javid shunt clamps or Rumel tourniquet. Disadvantages include damage to intima, air or debris embolus, and decrease in visualizing operative field.

Jaworski corpuscle: Spiral-shaped mucous collections found in gastric juice in hyperchlorhydria.

Jayle-Ourgaud syndrome: Internuclear ophthalmoplegia.

Jeanne sign: Positive for ulnar nerve paresis if metacarpophalangeal hyperextension occurs when patient tries gross grip with adduction.

Jeanselme nodules (Lutz-Jeanselme nodules, Steiner tumor): Nodules appearing on arms and legs near joints in advanced cases of yaws and tertiary syphilis.

Jebsen test: Used to measure range of motion, strength, stability, and standardized functional testing after hand/wrist surgery.

Jebsen-Taylor test: Used to measure hand function in performance of activities of daily living; uses 7 subtests.

Jefferson fracture: Fracture of posterior arch of atlas (1st cervical vertebra) caused by sudden axial load; results in separation and lateral spread of 2 lateral segments.

Jeliffe method: Technique for estimating creatinine clearance; equals 98—0.8 (age—20)/serum creatinine. (Value is reduced by 10% in women.)

Jellinek sign (Rasin sign): Brownish discoloration of edge of eyelids; seen in hyperparathyroidism.

Jendrassik maneuver: Reinforcement of patellar reflex by patients hooking their fingers with palms facing and pulling hard.

Jendrassik sign: Eye muscle paralysis occurring in Graves disease.

Jendrassik-Grof method: Determination of total bilirubin by adding Ehrlich diazo reagent and caffeine benzoate to specimen and taking spectrophotometric measurement.

Jennette syndrome (chloroquine nephropathy): Chloroquine-containing immune complexes causing nephron damage that mimics signs and symptoms of nephrotic syndrome; occasional spontaneous remission.

Jennings mouth gag: Device used to distract mandible 3–4 cm to provide exposure for transoral resection of small mouth tumors; also used for forcibly opening clenched jaws. Device incorporates ratchet mechanism with dental processes placed between upper and lower incisors.

Jennison-Turnbull modification: Variation of Brookmeyer-Crowley method for determining confidence limits for quartiles with right censored data.

Jensen classification: System used to describe intertrochanteric femur fractures. Type 1, stable, nondisplaced single fracture line; type 2, stable, displaced single fracture line; type 3, comminuted (not involving lesser trochanter) with possible instability; type 4, involving lesser trochanter with greater trochanter fragment attached to neck (risk of loss of reduction); type 5, unstable trochanteric fragments (highest loss of reduction).

Jensen disease (sarcoma): Malignant tumor in mice; important in cancer research, because transplantation of tumor cells causes tumor in recipient.

Jensen procedure: Method used in treatment of CN VI nerve palsy with associated impaired (saccadic velocity < 40% normal) lateral rectus muscle function. Temporal halves of superior and inferior rectus muscles are joined to split halves of lateral rectus muscle, part of vertical rectus muscle is temporally transposed, and medial rectus muscle recession is performed.

Jensen syndrome: Onset in infancy of sensorineural deafness followed by optic nerve atrophy in adolescence and dementia in adulthood; associated with severe calcification of CNS. Death usu. occurs by 40 years of age. Inheritance is X-linked.

Jervell syndrome (Lange-Nielsen syndrome): Rare association of cardiac conditions—prolonged QT intervals, T-wave abnormalities, relative bradycardia, and ventricular tachyarrhythmias—with sensorineural deafness. Patients present with episodes of seizures, syncope, or sudden death precipitated by intense emotion, exercise, or loud noises. Cardiac component of disorder is autosomal dominant, and deafness component is autosomal recessive.

Jessner-Cole syndrome: See Goltz syndrome.

Jeune dystrophy (infantile thoracic dystrophy): Variant of Ellis van Creveld syndrome; marked by severe, life-threatening deformity of thorax, misshapen iliac bones, elevated clavicles, notched ends of metacarpal and metatarsals, shortened fibula and ulnar bones, and abnormal ossification centers in sternum.

Jeune-Tommasi syndrome: Association of mental deficiency, cardiomyopathy with heart block, cerebellar ataxia, and sensorineural deafness. Condition is autosomal recessive and most commonly occurs in gypsies, with onset in childhood.

Jewett orthosis: Back brace that restricts spinal flexion; applies posterior pressure across thoracic-lumbar boundary and anterior pressure over symphysis pubis and sternum.

Jewett-Marshall system: System used to stage bladder cancer. Stage 0, mucosa involvement only (carcinoma in situ); stage A, lamina propria; stage B, muscle invasion; stage C, perivesicular fat involvement; stage D, lymph node or distant metastases.

Jewett-Whitmore classification: System used to define prostate cancer. *Stage A*—nonpalpable cancer; stage A1, < 5% of tissue and Gleason grade > 7; stage A2, > 5% of tissues or Gleason grade > 7; *stage B*—palpable nodule; stage B1, palpable nodule < 1.5 cm in diameter; stage B2, palpable nodule > 1.5 cm in diameter; *stage C*—extension beyond prostatic capsule without distant metastases; *stage D*—metastases; stage D1, metastases to regional lymph nodes; stage D2, metastases to bone or viscera.

Job syndrome: Hypereosinophilia with high serum levels of IgE (> 2000 IU/ml) and low *Staphylococcus aureus* IgA; defective T-cell suppressor activity and chemotaxis with recurrent skin abscesses and pneumonias, coarse facial features, and bone abnormalities. Condition is possibly mediated by histamine.

Jobe test: Used to evaluate anterior shoulder subluxation. Shoulder is abducted and externally rotated and posterior force is then applied to humerus. Test is positive if pain subsides when patient lies supine.

Jobst stockings: Graduated compression stockings.

Jodbasedow disease: Thyrotoxicosis that occurs secondary to iodine supplementation.

Joe's hoe: See Weinberg vagotomy retractor.

Joffroy sign: Absence of normal wrinkling of frontal muscles and skin when gaze is quickly moved upward; seen in Graves disease.

Johansson classification: System used to describe femoral fractures after total hip replacement. Type 1, fracture proximal to prosthesis; type 2, fracture running from proximal shaft to distal to prosthesis; type 3, fracture running distal to prosthesis.

John Henryism: Coping with psychosocial stressors using strong personality predisposition to hard work to overcome overwhelming obstacles.

Johnie syndrome: See Hurler disease.

Johns Hopkins gallbladder forceps: Locking forceps with ring-handle and curved tips; used in tissue dissection.

Johnson syndrome: Congenital alopecia, anosmia, hypogonadism, deafness, cleft palate, and heart abnormalities.

Johnson technique: Arthroscopic stapling technique for detached glenohumeral ligaments in traumatic unstable shoulders. Ligaments must be mobile to be effective. Loss of glenoid position is contraindication. Patient is placed in lateral decubitus position with affected arm suspended using skin traction.

joint of Luschka: Bony projection on superolateral edges of vertebral bodies that form articulations between adjacent vertebrae.

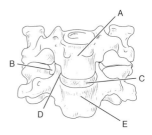

A. Vertebral body C4
B. Intervertebral foramen
C. Intervertebral disk
D. Joint articulation of Luschka
E. Vertebral body C5

Joint of Luschka

Jolliffe syndrome: Encephalopathy caused by deficiency of nicotinic acid; marked by cerebral focal demyelination and ganglion cell degeneration, cogwheel rigidity, and impaired sucking and grasping reflex. If condition becomes chronic, damage can be irreversible.

Jones criteria (revised): Guidelines for diagnosis of rheumatic fever. Major manifestations are carditis, polyarthritis, chorea, erythema marginatum, and subcutaneous nodules. Minor manifestations are fever, arthralgia, previous rheumatic fever or rheumatic heart disease, elevated sedimentation rate or positive C-reactive protein, and prolonged PR interval. Presence of 2 major criteria or 1 major and 1 minor criterion establishes diagnosis.

Jones fracture: Fracture line in base of 5th metatarsal from lateral edge towards proximal articulation of 4th and 5th metatarsal.

Jones procedure (wedge metroplasty): Technique for repair of double uterus. Biconcave uterine wedge from both sides of uterine septum is removed; length of incision is determined by length of septum. Stain is used to mark endometrial cavity, and vasopressin is injected into incision line to decrease bleeding. Myometrium is closed in 3 layers.

Jones syndrome (cherubism): Onset in early childhood of multilocular cystic disease of jaw, development of white line on sclera, and variable lymphadenopathy; usu. regresses somewhat in adolescence.

Jones towel clamp: Small, sharp-tipped, perforating metal surgical instrument used to fasten drapes on sterile field; applied by finger control of cross-action mechanism.

Jones tube (modified) [Putterman-Gladstone tube]: Variation of Jones tube with 2nd flange placed 4–6 mm from superior (top) flange to prevent movement within lacrimal canal; requires special dilator to insert.

Jones tube (standard): Small glass tube placed through lacrimal bone to open obstruction and correct epiphora. Diameter is 2.2 mm [top flange, 3–4 mm; flaring at distal (nasal) end, 2.8 mm].

Jones-Barnes-Lloyd and Roberts classification: System used to describe congenital anomalies of leg. Type 1a, absent tibia with hypoplastic lower femoral epiphysis, type 1b, absent tibia with normal femur; type 2, absent distal tibia; type 3, absent proximal tibia; type 4, diastasis.

Jonston alopecia (alopecia areata, Celsus alopecia): Patchy areas of baldness on scalp, eyebrows, and face; not associated with inflammation or infection.

Joseph rhinoplasty: Surgical technique to improve contour of nose by removing dorsal bony hump with saw.

Joussef fistula: Vesicovaginal fistula occurring after delivery, infection, tumors, or trauma.

Jordans anomaly: Rare congenital vacuolation of leukocytes marked by fat deposits in neutrophils; variably present in monocytes, eosinophils, basophils, and lymphocytes. Condition is usu. benign but has been associated with cardio-myopathy, muscular dystrophy, and ichthyosis.

Jorissen test: Used to detect formaldehyde in urine; positive if precipitate forms when 1 ml of sample is added to 0.5 ml of 1% phloroglucin and 10% sodium hydroxide.

Joubert facial anomalies: See Egger syndrome.

Joubert syndrome: Ataxia, abnormal eye movements, episodic hyperpnea, and mental retardation; autosomal recessive condition with onset in 1st 6 months of life.

Joubert-Bolthauser syndrome: See Egger syndrome.

Joussett disease: Development of vesicovaginal fistula after surgery, irradiation, or tumor. Treatment is surgery, with good results.

Juberg-Hayward syndrome: Congenital microcephaly, cleft palate, short stature, and hypoplasia of thumbs; autosomal recessive condition.

Juberg-Holt syndrome: Congenital dwarfism, malformed thumbs, waddling gait, and flattening of epiphyseal plates; autosomal recessive condition.

Juberg-Marsidi syndrome: Congenital microcephaly, mental retardation, deafness, flattened nasal bridge, and small genitalia; X-linked inheritance. Death occurs in boys in early childhood; condition is less severe in girls.

Judet view: Radiographic position used to detect acetabular fractures; pelvis is viewed bilaterally at 45° oblique angle.

Juhlin-Michälsson syndrome: Absence of basophils and eosinophils; marked by repeat infections, hemolytic anemia, alopecia, and warts.

Jung association test: Used to elicit personality traits. Patient is told word and asked to respond with 1st thought that comes to mind; there are no restrictions (e.g., opposite) on responses.

Jung muscle (pyramidal muscle of ear): Muscle fibers running from tragicus to spina helicis.

jungian psychology (analytical psychology, complex psychology): Modification of early Freudian principles; deemphasizes primacy of sex drive, broadens concept of the unconscious, highlights exciting causes for neuroses, and modifies techniques of dream interpretation.

Junius-Kuhnt syndrome: Age-related maculopathy.

Juzo stockings: Graduated compression stockings.

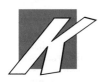

Kaes-Bekhterev line (stria, Vicq d'Azyr band): Fibrous lamina between external pyramidal and external granular layers in cerebral cortex.

Kaeser dystrophy (scapuloperoneal dystrophy): Degeneration of anterior horn motor neurons, causing atrophy of all muscles below knee except intrinsic muscles of foot; autosomal recessive condition. Atrophy of shoulder girdle develops some years later, with variable involvement of cranial nerves.

Kager triangle: Radiolucent area anterior to Achilles tendon seen on radiography.

Kahler disease: Multiple myeloma.

Kalamchi and Dawe classification: System used to describe congenital abnormalities of tibia. Type 1, complete absence; type 2, absence of distal tibia; type 3, severe ankle diastasis.

Kalicinski plication: Technique of ureteral imbrication for megaureter.

Kalicinski technique: Urethral imbrication for pediatric megaurethra using same surgical folding maneuver as in Kalicinski plication. Penile shaft is degloved, urethral lumen is downsized using running 6–0

horizontal mattress suture over 12F catheter, and this excluded segment is then folded over onto ventral urethra surface and secured with interrupted sutures.

Kallin syndrome: Autosomal recessive form of Cockayne-Touraine syndrome.

Kanavel cock-up splint: Appliance used to effect extension in finger contracture.

Kanavel sign: Positive for tendon sheath infection if there is point tenderness 2 cm proximal to base of 5th finger; alternately described as positive for pyogenic tenosynovitis if pain occurs on passive extension. Tendon sheath tenderness and diffuse enlargement of fingers also present.

Kanavel spaces: Anatomic areas separated by septum lying deep to long flexor tendons on palm; located at midpalm and in thenar area.

Kanavel triangle: Anatomic space in center of palm superficial to common tendon sheath of flexor tendons of finger.

Kandori syndrome (night blindness): Mild defect in dark adaptation without defects in acuity or visual field; large yellowish spots develop under retinal vessels. Etiology is unknown; condition affects both sexes equally.

Kaneda instrumentation:
Anterior spinal fixation device for thoracic and lumbar spine for treatment of kyphosis and burst fractures; allows ample room for bone graft placement. Dual-threaded rod is applied after surgical decompression for both distraction and compression, and bicortical screws are used to add stability.

Kanner syndrome (infantile autism, "wild boy of Aveyron" syndrome): Developmental disorder (more frequent in males) of intellectually normal children who have no interest in other people, intolerance to changed environment, and significant speech and motor development delays. Parents usu. have above-average intelligence and prestigious, desirable occupations. Etiology is unknown, possibly involving tryptophan derangement. Condition is associated with increased birth complications. Treatment is early, intensive psychiatric treatment and stimulation.

Kantor string sign: String-like appearance of contrast seen in contrast radiographic studies of colon; indicative of intra-luminal obstruction and suspicious for cancer.

Kapandji score: Measure of ability to oppose thumb (both base and tip) to palm and tips of other fingers.

Kaplan line: Imaginary line running between hook of hamate and 1st web space of hand and also running parallel to proximal transverse palmar

crease. Intersection with thenar skin crease marks origin of motor branch of medial nerve.

Kaplan-Meier method: Most commonly used life table; estimates percent survival at time of each outcome event (must be terminating), each with expressed degree of uncertainty. Technique generally underestimates late survival.

Kaposi sarcoma: Raised, painless purple-brown lesions occurring on skin, conjunctiva, lung, or in GI tract (including esophagus); may present with lymphadenopathy only. Disorder is found in HIV-infected men (homosexuals but not IV drug users and hemophiliacs); most commonly seen in North America in AIDS (50% incidence). Biopsy entails high risk of hemorrhage.

Kaposi syndrome: See Devergie syndrome.

Kaposi varicelliform eruption (eczema herpeticum): Primary infection in setting of chronic eczema; marked by fever and extensive skin vesiculation. Cause is herpesvirus type 1. Condition is rarely fatal.

Kappis disease: Aseptic necrosis of talus.

Kapsinow test: Used to detect bile pigments in urine; positive when sample is added to Obermayer reagent and heated and green color develops.

Kapur-Toriello syndrome: Congenital mental retardation,

cleft lip, long columella, iris coloboma, microphthalmia, intestinal malrotation, and congenital kidney and heart defects.

Karelian fever: See Sindbis virus.

Karev reconstruction: Digital pulley reconstruction technique used to maximize tendon excursion into finger flexion.

Karpati syndrome: Carnitine deficiency.

Karplus sign: Indicative of pleural effusion; vowel "U" spoken by patient is heard by examiner listening over site of effusion as "A."

Karsch-Neugenbauer syndrome: Congenital nystagmus.

Kartagener syndrome: Hypomotility of cilia; marked by chronic sinusitis, bronchiectasis, situs inversus, and dextrocardia.

Karydakis sliding flap: Procedure used to treat pilonidal cysts.

Kasabach-Merritt syndrome: Large, bluish, progressive vascular malformations in extremities; stagnant blood lesions can cause disseminated intravascular coagulation, platelet consumption, and bleeding. Condition mostly affects infants; sudden growth can cause drastic decrease in platelets. Treatment is steroids and low-dose radiation. Mortality is 30%.

Kasai procedure: Portoenterostomy performed in infants with biliary atresia; first described in 1959. Best results are obtained if procedure is done in first 8 weeks of life.

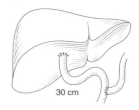

Kasai procedure

Kashida sign (thermic sign): Hyperesthesias and muscle spasms caused by applying cold or heat to affected muscle; occurs in tetany.

Katayama disease: Systemic schistosomiasis with fever, chills, headache, urticaria, organomegaly, lymphadenopathy, nausea, and vomiting; caused by *Schistosoma japonicum.* Serum IgE and IgG and eosinophils are increased.

Katz index: Assessment of activities of daily living; correlates with recovery from hip fracture, nursing home placement, and mortality.

Katzman test (infusion manometrics): Diagnostic test for normal-pressure hydrocephalus; fluid is infused into spinal subarachnoid space by lumbar puncture. Abnormal absorptive capacity is 300–600 mm of H_2O in 20 minutes.

Kaufman assessment battery for children: Intelligence evaluation for patients 2 1/2–12 years of age; useful in disadvantaged populations because it is independent of acquired knowledge.

Kaufman syndrome: Congenital mental retardation, stunted growth, hypotonia, respiratory distress, mongoloid eyes, ptosis of eyelids, sparse eyebrows, and lordosis.

Kaup index: Measure of body habitus; equals weight/body length squared.

Kawasaki disease: Disease of childhood with acute cervical adenitis; fever; myocarditis; conjunctivitis; and erythema of oral cavity, soles, and palms. Condition is also marked by desquamation of fingertips and coronary artery aneurysms in 25% of cases. Serial echocardiograms are used to follow disease. Early treatment is chronic aspirin.

Kayser-Fleischer rings: Brownish rings in cornea developing in some cases of Wilson disease.

Kazanjian T bar: Device for lip and jaw reconstruction; uses acrylic fastener to support soft tissues.

Kaznelson anemia: See Faber anemia.

Kearns-Sayres variant (of chronic progressive external ophthalmoplegia): Slowly progressive ptosis with cardiac conduction abnormalities and pigment changes of retina; due to mutations in mitochondrial DNA.

Kedani fever: Scrub typhus.

Keen sign: Increased ankle size at malleolus; occurs in Pott fibula fractures.

Kegel pelvic muscle exercises: Voluntary intermittent contractions of levator ani muscles; used to treat mild stress incontinence.

Kehr sign: Pain in top of left shoulder (referred from diaphragm irritation); sometimes occurs in splenic rupture.

Keith node (Keith and Flack node, Koch node, sinoatrial node): Bundle of specialized cells that make up "pacemaker" of heart; lies in upper posterior wall of right atrium.

Kelikan procedure: Technique used to correct congenital hallux varus, esp. severe conditions with very short 1st metatarsal. Incision is made between 1st and 2nd metatarsal with excision of joint capsule and suturing together of toes.

Kell blood group: Patients expressing Kell protein antigens. Kell antibodies in patients receiving Kell blood causes severe hemolytic reactions. Kell antigen subtypes have racial associations. Sutter antigen is found in 20% of blacks and is rare in whites, and Duffy antigen (4 alleles) is found in 90% of blacks and in 3% of whites.

Kell protein: Serum protein of 720 amino acids with immunogenicity slightly less than ABO and Rh antigens. Defects are associated with majority of chronic granulomatous diseases, acanthosis, and shortened RBC survival. Gene lies on X-chromosome.

Kellgren grade: System used to describe hip (and spine) osteoarthritis. Grade 1, osteophytes without joint space narrowing; grade 2, joint space narrowing and acetabular sclerosis (small osteophytes may be present); grade 3, joint space narrowing (osteophytes present); grade 4, femoral head deformed with sclerosis of acetabulum and femur.

Kelling-Madlener procedure: Truncal vagotomy and antrectomy with gastric ulcer (type 4) left in situ; must be accompanied by multiple biopsies to ensure lesion is benign.

Kellock sign: Positive for pleural effusion if placing left hand on chest wall just under nipple and firmly percussing ipsilateral side with right hand produces increased rib vibration.

Kelly abdominal retractor: Handheld retractor used during laparotomy.

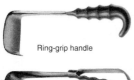

Ring-grip handle

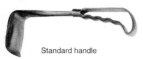

Standard handle

Kelly abdominal retractor

Kelly hemostatic forceps: Straight or curve-tipped, ring-handle, locking forceps placed on vessels to control bleeding or for tissue dissection; available with nontoothed or 1×2 teeth.

Kelly sign: Peristalsis of ureter when squeezed or pulled; performed intraoperatively to confirm anatomy.

Kelly-Kennedy plication: Transvaginal urethropexy.

Kelly-Seegmiller syndrome: Inborn partial deficiency in enzyme of purine metabolism hypoxanthine phosphoribosyltransferase (HPRT); causes hyperuricemia and tophi formation on extremity joints but lacks nervous system sequelae.

Kelman technique: Surgical method for treatment of cataracts; 1st reported (1967) cases of removal of crystalline lens through small incision. Technique involves nucleus subluxation followed by anterior chamber emulsion of nucleus. Procedure permits cataract extraction on outpatient basis and with no physical restrictions postop; most eye surgeons today use 1 of several modifications.

Kelvin thermometer: Instrument that measures temperature using Kelvin scale.

Kenawy sign: Louder venous hum on inspiration than expiration when stethoscope is placed just beneath xiphoid process; probably caused by engorgement of splenic vein. Sound can be found in splenomegaly caused by portal hypertension, esp. in bilharzial fibrosis of liver.

Kendall-Sheridan Laser-Trach tube: Copper foil–wrapped, fabric-covered tube for KTP and CO_2 lasers. Nonreusable tube must be soaked in saline before use.

Kendall-tau correlation: Type of nonparametric statistical analysis.

Kennedy bar: Metal retainer device used on lingual tooth surfaces.

Kennedy device (ligament augmenting device, LAD): Braided strip of polypropylene sutured to autogenous tissue to be repaired or to autologous graft; may be used with semitendinosus tendon, ilio-tibial band, patellar tendon, or retinacular tissue. One end of composite is sutured to bone and other end has tissue only sutured to bone.

Kennedy disease: See Currarino syndrome.

Kenny-Howard splint: Chest harness for anchoring, sling to push clavicle caudal, and separate sling to support elbow and wrist; used to stabilize acromioclavicular separations.

Kensey catheter: First atheroblation device in clinical use to remove intra-arterial blockages due to plaque; uses high-pressure water jet to rotate smooth cam. Limitations are larger-than-desirable fragments that travel downstream, iatrogenic vessel perforation, and

nonexpandability (requiring complementary balloon angioplasty).

Kent bundles: Myogenic tissue running directly from atria to ventricles, completely bypassing AV node and infranodal system; is anatomic basis of Wolff-Parkinson-White syndrome.

Kenya fever: Type of spotted fever caused by *Rickettsia;* transmitted by tick in family Ixodidae.

Kerandel sign: Profound pain and discomfort when even light percussion is directed at bony prominences; occurs in African trypanosomiasis.

Kerckring center (ossicle): Transiently occurring fetal ossification center in posterior foramen magnum.

Kerckring valves (plica circulares): Mucosal folds protruding in bowel lumen that slow food passage and increase absorptive surface.

Kergaradec sign: Uterine souffle.

Kerley B lines: Thickening of interlobular septa in pulmonary edema, which causes 1–3-cm chest radiograph shadows that run transverse and perpendicular to pleural surface; usu. seen at base of lungs when left atrial pressure is 25–30 cm H_2O or mitral valve area is 1.0 cm^2.

Kernig sign (test): Resistance to straightening knee after hip and knee have been flexed (or pain in lower back and posterior thigh with knee straightening); suggests meningeal irritation.

Kernohan grading system: Rating system for pathophysiology of astrocytic gliomas. Grade 1, pilocytic astrocytoma; grade 2, astrocytoma; grade 3, anaplastic astrocytoma; grade 4, glioblastoma.

Kernohan notch: Groove in cerebral peduncle that develops when it is displaced against tentorium; occurs in transtentorial herniation.

Kernohan notch sign: Fixed and dilated pupil ("blown pupil") on contralateral side of brain herniation, instead of expected ipsilateral side.

Kerr sign: Change in skin texture found below somatic level in spinal cord lesions.

Kersting-Hellwig tumor (spiradenoma): Well-defined, usu. single 1–3-cm diameter tumor that may be bluish yellow; onset in young adulthood. Treatment is local excision. Male-to-female ratio is 2:1.

Kesaree-Wooley syndrome (penta X syndrome): Phenotypic female (XXXXX); marked by stunted growth, mental retardation, camptodactyly, low-set ears, micromelia, radioulnar synostosis, congenital heart abnormalities (esp. patent ductus arteriosus), and ketotic hypoglycemia.

Keshan disease: Low serum levels of selenium associated with peripheral myopathies and multiple areas of myocardial necrosis; endemic in Keshan province of China where soil is deficient in selenium. Children and young women are most susceptible.

Kessler technique (modified): Surgical procedure used to correct finger flexor divisions.

Kestenbaum sign: Loss of arterioles that traverse optic disk margin; seen in optic atrophy.

Ketner syndrome: Congenital small tongue attached anteriorly to hard palate, small mandible, shortened digits, and lobster claw deformity; occasionally seen with facial or abducens nerve paralysis.

Kevorkian curette: Instrument used to obtain endometrial biopsy specimens.

Kew Gardens fever: Pox infection caused by *Rickettsia*.

Key-Conwell classification: System used to describe pelvic fractures. Type 1A, avulsion fractures of anterior spine or ischial tuberosity; type 2A, fracture of 2 ipsilateral rami; type 2B, fracture/subluxation of symphysis pubis; type 2C, fracture/subluxation of sacroiliac joint; type 3A, 2 vertical fractures of pelvic ring or straddle dislocation of pubis; type 3B, 2 vertical fractures of pelvic ring or Malgaigne ring dislocation; type 3C, multiple ring fractures; type 4A, acetabular fracture with nondisplaced pelvic fracture; type 4C, linear acetabular fracture with instability; type 4D, central acetabular fracture/dislocation.

Khoudadoust line: Leukocyte aggregation seen on posterior cornea; represents advancing endothelial corneal graft rejection.

Kidd antigen blood group: 2 allelic protein antigens containing intermittent level of immunogenicity; frequent cause of delayed hemolytic reactions when blood initially tests compatible.

Kidner procedure: Method involving transfer of flexor digitorum longus tendon to underside of navicular and medial cuneiform bones; treatment for posterior tibial tendon weakness (in absence of deformity).

Kienböck disease: Avascular necrosis of lunate bone in wrist; occurs without apparent injury. Condition is more common in patients with negative ulnar variance. Presenting features are tenderness over lunate bone (stage 1) that progresses to lunate collapse (stage 2) and arthritis (stages 3–4). Treatment is immobilization (stage 1), radial shortening (stages 2 and 3), and wrist fusion or carpectomy (stage 4).

Kiesselbach area (Little area): Area on anterior nasal septum lying superior to intermaxillary bone. This highly vascular zone (capillaries merge here) is common site of anterior nosebleed.

Killian area: Anatomic area between cricothyroid and cricopharyngeus muscles; site

where Zenker diverticulum develops.

Killian-Jamieson diverticulum: Pharyngeal pouch protruding laterally through muscle wall.

Kiloh-Nevin syndrome (chronic progressive external ophthalmoplegia): Progressive dystrophy of external ocular muscles due to fibrillary degeneration of striated muscles; marked by onset before 30 years of age, bilateral ptosis and diplopia, loss of facial expression, and occasional heart block.

Kimmelstiel-Wilson disease: Formation of hyaline nodules in glomerular loops and afferent and efferent arterioles of kidney.

Kimray-Greenfield filter: See Greenfield filter.

Kimura disease: Idiopathic inflammation of skin on head and neck; may involve orbit and lungs. Histopathology shows angiolymphoid hyperplasia with eosinophilia.

Kinkiang fever: Schistosomiasis japonica.

Kinsbourne syndrome (myoclonic encephalopathy of childhood): Myoclonus of limbs and torso, ataxia, and intention tremor with jerky eye movements and variable mental retardation; onset usu. at 1–3 years of age. Condition sometimes heralds neuroblastoma.

Kinyoun stain: Basic fuchsin, phenol crystals, alcohol, and distilled H_2O; combined with the

Ziehl-Neelsen stain to visualize acid-fast *Mycobacteria*.

Kirby-Bauer stain (disk–agar diffusion method): Qualitative method to determine which antibiotics are effective against which specific bacteria; involves placement of antibiotic-treated paper disks on agar surface containing bacterial species to be tested.

Kirghizian dermato-osteolysis: See Kozlova dermato-osteolysis.

Kirk arcade: Anastomosis of dorsal pancreatic artery with posterior-superior pancreaticoduodenal artery; present in 60% of individuals.

Kirkland classification: 1949 modification of Dukes classification for colorectal cancer. A, lesion confined to mucosa; B1, lesion extends into muscularis propia; B2, lesion penetrates muscularis propia into pericolonic fat.

Kirner deformity: Palmar and radial curvature of distal 5th finger with painless swelling; usu. seen in preadolescent girls. Treatment is wedge osteotomy or splinting.

Kirschner wire traction (K-wire): Traction using small wires attached to fractured bones to allow external traction device; used to treat hand and some pediatric fractures.

Kittner dissectors: 8×16–mm cylindrical, radiographically detectable sponges used to place blunt (but gentle) pressure on tissues; usu. held at tips of forceps.

Klatskin tumor: Cholangiosarcoma at junction of right and left hepatic bile ducts. Recent treatment approaches advocate aggressive resection of liver parenchyma (up to lobectomy) in an attempt for cure; clear microscopic margins are mandatory.

Klauder disease: See Baker-Rosenbach syndrome.

Klebs-Loeffler bacillus: *Corynebacterium diphtheriae.*

Kleihauer test (Kleihauer-Betke acid elution test): Most sensitive laboratory test used to confirm that blood sample is of pure fetal origin; requires 45–70 hours to complete and thus is not useful at bedside.

Kleine-Levin syndrome: Hypersexuality, hypersomnia, mood changes, and bulimia; occurs in young men. Etiology is unknown but condition is associated with trauma or acute illness. Interval between attacks may be months to years; episodes tend to disappear when full adulthood is reached. Treatment is lithium or amphetamines.

Kleinert rubber band traction: Traction used to effect primary finger flexor tendon repair.

Kleinman shear test: Used to detect triquetrolunate disease; positive if examiner's thumb is placed on lunate dorsum, and pain, crepitus, or significant movement occurs when pisotriquetral joint is given volar side pressure.

Kleinschmidt disease: 1940s term for respiratory distress secondary to influenza complications.

Klemm sign: Right lower quadrant abdominal distention on radiography; suggestive of chronic appendicitis.

Klenzak joint: Ankle/foot prosthesis with single-stopped ankle joint.

Klestadt cyst (nasoalveolar cyst, nasolabial cyst): Forms from caudal end of nasolacrimal duct at base of nostril and outside alveolar segment of maxilla and is often bilateral; occurs mostly in women.

Kliest sign: Positive for thalamic and frontal brain lesions if patient's finger "hooks" around examiner's finger when slightly elevated.

Klinefelter syndrome: 47 XXY syndrome (most common variant) with male phenotype; marked by male hypogonadism, infertility, eunuchoid body habitus, macrocephaly, long legs, gynecomastia, and atrophic testes. Condition is also associated with risk of male breast cancer and extragonadal germ cell tumors. Follicle-stimulating hormone is increased.

Klintworthe disease: Acute onset of myoclonic ataxia.

Klippel-Feil syndrome: Congenital abnormality of spine with failure of normal segmentation, resulting in mass of spine with no recognizable vertebrae; may affect any vertebra, although most common in cervical spine. Condition can range from lethal to asymptomatic and is associated with short neck, low posterior hairline, reduced lateral range of motion of neck, scoliosis (50%), hearing deficits (30%), renal abnormalities, and congenital heart defects. In children, bimanual synkinesias (mirror movements) may occur.

Klippel-Trenaunay syndrome: Large varicose veins on lateral calf and thigh and bone hypertrophy causing elongated leg and port-wine cutaneous hemangiomas.

Klippel-Weil sign: Positive is involuntary flexion and adduction of thumb when contracted fingers are passively extended; used to assess corticospinal tract functioning in arm.

Klumpke paralysis (Klumpke Dejerine palsy): Damage to lower (C8 and T1) roots of brachial plexus as result of jerking, upward traction on arm as seen in breech and arm presentation birth injuries; leads to loss of all intrinsic muscles in hand, with wasting.

Klüver-Bucy syndrome: Rare hypersexuality, hyperesthesias, aggressiveness, fearlessness, and inability to recognize known persons; caused by bilateral temporal lobe lesion.

Knapp iris scissors: Fine-tipped, ring-handled scissors used in eye surgery.

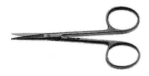

Knapp iris scissors

Knapp procedure (transposition): Surgical treatment of unilateral eye elevation defect caused by impaired elevating eye muscles (in absence of restrictive processes); uses 270° limbal peritomy to expose superior, medial, and lateral rectus muscles. Inferior border of rectus muscle is attached to nasal border of superior rectus muscle insertion. Upper border of medial rectus is attached slightly superior and nasal to inferior pole of medial rectus muscle. Lateral rectus muscle is then transposed to lateral border of superior rectus muscle. Procedure can correct 30–35 prism diopters of hypotropia.

Knapp streaks: Vascular-type linear lesions sometimes occurring in retina after hemorrhage.

Kneist syndrome (dwarfism): Craniofacial abnormalities, glaucoma, exophthalmos, variably detached retinas, shortened extremities at birth, joint swelling, lordosis, kyphoscoliosis, deafness, cleft palate, and altered gait.

Knies sign: Unequal pupillary dilatation sometimes seen in Graves disease.

Knoblock-Layer syndrome: Rare occipital encephalocele, detached retinas, and myopia; normal mental development.

Knodt distraction rod: Device used for stabilization of thoracic–lumbar spine.

Kober reaction: Colorimetric assay for detection of estrogen in blood or urine; most commonly used modification of Brown reaction. Acid (sulfuric or phenolsulfonic) hydrolysis of sample forms pink color.

Koch node: See Keith node.

Koch phenomenon (tuberculin hypersensitivity): Injection of tuberculoprotein or tubercle bacilli into tuberculous patients; leads to severe inflammatory reaction at skin injection site, with accompanying necrosis.

Koch postulates: Statements that clarify causative relationship between microorganism and disease. 1, microorganism must be routinely isolated from cases of illness; 2, microorganism must be grown in pure culture; 3, when pure culture of microorganism is inoculated into susceptible species, illness must result; 4, microorganism must be isolated from inoculated animal.

Koch-Mason dressing: Warm saline-soaked dressing placed on cellulitic limb.

Kocher approach (curved "L" approach): Technique for exposure of ankle, midtarsal, and subtalar joints; curved incision is made around lateral malleolus, peroneal tendons are retracted posteriorly, and calcaneofibular ligament is divided.

Kocher dilatation ulcer: Ulcer formed in distended bowel loops occurring in ileus.

Kocher fracture: Bone fragment of capitellum with entry into elbow joint.

Kocher hemostatic forceps: Straight, ring-handle, locking forceps with 1×2 teeth on tips; usu. placed on fascia and pulled upward for retraction.

Kocher incision: Right subcostal incision for cholecystectomy.

Kocher intestinal forceps: Long (279 mm), straight, locking, ring-handle forceps with long, thin jaws; nontoothed tip; and longitudinal serrations; used to clamp bowel.

Kocher maneuver: Surgical reflection of duodenum (by incising retroperitoneal attachments) medially to expose posterior pancreas, porta hepatis, aorta, and inferior vena cava.

Kocher maneuver: Procedure used to reduce anterior shoulder dislocation. Arm is abducted, externally rotated, adducted, and internally rotated.

Kocher sign: Positive for Graves disease if on quick upgaze superior eyelid moves faster than eyeball.

Kocher-Langenbeck approach: Acetabular exposure for posterior wall and posterior column up to sciatic notch. Patient is placed in lateral decubitus position or prone with ipsilateral knee flexed to 45° to relieve tension on sciatic nerve. Incision runs from superior edge of greater trochanter and is curved proximally to superior iliac spine. Gluteus maximus and fascia lata are then exposed, fascia lata is incised, and detachment of external rotators is performed, with retraction over sciatic nerve to expose posterior column.

Koch-Weeks bacillus: *Haemophilus aegyptius.*

Kock ileal neobladder: Spherical urinary reservoir formed using 60 cm of terminal ileum (2 22–25-cm segments of distal ileum and 1 17-cm segment of more proximal ileum) with intussuscepted afferent nipple valve to prevent reflux; used in women with cystectomy for transitional cell carcinoma of bladder.

Kock pouch (continent ileostomy): Several loops of ileum that serve as fecal reservoir to allow intermittent access and drainage; never used in Crohn's disease.

Koebner phenomenon (isomorphic phenomenon): Development of psoriasis (or lichen planus) on traumatized areas of skin.

Koehler disease (fracture): Avascular necrosis of tarsal navicular bone, often causing pain and swelling; usu. seen in boys 5–6 years of age. Condition is characteristic of "crushing"-type osteochondritis with necrosis in ossific nucleus. Spontaneous healing is norm.

Koehler-Stieda disease: See Pellegrini-Stieda syndrome.

Koenig-Schaefer technique: Medial approach to ankle for fractures/dislocations of talus and talar osteochondritis dissecans; high risk of tibial nerve and vessel injury.

Koeppe lens: Dome-shaped lens used intraoperatively to visualize "angle" of eye (interface between iris and cornea).

Koeppe nodule: Small punctate granulomatous keratoprecipitates on pupillary margin of iris.

Kohler disease: Aseptic necrosis of patella.

Kohler line: Imaginary line running from acetabular "tear drop" to most lateral tip of pelvic ring.

Köhler principle: Basis for adjustment of light source on microscope; makes it possible to illuminate only area to be studied.

Kohlrausch folds: See Houston valves.

Kohlrausch veins: Superficial veins draining underside of penis into dorsal vein.

Kohn pores: Microscopic openings in alveolar wall.

Kohnstamm phenomenon (aftermovement): Involuntary elevation of the arm after it receives firm pressure from hard object.

Kohs block design test: One of subtests of Arthur point scale of performance; used to evaluate intelligence, esp. in children who are deaf or non-English speaking. Patient must use blocks whose sides are printed with different colors to reproduce designs.

Köllicker membrane (reticular lamina, reticular membrane): Fine, web-like network of fibers lying over spiral organ; free ends of hair cells pass through openings.

Kolmer test: Complement fixation test used to detect spirochetes; based on reagin-containing sera that fixes complement in presence of cardiolipin antigen. Quantitative results may be obtained.

Kolmogorov-Smirnov test: Nonparametric statistical test that determines if 2 independently selected samples come from same population; sensitive to differences in skewness, scedasticity, and central tendency.

Kommerell diverticulum: Congenital dilation of left subclavian artery/descending aorta representing remnant of right dorsal aortic root; may be source of aberrant right subclavian artery. Esophageal compression requiring resection may result.

Kondo test: Used to detect skatole; positive if 1 ml sample added to 1 ml concentrated sulfuric acid and 3 drops formaldehyde produces yellow-brown color.

Kondo test: Used to detect indole; positive if 1 ml sample added to 1 ml concentrated sulfuric acid and 3 drops formaldehyde produces purple color.

Kondoleon operation: Staged mobilization of thick skin flaps with resection of underlying subcutaneous tissue to palliate congenital lymph-edema; medial limb flaps are fashioned 1st.

Konstram angle: Angle that defines gibbous deformity; formed by drawing lines from superior border of vertebral body and inferior border of vertebral body below it.

Koopmann technique (uvulopalatopharyngoplasty): Enlargement of airspace of oropharynx by eliminating redundant tissue of soft palate. Posterior superior part of posterior tonsillar pillar is retracted laterally and superiorly and secured with suture, anterior pillar is removed, and posterior pillar is then released and sutured into defect.

Koplik spots: Minute white specks surrounded by inflammation seen in buccal mucosa of children; strongly suggestive of prodromal measles if associated with fever and cough.

Kopp asthma (Miller asthma, Wichmann asthma): Acute onset of laryngeal spasm, noisy inspiration, and cyanosis; associated with laryngeal inflammation and rickets.

Korányi sign: Positive for pleural effusion if percussion of thoracic vertebral spinous processes causes increased resonance over dorsal surface.

Korean ginseng (Panax ginseng): Ginseng with macrophage-enhancing effect.

Korean hemorrhagic fever (Korin fever): Fever, hemor-rhage, vomiting, kidney failure, and systemic collapse; occurs in most severe forms in Korea, Japan, and northeastern China (Manchuria).

Korff fibers: Collagenous radial fibers at edge of tooth pulp that enter dentin and coalesce to form matrix.

Korin fever: See Korean hemorrhagic fever.

Korotkoff sounds: Sounds heard just distal to blood pressure cuff when noninvasive method of blood pressure mea-surement is used. Phase 1 is systolic pressure in adults; phase 2 is diastolic pressure in children; phase 5 is diastolic pressure in adults.

Korsakoff syndrome: Organic amnesia marked by confusion, memory loss, and confabulation; classically associated with thiamine defi-ciency in chronic and severe alcoholism.

Kossel test: Used to detect hypoxanthine; positive if red color results when sample is mixed with zinc, hydrochloric acid, and sodium hydroxide.

Koster-Collins operation: "Redo" operation for aortic aneurysm and dissection.

Kostmann syndrome: Congenital neutropenia (< 100 neutrophils/μl); manifests in early childhood and is often fatal.

Kostuick-Harrington instrumentation: Anterior spinal fixation device for thoracic and lumbar spine to correct kyphosis, burst fractures, and less frequently, tumors and degenerative disease; uses anterior Harrington distraction rod after corpectomy or diskectomy to reduce kyphosis and posterior Harrington compression rod to increase stability. Rods are connected via screws that pass through staple plates and into vertebral body.

Kovalevsky canal: See Braun canal.

Koyter muscle: Muscle fibers that act to draw eyebrows down and medially. Origin is medial superciliary arch, insertion is skin underlying eyebrows, and innervation is via facial nerve.

Kozlova dermato-osteolysis: Onset in infancy of recurrent skin ulceration, fistulous degeneration of joints, arthralgia, abnormal nails, fever, and visual impairment; autosomal recessive condition.

Krabbe disease: Globoid cell leukodystrophy marked by accumulation of galacto-cerebroside in brain causing blindness, optic atrophy, and death in first few years of life; autosomal recessive condition. Absent enzyme is galactosidase.

Krackow-Cohn technique: Procedure used for passing tendon or fascia through hole in bone. 2 sutures are tied in crisscross manner around distal end with ends in Chinese fingertrap suture to allow it to be pulled through.

Krackow-Thomas-Jones technique: Procedure for fixation of ligament or tendon (tibial collateral ligament, joint capsule, patellar tendon) to bone.

Kraemer disease: Suppurative scleritis caused by septic emboli to scleral vessels; marked by eye pain, tearing, and photophobia.

Kramer syndrome: See Ketner syndrome.

Krause end bulb (corpuscle): Sensory nerve ending (providing cold sensation) sheathed in connective tissue; found in skin, conjunctiva, mucosa, and heart.

Krause gland: Accessory lacrimal gland that lies beneath conjunctiva of the fornix.

Krause membrane: See Amici disk.

Krause valve: See Béraud valve.

Krause-Kivlin syndrome: Peter anomaly associated with short limb dwarfism; also with variable mental retardation, cleft palate, hydrocephalus, and failure to thrive.

Krause-Reese syndrome (ophthalmic dysplasia): Diagnosis of visual defects (ranging from minimal loss in 1 eye to total blindness), ptosis, strabismus, glaucoma, and hypoplasia of cerebellum and cerebrum.

Krebs cycle: Biochemical pathway of oxidative phosphorylation occurring in mitochondria.

Krebs-Henseleit cycle: Biochemical pathway found only in liver; contains enzymes that convert ammonia to urea.

Kreibig disease: Atherosclerosis of retinal arteries; associated with degeneration of optic nerve.

Kretschmer somatotype: 1920s theory that body morphology is associated with

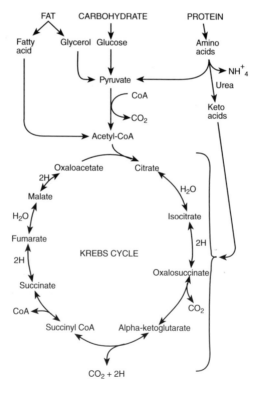

Krebs cycle

certain personality disorders (e.g., athletic build is associated with normal personality).

Kretz granule: Structure seen in cirrhotic livers.

Krimsky test: Used to measure strabismus by measuring strength of prism needed to move displaced central light reflex to pupil center; deviation given in prism diopters. Test is useful only in tropia (not phoria) and is more rapidly performed and more accurate than Hirschberg test.

Krisowski sign (Krisovski sign): Circular lines emanating from mouth in congenital syphilis.

Kroener fimbriectomy: Surgical procedure for sterilization.

Kronecker center (cardio-inhibitory center): Small area on vagus nerve partially responsible for inhibitory action on heart muscle.

Krönlein hernia: Hernia with both inguinal and properitoneal components.

Krönlein operation: Lateral orbitotomy; deep orbital tissues are approached through crescent-shaped incision lateral to orbit accompanied by lateral bone resection.

Kropp procedure: Technique of bladder neck reconstruction. Anterior bladder wall is exposed with anterior detrusor muscle flap developed and sutured temporarily over pubis; ureters are then dissected free of their attachments and reimplanted more laterally and cephalad

(thus freeing up space to make submucosal midline tunnel); anterior muscle flap is then released and rolled into tube to serve as new urethra, which is pulled through midline submucosal tunnel. A temporary suprapubic tube is then placed and bladder is closed primarily or with enterocystoplasty. Use of this technique for pediatric neurogenic bladder incompetence gives good results.

Krüger-Thiemer hypothesis: 1958 description of bactericidal effect of isoniazid on *Mycobacteria;* causes multiple metabolic disturbances in organism through formation of analog of NAD.

Kruis system: Scoring system used to distinguish organic GI disease from irritable bowel syndrome; involves patient history, physical exam, and laboratory values.

Krukenberg operation (kineplastic operation): Surgical procedure used to improve sensation and manipulative ability, in which forearm is fashioned into ulnar and radial pincers with distal amputation so it can accept myoelectrical prosthesis. Operation is cosmetically unappealing but useful in blind amputees in whom tactile sensation is at premium.

Krukenberg spindle: Pigmented lesions appearing on posterior corneal surface; seen in pigmentary glaucoma.

Krukenberg tumor: Metastatic disease found in ovaries,

which is classically described as originating in stomach; usu. produces excess androgens.

Krukenberg veins: Small veins in center of hepatic lobules that empty into hepatic veins.

Kruskal-Wallis statistical test: Nonparametric equivalent of ANOVA for > 3 groups.

Kubisagari disease: Myasthenia-like condition with bulbar weakness and ptosis in nutritionally deprived persons, esp. children.

Kuess disease: Chronic constipation.

Kufs disease (ceroid lipofuscinosis): Onset in adolescence of progressive loss of gait, seizures, dysarthria, ataxia, and spasticity; marked by deposits of lipopigments in all body tissues, esp. brain. Condition is autosomal recessive.

Kugel artery: Auricular anastomotic artery; 1st branch off left circumflex coronary artery.

Kugel repair: Technique for closure of inguinal hernia by using properitoneal approach to place synthetic patch.

Kugel-Stoloff disease: Idiopathic cardiomegaly.

Kugelberg-Welander disease (juvenile) [spinal muscular atrophy type 3]: Neuromuscular disorder due to neuron disease with slowly progressive proximal muscle weakness; onset begins after 2 years of age. Both autosomal

recessive and autosomal dominant forms are described.

Kuhelendahl syndrome: See Barré-Liéou syndrome.

Kühne phenomenon: Undulating movement in muscle from positive to negative pole when constant current is applied to muscle; occurs in EMG.

Kühne terminal plate: Endplates of nerve fibers in muscle spindles.

Kuhnt intermediary tissue (meniscus): Glial fibers found circumferentially around optic nerve; lie between nerve and retina.

Kuhnt postcentral vein: Vessel running posteriorly from center of optic nerve and draining into canalis opticus.

Kuhnt-Szymanowski procedure: Technique for repair of ectropion.

Kulenkampff-Toronow syndrome: Spastic muscles in mouth, pharynx, tongue, and neck secondary to chlorpromazine toxicity; may be associated with tachycardia and hypotension.

Kümmell disease: "Disappearing bone disease" of vertebral body; wedge-shaped collapse occurs due to linear fracture. On 2nd trauma (often minor), entire vertebral body disintegrates. Condition may be variant of Gorham disease.

Künnel spondylitis: Inflammation of vertebrae following compression fractures.

Kupffer cell: Stellate-shaped macrophages that phagocytize foreign particles and line walls of hepatic sinusoids.

Kupffer cell sarcoma: Angio-sarcoma of liver; associated with exposure to vinyl chloride, arsenic compounds, and thorium dioxide.

Kurtzke scale (expanded disability status scale): Used to measure neurologic defects and disability in multiple sclerosis; evaluates bowel, bladder, pyramidal, cerebellar, brain-stem, sensory, visual, and mental functions.

Kurz disease: Congenital blindness, wandering eye move-ments, and mental retardation.

Kurzbauer position: Lateral projection for radiologic imaging of unilateral sterno-clavicular articulation.

Kuskokwim syndrome: Congenital joint contractures, esp. of knees and ankles; sometimes associated with pigmented nevi and diminished corneal reflex. Patients tend to walk on knees or develop waddling gait.

Kussmaul respiration: Labored, rhythmic breathing, usu. associated with diabetic ketoacidosis.

Kussmaul sign: Absence of decrease or, presence of increase, in jugular venous pressure with inspiration; seen in restrictive cardiomyopathy and mediastinal tumor.

Kussmaul sign: Paradoxical pulse.

Küstner incision: Similar to Pfannenstiel incision; uses slightly transverse incision beginning just below anterior iliac spine on each side and runs to just below pubic hairline. Fascia is incised through midline (unlike transverse fascial incision in Pfannenstiel), rectus muscles are retracted laterally, and peritoneum is opened in midline.

Küstner sign: Cystic tumor on anterior median uterus in association with ovarian dermoid.

Küstner rule: In ovarian torsion, right ovary twists in clockwise manner and left ovary twists in counterclockwise manner.

Küttner ganglion (haupt-ganglion of Küttner): Lymph node located just below posterior digastric muscle at level of greater cornu of hyoid.

Kveim-Siltzbach test: Skin test for sarcoidosis performed by injecting suspension of sarcoidosis spleen extract intradermally; skin biopsy performed 4 weeks later shows sarcoid-like lesions in positive patients 70%–80% of time.

Kyasanur-Forest disease: Hemorrhagic disease occurring in India caused by tick-borne encephalitic flavivirus. Prophylaxis is inactivated vaccine.

Laband syndrome (Zimmerman-Laband syndrome): Congenital fibromatosis of gums, hirsutism, hypoplasia (or absence) of digits and nails, joint hypermobility, abnormalities of ears and nose, hepatosplenomegaly, abnormalities of 3rd and 4th ventricle, and variable mental retardation; unknown etiology and inheritance pattern.

Labbé syndrome: Severe hypertensive condition in pheochromocytoma.

Labbé vein: Vessel that connects superficial middle cerebral vein and transverse sinus.

Lachman test: Used to test for anterior cruciate ligament injury; positive if forward movement of tibia occurs when femur is placed in 15°–30° of flexion. If there is laxity with a fixed endpoint, tear is partial; if there is no endpoint, tear is complete.

La Crosse encephalitis (California encephalitis): Abrupt onset of severe bilateral frontal headache, high fever, vomiting, and convulsions; caused by arbovirus infection. Insect vector is unknown; condition occurs mainly in central, eastern, and southern U.S. Disease is rarely fatal.

lactated Ringer's solution: Na° 130 mEq/L, Cl⁻ 110 mEq/L, K⁺ 4 mEq/L, Ca²⁺ 3 mEq/L, lactate 28 mEq/L; most optimum initial resuscitation fluid.

Ladd band: Abnormal fibrous tissue running from abdominal wall over duodenum when cecum is malpositioned in right upper quadrant.

Ladd procedure: Counterclockwise surgical reduction of midgut volvulus, division of Ladd bands, appendectomy, and division of right colon and cecal retroperitoneal attachments.

Ladd syndrome: Duodenal stenosis presenting in 1st hours after birth to 1st feeding, usu. with bilious vomiting, upper abdominal distention, and lack of or small amounts of gas in intestinal lumen; may be due to atresia, stenosis, or extrinsic compression. Treatment is urgent duodeno- or gastro-jejunostomy.

Ladd-Gross syndrome: Congenital bile duct atresia presenting within 1st 2–3 weeks of life; marked by progressive jaundice, hepatosplenomegaly, and liver failure. Condition is caused by arrest of canalization of hepatic ducts (intrahepatic and/or extrahepatic); it is possibly related to intrauterine infection with *Listeria monocytogenes*. Treatment is Kasai procedure and (in liver failure) transplantation.

Ladd-Steritek system: Small, disposable pneumatic device placed in epidural space; frequency response wave produces intracranial pressure values close to intraventricularly placed devices.

Ladewig stain: Trichromic stain using iron hematoxylin that stains nuclei black; uses acid fuchsin–gold–orange that stains fibrin and muscle orange and aniline blue that stains mesenchyme and parenchyma grayish blue.

Laënnec cirrhosis: Stage of Laënnec disease with presence of small yellow nodules on liver surface.

Laënnec disease (Morgagni-Laënnec disease): Liver damage marked by slow progression to cirrhosis and failure; characterized by variable presence of anorexia, fatigue, abdominal pain, spider angiomata, ascites, encephalopathy, and gastric and esophageal varices. Onset of clinical signs occurs in 5th–6th decade. Liver becomes enlarged with smooth surface progressing to shrunken and nodular shape. Cause is toxic effect of alcohol in setting of dietary insufficiency.

Laënnec pearls (sign): Gelatin-like, oval bodies found in sputum in bronchial asthma.

Lafora bodies (amyloid inclusions): Circular inclusions found in cytoplasm of CNS neurons, esp. in patients with myoclonic epilepsy; thought to contain acid mucopolysaccharide.

Lafora body disease: Ataxic disorder marked by myoclonic epilepsy. Onset occurs at 6–16 years of age. Condition is autosomal recessive.

Lafora sign: Nosepicking in earliest stages of meningitis.

Lager syndrome: Psychiatric disorder experienced by patients rescued from severe persecution (e.g., concentration camp survivors, fugitives). Condition is marked by chronic tension, alertness, depression, agitation, headaches, and sweating. Patients tend to seek isolation and to suffer memory defects.

Lagos bat virus: Rabies-type virus occurring in Africa.

Lahey gall duct forceps: Curve-tipped, ring-handle, locking forceps used in tissue dissection; available with varying curvature of tips and longitudinal or cross serrations.

Lahey hemostatic forceps: Curved or straight-tipped, ring-handle, locking forceps placed on vessels to control bleeding.

Lahey syndrome (agitation): Phase of thyroid storm marked by tachycardia, sweating, flushed facies, and agitation.

Lahey syndrome (apathetic): Phase of thyroid storm marked by apathy and lethargy.

Lahore sore: See Aleppo boil.

Laignel-Lavastine-Viard syndrome: Identical to Barraquer-Simons syndrome with added excessive production of lower body subcutaneous fat.

Laimer-Haeckerman area:
Lower pharyngeal–upper esophageal region; most common site for diverticula of upper GI tract.

Laitinen stereoadapter:
Device that uses stereoguide and biopsy probe for brain surgery.

Laki-Lorand factor: Blood coagulation factor XIII that stabilizes clots; synthesized in liver and megakaryocytes/platelets and also found in placenta. Factor has 2 α chains and 2 β chains, and its half-life is 100 hours. Deficiency is rare and causes severe bleeding and poor wound healing; condition may be seen shortly after birth with bleeding from umbilicus. Disorder is autosomal recessive, with normal clotting tests. Adequate treatment/prophylaxis is 1 unit of blood or plasma.

Lamaze method (technique):
Popular method of birth delivery involving breathing exercises and relaxation techniques with supportive coaching from partner.

Lambert syndrome:
Intrahepatic biliary atresia, clubfoot, inguinal hernia, branchial dysplasia, macrostomia, and mental retardation; death usu. occurs by mid-childhood. Condition is autosomal recessive.

Lambert syndrome
(porcupine man): Ichthyosis hystrix.

Iambliasis: *Giardia lamblia* infection.

Lambling syndrome: Post-gastrectomy malabsorption marked by weight loss, diarrhea, nutritional derangements, and anemia.

Lambotte syndrome: Mental retardation, microcephaly, small birth weight, large pinna, and hooked nose; seen largely in persons of Arabic descent. Death occurs by 2 years of age. Condition is autosomal recessive.

lamellar injury of Werenskiold: Variation of type of epiphysis injury at ankle; marked by small, lamellar segment of metaphyseal bone separated by growth plate. Injury is caused by significant shear forces.

Lance disease: Aseptic necrosis of cuboid.

Lance-Adams syndrome:
Myoclonus, impaired speech, and ataxia developing after hypoxic encephalopathy; no symptoms are seen at rest.

Lance-Anthony syndrome:
Pain and tongue numbness when head is suddenly turned; due to C2 lesion.

Landolt ring: Visual test using series of cards printed with open rings; child must identify direction the apertures point.

Landry paralysis: See Guillain-Barré syndrome.

Landry-Guillain-Barré syndrome: See Guillain-Barré syndrome.

Landsmeer ligaments
(oblique retinacular ligaments):
Connective tissue that runs on
lateral sides of finger and
synchronizes distal joint motion.

Landström muscle: Scattered
muscle buried in fascia surrounding eyeball; extends to
eyelids and anterior orbital
fascia.

Landzert fossa (paraduodenal
fossa): Variably present space
present to left of 4th part of
duodenum; formed by peritoneal fold enveloping inferior
mesenteric artery.

Lane plate: Stainless steel
device with screw holes used to
internally fix bone fragments.

Langdon Down syndrome:
See Down syndrome.

Lange-Nielson syndrome
(Jervell syndrome): Hereditary
long QT syndrome associated
with deafness.

Langer muscle: Muscle
running over bicipital groove;
originates at insertion of
pectoralis major muscle and
inserts at latissimus dorsi.

**Langerhans cell histio-
cytosis** (histiocytosis X): Lytic
bone lesions (sometimes
diagnosed incidentally on radiography) are clinical hallmark;
also marked by diabetes insipidus, chronic otitis, fever, and
weight loss. Definitive diagnosis
requires presence of Birbeck
granule–positive cells in lesions
seen on electron microscopy.
Classically, when bone lesions
only are present, disease is
termed eosinophilic granuloma.

When bone lesions, diabetes
insipidus, and exophthalmos are
present, disease is termed Hand-
Schüller-Christian disease, and
disseminated form is termed
Letterer-Siwe disease.

Langerhans granules: See
Birbeck granules.

Langer lines: Connective
tissue alignment in dermis;
parallel incisions reduce scar
formation.

Langer-Giedeon syndrome:
Segmental monosomy of
chromosome 8; occurs only in
males.

Langer-Saldino syndrome:
Type of achondrogenesis.

Langhans cells: Giant multinucleated cells.

Langhans layer: Inner cellular
lamina of trophoblast.

Langley granules: Particles in
serous glands with secretory
functions.

Langley nerves: Individual
nerve fibers running to each hair
follicle; mediate piloerection.

Langoria sign: Relaxation of
extensor thigh muscles in
femoral intracapsular fracture.

Lanterman clefts (incisure,
Schmidt-Lanterman clefts):
Passages in myelin sheath
cytoplasm that provide connection to Schwann cell body.

Lanthony test: Test of color
vision used to detect saturation
discrimination by varying green-
ness of visual field.

Lanz point: See McBurney
point.

Lapicque constant: Value used in calculations to convert noninductive resistance values into direct current equivalent values; equals 0.37.

Lapides classification: Commonly used system of describing neuropathic voiding dysfunction; distinguishes between sensory neurogenic bladder, motor paralytic bladder, uninhibited neurogenic bladder, reflex neurogenic bladder, and autonomous neurogenic bladder.

Lapides vesicostomy: Urinary diversion technique that involves Pfannenstiel incision and cutaneous flap sewn to anterior bladder flap; used in adults with stomal appliance.

Laplace law: Expression stating that wall tension = radius × pressure; explains why viscus with larger distention (e.g., cecum) ruptures first.

Laquerrier-Pierquin position: Plain film radiographic technique using tangential projection to image scapular spine.

Laquesna-Deseze angle: Angle formed on lateral view of hip by center of femoral head and anterior acetabular rim; used to assess hip dysplasia.

Laron syndrome (dwarfism): Condition caused by defect in receptors for growth hormone.

Larrey cleft: Triangular space between pars costalis and sternal diaphragm; traversed by thoracic vessels before they become upper epigastric vessels.

Larrey spaces: Spatial division of diaphragm lying between attachments to ribs and sternum.

Larsen syndrome (McFarland syndrome): Anomalies of hands; face; upper spine; and joint articulations (dislocations of hip, knee and elbow). Characteristic facial features are prominent forehead, widened eyes, and hypoplastic nasal bridge. Spina bifida, clubfoot, platybasia, kyphosis and lordosis, mild mental retardation, and dwarfism also occur. Both autosomal dominant and recessive forms exist.

laryngeal cartilage of Luschka: Composed of laryngeal cartilages and articulations between them; includes 2 each of arytenoid, corniculate, and cuneiform cartilages, and 2 each of epiglottic, thyroid, and cricoid cartilages.

Lasègue sign: Diagnostic for hysterical anesthesia when patient has inability to move limb with closed eyes.

Lasègue sign: Used to distinguish sciatica from hip pain. In sciatica, flexion of thigh is painless and easily accomplished when knee is flexed. With hip pain, patient is unable to flex thigh when knee is flexed without feeling pain.

laser Doppler velocimetry: Measurement of flow of RBCs using laser light directed at microcirculation via fiberoptic probes.

Lash medium: Culture medium used to grow *Trichomonas*, esp. *T. vaginalis*. Vaginal specimens are placed in agar of beef blood, casamino acids, sugars, and salts and incubated at 37.5°C for 1–2 days.

Lash procedure: Preconceptual cerclage used to correct structural defect within cervical wall of uterus secondary to previous obstetric injury; rarely performed.

Lassa fever: Disorder marked by high fever, mouth ulcers, muscle aches, hemorrhagic skin lesions, and severe heart, lung, and kidney damage; caused by arenavirus. Transmission is via house rat and human-to-human contact. Mortality rate is 40%–60%.

Las Vegas voice: Voice fatigue, hoarseness; and dry, irritated throat caused by exposure to smoke or other irritants.

Lauge-Hansen classification: System used to describe ankle fractures. Categories are supination–eversion (external rotation), supination–adduction, pronation–abduction, and pronation–adduction.

Laugier fracture: Humeral fracture of trochlea.

Laugier hernia: See Velpeau hernia.

Laugier sign: Positive for displaced distal radial fracture if ulna and radial styloid process are at same level.

Laugier-Hunziker syndrome: Dark pigmentation developing on lips and oral mucosa and blackish streaks developing on nails; no associated systemic conditions.

Laumonier ganglion: See Bock ganglion.

Laurell technique: Method of electroimmunophoresis.

Lauren classification: System used to describe gastric cancers based on intestinal or diffuse-type histology; intestinal histology is associated with better prognosis and is also most prevalent in high-risk populations.

Laurence-Moon-Biedl syndrome: Obesity, short stature, spastic paraplegia, retinitis pigmentosa, polydactyly, skull deformities, and mental retardation; likely due to hypothalamic dysfunction.

Laurin angle: Angle formed by imaginary lines drawn from lateral inferior patella and to lateral edge of medial condyles.

Law position: Patient positioning technique used to obtain radiograph of petrous portion of temporal bone and lateral view of mastoid process. Film is placed parallel to median sagittal plane and 2 cm posterior to ear canal.

Lawrence position: Radiographic technique using inferosuperior axial projection of shoulder joint to image glenohumeral joint, lateral coracoid process, and acromioclavicular articulation.

Le Merrer syndrome:
Dwarfism with associated "gloomy" facies; autosomal recessive condition.

Leadbetter colon reimplant: Technique for ureterocolic anastomosis. Groove of 2–3 cm is made in antimesenteric tenia with incision made through muscularis and serosa but not mucosa. Small opening is then made through mucosa to allow urine to pass from spatulated ureter into colon lumen, and seromuscular layer is then loosely reapproximated over ureter.

Leadbetter ureterocolonic anastomosis: Surgical method to establish nonrefluxing ureterocolonic anastomosis in urinary diversion; ureter is implanted in submucosal tunnel of antimesenteric tenia.

Leadbetter-Politano procedure: Commonly performed technique for reimplantation of ureter or surgical correction of ureteral reflux. Ureter is intubated and mobilized, hiatus is dilated and retroperitoneal ureter mobilized, peritoneum is reflected from outer surface of bladder, neohiatus is created with internalization of ureter (with scissor dissection used to create channel) into bladder, and original hiatus is closed. Advantages are easily accessible ureteral orifices via cystoscopy and good tunnel length. Possible disadvantages are ureteral obstruction and inadvertent sigmoid colon injury if performed on left side.

Leaunois-Cléret syndrome:
See Froehlich syndrome.

Lebek test: Oxygen preference test used to separate *Mycobacterium tuberculosis* and *M. bovis* bacille Calmette-Guérin (aerobic) from *M. bovis* (microaerophilic).

Leber amaurosis (retinopathy): Congenital abnormality of both cones and rods causing severe vision defects or blindness; often associated with keratoconus.

Leber aneurysms (multiple miliary aneurysms:) Idiopathic retinal telangiectasia with segmentally dilated and leaky capillaries, fusiform aneurysms, and coarsening of remaining capillaries.

Leber corpuscle: See Hassall corpuscle.

Leber disease: Hereditary optic nerve disease marked by painless, central visual loss in 1 eye followed weeks later in other eye; transmitted from mother to all offspring but usu. apparent only in males. Cause is point mutation in mitochondrial gene for NADH.

Leber plexus: See Hovius plexus.

Lebert disease: See Biermer disease.

LeCompte maneuver: Division of ductus arteriosus and translocation of pulmonary artery bifurcation anterior to aorta; used as one phase in arterial switch procedure to correct transposition of great arteries.

LeCompte procedure:
Technique for correction of pulmonary artery stenosis in which left ventricle is connected to aorta and right ventricle to pulmonary artery without extracardiac conduit; used in patients in whom arterial switch operation or intraventricular tunnel repair is not possible.

Lederer anemia: Megalocytic anemia of alcoholics due to folic acid deficiency. Causes are alcohol toxicity on bone marrow, dietary deficiency, and insufficient conversion of polyglutamate monogluta-mate.

Lee ganglion: Collection of nerve cell bodies on uterine cervix.

Lee-Jones test: Rapid quantitative spot test performed on gastric aspirate. 5-ml sample is mixed with several crystals of ferrous sulfate and 4–5 drops 2% NaOH (this precipitates any iron present), boiled, and cooled; then 8–10 drops 10% HCl are added. Cyanide is present if precipitate intensifies or blue-green color develops. Purplish color indicates presence of salicylate without cyanide, and immediate formation of blue-green indicates presence of both salicylates and cyanide.

Lee-White clotting time: Normal value is 6–7 minutes.

Le Fort I fracture: Transverse maxillary and pterygoid plate fracture above tooth line, with mobile palate and stable nasal plate.

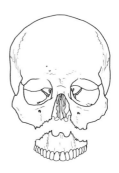

Le Fort I fracture

Le Fort II fracture: Fracture line running through orbital floor, pterygoid plate, and frontal process of maxilla.

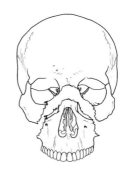

Le Fort II fracture

Le Fort III fracture: Fracture of midface with complete craniofacial disjunction.

Le Fort IV fracture: Infrequently used term for combined severe naso-orbitoethmoid fracture.

Le Fort I osteotomy: Transection of maxilla, advancement,

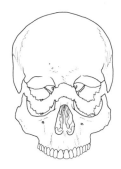

Le Fort III fracture

and rigid fixation with plates and screws.

Le Fort III osteotomy: Transection at pterygomaxillary fissure, lateral maxilla, orbital floor, and nasofrontal junction for advancement of midface in craniosynostosis.

LeFort fracture: Vertical fracture line in distal fibula running in anterior medial margin.

LeFort operation: Rarely used surgical correction of uterine prolapse; considered only when there is strong contraindication to 1 of the usual prolapse correction procedures. Permanent, almost complete closure of vagina is involved, with termination of intravaginal intercourse.

LeFort sound: Device with screw tip for attachment of filiform device; used to dilate tight strictures in urethra.

Legg-Calvé-Perthes disease: Aseptic necrosis of capital femoral epiphysis in children.

Legionnaire disease: Diarrhea, fever, nausea, vomiting, pneumonitis, and hyponatremia; occurs 2–10 days after infection with *Legionella*. Course is mild to fulminant.

Lehmann acoumeter: Early type of audiometer; device measured hearing ability by dropping pellets from different heights.

Leichtenstern sign: Positive for cerebrospinal meningitis if light tapping on bones of extremities causes sudden wincing.

Leiden mutation: Single nucleotide base substitution (Glu→Arg) at 1 of cleavage sites where factor V is cleaved by activated protein C; results in abnormal factor V. Mutation may be involved in 50% of unexplained cases of venous thrombosis and occurs in 95% of activated protein C resistance. Positive result should be viewed as risk for thrombosis (not absolute marker).

Leiden simulator: Anesthesia simulator using mannequin; capable of spontaneous ventilation and different critical clinical events.

Leigh disease: Ataxia, dysmetria, ophthalmoplegia, weakness, and epilepsy; onset in early childhood. Condition occurs due to defects in thiamine triphosphate, cytochrome disorders, or defects in pyruvate dehydrogenase. Disorder is autosomal recessive.

Leigh syndrome: Early onset of mitochondrial disorder marked by rapid degeneration of brainstem, basal ganglia, and diencephalon; caused by severe deficiency of cytochrome C oxidase (complex 4).

Leiner disease (erythroderma desquamativum): Severe, diffuse seborrheic dermatitis, recurrent infections (usu. gram-negative), severe diarrhea, and muscle wasting; onset in infancy. Familial form exists. Condition is associated with dysfunction of complement 5 but normal levels of IgE and absence of eosinophils.

Leipzig school of gestalt psychology (holistic psychology): Branch of psychology that advocates that all psychological phenomena should be included in Gestalt "idea of the wholes."

Leishman-Donovan body: Intracellular form of *Leishmania donovani, L. tropica,* and *Trypanosoma cruzii;* appears as small oval bodies in reticuloendothelial cells in liver and spleen in kala azar. Nucleus and kinetoplast together form distinctive complex.

Leishmania: Flagellate protozoa with amastigote and promastigote stages; needs both human and insect vectors.

leishmaniasis: Infection caused by *Leishmania tropica* and *L. braziliensis;* marked by chronic ulcerative granulomas on extremities (*L. tropica*) and skin lesions that spread to oral mucous membranes (*L. braziliensis*).

Leiter scale (international performance scale): Nonverbal intelligence test; gives mental age and extrapolated IQ score. Test is good for young children who are non-English speaking or mentally retarded.

Leitner syndrome: Loeffler syndrome in setting of TB.

LeJeune syndrome (cat cry syndrome, cri du chat syndrome): Chromosome abnormality on short arm of chromosome 5 causing high-pitched cry in infancy, severe mental retardation, variable heart anomalies, microcephaly, stunted growth, laryngeal anomalies and oblique palpebral fissures; usu. with reduced life span.

Leksell frame: Stereotactic frame using fiducial plates clamped to patient's head; used with CT-guided imagery in brain surgery.

Lemieux-Neemeh syndrome: Charcot-Marie-Tooth disease with associated sensorineural hearing loss and variable nephropathy.

Lemmon sternal approximator: Metal instrument with opposing C-shaped clasps that grab lateral edges of sternum to reapproximate bone after sternotomy.

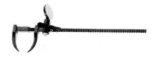

Lemmon sternal approximator

Lendrum stain: Meyer hematoxylin, phloxine solution, and tartrazine in Cellosolve; used to visualize acidophilic inclusion bodies. Inclusion bodies stain red, nuclei blue, and background yellow.

Lenegre disease: Rare sclerodegeneration of heart with damage limited to conduction system.

Lennert lymphoma: Type of low-grade non-Hodgkin lymphoma; tends to manifest in older women with cervical lymphadenopathy.

Lennhoff index: Measure of body habitus; equals 100 x distance between symphysis pubis and sternal notch/largest abdominal circumference.

Lennhoff sign: Indicator of echinococcal cyst in liver if tissue furrow occurs below 12th rib and liver edge on deep inspiration.

Lennox triad: Akinetic seizures, myoclonic jerks, and petit mal epilepsy occurring in same patient.

Lennox-Gastaut syndrome: Early childhood–onset epilepsy with tonic, akinetic, and tonic–clonic seizures that are refractory to anticonvulsant drugs; seen with mental retardation if presents before 2 years of age. Slow waves and spikes are seen on EEG.

Lenoble-Aubineau syndrome: Myoclonic jerks in trunk and extremities, hyperreflexia, hypospadias, asymmetrical facies, and malformed teeth; onset in 1st few years of life. Cold worsens symptoms. Condition is usu. not progressive.

Lenox Hill orthosis: Device used for support brace in injuries of anterior cruciate ligament and patella with tendency for lateral subluxation.

Lenz syndrome: See Wiedemann syndrome.

Lenz-Majewski syndrome (Braham-Lenz syndrome): Severe congenital mental retardation and connective tissue disorder marked by enlarged head, bulging scalp veins, floppy ears, choanal stenosis, wide-set eyes, syndactyly, hypotonic muscles, loose and wrinkled skin, and genitourinary malformations; associated with advanced paternal age.

Leonard catheter: Central indwelling catheter similar to Hickman and Broviac catheters.

Leonardo paradox: Ability of binocular vision to make viewed object transparent (i.e., more background is seen than with monocular vision); explains why paintings can never reproduce 100% of what is seen with binocular vision.

Leopold maneuver: Obstetric technique used during childbirth to assist movement of infant's head through pelvis.

Lepoutre syndrome (oxalosis): Accumulation of calcium oxalate in tissues leading to eventual kidney failure and cirrhosis. Type 1 defect (glycolic aciduria) is caused by abnormal 2-oxoglutarate/glyoxylate carboligase; type 2 defect (l-glyceric aciduria) is caused by abnormal d-glyceric dehydrogenase.

Leriche syndrome: Thigh and buttock claudication, impotence, loss of femoral pulses, and lower extremity atrophy; due to severe aortoiliac atherosclerosis.

Leri pleonosteosis: Premature bone ossification with onset in infancy; marked by increasing limitation of joint mobility, carpal tunnel syndrome, broadened digits, and usu. normal intelligence. Etiology is unknown. Condition is autosomal dominant. Treatment is multiple orthopedic surgeries.

Leri sign: Positive if normal elbow flexion is absent when hand and wrist on affected side are passively flexed; occurs in hemiplegia and lesions of corticospinal tract.

Leri-Joanny syndrome (flowing hyperostosis): Onset in childhood of abnormal bone growth along shaft and under periosteum; morphologically appears like melted wax (melorheostosis). Condition causes severe but diffuse pain. In advanced cases, limited limb motion can result if changes cross joint spaces.

Leri-Weill dyschondrosteosis: Short stature marked by skeletal dysplasia (including Madelung deformity); autosomal dominant condition.

Lermoyez syndrome: Onset in adulthood (30–40 years of age) of tinnitus initially followed by vertigo; thought to be caused by allergic reaction.

Leroy disease: See lilliputian syndrome.

Leroy I-cell disease (mucolipidosis type 2): Defect in phosphorylation of hydrolases caused by defective UDP-N-acetylglucosamine–lysosomal enzyme N-acetyl-glucosaminyl-1-phosphotransferase; functionally causes inactive lysosomes. Condition is marked by onset in early infancy of retarded development, recurrent lung infections, hip dysplasia, severe corneal clouding, rib cage deformities, gum hyperplasia, and restricted joint movements. Disorder most commonly occurs in Arabs with autosomal recessive inheritance.

Lesch-Nyhan syndrome: Complete inborn deficiency of enzyme hypoxanthine phosphoribosyltransferase (HPRT) in purine metabolism pathway; causes mental retardation, self-mutilation, choreoathetosis, and hyperuricemia. Disorder is invariably fatal in childhood.

Leser-Trélat sign: Sudden onset of multiple seborrheic keratoses in association with acanthosis nigricans and skin tags; heralds internal malignancy.

Lesieur sign: Decreased resonance over lower right posterior thorax; occurs in typhoid fever.

lesser fossa of Scarpa: Anatomic depression lying

between pectineus and iliopsoas muscles in floor of femoral triangle.

Lesshaft space (triangle): Anatomic area bounded by latissimus dorsi posteriorly, serratus posticus superiorly, and external oblique muscle superficially; lies deep to internal oblique muscle. Area almost exactly approximates Grynfeltt triangle; is prone to abscess formation.

Letournel approach (ilioinguinal approach): Surgical approach to anterior pelvic column and anterior acetabular wall. Indwelling Foley catheter is placed to decompress bladder. Curved skin incision is made medially from anterior iliac spine to 2 cm above symphysis pubis; aponeurosis of external oblique is incised from anterior iliac spine to midline and to 2 cm proximal to external inguinal ring; conjoined tendon is cut away from outer inguinal ligament, and iliopectineal fascia is divided with preservation of lacuna vasorum. Iliopsoas muscle is then bluntly dissected from pelvic ring, and spermatic cord and external iliac vessels are dissected free and retracted using encircling Penrose drains.

Letournel-Judet classification: System used to describe acetabular fractures according to anatomic position. Type A, posterior wall; type B, posterior column; type C, anterior wall; type D, anterior column; type E, transverse fracture; type F, posterior column and wall; type G, transverse and posterior wall; type H, T-shaped fracture; type I, anterior and posterior hemitransverse fracture; type J, complete fracture of anterior and posterior column.

Letterer-Siwe disease: Systemic histiocytosis; onset in infancy of hemorrhagic rash, lymphadenopathy, hepatomegaly, and bone involvement. Langerman granules are visible on electron microscopy. Condition is closely related to Hand-Schüller-Christian disease. Earlier presentation and systemic presentation lead to poorer prognosis.

Letts-Vincent-Gouw syndrome: Descriptive classification of pediatric tibia–femur fractures. Type A, both diaphyseal plates closed; type B, 1 metaphyseal and 1 diaphyseal plate closed; type C, epiphyseal and diaphyseal plates closed; type D, 1 open fracture; type E, 2 open fractures with soft tissue injury.

Leudet tinnitus: Crackling noise produced by tic of mandibular division of CN V, resulting in contraction of muscle; sometimes loud enough to be heard by examiner.

Leuven variant: Type of corticosteroid-binding globulin; has decreased cortisol-binding affinity caused by point mutation resulting in L93H substitution.

Lev disease (block): AV block, usu. occurs in elderly patients.

Levaditi stain (method): Reduced pyrogallic acid used to stain *Spirochaeta pallida* and

Listeria monocytogenes black on yellow-brown background.

LeVeen shunt (portovenous shunt): Open-end catheter used for control of intractable ascites; placed freely into abdominal cavity and traverses subcutaneous tissue to internal jugular vein to allow movement of ascites into intravascular space. Diuretics are given to facilitate renal excretion of fluid; palliative procedure only. Postprocedure replacement of ascites with lactated Ringer's solution or saline decreases risk of coagulopathy; not indicated in candidates for liver transplantation.

Levi disease: See Lorain disease.

Levin disease: Variant of osteogenesis imperfecta with multilocular lesions of jaws and associated frequent jaw infections (usu. with normal teeth).

Levine sign: Positive if patient places clenched fist over sternum when describing chest symptoms; seen in angina.

Levine-Drennan angle: Angle formed by imaginary lines drawn through distal lateral and medial parts of metaphysis and perpendicular to lateral tibial cortex.

Levine-Edwards classification: System used to describe fracture of atlas (C1). Type 1—through neural arch, < 3 mm displacement, no angulation; type 2—through neural arch with angulation and translation; type 2a—through neural arch, minimal translation, severe angulation; type 3—facet dislocation of C2–C3, severe angulation and displacement.

Lévy-Roussy syndrome: Type of hereditary ataxia.

Lewis acid (electrophile): Any molecular ion that acts as electron pair acceptor; forms coordinate covalent bond with unshared electron pair in another molecule or ion (Lewis base). Examples are protons and boron trifluoride.

Lewis antigen: Oligosaccharide.

Lewis base (nucleophile): Electron pair donor; equivalent to Brönsted-Lowry base.

Lewis phenomenon (hydrophagocytosis): Ability of macrophages to absorb surrounding plasma.

Lewis reaction: Onset of wheal-and-flare response in skin.

Lewis-Besant syndrome: Congenital absence of unilateral or bilateral diaphragm, abdominal organs resident in thorax, and hypoplastic lung; also associated with musculoskeletal defects. Treatment is mechanical respiration, surgery, and extracorporeal membrane oxygenation.

Lewy body: Eosinophilic hyaline body found in cytoplasm of pigmented neurons; composed of compact aggregations of fibrillary material. Structure is frequently seen in locus ceruleus and substantia nigra in Parkinson's disease but also in asymptomatic patients.

Lewy body disease: Parkinsonism, dementia, and diffuse neurologic deficits.

Leyden-Moebius type: Variant of Erb disease in which 1st group of muscles affected is in lumbosacral region.

Leydig cell (interstitial cell of Leydig): Polyhedral cell found in clusters around seminiferous tubules of testes, which synthesizes and secretes testosterone under influence of luteinizing hormone; contains prominent cytoplasmic crystals (of Reinke).

Leydig cell tumor (adenoma, interstitial cell tumor): Tumor of Leydig cell of testes and ovaries; usu. benign but can cause gynecomastia through hyperfunction. In females, it can result in virilization.

Leydig cylinders: Parallel muscle fibers grouped between areas of protoplasm.

Leydig duct: Embryonic duct that drains mesonephric tubules. In females, duct remains only in vestigial form; in males, it becomes ductus deferens.

Lhermitte sign (syndrome): Sudden transient electric-like shocks spreading down trunk and legs with neck flexion; seen in multiple sclerosis, cervical cord compression, Lyme disease, and mantle irradiation (15%). Condition usu. resolves over several months.

Lhermitte-Cornil-Quesnel syndrome: Neuropsychiatric condition with onset typically in middle or old age; gradual onset/progression of affective disturbances (agitation, depression, involuntary crying and laughing); neurologic disturbances of lower limb (pain, paresthesias, and rigidity); and abnormal hand posture (extension of wrist and finger joints, except flexion in metacarpophalangeal joint). Condition is associated with cases of epidemic encephalitis, but cause is unknown. Putamen shows reduction of cells and neuroglial overgrowth. Death occurs within 1 year.

Lhermitte-Levy syndrome (Lhermitte-Delthil-Garnier syndrome): Slowly progressive neurologic deterioration seen in some elderly patients after stroke; marked by choreiform movements of limbs progressing to paralysis and auditory and visual hallucinations. Likely cause is lesion in upper peduncle or subthalamic areas.

Lian-Siguier-Welti syndrome: Venous thrombosis in setting of diaphragmatic hernia or eventration.

Libian-Kozenitzki syndrome: See Perlman syndrome.

Libman-Sacks disease: Noninfective verrucous endocarditis occurring in lupus; vegetations are found on valves (usu. tricuspid and mitral) and chordae tendineae composed of fibrin strands with cellular infiltration. Lesions contain characteristic clumps of basophilic cellular debris (hematoxylin bodies).

Liche technique: Reimplantation of ureter into bladder.

Lich-Gregoir procedure:
Extravesicular reimplantation of ureters for correction of vesico-ureteral reflux; uses standard transverse incision and approach to prevesical space in supine patient. Ureters are identified and dissected from surrounding tissue and incised at level of bladder muscular wall, and opening of remnants of intravesical part of ureter is oversewn. Cut ends are then reimplanted into bladder; muscular wall is opened down to mucosa for 4–5 cm in cephalad line to ureter, with small opening made for new ureteral anastomosis; and freshly prepared muscle bed is then closed over ureters. Foley catheter can be removed 48–72 hours postop.

Lichtenstein repair: Plug repair for recurrent inguinal hernias originally conceived in 1960s; uses rolled-up "cigarette plug" of Marlex mesh wedged into hernia defect. Procedure is generally best used for recurrent direct and femoral hernias; minimizes overall dissection and "taking down inguinal floor."

Lichtenstein repair: Tension-free repair of inguinal hernia; Marlex mesh is stitched to aponeurotic tissue of pubic bone and along shelving edge of Poupart (inguinal) ligament. Mesh is split, and ends are passed around spermatic cord and overlapped and sutured together to tighten internal ring.

Lichtheim plaques: Focal areas of cerebral white matter degeneration occurring in pernicious anemia.

Lichtheim sign: Patient can indicate with upraised fingers how many syllables are in word that he or she cannot speak; seen in subcortical aphasia.

Lichtman classification: System used to describe avascular necrosis of lunate. Stage 1, no plain film evidence or only 1 linear line across lunate visible; stage 2, density changes evident; stage 3, collapsed lunate with proximal displacement of capitate; stage 4, stage 3 with addition of degeneration in carpus.

Lichtman test: Used to indicate ulnar midcarpal instability and atrophy of triquetrohamato-capitate ligament; positive if after flexing wrist with forearm pronated, "clunking" sound is heard as wrist is radially and then ulnarly deviated.

Liddle syndrome: Volume expansion caused by increased activity of collecting duct sodium channels; marked by normal aldosterone levels and hypokalemic alkalosis.

Liddle test: Dexamethasone suppression test; used to differentiate Cushing disease from ectopic ACTH source.

Lieberkuhn crypts (follicles, glands): Intestinal glands in lamina propria of jejunum and ileum, which open into lumen between villi; contain argentaffin cells.

Liebermann-Burchard reaction: Positive for cholesterol if addition of concentrated sulfuric acid in acetic anhydride to chloroform sample solution produces green color.

Liebermann-Cole syndrome: See Goltz syndrome.

Liebermeister grooves: Anterior-posterior depressions seen on liver surface; due to irregular growth.

Liepmann disease: Construction subtype is inability to assemble pieces into a whole; usu. cause is right hemisphere lesion. Ideational subtype is inability to plan coordinated actions; cause is diffuse bilateral disease or toxic state. Ideo-kinetic subtype is inability to link ideation and motor performance; cause is lesion in sub-marginal gyrus. Kinetic subtype is inability to use one hand or arm to perform manual tasks; cause is focal lesion of pre-central contralateral cortex.

Liesegang rings: Laminated, acellular structures that stain acidophilic; associated with endometrioid, renal, or synovial cysts.

Lieutaud trigone: Triangular area at inside base of bladder bordered by orifices of ureters and urethra; mucosa is pale and nonredundant.

Li-Fraumeni cancer syndrome: Familial clustering of sarcoma, breast, leukemia, bone, brain, and adrenal tumors; associated with p53 mutation. 50% of patients have malignant degeneration by 30 years of age.

Lifton syndrome: Hyperaldosteronism due to gene duplication, leading to abnormal aldosterone synthase coding sequences; severe hypertension results. Condition is autosomal dominant. Treatment is spironolactone.

ligament of Scarpa: Proximal falciform margin of saphenous hiatus.

Lightwood-Albright disease: Early term for renal tubular acidosis.

Lijo syndrome: Visual deficits, optic atrophy, vertigo, psychiatric conditions, and headaches. Condition is more common in women; etiology is unknown. Treatment is gonadotropic hormone.

Liley zone: Indicator of severity of hemolytic disease in erythroblastosis fetalis; measures spectrophotometric values of amniotic fluid containing bilirubin that must be shielded from direct light. Larger deviation from straight line on chart at optical density of 450 nm (ΔOD) means more severe hemolysis.

Lilienfeld position: Radiographic technique using posterior oblique projection to image scapula.

lilliputian hallucination: Visual hallucination in which objects are extremely small; occurs in febrile episodes and psychosis.

lilliputian syndrome (Leroy disease): Visual hallucinations of small people, usu. with belligerent attitude; occurs in toxic delirium from drugs or alcohol, traumatic brain injuries, and severe febrile states. Condition is also associated with left hemianopia and deviation of eyes and head to left.

limbal palisades of Vogt: Pigmented conjunctival epithelium at limbus; arranged in radial spokes extending into subepithelial connective tissue and flanked by vascular connective tissue.

Linch-Clark syndrome: Many large (> 2 cm) dysplastic nevi with irregular borders, notching, and associated inflammation. Lifetime risk of developing malignant melanoma is 5%–15%. Treatment is periodic photographic surveillance and excision of changing lesions.

Lincoln-Oseretsky motor development scale: Test used to assess general motor skills of children 6–14 years of age; contains 36 items.

Lind fundoplication: Surgical treatment of gastroesophageal reflux disease; may be performed laparoscopically.

Linder sign: Positive for sciatica if passive flexion of head causes lumbar or leg pain in patient with outstretched legs.

line of Gennari (band of Gennari, striate cortex, stripe of Gennari): Most prominent and highly visible part of external portion of band of Baillarger; lies near calcarine sulcus in brain.

lines of Park: Usu. multiply occurring transverse lines seen on radiography of metaphyses of long bones; found in both ill and healthy children of all ages.

lines of Retzius: Incremental growth lines of tooth; seen on longitudinal section as dark striae.

Lineweaver-Burk equation (plot): Linearized form of Michaelis-Menten equation where both sides are put in reciprocal form and equated. $1/V = (K_m/V_{max})(1/[S] + 1)V_{max}$, where V is reaction velocity, [S] is substrate concentration, and K_m is Michaelis-Menten constant. Y-intercept allows calculation of V_{max}, and x-intercept allows calculation of K_m.

Link trainer (flight simulator): Device for training pilots or other highly skilled equipment operators in virtual environment.

Linton procedure: Subfascial interruption or ligation of perforator veins to palliate venous ulceration. Traditionally performed in open approach but some reports describe good results using minimally invasive techniques.

Lipschutz disease: See Afzelius disease.

Lipschütz ulcer (disease): Shallow ulcer on vulva of nonvenereal origin; occurs in association with fever.

liquor of Scarpa: Viscous fluid secreted by membranous labyrinth of inner ear.

Lisch nodules: Minute melanocytic hamartomas occurring on irides in neurofibromatosis.

Lisch syndrome: Horizontal nystagmus, pellucid iris, and variable fundus flavimaculatus; autosomal dominant condition.

Lisfranc amputation: See Dupuytren amputation.

Lisfranc amputation (Hey amputation): Disarticulation through metatarsal–tarsal or metatarsophalangeal joints with removal of part of medial cuneiform bone; prosthesis is foot plate with toe filler.

Lisfranc fracture: Fracture/dislocation of proximal metatarsal or tarsometatarsal joint.

Lisfranc joint: Articulation between midfoot (navicular, cuboid, and cuneiform) and forefoot (metatarsals and phalanges).

Lisfranc tubercle: Bony prominence on upper surface of 1st rib; acts as insertion point of anterior scalene muscle.

Lisker disease: Neurologic deterioration presenting in childhood with slowly progressive distal muscle weakness, followed by onset of autonomic deterioration with achalasia, profuse sweating, digit cyanosis, and orthostatic hypotension; due to defect in cholinergic innervation. Both autosomal dominant and recessive inheritance patterns exist. Treatment is supportive and involves surgical palliation of achalasia.

Lissauer tract: Dorsolateral fasciculus of cervical spinal cord.

Lister reconstruction: Digital pulley reconstruction to provide optimal transformation of tendon excursion into finger flexion.

Lister tubercle: Bony prominence of dorsal surface of distal radius; tendon of extensor pollicis longus muscle runs on surface.

Listerosis: Mild, acute febrile illness with headaches, chills, and myalgias; due to infection with *Listeria monocytogenes*. Disorder can cause spontaneous abortions in pregnancy.

Litten sign: Indication of intact phrenic nerve innervation to diaphragm; positive is retraction of lower intercostal spaces in inspiration in top-down succession.

Little area: See Kiesselbach area.

Littre glands: Branched, tubular glands found in penile urethra.

Littre hernia: Incarcerated Meckel diverticulum (sole component); difficult to diagnose secondary to lack of obstructive symptoms. Presenting complaints are pain, abscess, or fistulization.

Litzmann obliquity: Slanting of fetal skull that allows posterior parietal bone to contact birth canal during delivery.

Livaditis myotomy: Circular cutting of proximal esophageal pouch to effect lengthening in repair of esophageal atresia.

Liverpool prosthesis: Knee replacement with maximum freedom of joint motion; requires good soft tissue stability.

Livierato sign: Systemic vaso-constriction caused by percussion along xiphoumbilical line.

Lloyd sign: Positive for kidney stones if deep flank percussion causes pain in groin area when pain is not elicited by palpation.

Lloyd syndrome: Multiple endocrine neoplasia type 1 (MEN-1); with association of pancreatic islet cell tumors, parathyroid adenomas, and pituitary tumors.

Lloyd-Davis stirrups: Apparatus used to place patient in lithotomy position in operating room.

Lobstein ganglion (splanchnic thoracic ganglion): Small collection of nerve bodies on greater thoracic splanchnic nerve near T12.

Lockhart-Mummery excision: Extended perineal excision used in early 1900s for resection of rectal carcinoma.

Loeb decidual reaction: Mechanical irritant of uterine mucosa causing formation of small deciduoma; requires presence of normally developing corpora lutea.

Loeffler disease (eosino-philia): Infestation of lung parenchyma with parasites (usu. *Ascaris lumbricoides, Trichinella, Ancylostoma duodenale*); eggs hatched in lumen of gut with larval migration to lung tissue, causing eosinophilia. Treatment is mebendazole.

Loefgran disease: Variant of erythema nodosum.

Loehr-Kindberg syndrome: Variant of Loeffler syndrome; occurs mostly in women. Condition is marked by allergic-type pneumonitis, malaise, fever, coughing, and variable hemoptysis. Treatment is corti-costeroids with good results.

Loewenthal disease (myosclerosis): Congenital flaccid muscles, hyperextensible joints, contractures, hyperhidro-sis, and blepharoptosis.

Loewenthal tract (bundle): Tectospinal tract running in lateral spinal cord.

Löffler endocarditis (con-strictive endocarditis): Fibrotic thickening of endocardium, eosinophilia, congestive heart failure, tachycardia, hepato-splenomegaly, pleural effusions, and limb edema.

Lofgren syndrome: Subtype of acute sarcoidosis with erythema nodosa and bilateral hilar adenopathy; more prevalent in women, esp. during pregnancy.

Lohlein syndrome (Rich syndrome): Focal glomerular sclerosis.

Löhlein-Baehr lesion: Focal glomerular necrosis and hyalinization seen in kidneys of patients with bacterial endocarditis; possibly embolic in origin.

Lohmann reaction: Transfer of ATP high-energy phosphate bond to creatine to form creatine phosphate; catalyzed by creatine kinase. Reaction occurs in muscle and is easily reversible.

Lomadtse sign (distant toe flexor reflex): Positive finding is plantar flexion of toes after pressure on anterior tibial area; may be seen in extrapyramidal dysfunction.

Lombard effect: Tendency to increase vocal effort in response to increased background noise.

Lombardi sign: Varicose veins in C7–T3 spinous process area; occurs in early lung TB.

Londsdale-Blass syndrome: Deficiency in pyruvate dehydrogenase marked by small head, intermittent ataxia, choreoathetosis, inability to metabolize carbohydrates, failure to thrive, optic atrophy, and blindness. Treatment is low-carbohydrate diet and thiamine. Life expectancy ranges from death in 1st decade to normal lifespan.

Lone Star tick: *Amblyomma americanum*; one of primary vectors of Rocky Mountain spotted fever. Tick is found in southern U.S.; infects humans in multiple stages of life cycle. Host animals include dogs and farm animals.

Long-Evans rat: Commonly used experimental animal.

loop of Henle: Basic unit of solute transfer in kidney.

Looser zone: Virtually pathognomonic for osteomalacia; transverse band on rarefaction secondary to poorly healed stress fracture seen on radiography.

Lorain disease (Brissaud disease, Levi disease, Lorain-Levi dwarfism): Dwarfism due to pituitary deficiency (specifically growth hormone) in childhood; results in epiphyseal growth retardation. Causes are craniopharyngioma, pituitary fibrosis, and suprasellar cysts.

Lorenz operation (Hoffa-Lorenz operation): Rarely performed surgical treatment of congenital hip dysplasia. Dislocation is reduced, and primitive acetabulum is fashioned into more complete socket by having femoral head exert direct pressure.

Lorenz position: Radiographic technique using posterior oblique projection to image scapula.

Lorenz sign: Spinal column rigidity (esp. lumbar and thoracic) in ankylosing spondylitis.

Lortat-Jacob-Degós syndrome: Variant of Duhring-Brocq disease, with chronically appearing bullae and subsequent erosions on mucosa and skin surrounding body orifices; strongly associated with gluten-sensitive enteropathy. Condition is usu. seen in elderly women. Treatment is gluten-free diet, dapsone, and sulfapyridine.

Los Angeles disease: Variant of Mason-Turner syndrome.

Loschmidt number: See Avogadro number.

Lostorfer corpuscle (bodies): Granular inclusions occurring in serum in syphilis infections.

Lou Gehrig disease (amyotrophic lateral sclerosis, ALS): Degeneration of anterior horn motor neurons causing progressive destruction of anterior horn cells with muscle weakness initially in extremities (usu. arms); almost always fatal. Although controversial, a small number of clinicians believe some cases may be caused by an infectious agent, esp. *Borrelia* (Lyme Disease), that may respond to antibiotic treatment.

Louis-Bar syndrome (disease; ataxia–telangiectasia, Border-Sedgwick disease): Rare ataxia manifesting at onset of walking, abnormal eye movements, telangiectasias of face and conjunctiva (presenting at 3–6 years), increased risk of infection and neoplasm, variable choreoathetoid movements, and mental retardation. Death usu. occurs by 10 years of age. Defect in DNA repair causes abnormal immunoglobulins. Elevated α-fetoprotein is diagnostic serum marker. Condition is autosomal recessive.

Loutit disease: 1940s term for autoimmune hemolytic anemia.

Love test: Used to suggest presence of glomus tumor on finger. Head of pin is pressed around area of pain, and extreme tenderness is elicited only when pressure is directly placed on insignificant tumor mass.

Lovelace gallbladder forceps: Curve-tipped, ring-handle, locking forceps used to provide tissue traction; tips are shaped in open triangular fashion.

Lovett test: Used to detect boutonnière deformity; positive if proximal interphalangeal joint strength is less than contralateral side with wrist and metacarpophalangeal flexion.

Lovibond angle: Angle between nail plate and proximal nail fold ($> 180°$ indicates clubbing).

Löw-Beer position: Radiographic technique used to image petrous portion (apex, labyrinthine, and antral areas) of temporal bone, mastoid cells, and internal auditory canal. Temporal area is placed on table with central ray positioned 10° cephalad and 33° anteriorly.

Lowe syndrome (Lowe-Bickel syndrome, oculocerebrorenal dystrophy): Onset in early infancy of mental retardation, hypotonia, screaming, choreoathetoid movements, hypermobile joints, cryptorchidism, renal failure in 3rd decade, and cataracts; X-linked inheritance. All patients have blond coloring.

Löwenberg sign: Positive for thrombosis of deep calf veins if immediate pain occurs when blood pressure cuff placed around calf is inflated to 80 mm

Hg; occurs in only 1/3 of cases of actual deep venous thrombosis.

Lowenberg-Hill syndrome [Pelizaeus-Merzbacher type 4 (adult-type)]: Onset in adulthood of incomplete patchy demyelination causing a slowly progressive tremor of limbs, head, and jaw; death occurs approximately 20 years after onset.

Lower tubercle: Anatomic structure on posterior wall of fetal right atrium separating flow from superior vena cava and inferior vena cava.

Lowry syndrome: Rare congenital craniosynostosis and absent fibula; autosomal recessive condition.

Lowry-Wood syndrome: Congenital small head, stunted growth, mental retardation, and nystagmus; autosomal recessive condition.

Lubarsch-Pick disease: Enlarged tongue in setting of amyloidosis.

Lubinsky syndrome: Nephrocalcinosis, chronic nighttime urination, and incomplete enamel formation on teeth; autosomal recessive condition.

Lubinus prosthesis: Knee replacement with maximum freedom of joint motion; requires good soft tissue stability.

Lubs phenotype: Male pseudohermaphroditism; marked by enlarged clitoris, labia-containing testes, large female breasts, and female hair pattern. Treatment is removal of testes and adoption of female identity.

Lubs syndrome: See Gilbert-Dreyfus syndrome.

Lucas sign: Abdominal distention sometimes seen in early rickets.

Lucey-Driscoll syndrome: Rapidly progressive neonatal jaundice leading to kernicterus and death within 7–10 days if untreated; due to presence of inhibitor substance of uridine diphosphate glucuronylsyltransferase. Condition is autosomal recessive. Treatment is phototherapy and exchange transfusion.

Lückenschädel deformity (craniolacunia): Radiographic skull deformity seen in most children with myelomeningocele.

Lucké virus: Herpesvirus (DNA virus) that causes adenocarcinoma in frogs.

Ludloff sign: Patient in sitting position cannot flex thigh and develops ecchymosis and swelling at base of Scarpa triangle; seen in avulsion of lesser trochanter.

Ludwig angina: Life-threatening cellulitis of submandibular and sublingual spaces; usu. starts in infected lower molar and involves connective tissue, fascia, and muscles. Brawny, painful edema occurs. Condition is seen in abscess, trauma, posterior lower molars, lupus, alcoholism, and immunodeficiency. 1/3 of patients need intubation or tracheotomy. Operative drainage should be done on an emergent/urgent basis with control of the airway on the first attempt critically important to eliminate life-threatening laryngospasm and edema with excessive manipulation.

Ludwig classification: System used to describe alopecia in females.

Ludwig classification: System used to describe staging of primary sclerosing cholangitis. Stage 1 (portal stage)—inflammation, ductal proliferation, and portal edema; stage 2 (periportal stage)—periportal fibrosis with variable ductular proliferation and piecemeal necrosis; stage 3 (septal stage)—septal fibrosis present; stage 4 (cirrhotic stage)—frank biliary cirrhosis.

Ludwig disease: Parapharyngeal abscess; occurs in childhood and is more common in boys. Complications include jugular thrombosis, mediastinitis, and meningeal infection. Treatment is antibiotics and surgery.

Lueers-Spatz syndrome: Atrophy of frontal lobes of brain.

Lujan-Fryns syndrome: X-linked mental retardation associated with marfanoid body habitus.

Lukianowicz phenomenon: Double vision with gray-white image; associated with schizophrenia, seizures, migraine, and depression.

Lumsden center (pneumotaxic center): Area in superior pons partially responsible for inhibition of inspiration; acts independently of vagal action.

Lund-Browder method: System used to determine skin surface area; accounts for differences in body surface area by age.

Lundbaek syndrome: Pain, paresthesia, and stiffness of hands developing in long-term diabetes mellitus; caused by vascular compromise.

Lundberg syndrome: Development in childhood of ataxia, pyramidal tract signs, and optic atrophy; autosomal dominant condition.

Lundberg syndrome: Development in childhood of mental retardation; myopathy (usu. involving proximal limb muscles, external ocular muscles, and masticatory muscles), cataracts, and hypergonadotropic hypogonadism. Condition is autosomal recessive.

Luse bodies: Long, sparse collagen fibrils seen in Schwann cells in neurilemmoma on electron microscopy.

Luschka bursa: Variably present fluid-filled sac superior to pharyngeal tonsils and midline in posterior nasopharyngeal wall; represents embryonic remnant connecting pharynx and anterior notochord.

Luschka cartilage (sesamoid cartilage): Variably present small cartilage found within ligaments of vocal structures.

Luschka fossa: Anatomic space located deep and inferior to peritoneal cecal fold, medial to ascending colon, and superior to ileum.

Luschka tubercle: Rugae-type mucosal folds in lower, anterior vagina, just beneath urethral opening.

Luschke crypts: Aberrant bile ducts that occur in wall of gallbladder.

Lust phenomenon: Foot eversion and dorsiflexion caused by tapping over common peroneal nerve on upper, outer shin; occurs in tetany.

Lutembacher syndrome: Acquired mitral stenosis (usu. due to rheumatic fever) with congenital atrial septal defect, which worsens hemodynamic consequences of defect. Treatment is surgery.

Lutheran blood group: Minor blood antigens with 2 alleles Lu^a and Lu^b; clinically insignificant unless isoimmune antibodies develop.

Lutz-Jeanselme nodules: See Jeanselme nodules.

Lutz-Miescher disease (porokeratosis): Areas of skin perforation forming narrow canals with keratin plugs; usu. affects neck and may be symmetrical. Lesions start with slight pruritus and progress to papules and then to perforation. Condition is more prevalent in males.

Lutz-Richner syndrome: Biliary malformation and cholestatic jaundice in setting of renal tubular insufficiency; also with variable presence of clubfoot, arched palate, micrognathia, and low-set ears. Condition is autosomal recessive.

Lutz-Splendore-Almeida disease: See Almeida disease.

Luys body: Hypothalamic nucleus located on basilar lateral and anterior nuclei of thalamus; represents anterior continuation of substantia nigra.

Lyle disease: Bilateral mydriasis in setting of bilateral nerve palsy; also with variable occurrence of vertical gaze disturbances and somnolence. Condition is considered variant of Bickers-Adams syndrome. Cause is lesion involving cerebral aqueduct.

Lyman-Smith traction: Stabilization of distal humeral fractures with overhead traction and olecranon pin.

Lyme disease: Tick-borne infection caused by spirochete *Borrelia burgdorferi*. Classic target rash (primary erythema chronicum migrans) at site of tick bite occurs in < 50% of patients; sometimes followed by a secondary annular nonpruritic, nonpainful rash several weeks to months later at distant site, heralding systemic spread of spirochete. Physician confirmation of either type of rash mandates immediate treatment without delay. Signs and symptoms are multiple, with initial presentation possible in disseminated form. Disease may mimic multiple sclerosis (with pattern of demyelinated plaques in CNS indistinguishable from multiple sclerosis), juvenile rheumatoid arthritis, and Parkinson's disease. Antibody tests (including Western blot) are notoriously unreliable and should *never* be used to rule out Lyme disease. PCR, urine, antigen, and culture tests are being used with increasing frequency but controversy remains regarding specificity and sensitivity. Diagnosis of Lyme disease mandates evaluation for ehrlichiosis and babesiosis coinfections. Controversy also exists regarding treatment protocols. Growing minority of Lyme experts favor prolonged, multiantibiotic regimens (doxycycline, cefuroxtime, azithromycin, ceftriaxone, metronidazole) for up to 18 months or until symptoms abate and ascribe existence of post-Lyme syndrome to inadequate treatment. Use of antibiotics usu. causes worsening of symptoms and excessive fatigue (Jarisch-Herxheimer reaction). Some clinicians treating this disease consider the lingering symptoms of "chronic Lyme" to be

mediated by a Borrelia neuroloxin. They have reported success in blocking α-TNF release using an initial 10-day course of Actos, followed by several weeks to months of daily oral Questran (cholestyramine).

Lynch syndrome: Predisposition for early-onset, hereditary, nonpolyposis (usu. right-sided) colorectal carcinoma; type 1 is site specific and type 2 is associated with other adenocarcinomas (i.e., stomach, breast, ovary, endometrium). Condition is autosomal dominant and is associated with DNA mismatch repair genes MSH2, MLH1, PMS1, and PMS2. Surveillance colonoscopy should begin at 25 years of age. Surgical treatment for index cancer is subtotal colectomy. Carcinoma has better prognosis, stage-for-stage, than sporadic, colorectal cancers.

Lyon disease: Recurrent pain in testis caused by injury to genitofemoral nerve.

Lyon rat: Derived from Sprague-Dawley rat; used as animal model to study sensitivity of blood pressure to oral Ca^{2+}.

Lysholm method: Radiographic positioning technique for viewing petrosa, internal auditory canal, carotid canal, and mastoid cells. Temporal area of head is placed on table with tilt of 15° and central ray is placed at 30° from upright.

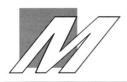

Ma-Griffith technique: Surgical repair for acute closed rupture of calcaneus tendon. Small stab wounds are made 2.5 cm proximal to proximal end of rupture, tendon is dissected free from subcutaneous tissue, straight needle is used to puncture tendon and passed back in crisscross manner on proximal rupture, second suture is placed distal to rupture through small stab wounds, and 2 sutures are tied together to cinch ruptured ends together.

Macalister tubercle: Amygdala; this complex of nuclei is located in tip of temporal lobe.

Macchiavello stain: Rickettsial stain.

MacConkey agar: Medium used to grow and identify enteric bacteria.

Macdowel frenum: Fibrous attachment of tendon of pectoralis muscle; adds strength to intermuscular fascia.

Macewen sign: Percussion of parietal bone producing "cracked jar" sound before closure of skull sutures in normal infants; after infancy, sign indicates increased intracranial pressure due to separation of cranial sutures. Condition is seen in brain tumors, abscesses, hydrocephalus, and lead encephalopathy.

Macewen triangle: Area of middle ear bounded superiorly by linea temporalis, anteriorly by posterior upper wall of meatus, and posteriorly by imaginary line running downward to posterior border of meatus and perpendicular to linea temporalis.

Macewen-Shands operation: Osteotomy for treatment of congenital coxa vara.

MacFee incision: Incision used for exposure of anterior neck and lower mandible.

Mach bands: Optical effect mimicking fracture line sometimes seen on radiography over dens on open-mouth view; due to line shadow cortical bone superimposed on another bone.

Machado-Joseph disease: Type of neurodegenerative disorder with ataxia, dystonia, rigidity, and ophthalmoparesis; similar to spinocerebellar ataxia type 3. Defect is in MJD1 gene. Condition is autosomal dominant.

Machray catheter: Rubber balloon catheter.

Macintosh laryngoscope blade: Curved metal blade used to intubate trachea; available in adult and pediatric sizes.

MacKay-Marg electronic tonometer: Applanation

device with flat surface placed directly onto eyeball to measure intraocular pressure.

Macready "masked" hernia: Incarcerated Spigelian hernia mistaken for tumor mass on palpation.

Madelung deformity: Dorsal dislocation of distal ulna; causes hand to deviate toward radial side.

Madelung disease: Development of multiple lipomas on neck, shoulders, and back.

Madlener procedure: Surgical technique for tubal ligation.

Madura foot: Severe fungal infection of foot.

Maeda disease: See Harrison disease.

Maffucci syndrome (blue rubber bleb syndrome): Dyschondroplasia seen with hemangioma; presents as nodule on digits in childhood with tumors occurring symmetrically through young adulthood. Sarcomatous changes are common. Walls may be calcified on radiograph.

Magendie foramen: Anatomic opening between 4th ventricle and subarachnoid space that allows flow of CSF.

Magendie sign (Magendie-Hertwig sign): See Hertwig-Magendie position.

Magendie spaces: Areas lying between arachnoid and pia that correspond to major sulci of brain.

Magill catheter: Rubber balloon catheter.

Magill circuit: "Noncircle-type" anesthesia breathing system.

Magnan sign ("coke bugs"): Tactile hallucinations and formication in cocaine-induced acute psychoses.

Magnus syndrome (erythropoietic protoporphyria): Hypersensitivity (swelling, itching, redness) of skin to sunlight that lasts 1–2 days; associated with increased protoporphyrin in bone marrow and decreased ferrochelatase activity and possible liver damage leading to organ failure. Treatment is cholestyramine, beta carotene, iron, and liver transplantation.

Magnuson-Stack procedure: Advancement of subscapularis tendon from lesser tuberosity to greater tuberosity; used to repair recurrent anterior dislocation of glenohumeral joint.

Mahaim bundles: Myogenic tissue originating from either AV node and His bundle or its branches and inserting into ventricles in septal region.

Mahler sign: Increase in pulse rate seen in thrombosis (in absence of fever).

Mahorner retractor: Self-retaining metal retractor; often used in thyroid surgery.

Mahurkar catheter: Double-lumen catheter; percutaneously placed into central vein used for venovenous hemodialysis.

Mainz pouch: Extension and modification of Mitrofanoff technique for continent urinary diversion using an appendiceal/bladder anastomosis. Appendix is left in situ; bowel loops are opened and sewn back together to form high-capacity, low-pressure reservoir pouch; both ureters are implanted into large bowel end of pouch with generous submucosal tunnels to retard reflux; and in situ appendix is then embedded in cecum.

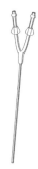

Mahurkar catheter

Maisonneuve fracture: Spiral fracture of proximal fibula, usu. seen with tear of anterior tibiofibular ligament and resulting unstable ankle joint. Injury can be difficult to detect if there is no accompanying ankle fracture. Cause is severe external rotation of foot. Fracture should be suspected if there is medial or posterior malleolar fracture in absence of lateral malleolar fracture or widened joint space between talus and medial malleolus in absence of distal fibular fracture. Break is also associated with rupture of deltoid ligament.

Maisonneuve sign: Hyperextensible wrist and hand occurring in Colles fracture.

Maissiat band (ligament, tract): Iliotibial tract; part of fascia lata running on lateral thigh from tensor muscle to lateral tibial condyle.

Majewski syndrome: Congenital short tibia, cleft palate, hydrops, malformed rib cage, and multiple visceral anomalies; autosomal recessive condition. Cause is defective cartilage malformation. Death occurs shortly after birth.

Majocchi disease (granuloma): Small circular lesions (yellow-purple) usu. occurring in adolescence or early adulthood; associated with hemosiderin deposits or telangiectasias. Lesions may appear anywhere on body.

Makai-Rothman lipogranulomatosis: Inflammation of subcutaneous fat in absence of systemic symptoms.

Malamud-Cohen disease: Type of cerebellar ataxia; X-linked inheritance.

Malassez rest: Scattered root sheath cells located in periodontal ligament; occasionally persist and organize into dental cyst.

Malayan filariasis: See Brug filariasis.

Malecot catheter: Flexible rubber or Silastic catheter used for drainage in abdominal surgery; has syringe-activated extendable "wings."

Malgaigne fracture: Supracondylar fracture of humerus.

Malgaigne fracture: Unstable pelvic fracture running

through sacrum or ilium and ipsilateral pubic rami. Condition is frequently associated with internal organ injury, and 50% of patients have residual neurologic damage.

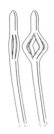

Malecot catheter

Malgaigne triangle (carotid triangle): Anatomic area bordered by anterior midline of neck, sternocleidomastoid muscle, and posterior digastric muscle belly.

Malherbe epithelioma (Malherbe-Chenatais syndrome, pilomatrixoma): Firm, nonmobile, calcified tumor of hair follicle (usu. benign); occurs on face, neck, and scalp. Condition is more common in females and generally occurs in myotonic dystrophy.

Mali disease (pseudo-Kaposi disease): Purplish lesions (sometimes ulcerated) on extensor surface of toes and foot; seen in chronic venous insufficiency.

Mall ridge (pulmonary ridge): Embryonic fold next to fetal common cardinal vein; develops into pleuropericardial membrane.

Mallinckrodt tube: Double-lumen plastic endotracheal tube with 2 air channels of unequal length; used for selective lung intubation. After proper positioning, shorter channel lies in trachea, and longer channel lies in left or right bronchus. Both lumens/air channels have inflatable cuffs with pilot balloons.

Mallorca acne: Facial pustules/papules that develop following chronic sun exposure.

Mallory bodies: Cytoplasmic hyalinization of hepatocytes; seen in fat hepatitis due to alcohol injury. Structures appear focal and horn-shaped under light microscopy.

Mallory classification: System used to describe femoral shaft fractures occurring during total hip arthrodesis. Type 1, involves lesser trochanter and calcar; type 2, extends through lesser trochanter and 4 cm proximal to prosthesis; type 3, extends through lesser trochanter and > 4 cm proximal to prosthesis.

Mallory leukemia: Leukemia caused by carcinogens benzol, indole, and tar.

Mallory-Azan stain: Material used to visualize bone, heart, and nerves; stains Purkinje fibers pale red; nuclei, axons, and neurokeratin red; and neurolemma (nervous tissue) pale blue.

Mallory-Weiss tear: Longitudinal tear in gastroesophageal junction due to vomiting; unrelated to ulcer disease. Risk factors are hiatal hernia, alcohol abuse, and pregnancy. Bleeding is arterial. Lavage and nasogastric decompression stops most bleeding; 2nd-line procedures are vasopressin infusion, endoscopic ablation, and angiographic embolization. Mortality (5%–10%) is largely function of underlying cirrhosis.

Malloy-Evelyn method: Measurement of conjugated bilirubin; involves taking spectrophotometric reading 1 minute after Ehrlich diazo reagent is added to specimen. Measurement of total bilirubin is done by taking spectrophotometric reading 15 minutes after methanol is added to sample.

Maloney dilator: Mercury-filled rubber device used to enlarge esophageal strictures.

Malouf syndrome: Ovarian dysgenesis and cardiomyopathy.

malpighian corpuscle: Renal filtering structure formed from glomerulus and capsule.

malpighian corpuscle: Clusters of lymphocytes around arteries in splenic white pulp.

Malpuech disease: Facial cleft, small penis, hypospadias, and mental retardation; most commonly seen in males of gypsy descent.

Mancall-Rosales syndrome: Necrotic brain lesion associated with visceral carcinoma; marked by striking absence of metastatic or neoplastic cells in CSF.

Manchester classification: Description of breast carcinoma.

Manchester operation (Fothergill operation): Surgical correction of uterine prolapse and cystocele. Bladder is dissected away from cervix; circular incision is made on cervix with mucosa being dissected free to expose base of cardinal ligament, which is clamped and cut; cervix is amputated after each uterine artery is ligated with mucosa sutured to posterior lip and broad ligament base sutured to anterior lip; pubovesicocervical fascia is approximated in midline beneath urethra; and excess vaginal mucosa is resected.

Manchester technique: Intrauterine application of cesium or radium (intracavitary brachytherapy) for treatment of cancer of cervix; produces constant isodose patterns regardless of size and shape of organ.

Mann procedure: Transvaginal approach for dissection of scarred or shortened cervix that permits placement of suture at level of internal os; rarely performed preconceptual cerclage.

Mann sign: Apparent unequal level of eyes, sometimes occurring in Graves disease.

Mann-Whitney test: Nonparametric test that requires independence of samples; yields results identical to Wilcoxon test.

Mann-Williamson ulcer: Peptic ulcer induced in experimental animals by gastric resection.

Manning criteria: 6 cardinal symptoms of irritable bowel syndrome; abdominal distenon, mucus in stool, sensation f incomplete bowel emptying, ain relieved by bowel movement, looser stools at onset of ain, and more frequent stools t onset of pain. Sensitivity and pecificity are 85%–90% for presnce of 3 or more symptoms.

Mannkopf sign: Used to disnguish true pain from malinering; palpation of truly painful rea causes increase in pulse ate.

Manson larval tapeworm: *Diphyllobothrium latum*; uman pathogen.

Mapleson anesthesia circuits: "Semiopen" anesthesia reathing circuits; classified as Mapleson A–F based on position f components. Advantages are mplicity, lightness, and easy leaning. Disadvantages are

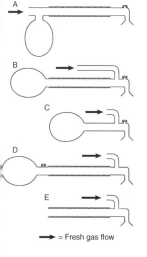

→ = Fresh gas flow

Mapleson anesthesia circuits

wasteful gas usage, potential CO_2 rebreathing, and relatively heavy valve positioned over patient's face. *Mapleson A circuit*—"noncircle" anesthesia breathing system used in pediatrics; advantages are relative inexpensiveness and valvelessness. *Mapleson D circuit* (Bain circuit)—widely used "noncircle" anesthesia breathing system with single tube-inside-a-tube design. It is valveless with no CO_2 absorber.

Maranon syndrome: Symmetric, diffuse muscle lipomas seen occasionally in wrestlers.

Maranon syndrome: Spinal anomalies and flat feet seen in ovarian insufficiency.

Maranon syndrome: Early term for association of testicular hypertrophy and gynecomastia.

Maranon syndrome: Early term for association of thyrotoxicosis, fever, and obesity.

Marchand adrenals: Small deposits of adrenal tissue found in broad ligament.

Marchand disease: Macronodular type of liver cirrhosis marked by liver nodules surrounded by collagen bands with bile retention in hepatocytes. Etiologies include hepatitis B, α-antitrypsin, and hemochromatosis.

Marchand disease: Hepatosplenomegaly, cyanosis, and clubbing caused by hepatosplenic infestation with schistosomiasis; results in portal hypertension and AV fistulas in lung parenchyma.

Marchesani syndrome: Condition marked by lens subluxation.

Marchi globule: Myelin debris visualized by Marchi stain in degenerated spinal cord diseases.

Marchi reaction: Absence of staining when demyelinated nerve is treated with osmic acid.

Marchiafava-Micheli syndrome (paroxysmal nocturnal hemoglobinuria): RBC anemia, episodic hemoglobinuria, variable leukopenia, and thrombocytopenia with infections and thrombosis; due to red cell membrane abnormality leading to lysis by complement.

Marcus Gunn dot: See Gunn dot.

Marcus Gunn phenomenon (jaw-winking sign): Opening and closing the mouth, causing slight ptosis together with protruding jaw (or moving side-to-side), with resultant elevation of affected lid; usu. congenital (autosomal dominant), but can be acquired in trauma or infection. Condition is more common in left eye and in males.

Marcus Gunn pupil: Pupillary accommodation without significant reaction; seen in optic nerve injury and possibly in congenital syphilis. Patient fixes gaze at distance; light is shone into normal eye, with contraction of both pupils; light is then moved to affected eye with brief dilation of both pupils; and finally, light is returned to normal eye, and both pupils contract and remain that way.

Marcy plication: Method of closure of inguinal ligament.

Marden-Walker syndrome: Congenital fixed facial expression, cleft palate, pectus carinatum, kyphoscoliosis, atrophic skeletal muscles, skeletal contractures, microcystic kidney disease, and cardiac anomalies; closely related to Schwartz-Jampel syndrome but has no pulmonary anomalies and is present from birth.

Marek disease: Highly contagious type of herpesvirus that causes lymphoproliferative disease in chickens; existing vaccine is effective.

Marfan sign: Reddish spot at tip of coated tongue is positive for typhoid fever.

Marfan syndrome: Hereditary cystic medial necrosis of aorta, esp. in ascending aorta, with resulting dissection; marked by long limbs in proportion to torso, lens subluxation, slender and elongated digits, scoliosis, slipped upper femoral epiphysis, joint laxity, hernias, and retinal detachment. Condition is autosomal dominant in 80% of cases and sporadic in 20% of cases; defect is on 15q21.

Marghescu syndrome (Braun-Falco syndrome): Congenital bullous poikiloderma (variable pigmentation and telangiectasias of skin).

Marie disease: Gigantism.

Marie sign: Extremity or whole body tremors sometimes seen in Graves disease.

Marie syndrome: Type of hereditary cerebellar ataxia.

Marie-Bamberger disease: Lung disease and hypertrophied joints.

Marie-Foix sign: Occurs in leg paralysis when forced flexion of toes or transverse tarsal pressure causes ipsilateral involuntary leg withdrawal.

Marie-Leri syndrome: Hand deformity in which fingers can be telescoped on themselves; associated with Ehlers-Danlos syndrome, rheumatoid arthritis, Thevenard syndrome, and congenital indifference to pain syndrome.

Marie-Strümpell disease (ankylosing spondylitis): Arthritic degeneration of lower spine and sacroiliac joints with eventual ossification of lower spinal ligament.

Marinesco succulent hand: Swelling, paleness, and coldness of hand seen in syringomyelia.

Marinesco-Radovici sign (palmomental reflex): Positive finding is slight ipsilateral contraction of corner of mouth and eyebrow lift when thenar area of hand is stimulated; seen in corticospinal tract lesions, frontal lobe lesions, and in diffuse white matter disease, as well as in normal patients with anxiety.

Marinesco-Sjögren syndrome: Ataxia, cataracts, and dementia; metabolic error is unknown. Onset is birth to 6 months of age. Condition is autosomal recessive.

Mariotte law: See Boyle law.

Mariotte spot: Early term for blind spot.

Marjolin ulcer: Squamous cell carcinoma arising in burn scar; may occur 15–20 years postinjury.

Markle sign: Positive is abdominal tenderness when standing patient raises onto toes and lets heels fall suddenly; seen with peritoneal irritation and acute abdomen.

Marmor prosthesis: Knee replacement with maximum freedom of motion; requires good soft tissue stability.

Maroteaux-Lamy syndrome (mucopolysaccharidosis type 6): Deficiency in lysosomal enzyme N-acetylgalactosamine-4-sulfatase (arylsulfatase B); results in deficient degeneration of keratan sulfate. Condition is autosomal recessive. Onset occurs at 2–4 years of age, with aortic valve degeneration and dyostosis multiplex. Disorder may be mild (relatively long survival) or severe (death by 30 years of age).

Marshall fold: Visceral pericardial fold (embryonic remnant) surrounding ligament of left vena cava lying between left pulmonary artery and left pulmonary vein.

Marshall oblique vein: Small vein sometimes found on posterior of left atrium emptying into coronary sinus; represents remnant of left superior vena cava.

Marshall-Marchetti-Krantz procedure: Transabdominal retropubic urethropexy.

Marshall-McIntosh technique: Surgical repair of tears on anterior cruciate ligament using patellar tendon and aponeurosis.

Marshall-Smith syndrome: Overly rapid physical growth and bone maturation, usu. starting in utero; marked by respiratory difficulties and mental retardation.

Martin-Gruber anastomosis: Anatomic anomaly of motor fibers of ulnar nerve, which join from median nerve or interosseous nerve in forearm instead of coursing entire length in ulnar pathway. Proximal median nerve injury causes total motor loss in hand.

Martin-Lester agar: Modification of chocolate agar with addition of antibiotics; used to isolate *Neisseria gonorrhoeae* and *N. meningitidis*.

Mason classification: System used to describe fractures of radial head. Type 1, nondisplaced marginal fracture; type 2, segmental displacement of fragment; type 3, comminuted fracture; type 4, posterior elbow dislocation with comminuted fracture.

Mason-Goldner stain: Trichromic stain using iron hematoxylin to stain nuclei black, light green to stain mesenchyme green, and azofuchsin to stain fibrin and parenchyma orange.

Mason-Pfizer virus: Retrovirus (RNA virus) that causes breast tumors in monkeys.

Mason-Turner syndrome (transferase deficiency galactosemia): Inability to metabolize galactose with hypoglycemic crises, diarrhea, vomiting, dehydration, cataracts, hepatomegaly, and ascites; due to deficiency of galactose-1-phosphate uridyltransferase. Onset is shortly after birth, with severity ranging from milk intolerance to significant deterioration and death. Treatment is galactose-free diet and (in severe cases) liver transplantation.

Masserman test (CSF formation test): Used to estimate rate of CSF formation; most common version estimates amount of fluid that must be removed to decrease intraspinal pressure to 60 mm H_2O divided by time needed to restore opening pressure on lumbar puncture.

Masshof lymphadenitis: Mesenteric lymphadenitis caused by *Yersinia pseudotuberculosis* or *Y. enterocolitica*; benign, self-limited condition that may mimic appendicitis.

Masson body: Cellular material found in pulmonary alveoli in rheumatic pneumonia similar to Aschoff bodies.

Masson disease: Benign congenital or childhood onset of multiple, usu. painful, blue-black skin lesions on head, neck, thigh and buttocks; formed by layers of glomus cells interspersed by nerve fibers and hemangiomas. Disorder may be associated with other malignancies. Treatment is excision.

Masson hemangioma: Intravascular papillary endothelial hyperplasia.

Masson-Fontana stain: Ammoniacal silver stain.

Mast-Spiegel-Pappas classification: System used to describe distal tibial fractures. Type 1, through malleolus with posterior plafond fragment; type 2, spiral fracture of shaft; type 3a, fracture of articular surface with no displacement; type 3b, fracture/dislocation of articular surface; type 3c, fracture/dislocation of articular surface with comminution and impaction.

master knot of Henry: Area on medial foot where tendons of flexor digitorum longus cross with tendons of flexor hallucis longus.

Masters intestinal clamp: Long (273 mm) curved, ring-handle, locking forceps, with long jaws and longitudinal serrations; used to occlude bowel.

Masters-Schwartz liver clamp: Long (305 mm) ring-handle, locking clamp, with long (191 mm), thin, concave jaws; used to compress liver parenchyma during liver dissection.

Mathison technique: Method of ureteral reimplantation using submucosal bladder tunnel and enlargement of hiatus.

Mattox maneuver: Surgical technique of exposing aorta by reflecting intraperitoneal contents to the right.

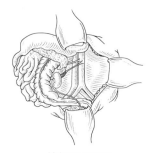

Maltox maneuver

Maumenee dystrophy (Stocker-Hall disease): "Birdshot" retinochoroidopathy marked by discreet yellow plaques confined to macula and radiating from fovea.

Maurer dots (Christopher spots): Fine cytoplasmic inclusions occurring in RBCs of malaria patients infected with *Plasmodium falciparum*.

Mauriac syndrome: Severe, "brittle" juvenile diabetes associated with dwarfism, obesity, organomegaly, and colicky abdominal pain; best to use longer-acting insulin to control glucose level.

Mauriceau maneuver: Technique used in breech deliveries to extract aftercoming head. Delivering physician cradles infant's chest in palm and applies traction to infant's shoulders using 2nd and 3rd fingers. Assistant maintains flexion of head by external suprapubic pressure.

Mauthner membrane (axolemma): Plasma sheath surrounding axons.

Maxwell spot: Yellowish depression located on retina lateral and inferior to optic disk; absorption site of short light wavelengths.

May-Grünwald-Giesma stain: Bichromic stain in which azure–eosin stains eosinophils, collagen fibers, and cytoplasm red, and methyl violet stains nuclei and basophilic substances blue; also stains mast cells violet and melanin green.

May-Hegglin anomaly: Rare triad of poorly granulated enlarged platelets; abnormally large, ovoid Döhle bodies in granulocytes; and variable thrombocytopenia. Disorder may be asymptomatic or marked by abnormal bleeding and postoperative hemorrhage, gingival oozing, and menorrhagia.

Mayaro virus: Alphavirus transmitted from monkeys to humans by *Haemagogus* mosquito in Bolivia and Brazil; leads to sudden onset of headache, fever, dizziness, chills, and arthralgias in small joints.

Mayer reflex: Patient's hand is held palm up with fingers slightly bent, and 3rd and 4th fingers are flexed at metacarpophalangeal joints until fingers touch palm. In normal patients, ipsilateral thumb adducts, flexes at metacarpophalangeal joint, and extends at interphalangeal joint. Reflex is absent in corticospinal tract lesions, hypotonia, peripheral nerve lesions, and sometimes bilaterally in normal patients, but it is exaggerated in brain tumors and meningitis.

Mayer waves: Recurring variation in blood pressure caused by altered homeostasis due to vasopressor activation or perturbations in baroreceptor system.

Mayer-Rokitansky-Kuster-Hauser syndrome: Congenital absence of vagina.

Mayfield aneurysm clip: Small metal device used to obliterate brain aneurysms.

Maylard incision (Maylard-Bardenheurer incision): Transverse incision of all layers of lower abdominal wall in pelvic and gynecologic surgery; provides excellent exposure but requires ligation of inferior epigastric vessels.

Mayne sign: Positive is decrease of 15 mm Hg in diastolic pressure when arm is raised from heart level to above head; occurs in aortic regurgitation.

Mayo ankle prosthesis: Used for replacement of ankle joint; usu. less successful than other joint replacements.

Mayo approach: See Bryan-Morrey approach.

Mayo classification: System used to describe olecranon fractures. Type 1a—nondisplaced, noncomminuted; type 1b—nondisplaced, comminuted; type 2a—displaced, noncomminuted (but stable); type 2b—displaced, comminuted (but stable); type 3a—unstable, noncomminuted; type 3b—unstable, comminuted.

Mayo kidney clamp (Guyon clamp): Long (229 mm), ring-handle, locking clamp; shaft has slight S-shape with nontoothed, curved tips.

Mayo-Gibbon heart–lung machine: Prototype pump oxygenator that uncoupled flow pressure to and from patient; device helped pioneer open cardiac surgery.

Mayo-Robson intestinal forceps: Long (241 mm), curved, ring-handle, locking forceps, with long jaws and longitudinal serrations; used to occlude bowel.

Maze procedure: Surgical treatment for refractory atrial fibrillation; uses surgical incisions made in cardiac muscle to prevent reentrant mechanism.

Mazzotti reaction: Pruritic maculopapular rash developing after test dose of diethylcarbamazine citrate is given to patients heavily infected with onchocerciasis.

McArdle disease (muscle phosphorylase deficiency): Type glycogen storage disease; deficiency of enzyme phosphorylase inhibits formation of ATP by glycogenolysis with glycogen accumulation. Disorder results in exercise intolerance with adult onset (patients report "second-wind" phenomenon). 50% have myoglobinuria after exercise.

McBurney point: 1/3 distance from anterior iliac spine to umbilicus; approximates position of appendix.

McBurney sign: Tenderness on palpation at McBurney point; occurs in appendicitis.

McCall procedure (modified) [McCoy procedure]: Technique that uses culdoplasty sutures to support vaginal vault mechanically and to close cul-de-sac in vaginal hysterectomy. Absorbable suture is placed intravaginally through vaginal wall and as high as possible on lateral fornix. Then it is passed through ipsilateral sacrouterine area and cardinal ligament and through contralateral sacrouterine and cardinal ligament tissues and brought out 1 cm from entry point. Second suture is placed identically from opposite side and tied after peritoneal cavity is closed with 2 purse-string sutures.

McCarey-Kaufman medium: Standard tissue medium (TC 199), 5% dextran, and gentamicin; used to store cornea tissue for transplantation. Preservation time is 3–4 days.

McCarthy-West syndrome (ablepharon–macrostomia syndrome): Absence of eyelids, macrostomia, triangular face, malformed ears, hypertrichosis of skin, and mental retardation.

McCune-Albright syndrome: Fibrous dysplasia with skeletal lesions causing localized pain, deformities, and fractures; seen with "coast of Maine" café au lait spots.

McCune-Albright syndrome: Precocious sexual development associated with hyperthyroidism (multinodular goiters); caused by missense mutation in gene for α subunit of G-protein that stimulates cAMP production.

McDonald dissector: Blunt, flat surgical instrument.

McDonald procedure (cerclage): Technique that partially closes incompetent cervix in pregnancy, using 4 sutures in diamond shape. Contraindications include uterine bleeding, uterine contractions, cervical dilation > 4 cm, or known fetal anomaly.

McDonald sign: Easily flexed cervical fundus occurring in 7th–8th week of pregnancy.

McDowell solution: Phosphate-buffered 1% glutaraldehyde with 4% formaldehyde solution; suitable fixative for both electron and light microscopy.

McFadden aneurysm clip: Small metal device used to occlude brain aneurysms.

McFarland syndrome: See Larsen syndrome.

McFee-type incision: Horizontal incision made just above clavicle; used in surgical approach to posterior tongue. Can be combined with stair-step incision.

McGinn-White sign: Clinical signs of cor pulmonale, with inverted T waves in V2 and V3, both Q wave and inverted T waves in III, and low T wave and ST intervals in II; suggests massive pulmonary embolism.

McGoon technique: Method used to avoid heart block in AV canal repairs; patch suture line is kept to left and superior to A node and His bundle.

McGovern sutureless valve Similar to Starr-Edwards ball-cage valve except ring is seated into annulus without need for anchoring stitches.

McGregor line: Imaginary lin at base of skull running betwee most caudal part of occipital curve and hard palate.

McIndoe procedure (Abbe-Wharton-McIndoe procedure): Surgical reconstruction of vagina in congenital absence; 1st described in 1938. 2 elliptic incisions are made in perineum with initial sharp dissection an then finger dissection to create space for placement of foam rubber mold. Labia are sewn shut over it with 3–4 sutures fo 7 days, with removal and place ment of #5 Young rectal dilator into neovagina for 6 months.

McKees Rock hemoglobin: High-oxygen-affinity hemoglobin with amino acid deletion in C-terminal region; results in hemoglobin of 18–21 g/dl.

McKusick chondrodysplasi (cartilage-hair hypoplasia, CHH):Abnormal development from birth of cartilage structures and hair growth, with shortened limbs, joint hypermobility, telescoping of fingers short and wide fingernails, inverted foot, protuberant abdomen, and sparse and silky hair; normal intelligence. Life expectancy is reduced. Condition is autosomal recessive.

McKusick-Kaufman syndrome: Rare congenital heart

defects, vaginal atresia with hydrometrocolpos, and post-axial polydactyly; autosomal recessive condition. Diagnosis is usu. made in infancy, with occasional misdiagnosis of Bardet-Biedl syndrome.

McLaughlin technique: Surgical repair of ruptured rotator cuff; uses anterior approach to shoulder with crescent-shaped resection of damaged tissue starting medially on shoulder. "Shoelace" suture is placed and pulled up tight (to point of tension) with arm placed by side. Small holes are drilled in tuberosity to pass suture ends through, and knot is then tied.

McLean tonometer (impression tonometer): Device placed directly on eyeball to measure intraocular pressure.

McLeod phenotype: Rare absence of Kell protein precursor, causing acanthocytosis, shortened RBC survival, and cardiac defects; associated with progressive muscular dystrophy.

McMurray test (test): Positive finding is "clicking" evident when examiner manipulates knee joint. Condition is seen in injury to meniscus in knee. Patient is placed supine and knee is flexed 90° with foot rotated in and then out, and then knee is extended.

McNemar test: Statistical test used for 2 related measures in same sample population; modification of chi-square test for paired t-test.

McVay operation: Technique for hernia repair involving trans-versus abdominis aponeurosis approximated to Cooper ligament; useful in repair of femoral hernias because space is closed by inguinal ligament and iliopubic tract (see Cooper ligament hernia repair).

MD Anderson system: System used to describe melanoma. Stage 1, lesion isolated to skin; stage 2, regional lymph node involvement; stage 3, distant metastasis.

Meadows disease: Dilated cardiomyopathy occurring in women 2 weeks–2 months postpartum; characterized by embolism, cough, chest pain, hemoptysis, and hepatomegaly. Left-sided failure precedes right-sided failure. Etiology is possibly autoimmune or viral. Treatment is bed rest, diuretics, and digitalis, with 65% of patients making complete recovery. Recurrence is common.

Mean sign: Slowness of upward eyeball movement seen in Graves disease.

Means-Lerman sign: Sign of thyrotoxicosis in which scratchy, systolic murmur is auscultated over left sternal border at base of heart.

mechanism of Schultze: Most common type of placental extrusion, in which placental separation occurs in center with fetal surface presenting first; no escape of placental blood occurs until after extrusion.

Mecke reagent: Solution made of 200 parts concentrated sulfuric acid and 1 part selenious acid.

Meckel cartilage (rod): Cartilage of 1st branchial arch, which lies below and medial to dentary plate. Inferior alveolar nerve runs on surface. Investing fibrous tissue surrounding cartilage ossifies during development to form mandible.

Meckel caves (spaces): Two cleft-like spaces that lie bilaterally in trigeminal impression on apex of petrous portion of temporal bone; houses semilunar (gasserian) ganglion.

Meckel diverticulum: Congenital true diverticulum of small bowel, resulting from incomplete closure of vitelline duct or omphalomesenteric duct (embryonic yolk stalk and sac); usu. found within 24–36 in. of ileocecal valve. Presenting features are usu. bleeding (most common cause of bright red blood per rectum in young people) or obstruction, but condition can mimic appendicitis. Diverticulum sometimes contains heterotopic gastric tissue, which is diagnosed with technetium pertechnetate scan. Incidental, noninflamed diverticula are not removed in adults.

Meckel ganglion: Collection of parasympathetic nerve cell bodies located in pterygopalatine fossa; preganglionic fibers derive from facial nerve and nerve of pterygopalatine canal and postganglionic fibers supply palatine, nasal, and lacrimal glands.

Meckel tubercle: Greater tubercle of humerus; serves as attachment for infraspinatus and supraspinatus.

Medi stockings: Graduated compression stockings.

Mediterranean familial fever: Recurrent episodes of severe abdominal pain, tachycardia, tachypnea, abdominal tenderness (esp. in epigastrium), and sometimes chest pain preceding fever (temperature up to 103°F); disorder mimics acute surgical abdomen (patients often have previous laparotomy). Disease is seen in people of Armenian or Jewish (Sephardic) descent.

Medusa head: Any structure or organism that morphologically resembles mythological female head with multiple snakes (e.g., *Bacillus anthracis*).

Mees line: Horizontal white lines on fingernails that appear several weeks after exposure to arsenic and heavy metals.

Meesman corneal dystrophy (juvenile epithelial corneal dystrophy): Multiple, pinpoint cysts in corneal epithelium, with no significant visual loss; autosomal dominant condition.

Mehlis gland: Structure surrounding trematode ootype.

Mehta angle difference (rib-vertebral angle difference): Angle of convexity—angle of concavity of spine; usu. ≥ 20° in idiopathic infantile scoliosis. Likely indication of poor prognosis and need for aggressive bracing.

Meibomian glands: Specialized sebaceous glands embedded in tarsal fibrous tissue. Alveoli open into central duct running parallel to conjunctival surface.

Meig syndrome: Benign ovarian tumors, ascites, and hydrothorax. Resection of involved ovary is curative.

Meige syndrome: Familial form of lymphedema occurring at onset of puberty.

Meige syndrome: See Brueghel syndrome.

Meissner corpuscle: Specialized nerve endings in papillae of corneum in hands, feet, and lips that are responsible for tactile sensation.

Meissner plexus (ganglion): Submucosal termination of preganglion fibers of autonomic nervous system in GI tract; occurs from esophagus to large bowel.

Melendez virus: Herpesvirus that causes lymphomas in monkeys.

Meleney gangrene: See Fournier gangrene.

Meleney ulcer: Slowly expanding gastric ulcer, usu. beginning at site of surgery or trauma; may be due to infection.

Melkersson-Rosenthal syndrome: Rare recurrent facial paralysis, recurrent and progressive facial and lip edema, and variable plication of tongue; unknown etiology.

Melzer disease: Cryoglobulinemia with renal failure; associated with liver, autoimmune, or lymphoproliferative disorders.

Meltzer sign: Loss of 2nd heart sound on swallowing; suggests lower esophageal contraction or occlusion.

Meltzer-Lyon test: Examination of bile for presence of birefringent and notched calcium bilirubinate or cholesterol crystals. Bile is aspirated during upper endoscopy after biliary tract is stimulated with cholecystokinin injection and immediately viewed at room temperature under microscope. Test is used in patients with biliary colic in absence of cholelithiasis to predict good prognosis for symptom resolution after cholecystectomy.

Mende syndrome: Variant of Klein-Waardenburg syndrome, with partial albinism, lanugo-type hair, small stature, congenital deafness, cleft lip, and variable mental retardation.

Mendel-Bechterew reflex (dorsocuboidal sign, tarsophalangeal reflex): Positive if tapping or stroking skin over cuboid bone or 4th or 5th metatarsal produces rapid plantar flexion of toes, esp. 4th and 5th; seen in most corticospinal tract lesions but may also occur in normal patients with hyperreflexia.

Mendeléev table: Periodic table of elements.

Mendelson syndrome: Aspiration of stomach contents, causing chemical pneumonitis; pH must be < 2.5 for development of clinical sequelae of tachycardia and hypoxia. Superior segmental bronchi of left and right lower lung lobes are most commonly involved.

Ménétrier disease: Large, thickened, tortuous mucosal folds in stomach with glandular atrophy that leak proteins into lumen, with resulting protein malnutrition, weight loss, and diarrhea; can mimic cirrhosis. Most common presenting feature is pain. Disorder is associated with increased risk of gastric cancer. Men older than 50 years are most commonly affected; occurrence in children may result from cytomegalovirus infection. Treatment is H_2 blockers, anticholinergics, and nutritional supplementation.

Menge pessary: Ring-shaped instrument with rigid cross-bar and detachable stem; inserted into vagina to prevent deviation of uterus.

Menghini needle: Used to obtain liver biopsies.

Meniere syndrome: Sudden, recurrent onset of vertigo with gradually progressive tinnitus and sensorineural hearing loss; associated with nausea, vomiting, and fullness in affected ear.

Menkes disease: Ehlers-Danlos syndrome type 9, with kinky hair, vascular aneurysms, cutis laxa, hypopigmentation, neurologic degeneration, and mental retardation; due to copper transport disorder. Inheritance is X-linked recessive. No liver sequelae occur.

Mennell sign: Indicator of etiology of sacral pain. If pain occurs with pressure over posterosuperior sacral spine, problem is lesion or deposit in gluteal structures of posterosuperior spine. If pain occurs more medially than posterosuperior sacral spine, problem is probably injury of superior ligament of sacroiliac joint.

Menzies method: Staining technique used to visualize cardiac and skeletal muscle striations; involves bromphenol blue, dilute acetic acid, and Scott tap water substitute, with viewing under oil immersion.

Mercedes-Benz sign: Radiographic shadow shaped like car symbol; seen in gallstones with fissures.

Mercier bar (interureteric ridge): Mucosal fold running transversely between ureteral orifices in bladder.

Merkel cell tumor: Growth that may occasionally be mistaken for chest wall metastasis.

Merkel muscle: Ceratocricoid muscle; fibers originate from cricoid cartilage and insert on inferior cornu of thyroid cartilage.

Merkel tactile cell (corpuscle, disk): 1 of 4 cell types in dermis; found in hard palate, hair follicles, and deep dermis. Each small, cup-shaped cell, which originates from neural crest cell, is in contact with one specialized epithelial cell.

Merril-Palmer test: Test of cognitive ability in children.

Merritt-Kasabach syndrome: Infantile hemangioma sometimes detectable on physi-

al exam as subcutaneous hard
mass; marked by decreased
platelets, decreased fibrin, and
increased fibrin split products.
Treatment options include
steroids, radiation, or endovas-
ular obliteration.

method of Spälteholz:
Method of bone specimen
preparation using wintergreen.

**Metzenbaum dissecting
scissors:**

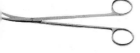

Metzenbaum dissecting scissors

Meunier sign: Daily weight
loss that occurs between incu-
bative and eruption stage in
measles.

Mexican hat sign: Sombrero-
shaped shadow seen on colon
contrast studies; caused by inferior wall pedunculated polyp.

**Meyenburg-Altherr-
Uelinger syndrome** (Altherr
syndrome, polychondritis, von
Meyenburg syndrome): Recurrent inflammation of cartilage
causing eventual degenerative
disease; results in "floppy" ears,
trachea, and larynx, as well as
saddlenose deformity. Condition may also involve aortic
heart valve and eyes. Treatment
is steroids or, in severe cases,
other immunosuppression.

Meyer hemalum: Staining
method used to visualize nuclei
of hepatocytes. Liver tissue is

stained with Best carmine stain;
nuclei appear violet.

Meyer sinus: Groove in floor
of external auditory canal lying
at base of external surface of
tympanic membrane.

Meyer theory: Etiology of
endometriosis involves delayed
differentiation into endometrium of congenitally present
pluripotential tissue.

Meyerding retractors: Handheld devices used to retract
small amounts of tissue.

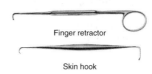

Finger retractor

Skin hook

Meyerding retractors

**Meyers-McKeever classifica-
tion:** System used to describe
pediatric intercondylar tibial
fractures. Type 1, nondisplaced
avulsion; type 2, posterior rim
intact and anterior rim partially
separated; type 3, total displacement.

**Meyers-Schwickerath syn-
drome:** See Fraser syndrome.

Meynert commissure: Tract
of nerve fibers running transversely that connects globus
pallidus on each side with fibers
running to subthalamic nucleus;
enlarged in Arnold-Chiari malformation.

Meynert fasciculus (retro-
flexus fasciculus): Nerve tract
largely arising from habenular

nucleus; passes obliquely through red nucleus.

Meynert layer: Layer 3 of cerebral cortex (external pyramidal layer); has inner zone of slightly smaller-size pyramidal cells and an outer zone with large pyramidal cells and cells with processes that extend outside this layer.

Meynet nodules: Lesions developing on tendons in rheumatic disease.

Mibelli angiokeratoma: Rare, reddish papules occurring on knees, elbows, and back of hands in young women; most cases are associated with history of frostbite, cold sensitivity, or chilblains. Familial condition is autosomal dominant.

Michaelis constant (Michaelis-Menten constant): Measure of enzyme/substrate affinity; equals concentration of substrate at which V is $V_{max}/2$, where V is initial reaction velocity and V_{max} is maximal reaction body.

Michaelis rhomboid: Area formed by imaginary lines drawn between points formed by edge of gluteal muscles, groove at distal vertebral column, and posterior superior iliac spines.

Michaelis-Gutmann bodies: Basophilic structures appearing in nuclei with "target" morphology; closely associated with cells found in malacoplakia lesions, esp. bladder lesions. Structures also stain positive for calcium and iron.

Michaelis-Menten equation: Expression that describes rate of reaction catalyzed by enzyme involving single substrate and product. Equation is $V = V_{max}[S]/(k_m + [S])$, where V is initial reaction velocity, [S] is substrate concentration, k_m is Michaelis constant (measure of enzyme/substrate binding), and V_{max} is maximal reaction velocity.

Michel forceps: Small, scissor-shaped forceps used to remove Michel wound clips; available with spring-action or ring handles.

Michel wound clips: Nickel-silver surgical staples varying in size from 11–22 mm; used for securing small amounts of tissue or approximating skin edge when closing wounds.

Michelin tire baby: Congenitally present multiple redundant skin folds; occurs in otherwise healthy infants or with multiple other abnormalities.

Michigan alcoholism screening test (MAST): List of 10 yes–no questions concerning drinking habits and history; performance rated on scale of 2–5. Score > 5 indicates alcoholism.

Michotte syndrome: See Baastrup syndrome.

Middlebrook agar: Culture media. Type 7H10 is used to isolate and test antibiotic sensitivity to mycobacteria. Type 7H11 is similar to 7H10 but with dilute casein hydrolipate substituted for glucose.

Miehlke-Partsch syndrome: Variant of Wiedemann disease with thalidomide-induced defects limited to palsy of abduction muscles and abnormalities of ears and face.

Mietens-Weber syndrome: Dwarfism, mental retardation, corneal opacity, elbow contractures, nystagmus, ear abnormalities, and hypertrichosis.

Mikasa technique: Procedure used in subacromial bursography to investigate partial-thickness rotator cuff tears on bursa side. 38-mm, 25-gauge fluoroscopy needle is inserted into supine patient 1.5 cm distal to anterolateral border of acromion and directed upward toward glenohumeral interval until tip is 2 mm medial to lateral edge of acromion. 6 ml of 1% lidocaine is injected with 4, 6, 8, and 12 ml of contrast material in series of 4 injections, with radiologic views taken in anterior-posterior direction with humerus in rotation. Tear is detectable as extravasation of dye.

Mikulicz aphthae (minor aphthous ulcer): Small, recurrent painful ulcers (< 1 cm) in oral, anal, and GI tract mucosa, likely due to trauma; more common in women.

Mikulicz cells: Foamy histiocytes.

Mikulicz drain: Fashioned by layering gauze strip onto wound, with use of additional pieces of gauze placed on top as "plunger" to push initial strip deep into wound.

Mikulicz sack: Surgical technique used to drain peritoneal cavity, sometimes following anastomotic leakage after bowel resection.

Mikulicz syndrome: Granulomatous or lymphocytic unilateral or bilateral inflammation of lacrimal and submandibular glands; seen in sarcoidosis.

Milan rat: Laboratory animal; both hypertensive and normotensive strains used as animal models for studying alterations in calcium regulation.

Milch classification: System used to describe pediatric condylar fractures of humerus. Type 1, fracture runs from trochlear sulcus to medial superior eminence or from trochlear sulcus to lateral superior eminence (usu. due to compression); type 2, fracture runs from trochlear sulcus to lateral superior eminence or trochlear groove to medial superior eminence (usu. due to compression or dislocation).

Milian erythema: Scarlet fever–type rash with malaise and fever 7–9 days after injection of drugs or arsphenamine; reaction to drug administration.

Milker nodule: Skin lesion that progresses from red nodules to purple papules; contracted via contact with cows infected with parapoxvirus.

Milkman syndrome: Multiple stripes seen in bones on radiographs; caused by defective phosphate reabsorption in renal tubules.

Millard-Gubler syndrome:
Injury to lateral pons with involvement of CN VI, causing ipsilateral palsy; CN VII, causing ipsilateral facial weakness; and corticospinal tract, causing contralateral hemiplegia.

Milledgeville hemoglobin:
High-oxygen-affinity hemoglobin with replacement of proline by leucine in $\alpha_1\beta_2$ contact region; results in hemoglobin of 15.6–18.1 g/dl.

Miller asthma: See Kopp asthma.

Miller body splint: Straight board used to stabilize position of injured patient in the field for transport.

Miller laryngoscope blade:
Straight metal blade used to intubate trachea; available in adult and pediatric sizes.

Miller vein patch (collar):
Short, cylindrical piece of vein sutured between native vessel and distal prosthetic graft; minimizes anastomotic intimal hyperplasia.

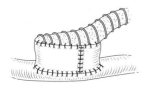

Miller vein patch

Miller-Abbott tube (Abbott tube): Double-lumen long intestinal tube inserted through nose and allowed to travel to intestines. Tip is weighted and carried distally via peristalsis (thus not indicated in ileus). Tube is used in recurrent small bowel obstructions secondary to adhesions (esp. in radiation enteritis) and sometimes when obstruction is secondary to malignancy.

Miller-Fisher syndrome:
Variant of Guillain-Barré syndrome, with descending rather than ascending paralysis; commonly misdiagnosed as botulism.

Miller-Gallante prosthesis
(MG prosthesis): Knee replacement with maximal freedom of motion of joint; requires good soft tissue stability.

Mills maneuver: Positive for tennis elbow (throbbing pain on lateral side of elbow) if pain results when patient has flexed wrist and straightened elbow and examiner pronates forearm.

Milroy disease: Familial form of congenital lymphedema.

Milton disease: See Bannister disease.

Milwaukee brace: Device used to treat scoliosis of spine. Brace is worn under clothes and has thoracic and lumbar pads, and molded pelvic section has one anterior and two posterior upright parts that connect to neck ring.

Minamata disease: Chronic, low-level mercury ingestion causing mental deterioration, paresthesias, tremors, ataxia, and excessive sweating and salivation.

Minkowski figure: Glucose-to-nitrogen ratio (2.8:1) in urine on fasting or pure protein diet.

Minnesota test for differential diagnosis of aphasia (MTDDA): Used to evaluate, classify, and locate aphasias, esp. simple aphasia with visual involvement.

Minnesota tube: Device similar to Sengstaken-Blakemore tube, except with 4th port that allows lavage of esophagus when balloons are inflated.

Minor sign: Characteristic rising from sitting position seen in sciatica; patient shifts weight onto pain-free side with hand supporting back and bends affected leg while rising.

Mirchamp sign: Positive for sialadenitis when vinegar placed on tongue causes painful reflex secretion of saliva.

Mirrizzi syndrome: Cystic duct stone that causes external impingement of common bile duct; can cause acute cholangitis.

Mitchell disease type 2: See Barraquer-Simons syndrome.

Mitchell modification: Penile elongation and urethroplasty used in boys with epispadias and bladder exstrophy; uses total penile disassembly with division of glans penis.

Mitrofanoff technique: Creation of catheterizable continent bladder using appendix–bladder anastomosis.

Mittendorf dot: Small, rounded opacity in inferior nasal portion of posterior lens capsule seen on ophthalmoscopic exam; represents attachment of hyaloid artery to posterior aspect of lens. It does not affect vision.

Mixter gallbladder forceps: Curve-tipped, ring-handle, locking forceps used for tissue dissection.

Miyasato disease: α_2-antiplasmin deficiency with congenital, severe, recurrent, hemorrhaging originating from umbilical cord. Condition manifests as joint hemorrhages and hemothorax in adults. Treatment is antifibrinolytic agent tranexamic acid.

Moberg flap: Advancement flap used to close palmar-angled loss-of-tissue wound on thumb via "dog-ear" closure and Kirschner wire to maintain interphalangeal flexion of thumb during healing.

Mobin-Uddin filter: Early intravascular, umbrella-type prosthesis made of 6 struts of stainless steel and perforated Silastic membrane. Disadvantages were caval thrombosis and too-frequent migration to right atrium.

Mobitz heart block (type 1) [Wenckebach block]: Condition marked by progressive PR lengthening culminating in "dropped" P wave; followed by identical cycle or sometimes escape AV junctional beat before repeating cycle. Block is usu. located in AV junction. Causes include digoxin toxicity, acute myocardial ischemia, calcium deposits in conducting tissue, and excessive vagal stimulation. Temporary or permanent pacing is not necessary.

Mobitz heart block (type 2): 2nd-degree AV heart block; represents intraventricular block and is marked by widened QRS on ECG. PR interval is constant but there are multiple P waves for each QRS. Causes are acute MI, myocarditis, and calcium deposition in conducting system. Immediate temporary pacing is necessary until cardiac pacemaker can be permanently implanted.

Möbius I syndrome: Atrophy of tongue and dysfunction of CNs VI and VII.

Möbius sign (Moebius sign): Defective functioning of internal rectus muscles in Graves disease; results in inability to converge eyes.

modified Fontan procedure: Last stage of 3-stage reconstruction of hypoplastic left heart; performed at 18–36 months of age.

Moe plate: Stainless steel device used to fix intertrochanteric femur fractures internally.

Mohs scale: Measure of hardness of material; comparison of ability to resist scratching to standards with known abrasive characteristics.

Mohs surgery: Microsectioning of superficial lesions and examination using grid system to determine areas of invasion to minimize resection and tissue loss; used today mostly by dermatosurgeons. Technique is best for lesions of face.

Mokola virus: Serotype of lyssavirus similar to rabies virus; isolated from animals in Africa.

Moll glands (ciliary glands): Sweat glands found between eyelash hair follicles; run parallel to bulbs of eyelashes.

Mollaret syndrome: Recurrent, benign, aseptic meningitis with presence of large endothelial cells in CSF during attacks.

Monafo formula: Expression that calculates amount of fluid needed to resuscitate burn patients; uses hypertonic saline input ($\sim$ 50 mEq/L) sufficient to maintain urine output of 30 ml/hr.

Mönckeberg sclerosis (medial calcinosis): Ring-like calcifications forming in media of ulnar, radial, tibial, and femoral arteries; unknown etiology. Condition is usu. not clinically significant.

Mönckeberg syndrome: Ulcers of upper and lower distal extremities found in hypertension.

Mondini deformity: Thinwalled, CSF-filled cyst that originates from oval window and bulges into middle ear; usu. associated with footplate perforation in deformed stapes along with profound unilateral vestibular and sensorineural hearing loss.

Mondor disease: Superficial phlebitis of thoracoepigastric vein, which runs from axilla to lateral edge of breast to subareolar area to epigastrium; may occur after any breast surgery, trauma, or radiation. Treatment is usu. close observation after negative mammogram is obtained to rule out breast cancer.

Monfort approach: Umbilicus preservation in abdominal wall reconstruction in Eagle-Barrett syndrome (prune-belly syndrome). Midline skin incision is made from xiphoid to pubis with elliptical incision around umbilicus, and skin flaps are raised laterally just superficial to fascia. Incisions are made in peritoneum lateral to epigastric vessels on each side, with fascia brought toward center from each side and secured with running stitch, and ending with overlapping reinforced fascial wall. Skin flaps are then trimmed, if needed, and reapproximated in midline.

Moniz sign: Corticospinal tract response with dorsiflexion of toes elicited by forceful passive ankle flexion.

Monod sign: Radiolucent crest seen over round, uniform shape of *Aspergillus* fungus balls on lung radiograph.

Monro bursa: Fluid-filled sac within triceps tendon close to its insertion.

Monro line: Imaginary line between anterior superior iliac spine and umbilicus.

Monro-Kellie doctrine: Total volume of cranium and spinal canal is constant; increase in volume of nervous tissue, CSF, or blood displaces others substances and structures inside cranium.

Monro-Richter line: Imaginary line between left anterior superior iliac spine and umbilicus.

Monteggia fracture ("nightstick" fracture): Fracture of ulna with displacement of radius; fragments may override radial head.

Monteggia fracture: Dislocation of femoral head in direction of anterosuperior iliac spine.

Montercaux fracture: Fracture of proximal fibula; associated with ankle diastasis.

Montgomery glands: Sebaceous glands on areola that appear as small elevations.

Montgomery tubercles: Greatly enlarged Morgagni tubercles (sebaceous glands) of areolar tissue of nipple; seen in pregnancy.

Montreal platelets: Congenitally enlarged platelets associated with thrombocytopenia and prolonged bleeding time; show aggregation with ristocetin but not with thrombin.

Moon teeth: Dome-shaped 1st molars sometimes seen in congenital syphilis.

Moore fracture: Distal radius fracture and fracture of ulnar styloid with dorsal displacement of ulna and entrapment of annular ligament.

Moore lightning streaks: Vertical light seen in peripheral visual fields when eyes are moved laterally; clinically benign.

Moore procedure: Technique for surgical correction of rectal prolapse.

Mooren ulcer: Usu. chronic bilateral ulcers that form at marginal side of cornea.

Mooser body: Rickettsial-like structure sometimes seen in typhus and in epithelial cells from tunica vaginalis exudate.

Moran method (uvulopalatopharyngoplasty): Technique used to enlarge oropharyngeal airspace by resecting soft tissue in palate and pharyngeal sidewall; involves almost complete excision of anterior pillars via vertical incision along lateral anterior pillar border to musculocutaneous part of soft palate, where horizontal incision is made. Similar incision is made for posterior pillar with partial resection and lateral mucosal flap over posterior musculature to remucosalize tonsils and eliminate posterior corrugations. Small incision is made at base of tongue to promote scarring and prevent tongue from falling back into airway.

Morand foot: Foot with 8 toes.

Morel ear: Large, deformed ear lobe with obliteration of ear folds and thin edge.

Morel-Wildi syndrome: Asymptomatic nodular morphology of frontal cortex.

Morgagni disease (hyperostosis frontalis interna): Obesity due to fat metabolism defects and endocrine defects.

Morgagni foramen of tongue: Foramen cecum of tongue; slight depression on back of tongue marking original opening of thyroglossal duct.

Morgagni glands (Littre glands): Mucus-secreting glands lining urethral lumen in males.

Morgagni globule: Cell fragments found in lens cortex seen in mature cataracts.

Morgagni hernia: See foramen of Morgagni hernia.

Morgagni hydatid (appendix testis): Variably occurring 3–8-mm body of connective tissue found on upper extremity of testis; little clinical significance.

Morgagni lacunae: Numerous small invaginations found in urethra mucous membrane into which glands of Littre open.

Morgagni nodule: See Arantius nodule.

Morgagni prolapse: Chronic inflammation of mucosa and submucosa in laryngeal saccule.

Morgagni tubercle: Small nodules on areolar surface of breast; represent large superficial sebaceous glands.

Morgagni-Adams-Stokes syndrome: See Adams-Stokes syncope.

Morgenstern needle (Morgenstein needle): Stabilizing needle used during brachytherapy for prostate cancer.

Moritz reaction: See Rivalta reaction.

Moritz syndrome: Extrinsic compression of common bile

duct due to inflamed, enlarged gallbladder.

Mörner reagent: Solution of 45 parts distilled H_2O, 55 parts concentrated sulfuric acid, and 1 part formalin; used to detect tyrosine.

Moro response (startle reflex): Brisk abduction of arms with extension and opening of palms and abduction and flexion of legs in infant in response to loud noise; reaction also elicited by allowing head to drop from 30° to 10° angle.

Morquio syndrome: Resistance to attempts to raise to sitting position from supine position, until knees are passively flexed; seen in poliomyelitis.

Morquio syndrome type A: Mucopolysaccharidosis type 4; deficiency of *N*-acetylgalactosamine-6-sulfatase with defective degeneration of keratan sulfate or chondroitin-6-sulfate. Characteristic features include distinctive skeletal abnormalities, hypoplastic odontoid, aortic insufficiency, and normal intelligence. Death usu. occurs by 30 years of age. Condition is autosomal recessive.

Morrow myomectomy: Surgery for treatment of idiopathic hypertrophic subaortic stenosis.

Morrow-Brooke acne (chloracne): Acute outbreak of erythematous papules with degeneration to comedo and follicular cysts, which may become confluent with resultant keratinized plaques. Suspected etiol-

ogy is exposure to toxins, esp. chlorinated compounds.

Morscher plate (AO-Morscher plate): Internal fixation device for anterior cervical fusion.

Morton disease: Shortened 2nd metatarsal bone causing pain in area of 2nd and 3rd metatarsals.

Morton disease: Neuroma secondary to trauma located between 3rd and 4th toes; forms on common digital nerves running between metatarsals. Weight-bearing is painful. Disorder often recurs after excision.

Morton foot (Grecian foot): Length of 2nd toe greater than length of 1st toe; occurs in 22% of U.S. general population. Increased stress occurs on 2nd toe, with 1st toe tending to be hypermobile.

Morton test: Increased pain, esp. between 2nd and 3rd metatarsals, caused by transverse pressure on dorsum of foot; occurs with chronic metatarsal pain.

Morvan disease (chorea): Painless finger ulceration in setting of syringomyelia.

Moschowitz syndrome (thrombotic thrombocytopenia purpura, TTP): Microangiopathy, thrombocytopenia, hemolytic anemia, fever, renal failure, and fluctuating neurologic defects. Survival is < 10%.

Moschowitz technique (single): Culdoplasty (obliteration of cul-de-sac) using concentric purse-string sutures in conjunction with hysterectomy;

performed with interrupted purse-string sutures that plicate uterosacral ligaments. Procedure is associated with risk of ureteral injury or entrapment.

Moschowitz technique (hemi): Culdoplasty (obliteration of cul-de-sac) using concentric purse-string sutures in conjunction with hysterectomy; reinforced over top by interrupted sutures that plicate uterosacral ligaments posterior to vagina. Procedure is performed on both sides of vagina to avoid risk of entrapment of ureters.

Moschowitz test (hyperemia test): Positive for arteriosclerosis; delayed return of normal tissue color occurs after blood flow to limb is impeded using Esmarch bandage for 5 minutes and released. Reestablishment of color occurs in several seconds in normal patients.

Mose concentric ring classification: System for description of avascular necrosis of femoral head using malformation of imaginary concentric ring tracings with 2-mm separations on outline of femoral head. Good, both hips form perfect circles; fair, deviation ≤ 2 mm; poor, deviation > 2 mm.

Mosler sign: Sternal tenderness occurring in acute myelogenous leukemia.

Moss cage: Anterior thoracic and lumbar spinal fixation device made of titanium mesh formed into cylinder; inside is packed with autologous bone to serve as both graft and interbody support.

Mosse disease: Polycythemia in association with liver cirrhosis.

Mostellar equation: Estimate of body surface area (m²); equals $\sqrt{\text{weight} \times \text{height}/3600}$.

Mostofi system: Grading scheme (papilloma and grades 1–3) for transitional cell carcinoma.

Mott body: Inclusions filled with clear gelatin-type material in cytoplasm of multiple myeloma plasma cells.

Mouchet fracture: Humeral fracture through capitellum.

Mouchet syndrome: Paralysis of cubital nerve in setting of fracture of external humeral condyle.

Mouchet-Belot syndrome: See Trevor syndrome.

Moyamoya disease: Rare progressive stenosis of arteries of circle of Willis, which initially involves cerebral hemisphere vessels bilaterally and then progresses to unilateral or bilateral involvement of middle and posterior cerebral arteries. To compensate, abnormal capillary network develops at base of brain. Condition is most common in Orientals; its cause is unknown. Results include ischemic strokes in children and cerebral hemorrhage in adults. Name is not true eponym.

Moyer line: Imaginary line between middle of 3rd sacral vertebrae to point midway between anterior superior iliac spines.

Moynahan syndrome (alopecia): Congenital alopecia, mental retardation, seizures, and variable microcephaly, with delayed hair growth until 2–4 years of age.

Moynahan syndrome (xeroderma): Congenital cleft palate, hypohidrosis, defective teeth and hair, skin bullae, and no eyelashes on lower lid; autosomal dominant condition.

Moynihan gallbladder forceps: Relatively blunt, curved-tipped, ring-handle, locking forceps used for tissue dissection.

Moynihan method: Technique used to elicit Murphy sign in acute cholecystitis. Fingers of left hand are placed on rib with left thumb placed over fundus of gallbladder in subcostal area.

Moynihan test: 2 parts of Seidlitz powder are given separately. In hourglass configuration of stomach, components appear as 2 different abdominal wall protrusions on radiology.

Mozart ear: Congenitally fused helix and anthelix.

Much granules: Modified tubercle bacilli seen in sputum from TB patients; stain gram-positive and non–acid-fast.

Mueller-Hinton agar: Medium used to isolate *Neisseria gonorrhoeae* and *N. meningitidis* and for sulfonamide and antibiotic susceptibility testing.

Muenzer-Rosenthal triad: Catalepsy, anxiety, and hallucinations in psychiatric conditions.

Muir-Torre syndrome: GI polyposis, epidermoid cysts, sebaceous adenomas, desmoid tumors, fibromas, and lipomas; also with significantly increased risk of fibrosarcomas and solid organ tumors.

Muller cells: Specialized neuroglial cells found in retina that have elongated inner and outer processes contributing to different layers of retina.

Müller fibers: Specialized nerve cells in retina.

Müller maneuver: Technique used to stop paroxysmal atrial tachycardia.

Müller sign: Positive for aortic insufficiency when heart action is synchronous with erythema of tonsils and pulsation of uvula.

Müller technique: Surgical intertrochanteric varus osteotomy. 2 Kirschner wires, inserted anterior to femoral neck and through greater trochanter, are used as guides for wedge cut of femoral bone. These 2 surfaces are then opposed and secured with plate. No weight-bearing is allowed for 3–4 months.

Müllerian duct: Embryonic structure formed from invagination of each wolffian body peritoneum near its cranial end; it lies parallel to wolffian duct. Ducts grow posteriorly and fuse at the distal end and open through one ostium into urogenital sinus.

Munchausen syndrome: Psychiatric illness manifested by self-infliction of harm to induce injury or illness. Patients are extremely difficult to treat both emotionally and physically.

Munchausen-by-proxy syndrome: Psychiatric illness manifested by infliction of harm on another person to cause repeated illness and hospitalization. Parent inflicting harm on child is common scenario.

Munro microabscess: Focal collection of neutrophils located in parakeratotic part of stratum corneum; occurs in psoriasis, seborrhea, and Reiter disease.

Munro point: Landmark used for performing abdominal puncture; midway between left anterior superior iliac spine and umbilicus.

Munro-Kerr incision: Transverse opening of uterus performed in cesarean section.

Munson sign: Lower eyelid bulging on downward gaze caused by abnormal corneal curvature (keratoconus).

Münster disease: Variant of Mason-Turner syndrome.

Munster socket: Prosthesis for below-the-elbow amputations that uses myoelectrically controlled terminal device; no suspension harness or control cable is needed.

Murat sign: Sensation of vibration and discomfort occurs on affected side of chest when speaking; occurs in lung TB.

Murphy button: Internal stent that brings bowel ends together in anastomosis without sutures; devised in 1892.

Murphy eye endotracheal tube: Tube with small side opening at distal end.

Murphy position: Left or right lateral decubitus position with legs tilted lower than head; positioning technique for patients on operating room table.

Murphy sign: Sharp tenderness elicited by deep palpation in right upper quadrant with cessation of inspiration; indication of acute cholecystitis or hepatic inflammation (if tenderness is less localized).

Murray disease: See Jackson-Lawler syndrome.

Murray syndrome: See Puretic syndrome.

Murri syndrome: Gradual onset of cerebellar ataxia; usu. confined to legs; most commonly seen in men in 4th–7th decade. Etiology includes alcohol abuse, cerebrovascular accident, malignancy, and possible nutritional deficits. Treatment is symptomatic support and alcohol abstinence.

muscle of Muller: Superior tarsal smooth muscle.

Muskowitz procedure: Surgical prevention of enterocele performed as part of Burch procedure; pouch of Douglas is obliterated by intraperitoneal sutures placed at different levels.

Musset sign: Slight rhythmic jerking of head; seen in aortic insufficiency and aneurysm.

Mustard operation: Procedure for repair of transposition of great arteries; uses longitudinal incision in right atrium, partial excision of atrial septum, and placement of coronary sinus into left atrium. Baffle is then constructed to divert pulmonary vein return to tricuspid valve and caval return to mitral valve.

Mustarde cheek flap: Transposition flap used to reconstruct 50%–100% defect of lower lid surgically; involves lateral orbital and zygomatic incision to provide muscularized skin. Dissection plane must be super-ficial to zygomatic branch of facial nerve. To prevent ectropion, flap should be sutured to lateral orbital periosteum.

Myerson sign: Positive for Parkinson's disease when tapping frontalis muscle causes eyelid spasm.

Myhre syndrome: Extremely short stature, mental retardation, early onset deafness, muscle hypertrophy, stiff joints, cardiac abnormalities, and maxillary hypoplasia.

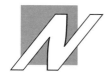

nabothian cyst (Montgomery follicle): Occluded, distended glands in uterine cervix mucosa.

Nadbath-Rehman technique: See O'Brien block (modified).

Nadi reaction (indophenol test): Used to detect presence of oxidizing enzymes in cells (myeloblasts, myelocytes, and neutrophils). Cell specimens are fixed in alcohol and floated face down for 15 minutes in Nadi reagent, rinsed, and mounted in glycerin; positive result is blue color.

Nadler-Egan syndrome: Familial deficiency of lysosomal acid perosphatase.

Naegeli leukemia: Acute myelogenous leukemia.

Naegeli syndrome (Franceschetti-Jadassohn syndrome): Rare onset of fine reticular pigmentation of skin, palmoplantar hypohidrosis, yellow spotting of teeth, nystagmus, and optic atrophy. Etiology unknown; inheritance is autosomal dominant.

Naegleria: Free-living freshwater and soil ameboflagellates that cause amebic meningitis. Organisms enter nose when individuals swim in contaminated water.

Naffziger test: Used to detect herniated nucleus pulposus; positive if pain results when external jugular vein area is compressed.

Nagamatsu incision: Surgical approach to kidney using subpleural, retroperitoneal dissection through curved flank incision.

Nägele pelvis (obliquity): Anatomically asymmetric pelvis; marked by rotation of symphysis pubis, underdevelopment of lateral half of 1 sacrum, rotation of sacrum to that side, and ankylosis of sacroiliac joint.

Nager-Reynier syndrome (Nager acrofacial dysostosis): Congenital hypoplastic mandible, temporomandibular joint aplasia, cleft palate, malformed ear canal, and hypoplastic or absent thumb, radius, and ulna.

Nagler reaction: Positive for *Clostridium perfringens* if colonies on egg yolk agar develop opaque zone that circles bacteria; caused by diffusable lecithinase.

Najjar syndrome: Congenital cardiomyopathy, mental retardation, and hypoplastic penis and scrotum.

Nakagawa syndrome: Benign progressive capillary hemangioma with finger-like projections ("cannonball pattern") occurring largely on neck and torso in infants and small children. Treatment is surgery (frequent recurrence), electrocautery, and lasers.

Nakata index: Cross-sectional area index.

Nakayama reagent: Solution made of 99 parts 95% alcohol, 1 part concentrated hydrochloric acid, and 0.4 g ferric chloride.

Namaqualand dysplasia: Degenerative hip arthritis and pain in African children; growth defect is in femoral epiphysis.

Nance leeway space: Enlargement of space occupied by 3 deciduous teeth (canine, 1st molar, and 2nd molar) as compared to same 3 permanent teeth; 1.7 mm on each side of dental arch is normal.

Nance-Horan syndrome: Congenital onset of progressive punctate cataracts, extra central incisors shaped like screwdrivers, and hypoplastic 4th metacarpals; X-linked inheritance. Gene defect is at X21.1-p22.3.

Nashold electrode (El-Naggar electrode): Device used in neurosurgical relief of pain in nucleus caudalis dorsal root entry zone (DREZ) ablation via coagulation; uses 2 electrodes for varying sizes of nucleus caudalis and right-angle bend to place ablative lesions accurately.

Natal sore: See Aleppo boil.

Naughton protocol: Exercise tolerance test best used in

patients with decreased cardiac reserve or disability.

Neal-Robertson litter: Spine board used for field transport of spinal trauma patients.

Neer classification: System used to describe location of fracture of humeral head as located in anatomic neck, surgical neck, greater tuberosity, lesser tuberosity, anterior fracture/dislocation, or posterior fracture/dislocation.

Neer sign: Positive for rotator cuff injury if pain occurs when examiner simultaneously depresses scapula and elevates humerus.

Neer-Horowitz classification: System used to describe pediatric proximal fractures through humeral physeal. Grade 1, < 5-mm displacement; grade 2, < 1/3 shaft width displacement; grade 3, 1/3–2/3 shaft width displacement; grade 4, > 2/3 shaft width displacement.

Negri bodies: Spherical inclusion bodies occurring in nerve cells of rabid animals or cytoplasm of humans; pathognomonic for rabies.

Negro disease: Variant of Mason-Turner syndrome.

Negro sign: Cogwheel rigidity.

Neill-Mooser body (reaction): Mononuclear cells with cytoplasmic rickettsiae taken from scrotal edema fluid in laboratory animals infected with murine typhus.

Neisseria: Gram-negative cocci, which usu. appear in pairs; generally cultured on Mueller-Hinton or modified Thayer-Martin agar. *N. gonorrhoeae* and *N. meningitidis* are pathogenic in humans.

Nélaton disease: Displacement of talus between tibia and fibula.

Nélaton fold: Transverse mucosal fold at junction of middle and lower third of rectum.

Nélaton line: Imaginary line drawn from ischial tuberosity to anterosuperior iliac spine; forms 1 side of Bryant triangle.

Nelson method: Specialized life table method in which outcome events may happen more than once (e.g., MI or transplant rejection).

Nelson syndrome (Nelson-Salassa syndrome): Development of ACTH-secreting tumors in patients with Cushing disease following bilateral adrenalectomy.

Nelson syndrome: Functioning pituitary tumors arising in 10% of bilateral adrenalectomies; marked by hyperpigmentation, vision abnormalities, and amenorrhea. Condition is now rare.

Neri sign: See Strümpell sign.

Neri sign (combined flexion sign): Indication of unilateral corticospinal tract paresis of leg. Patient bends forward from standing position, and flexion at knee in paretic leg occurs. In normal patient, extension is maintained.

Nernst equation: Expression used to calculate electrode potential.

Nernst potential: Voltage that exactly opposes movement of an ion across a membrane.

nerve of Latarjet (left): Branch of left vagus nerve running on lesser curvature and terminating in anterior crow's foot; supplies motor function to pylorus and terminates in pyloroantral area. Selective vagotomy is division distal to hepatic branches, and highly selective vagotomy is division of individual branches with preservation of crow's foot.

nerve of Latarjet (right): Branch of right vagus nerve running on posterior lesser curvature and terminating in pyloroantral area; gives off small branches to proximal "criminal nerves" on posterior of stomach that must be transected to achieve complete vagotomy. Selective vagotomy is division distal to celiac branches, and highly selective vagotomy is division of individual branches with preservation of crow's foot.

nerve of Luschka: Posterior ethmoid nerve that carries sensory fibers; is formed from branches of ophthalmic and nasociliary nerves and supplies sphenoid sinus and posterior ethmoid cells.

nerve of McCrea: Separate pyloric nerve branching off anterior nerve of Latarget.

nerve of Willis (spinal accessory nerve): CN XI, which carries motor and parasympathetic fibers.

nerves of Lancisi: Thin, myelinated nerve tracts running on superior aspect of each corpus callosum.

nerves of Luschka: Meningeal nerves that branch off each spinal nerve and reenter spinal canal through vertebral foramen; supply vertebrae, ligaments, and dura.

Nesbit procedure: Early surgical technique for correction of Peyronie disease.

Nessler reagent: Aqueous solution made of 16% potassium hydroxide, 5% potassium iodide, and 2.5% mercury bichloride; used to detect ammonia.

Netherton syndrome: Ichthyosis, atopy, and trichorrhexis invaginata (bamboo-like hair shafts).

Nettleship-Falls syndrome: Ocular albinism (heterozygotes), with reduced iris pigmentation, photophobia, defective visual acuity, strabismus, nystagmus, and head nodding (homozygous males). Inheritance is X-linked.

Neubauer artery: Variably present lowest thyroid artery; originates as direct branch off aorta or alternately right brachiocephalic trunk or subclavian artery.

Neuhauser sign (soap-bubble sign): Ground-glass appearance seen on plain radiograph in lower right quadrant of neonates; represents viscid meconium mixed with air. Conlition is seen in meconium ileus nd colon atresia.

Neviasser test: Used to detect proximal triceps tendonitis; positive if pain occurs when shoulder is adducted and elbow is extended against force.

Nevin system: Staging system used for gallbladder cancer. Stage 1, confined to mucosa; stage 2, extending into muscularis; stage 3, transmural with extension into serosa; stage 4, all layers involved; stage 5, invasion into adjacent tissues or distant metastases.

nevus of Ota: Unilateral pigmented conjunctival lesion; rarely malignant.

Newcastle disease: Conjunctivitis, eyelid edema, and inflammation caused by human infection by avian virus; usu. spontaneous recovery in 10–14 days.

Newman D2C: Substance used in staphylococcal clumping test.

Newman projection: Convention used to represent 3-D molecule in 2 dimensions.

Newman-Keuls test: Statistical measure of whether differences of means obtained in ANOVA are statistically significant.

newton: Unit of force in International System (SI) equal to 1 kg-m/sec^2.

Newton color circle: Earliest color circle construction. Complementary colors whose mixtures result in white and gray are arranged 180° across from each other, with white at center.

Newton law: Temperature change of object per unit time is directly proportional to temperature difference between object and surroundings.

Newton law: If 2 color mixtures produce identical color sensation, then combination of mixtures will produce that same color sensation.

Newton prosthesis: Ankle replacement.

newton-meter (N-m): Unit of torque; dimensionally equivalent to joule (J).

newtonian aberration: Different colors appearing on periphery of images caused by unequal deviation of wavelengths of light passing through refractive medium.

New York heart association classification: System used to describe degree of impairment in heart disease. Class I—no limitation, ordinary physical activity does not cause symptoms; class II—slight limitation, ordinary activity does not cause symptoms (comfortable at rest); class III—marked limitation, less-than-ordinary activity causes symptoms (comfortable at rest); class IV—inability to carry on any physical activity.

New Zealand mouse (black) [NZB]: Inbred mouse strain that spontaneously develops autoimmune diseases; also has premature development and abnormal functioning of B and T cells. Mouse is animal model for human systemic lupus erythematosus.

New Zealand mouse (white) [NZW]: Inbred mouse strain that is cross-bred with New Zealand black mouse, producing offspring with severe autoimmune disease.

New Zealand rat: Both hypertensive and normotensive strains are used as animal models in study of human essential hypertension.

Nezelof syndrome: T-cell deficiency, variable B-cell deficiency, and recurrent bacterial, fungal, viral and protozoal infections. Condition is also marked by lymphadenopathy, liver and spleen enlargement, eczematous rashes, and increased serum IgE concentration. Risk of malignancy is increased.

Nezelof type: Thymic alymphoplasia with disordered immunoglobulin synthesis.

Niagara blue: See Congo blue.

Nicoladoni sign: See Branham reaction.

Niemann-Pick disease (sea-blue histiocyte syndrome): Deficiency of lysosomal enzyme sphingomyelinase with accumulation of sphingomyelin and cholesterol in reticuloendothelial system; marked by foam cells, hepatomegaly, splenomegaly, and alveolar proteinosis in lungs. Condition occurs mostly in Jewish infants.

Nierhoff-Huebner syndrome (endochondral dysostosis): Variant of Morquio

syndrome with onset of flaccid muscles, convulsions, somnolence, dilated heart ventricles, dehiscence of cranial sutures, and abnormal calcification of epiphyses and metaphyses in 1st weeks of life. Death usu. occurs in 1st few months.

Nievergelt syndrome: Congenital joint contractures, esp. of knees and ankles; patients tend to walk on knees or develop waddling gait. Condition is sometimes associated with pigmented nevi and diminished corneal reflux.

Nigerian neuropathy: Condition marked by segmental nerve demyelination, ataxia, optic atrophy, deafness, stomatitis, and glossitis; prevalent in areas where cassava, which contains a cyanogenic glycoside, is principle component of diet.

Nigro protocol: 5-fluorouracil, mitomycin C, and radiation therapy; used as 1st-line treatment (supplanting abdominoperineal resection) of cloacogenic anal carcinoma.

Nikaidoh procedure: Method used in repair of Taussig-Bing malformation with pulmonary stenosis. Aortic root is severed from right ventricle and posteriorly translocated (this functionally closes ventricular septal defect), and transection of pulmonary artery to right ventricle is performed.

Nikolsky sign: Lateral pressure on skin lesion causing erosions and blister extension; suggests pemphigus vulgaris, scalded skin syndrome, thermal burn injuries, and toxic epidermal necrolysis.

Nissen fundoplication:
Antireflux procedure using 360° wrap of gastric fundus around esophagus and fixture to medial arcuate ligament; involves transabdominal (more common) or transthoracic approach using open or laparoscopic technique. Most common early postop complaint is dysphagia. Success rate is > 90%.

Nissen-Rossetti procedure:
Variation of Nissen fundoplication using mobilization of stomach fundus without cutting short gastric vessels; usu. performed laparoscopically.

Nissl body: Coarsely granular chromophilic material found in neuron cytoplasm; composed of rough endoplasmic reticulum and free ribosomes.

Nissl stain: Basic aniline stain of chromophilic gray matter; stains cytoplasm of nerve cell body bright blue.

Nitabuch layer: Fibrinoid material in placenta located at decidua/trophoblast junction.

Noack syndrome (Pfeiffer type): Acrocephalopolysyndactyly type 1; autosomal dominant condition.

Nobel prize: Awards now given in Chemistry, Physics, Medicine and Physiology, Economics, Literature, and Promotion of World Peace; first given in 1901.

Noble procedure: External plication of small bowel and mesentery to prevent episodes of obstruction in multiply recurrent bowel obstruction; mostly abandoned technique.

node of Aschoff and Tawara: See Aschoff node.

node of Rouvier: Lateral group of retropharyngeal lymph nodes.

Noguchi reagent: Solution made of 90 parts 0.9% sodium chloride and 10 parts butyric acid.

Nonne test: See Ross-Jones test.

Nonne-Milroy-Meige syndrome: See Milroy disease.

Noonan syndrome: Increased risk of schwannoma and myelodysplasia.

Norman-Wood disease: Congenital small brain, blindness, seizures, and rigidity; lethal shortly after birth. Etiology is unknown.

North American blastomycosis: Chronic granulomatous disease in skin and pleural cavity caused by dimorphic fungus *Blastomyces dermatitidis;* can mimic bronchogenic carcinoma. Disease occurs in central U.S., Canada, Central America, and Africa. Diagnosis is made by serum testing and Papanicolaou sputum smears. Treatment is itraconazole (mild-to-moderate disease) and amphotericin B (severe disease).

North Asian fever (tick typhus): Illness similar to Rocky Mountain spotted fever, with rash starting on extremities and moving centrally. Cause is *Rick-*

ettsia sibirica; disease is found in Siberia and Mongolia. Vector is tick belonging to family Ixodidae.

North Queensland fever (tick typhus): Illness similar to Rocky Mountain spotted fever. Cause is *Rickettsia australis.* Vector is tick belonging to family Ixodidae.

Norton laser endotracheal tube: Cuffless, spiral-wound, stainless steel device prone to leakage of anesthesia gases.

Norwalk agent: Viral particle of several strains that causes epidemic gastroenteritis in children and young adults; characterized by rapid onset and recovery.

Norwood operation: 1st stage (of 3) in surgical correction of hypoplastic left heart syndrome; requires deep hypothermia and bypass. Excision of interatrial septum, ligation of branch pulmonary arteries, and division of ductus arteriosus is performed. Main pulmonary artery is transected and anastomosed to underside of aortic notch, and artificial tube graft is interposed between proximal right pulmonary artery and innominate artery. It is critical to maintain adequate systemic perfusion postop and to limit pulmonary blood flow.

Nothnagel bodies: Spherical bodies 15–50 μ in diameter; sometimes appear in feces of patients who consume large amounts of meat.

Nothnagel sign: Facial muscle paralysis, esp. when attempt to move the muscle is due to emotional expression; seen in patients with tumors of thalamus.

Nothnagel syndrome (acroparesthesia): Pain, paresthesia, and numbness occurring while lying down; usu. affects dominant hand with absence of objective signs. Condition is most common in middle-aged women. Causes are multiple myeloma, amyloidosis, rheumatoid arthritis, and myxedema. Disorder is rarely idiopathic.

Nothnagel syndrome: Ipsilateral oculomotor palsy and contralateral cerebellar ataxia due to injury to superior cerebellar peduncle.

Novy-MacNeal blood agar: Medium for culture and identification of trypanosomes; contains nutrient agar with defibrinated rabbit's blood.

Nuck canal: Unobliterated processus vaginalis in females through which inguinal hernias occur; alternately described as sac-like extension of peritoneum associated with testis or round ligament in inguinal canal.

Nuel spaces (outer tunnel): Anatomic, fluid-filled cavities in organ of Corti lying between outer hair cells.

Nyhus hernia repair: Method using preperitoneal midline approach to place mesh with resulting fibrosis and obliteration of hernia space.

Nyhus classification: System used to describe inguinal hernias. Type 1, indirect with normal internal inguinal ring; type 2, indirect with dilated internal inguinal ring; type 3A, direct; type 3B, complex indirect (pantaloon/sliding); type 3C, femoral; type 4, recurrent direct.

Nylen-Bárány test: Positive finding is nystagmus when supine patient extends head 45°

over edge of examining table and turns from side-to-side.

Nyquist sampling theorem: Tenet used in spatial resolution models, which states that image should be sampled at least 2 times minimum of highest spatial frequency in original image to preserve all original information.

O'Brien block (akinesia, Nadbath-Rehman technique): Method used to anesthetize facial nerve before cataract surgery to achieve akinesia of orbicularis oculi muscle and provide better eyeball exposure; sometimes does not provide adequate blockade of lower portion of peripheral facial nerve because of injection site over orbital branch. Injection is just anterior to tragus of ear above mandibular condyle process.

O'Brien syndrome (actinic granuloma): Chronic progression of coalesced lesion formed from papular rash seen in fair-skinned patients with excessive sun exposure; usu. develops annular inflammation with thickened edge and atrophic center. Treatment is avoidance of sun

exposure and corticosteroids injected into thickened area.

O'Connor operation ("cinch" operation): Procedure used as alternative treatment in surgical correction of strabismus; involves "cinch" stitch in lateral rectus muscle that strengthens musculature and provides for adjustable alignment of globe postsurgery. Operation can lengthen rectus muscle but cannot shorten it. Procedure is useful in children because it is technically easy to perform.

O'Connor scope: Device used in arthroscopy; has 90° angle and instrument channel allowing for insertion of 3.4-mm instruments into joint.

O'Connor wiggly block: Used to test spatial ability. Block with wiggly lines, cut into 9 pieces, is disassembled, and patient is timed during reassembly.

O'Sullivan-O'Connor abdominal retractor: Ring-like retractor with self-retaining blades; used chiefly by gynecologists.

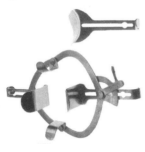

O'Sullivan-O'Connor abdominal retractor

Ober test: Used to detect contracture of iliotibial band. Patient lies in lateral decubitus position with side to be tested facing up, and lower leg is extended and upper leg is flexed at knee and abducted. If contracture is present, leg will not drop when released by examiner.

Occam razor (principle of parsimony): Concept largely synonymous with principle that explanations formulated with least number of assumptions are superior to those based on more numerous assumptions; initially conceived in Middle Ages.

Ochoa syndrome: Rare familial occurrence of congenital urinary obstruction associated with facial expression of emotion (e.g., grimacing, crying, smiling); associated with cryptorchidism (100%), neurogenic bladder, enuresis, frequent urinary tract infections, and constipation (65%).

Ochsner muscle: Variably present thickening of duodenal wall muscles just distal to common bile duct.

Ockelbo disease: See Sindbis virus.

Ockuly-Montgomery syndrome (lichenoid tuberculid): Sudden eruption of brown, nodular lesions in upper dermis on limbs; possibly similar to sarcoidosis and occasionally occurs in systemic TB.

Odland body: Keratinosome; spherical granule formed in upper layers of skin near Golgi apparatus, which migrates into cytoplasm and fuses with cell membranes to discharge acid phosphates, glycoproteins, and phospholipids.

Odland prosthesis: Type of ankle replacement.

Ogden classification: General description of fractures. Type 1, entirely through physeal plate; type 2, through provisional calcification and hypertrophic zone and into metaphysis; type 3, from articular surface through epiphysis and up to physis; type 4, from articular surface through epiphysis and physis up to metaphysis; type 5, involving germinal layer with no bony fracture; type 6, local contusion in zone of Ranvier; type 7, intraepiphyseal; type 8, involving metaphyseal growth plate.

Ogden classification:
Description of fractures of tibial tuberosity in children. Type 1a—distal fracture, slight displacement, may extend into primary ossification center; type 1b—fragments off metaphysis, variable separation from secondary ossification center; type 2a—noncomminuted fracture at ossification center; type 2b—comminuted fracture of ossification center; type 3a—disruption of articular surface under anterior attachments of medial and/or lateral meniscus, 1 displaced fragment; type 3b—type 3a with comminuted distal fragments.

Ogilvie syndrome (adynamic colonic ileus): Pseudo-obstruction and dilation of colon; underlying contributing factors can be electrolyte abnormalities and drugs. Classical treatment is mechanical decompression. New treatment is neostigmine.

Ogston line: Imaginary line between intercondylar notch and femoral tubercle.

Oguchi syndrome: Variant of night blindness with reduced visual acuity and dark adaptation fields; marked by gray to yellow fundus and thinning in pigmented epithelium of fundus. Condition is autosomal recessive and most commonly occurs in Japan.

Ohdo syndrome (blepharophimosis): Mental retardation, deafness, blepharophimosis, ptosis, and dental hypoplasia; also marked by variable scrotal hypoplasia and cryptorchidism in males.

Ohm acoustic law: Complex sounds are broken down by ear into simple harmonic components that are identical to sine wave components in Fourier analysis of complex sounds.

Okuda groups: Stages used to describe prognosis of liver cancer based on occurrence of 4 adverse criteria: bilirubin > 3 g/dl, albumin < 3 g/dl, tumor > 50% of liver volume, and presence of ascites. Stage 1, presence of 0–1 criteria; stage 2, presence of 1–2 criteria; stage 3, presence of 3–4 criteria.

Ollier approach: Surgical approach to ankle midtarsal and subtalar joints; involves incision over dorsolateral talonavicular joint, medial retraction of long extensor toe tendons, inferior retraction of peroneal tendons, and division of origin of extensor digitorum brevis muscle.

Ollier disease (enchondromatosis): Abnormal development of growth plate with defective resorption of hypertrophic cartilage and benign bone tumor; most common in ends of long bones.

Ollier layer: Innermost periosteal lamina.

Ollier retractor: Handheld device used to retract muscle and soft tissue.

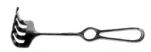

Ollier retractor

Olshausen suspension: Uterine suspension technique; involves shortening round ligament to "hitch up" uterus to undersurface of abdominal wall. Opening is made lateral to attachment site of round ligament to abdominal wall to allow round ligament to be passed through opening.

Ommaya reservoir: Device placed intrathecally through which chemotherapy can be infused to treat meningeal carcinomatosis.

Omsk fever: Hemorrhagic disease caused by tick-borne encephalitic flavivirus seen in butchers in Middle East; closely related to Kyansur Forest disease.

Onanism (coitus interruptus): Withdrawal of penis from vagina during sexual intercourse before occurrence of ejaculation.

Ondine curse: Ventilatory deterioration with frequent apneic episodes; occurs during sleep in patients with primary alveolar hypoventilation.

Onuf nucleus (Onufrowicz nucleus): Structure holding motor neuron bodies for striated external urethral and anal sphincter muscles; located at ventral horn at S1–S2.

Opitz syndrome (C-trigonocephaly syndrome): Congenital misshaped anterior skull, mental retardation, frontal cortex anomaly, short nose, short limbs, joint abnormalities, congenital heart defects, lobulated viscera, and hypotonia; auto

somal recessive condition with 50% death rate in 1st year.

Opitz syndrome: See Cauchois-Eppinger-Frugoni syndrome.

Oppel illusion (Oppel-Kundt illusion): Illusion that size of filled space seems larger than unfilled space of same size.

Oppenheim reflex: Flexion of big toe in response to downward stroking of inside of calf; seen in corticospinal tract lesions.

Oppenheim sign: Stroking ankle to determine direction of plantar response; seen in corticospinal tract lesions and used in patients who voluntarily withdraw during plantar stroking.

Oppenheim-Scholz-Morel syndrome (dysphoric angiopathia): Abnormal permeability of arteriolar walls with transudation and deposition of amyloid-type material in parenchyma, esp. occipital area; usu. detected at autopsy.

Oppenheim-Urbach syndrome (necrobiosis lipoidica): Rare onset of purple-red plaques on dorsal hands and feet with variable involvement of tongue, ears, and chest, and variable hepatomegaly. 75% of patients have coexistent diabetes, but condition develops in only 0.25% of all diabetic patients.

Orbison illusion: Illusion in which square is drawn on set of equally spaced, same-size circles. If center of square overlays center of circles, sides of square appear concave.

Oregon Polyz prosthesis: Type of ankle replacement.

Oregon prosthesis: Type of ankle replacement.

Oreopoulos-Zellerman disc: Dual-cuffed intraperitoneal dialysis catheter.

Orestes complex: Tenet in psychoanalysis that son represses desire to kill mother in outcome of Oedipus complex.

organ of Corti: Specialized hair cells that receive sound vibrations and transmit them as nerve impulses to brain; located on basilar membrane of inner ear in 2 rows sloping against one other. Cells are widest at helicotrema, where low-frequency sounds are received, and narrowest at base, where high-frequency sounds are heard.

organ of Giraldès (paradidymis): Whitish body located above head of epididymis; composed of irregularly coiled tubules with blind ends, which are probably efferent ducts that have failed to connect with each other.

organ of Rosenmüller (epoophoron): Structure comprised of series of narrow, vertical tubules lined by ciliated epithelium found in loose connective tissue in broad ligament; located in cranial part of parovarium.

organ of Zuckerkandl: Small amount of chromaffin tissue at aortic bifurcation; possible site of development of pheochromocytomas.

Oriental boil: See Aleppo boil.

Orkel syndrome (multiple epiphyseal dysplasia type 4): Ambulation deficits, ankle deformities, bowleg, and widened hip joint; possibly autosomal recessive condition. Defect occurs on chromosome 19q12. Onset occurs at 4 years of age, and retinitis pigmentosa and paraparesis develops in adolescence.

Ormond disease: Back pain, nausea, vomiting, anorexia, and constipation or diarrhea; occasionally associated with diabetes insipidus. Cause is fibrotic band constricting ureter or sometimes aorta or iliac artery. Condition is more common in men. Treatment is surgical removal of fibrous band.

Oropouche fever: Fever, rash, and meningitis; often confused with malaria. Cause is member of Simbu serologic group of bunyaviruses. Insect vector is *Culicoides paraensis.* Fever occurs only in Brazil and Trinidad.

Oroya fever: Severe anemia secondary to hemolysis, enlargement of spleen and liver, and hemorrhagic lymph nodes; 1st of 2 stages of bartonellosis. Cause is gram-negative bacteria *Bartonella.* Insect vector is sandfly. Fever occurs in Peru, Ecuador, and Colombia. Treatment is penicillin, streptomycin, chloramphenicol, and transfusion.

Orringer procedure: Transhiatal esophagectomy; uses abdominal and left neck incisions to approach esophagus. After stomach has been mobilized and esophagus bluntly dissected free from above and below and resected, stomach is pulled up through chest and anastomosed via left neck incision. Right gastroepiploic artery is only vascular supply of stomach left intact.

Orrunga treatment: Type of orbivirus transmitted by mosquitoes in Africa; causes febrile illness.

Ortner syndrome: Hoarseness, mitral stenosis, coronary artery disease, hypertension, congenital cardiac abnormalities, and left vocal cord palsy. Cause is left laryngeal nerve compression between pulmonary artery and aorta.

Ortolani sign: "Clicking" felt on flexing and externally rotating neonate's legs; positive for congenital dislocation of hip.

Orzechowski syndrome: Self-limiting onset of involuntary oscillations of eyes, postural tremulousness of body, fever, and benign-type encephalitis; usu. follows upper respiratory infection and resolves without sequelae.

Osborne wave (J wave): ECG deflection between QRS complex and ST segment caused by hypercalcemia or lowered body temperature.

Osebold-Remondini syndrome (type 6 brachydactyly): Congenital short stature, mesomelic shortening of limbs, fused hamate and capitate bones, hypoplastic middle phalanges, numbness, and bipartite calcanei; autosomal dominant inheritance.

Osgood-Schlatter disease: Osteochondrosis of tibial tuberosity.

Osler disease: Mobile gallstones in common bile duct acting in ball-valve manner; leads to recurrent episodes of colicky right upper quadrant pain, fever, and jaundice.

Osler nodes: Small, tender nodules appearing on fingers and toes; common in endocarditis and also seen in typhoid fever and collagen vascular disease.

Osler-Vaquez disease: Polycythemia vera.

Osserman classification: Description of symptoms of myasthenia gravis. Group 1, ocular symptoms only; group 2, mild generalized symptoms; group 2b, moderately severe generalized symptoms; group 3, acute fulminant onset of symptoms; group 4, late stage of disease with severe symptoms.

Ossoff-Pilling microlaryngoscope: Modification of Holinger laryngoscope; permits binocular vision. Instrument is useful in providing good exposure of anterior commissure in retrognathic patients when performing endoscopic partial laryngectomy at glottis.

Ostertag disease: Variant of familial amyloidosis with striking amount of deposition in kidneys; also with variable cirrhosis.

Ostertagia: Nematodes that are parasitic largely in herbivorous animals. 2 species are known to be transmitted to humans by eating undercooked abomasums of cattle and sheep.

Ostrum-Furst syndrome: Related to Bremer disease.

Ostwald color atlas: Addition of neutral colors ranging from black to white to each of 24 hues on color spindle; produces gradations of lightness and darkness.

Osuntokun disease: Rare association of indifference to pain and deafness.

Ota disease: Onset in childhood of bluish lesions developing on sclera, periorbital tissues; variable involvement of facial cheeks, earlobes, nose, and forehead. Occurs most commonly in Japanese.

Othello syndrome: Overwhelming jealousy and belief that spouse is unfaithful; usu. affects middle-aged men. Condition is often resistant to treatment.

Otis quick scoring mental ability tests: Series of intelligence tests designed for 3 different levels of schooling.

Otto Bock hand: Myoelectric hand prosthesis with good cosmetic results; may require additional removal of tissue from forearm stump for optimal fitting.

Otto disease: See Guérin-Stern disease.

Otto disease: Hip dislocation marked by gradual displacement of femur; unknown etiology.

Ottoson potential (electro-olfactogram): Production of negative deflection from electrode in contact with olfactory system when odorant is blown past epithelium.

Ouchterlony immuno-diffusion (double diffusion technique): Method of antigen analysis using double-diffusion, 2-D immunogel assay comparing 2 antigens. Antibodies and antigens are combined to form stable complexes, and diffusion of complexes through agar forms precipitin bands in 1 of 4 patterns.

Oudin immunodiffusion (single diffusion technique): Method for detection of antigen–antibody reactions in agar; uses single diffusion period of 2 days for antibody–antigen complex. Number of bands formed indicates minimal number of antigen–antibody systems present.

Owen lines: Interglobular spaces in dentin located in tooth crown; seen on longitudinal section.

Owren disease (parahemophilia): Congenital factor V deficiency; causes mild bleeding with PTT and PT. Treatment is fresh plasma replacement.

Ozeran technique: Surgical procedure used to repair brachioaxillary bridge fistula.

Ozzard filaria (*Mansonella ozzardi*, mansonelliasis): Non-pathogenic organism in peritoneal cavity and blood; found in persons in equatorial regions.

pacchionian bodies (arachnoid granulations): Villous type projections of subarachnoid tissue, esp. along margins of longitudinal fissure in frontal lobes; first appear in childhood and increase throughout life.

Pacinian corpuscle (lamellar corpuscle, Pacini body, Vater-Pacini corpuscle): Nerve endings in deep dermis and subcutaneous tissue that detect pressure and deep touch.

Packard-Wechsel syndrome: Chronic addisonian state.

Page syndrome (hypertensive diencephalon syndrome): Episodes of perspiration on face and chest with blotchy areas of skin and cold, mottled limbs; also with polyuria, headache, tachycardia, and GI distress. Condition affects young to middle-aged females. Histamine precipitates attack.

Paget abscess: Residual or recurring abscess due to persistence of microbes and purulent material.

Paget disease: Osteitis deformans with accelerated bone turnover; thickening, softening, and deformation of bone with late ossification. Condition is characterized by high alkaline phosphatase and 10% occurrence of sarcomatous changes. Treatment of pain symptoms is calcitonin.

Paget disease: Infiltrating ductal or intraductal carcinoma of nipple. Initial symptoms are usu. burning and itching of nipple, with eventual superficial erosion or ulceration, frequently without palpable mass (presence of mass confers better prognosis).

Paget disease: Intensely pruritic malignant neoplasm of intraepidermal portion of apocrine glands of perineum; appears as red-gray, plaque-like, crusted lesion found in vulvar and perineal area. Condition is usu. not associated with invasive malignancy. Cells stain with periodic acid–Schiff stain, unlike those in Bowen disease.

Paget-von Schrötter (Schroetter) syndrome: Primary deep vein thrombosis in subclavian or axillary veins with swelling and discomfort in arm; due to direct blow, major surgery, prolonged pressure, or excessive stretching and effort. All pulses are present.

Pagon syndrome: Congenital anemia with onset of ataxia by age 1 year; associated with increased iron levels in tissues. Condition is X-linked recessive.

Pahvant Valley fever: Tularemia.

Paine syndrome: Microcephaly, mental retardation, stunted growth, seizures, and poor swallowing. Generally, death occurs within 1st year of life, usu. from pulmonary complications. Condition is X-linked recessive.

Paine-Efron syndrome: Variant of ataxia–telangiectasia syndrome with milder symptoms and much slower progression; marked by onset in adolescence of pain in legs and lower back, slowly progressive ataxia, heavily pigmented nevi, and late onset of diffuse telangiectasia. Condition is autosomal dominant.

Pal modification: Variation of Weigert myelin sheath stain; specimen is placed in potassium bichromate solution for several weeks.

Pancoast syndrome: Weakness of muscles of arm and hand, pain, and sensory deficits seen with tumor in lung apex (usu. bronchogenic carcinoma); due to neoplastic involvement of brachial plexus and sympathetic (inferior cervical) ganglia. Condition may be seen with Horner syndrome.

Pander layer: One of pleural layers of mesoblast.

Paneth cell: Pyramid-shaped epithelial cell found in base of small intestine crypt (sometimes in colon); secretes peptidase and lysosyme.

Panner disease: Aseptic necrosis in ossific nucleus of humeral capitellum; usu. occurring in adolescence. Treatment is analgesics and splinting.

Panse flap (method): Procedure performed after exentera-

tion of middle ear. T-incision is made in concha to create skin flaps to cover bony surface.

Panum area (fusion area): Retinal area over which pinpoint-sized object can be moved and still maintain stereoscopic image with stimulus of contralateral area.

Panum phenomenon: Optical illusion produced in stereoscopic imaging. 2 identical, parallel lines are viewed with 1 eye; 3rd equal parallel line is viewed with other eye; and single line is then moved to overlap 1 of 1st 2 lines. Combined line appears closer.

Papanicolaou smear: Cytology specimens most commonly obtained from cervical exam. Most techniques involve endocervical swab, cervical scrape, or vaginal swab of posterior fornix.

Papanicolaou stain: Commonly used method of staining smears of cells from respiratory, genitourinary, and GI tracts. Smears are fixed in alcohol and ether, hydrated through graded alcohols, stained with Harris hematoxylin, and differentiated in hydrochloric acid or Meyer hematoxylin. Stain colors nuclei blue and cytoplasm orange, yellow, pink, green, and blue.

Papez-MacLean theory of emotions: Limbic system is center of emotion; stresses importance of hippocampus, amygdala, and hypothalamus in processing sensory inputs in emotional arousal.

Papillon-Lefèvre syndrome:
Hyperkeratosis of soles and palms, excessive and foul-smelling sweat production of feet, swelling and bleeding of gums with abscesses, halitosis, and eventual tooth loss; occurs early in childhood with repeating clinical course involving permanent teeth. Condition is autosomal recessive and is associated with mutations in gene coding for cathepsin C. Treatment is vitamin A, antibiotics, and dentures.

Papillon-Lége and Psaume syndrome (Gorlin syndrome, orodigitofacial syndrome): Rare congenital tremors, mental retardation, cleft palate and tongue, finger abnormalities (clinodactyly, syndactyly, brachydactyly), alopecia, and CNS abnormalities.

Pappenheim stain: Early stain for RBCs, RNA, and DNA; uses methyl green–pyronine stain technique.

Pappenheimer body: Phagosome occurring in RBCs that contains iron-bearing granules; stains basophilic with Giemsa stain and positive with Perls reaction.

Pappenheimer method: Combination of May-Grunwald and Giemsa stains used to visualize blood smears; stains nuclei purple, azurophilic granules brilliant purple, neutrophilic granules violet, eosinophilic granules red-orange, basophilic granules dark violet, basophilic cytoplasm blue, and acidophilic cytoplasm varying shades of red.

Paquin procedure: Commonly performed correction of ureteral reflux; main advantage is usefulness during complex reconstructive procedures.

Parenti-Fraccaro syndrome: [Fraccaro syndrome (type 1A), Houston-Harris syndrome (type 1B)]: Congenital dwarfism, heart malformations, cleft palate, and urogenital malformations.

parietal vein of Santorini: Vessel connecting superficial temporal veins and superior sagittal sinus; runs through parietal foramen of skull.

Parinaud disease: Tenderness and erythema at scratch site associated with conjunctivitis, parotid swelling, and anterior cervical lymphadenopathy. Infectious causes include sporotrichosis, sarcoidosis, tularemia, catscratch fever, and leptotrichosis.

Parinaud syndrome (dorsal midbrain syndrome): Loss of up-gaze, nystagmus, lid retraction, downward ocular deviation, and pseudoabducens palsy; often due to hydrocephalus from stenosis of aqueducts or pineal tumors.

Paris classification (chromosome band, nomenclature): System used to identify human autosomes; uses distinct band patterns to assign numbers (1–22) by decreasing size.

Paris green: Mixture of arsenic and cupric acetate; kills mosquitoes at larval stage.

Paris technique (intracavitary brachytherapy): Intrauterine application of radium (or cesium) for treatment of cervical cancer. Probes are left in place for 12–36 hours 2–3 times per week for several weeks; no radium probes are placed in lower cervical canal.

Parker disease: Familial occurrence of normal tone and volume of voice deteriorating into whisper in early childhood; voice becomes normal during sleep and stress. Condition is most common in Australia and occurs in isolation or with other dystonic symptoms (e.g., torticollis, tics).

Parker disease: Adrenal medullary neuroblastoma or malignancy of sympathetic chain ganglia; occurs in childhood with abdominal pain, back pain, failure to thrive, anorexia, and change in bowel habits. Condition is rapidly progressive; spontaneous regression is very rare. Treatment is chemotherapy and radiation therapy.

Parker retractor: Handheld, double-ended retractor.

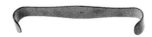

Parker retractor

Parkes-Weber syndrome: Fistula-type connections in deep venous drainage system of legs that can be demonstrated angiographically.

Parkinsonian gait: Short shuffling steps with arms flexed at elbows and wrists and decreased arm swings.

Parkinson's disease: Gradual onset in 5th and 6th decades of tremors in hands and upper limbs; occur mostly at rest with onset initially unilateral. Condition is also marked by muscle rigidity, slowed voluntary movements, myalgia, mask-like facies, short steps with shuffling gait, bent torso, cogwheel jerks, and "pill-rolling" movements of hands. Patient writes in increasingly small script, and voice loses intonation. Brain shows degeneration of substantia nigra and globus pallidus. Medical treatment includes levodopa, belladonna, benztropine, bromocriptine, pergolide, and ethopropazine. Minority of Lyme disease experts believe that infectious agent *Borrelia* may be somehow implicated in this condition.

Parkinson's facies: Mask-like facial features with infrequent blinking seen in some forms of Parkinson's disease.

Parkland formula: Estimate of fluid requirement in adults after burn injuries. In 2nd- and 3rd-degree burns, Ringer's lactate 4 ml/kg/% body surface area is given in 1st 24 hours after burn is sustained (*not* when treatment is started). Half of total fluid is given in first 8 hours and balance is given in remaining 16 hours, assuming signs of resuscitation (urine output, blood pressure) are adequate.

Parkland regimen: Treatment protocol for management of eclampsia that involves magnesium sulfate (IV loading dose and periodic IM injections) to control convulsions, IV hydralazine to lower blood pressure (if diastolic blood pressure > 110 mm Hg), avoidance of diuretics and hyperosmotic agents and IV fluids, and steps to effect prompt delivery of infant once mother is stabilized.

Parkland tubal ligation: Commonly used method of tubal sterilization.

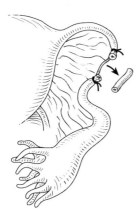

Parkland tubal ligation

Parks classification: Description of anal fistulas as intersphincteric, transsphincteric, suprasphincteric, or extrasphincteric.

Parodi device: Endovascular stent design used for treatment of aortic aneurysms outside of U.S.; Palmaz stent is sewn to each end of prosthetic graft of appropriate size, which is placed using angioplasty balloon.

Parrot disease: Infantile failure to thrive, emaciation, hypotonic muscles, listlessness, and hypothermia. Cause is multifactorial (inappropriate feeding, maternal neglect, metabolic abnormalities). Condition is reversible over several months with appropriate intervention.

Parrot nodes (sign): Bony protuberances seen in congenital syphilis.

Parrot pseudoparalysis (Bednar-Parrot disease, Wegner disease): Periarticular swelling and immobilization of involved limbs in early congenital syphilis (3 weeks–3 months of age).

Parrot sign: Ciliospinal reflex.

Parry disease: See Graves disease.

Parsonage-Turner syndrome: Sudden onset of pain followed by constant severe ache across shoulder girdle, generally accompanied by lower motor neuron paralysis with flaccidity and wasting. Etiology is unknown; condition typically occurs after injection of some kind. Pain usu. improves with onset of paralysis. Majority of patients recover completely over several years.

Partington syndrome: Low birth weight, asthma, and triangular café au lait spots developing on trunk in 1st 2 years of life; more severe in males.

parvilocular tumors of Schiller: Benign clear cell adenofibroma of ovary.

Pascal triangle: Triangular matrix that permits determination of binomial coefficients for binomial expansion without actual calculation.

Pascheff disease: Suppurative, necrotic conjunctivitis caused by *Microbacillus polymorphium necroticans*.

Pascheff disease: Coalescence of conjunctival trachoma lesions into tumor-like plaque; caused by *Chlamydia trachomatis*.

Paschen body: Cytoplasmic inclusions in cells infected with variola and vaccinia.

Pasini disease: Variant of epidermolysis bullosa with appearance of small, whitish perifollicular lesions; often first seen in lumbosacral area with progression to blistering; results in keloids after healing. Cause is derangement of glycosaminoglycan metabolism. Treatment is skin protection, antibiotics, local steroids, and phenytoin.

Passavant bar (cushion, pad, ridge): Transverse ridge on posterior pharyngeal wall seen during normal swallowing and in speech with cleft palate; due to contraction of palatopharyngeal sphincter.

Passy-Muir valve: Device with 1-way valve that fits into opening of tracheostomy tube; used to produce speech in postlaryngectomy patients.

Pastia sign: Linear petechiae on lower torso and thighs in scarlet fever.

Patau syndrome: Trisomy 13.

Patein albumin: Protein similar to serum albumin but soluble in acetic acid.

Paterson nodule: Early term for molluscum body.

Paterson-Kelly syndrome: See Plummer-Vinson syndrome.

Patey mastectomy: Modified radical mastectomy with excision of pectoralis minor muscle, allowing for more complete level 2 and 3 node dissection. Routinely sacrificed nerves include lateral pectoral and intercostobrachial nerves.

Patil frame: Stereotactic system used in brain surgery.

Patrick test (Faber test): Used to detect hip arthritis. Positive outcome occurs if supine patient places ankle to opposite knee; flexed knee is depressed; and pain, decreased range of motion, or hip spasm results. Sacroiliac pathology is likely if sudden pressure on contralateral hip or abducting flexed hip causes back pain.

Patterson test: Used to detect uremia; positive if blood spot on white filter paper turns green when drop of Ehrlich reagent is added.

Patterson-Parker technique: Peripherally weighted pattern of seed loading in radiation treatment of prostate cancer, with 60%–70% of total seed activity at edges of gland.

Pauchet procedure: Type 4 gastric ulcer removal (very proximal) using vertical extension of resection along lesser curvature that includes ulcer.

Paul-Bunnell antibodies: Heterophil antibodies (IgM) occurring in 60% of mononucleosis patients in 1st 2 weeks and up to 90% in 1st month; highly suggestive of Ebstein-Barr virus, but not pathognomonic.

Paul-Bunnell test (Monospot test): Heterophil agglutination in infectious mononucleosis; determines the most dilute serum still capable of agglutinating sheep RBCs.

Paul-Bunnell-Davidsohn test: Variation of heterophil agglutination test; used to differentiate agglutinins associated with infectious mononucleosis, antibodies against Forssman antigen, and serum sickness.

Pautrier microabscess: Focal collection of mycosis cells found in intraepidermal vesicles in T-cell lymphoma and mycosis fungoides.

Pauwels classification: System used to describe femoral neck fractures (angle of fracture line from horizontal). Type 1, 30°; type 2, 50°; type 3, 70°.

Pauwels osteotomy: Compression osteosynthesis in femoral neck fracture.

Pavlik harness: Prosthesis for infants for maintenance of leg abduction in congenital hip displacement.

Pawlik triangle: Anatomic area in vagina corresponding to trigone of bladder, with Pawlik folds as lateral borders.

Pavy test: Used to detect glucose in urine; positive if color change occurs if sample is boiled with mixture of 1000 ml H_2O, 400 ml sodium hydroxide solution, 200 ml ammonia, and 120 ml Fehling solution.

Payr pylorus clamp: Long (203–279 mm), thin clamp with pliers-type handle and longitudinal serrations on tip; used on bowel.

Payr sign: Evidence of impending thrombosis if palpation of medial foot causes tenderness.

Peabody individual achievement test: Academic achievement test used in kindergarten–12th grade in which responses require pointing only; good for use with disabled.

Peabody picture vocabulary test: Language skills test used in children 2 1/2–18 years of age with motor and speech difficulties.

Pean hemostatic forceps: Locking, ring-handle, curve- or straight-tipped forceps with long (229–305 mm) jaws; placed on vessels to control bleeding.

Pearson correlation (product moment correlation coefficient): Measure of intensity of linear association between 2 variables; assesses agreement among observers and relationship of experience when evaluating observations.'

Pearson position: Radiographic technique using bilateral frontal projection to image bilateral acromioclavicular articulations.

Peers towel clamp: Blunt-tip, nonperforating, ring-handle surgical instrument used to fasten drapes on sterile field.

Pel-Ebstein fever: Classic fever seen in lymphoma with 3–10-day febrile periods alternating with 3–10-day afebrile periods.

Pelger-Huët anomaly: Benign congenital variation in normally functioning granulocytes marked by failure of normal nuclear lobe formation during terminal differentiation, with "pince-nez" bridge between lobes and coarse nuclear chromatin clumping. Condition is autosomal dominant, with incidence of 1:6000.

Pelger-Huët pseudoanomaly (acquired Pelger-Huët anomaly): Morphologically similar granulocytes to those in Pelger-Huët anomaly that develop transiently in acute and chronic myeloproliferative diseases and with use of colchicine, alkylating agents, and sulfonamides.

Pelizaeus-Merzbacher disease (sudanophilic leukodystrophy): Ataxic disorder with seizures and dementia, with onset at 6–16 years of age. Metabolic defect is unknown. Condition is X-linked recessive.

Pelizzi syndrome: Lesion in pineal gland (e.g., teratoma, glioma, necrosis) in precocious puberty and increased growth; possibly related to mechanical pressure on pituitary and hypothalamus, causing increased gonadotropins.

Pellegrini-Stieda syndrome (Koehler-Stieda syndrome): Calcification of medial collateral ligament; marked by knee pain and stiffness and variable swelling.

Pelorus frame: Stereotactic system used in brain surgery.

Pélouse-Moore test: Used to detect glucose in urine; positive if "burnt sugar" smell develops when sample is boiled after potassium hydroxide solution is added, mixture is cooled, and 1 drop of concentrated potassium hydroxide is added.

Pemberton operation: Suspension–fixation operation for treatment of rectal prolapse; 25%–30% recurrence rate.

Pena procedure (Pena-De Vries procedure): Posterior sagittal anorectoplasty for correction of high anorectal malformations or imperforate anus; uses transsphincteric approach.

Pena-Shokeir syndrome (type 1): Congenital underdevelopment of lungs, joint contractures, global muscle atrophy, camptodactyly, and facial abnormalities; death occurs in 1st days of life due to respiratory infection.

Pena-Shokeir syndrome (type 2) [cerebro-oculofacioskeletal, COFS]: Congenital knee and elbow contractures, camptodactyly, longitudinal foot groove, scoliosis, kyphosis, and osteoporosis; possibly different degree of expression of type 1 syndrome. Condition is autosomal recessive, with death occurring by 3 years of age.

Pende sign: See André Thomas sign.

Pendred syndrome: Genetic disease with deafness or severe hearing defect developing in infancy or early childhood and goiter developing in middle childhood. Cochlea exhibits Mondini defect.

Penfield epilepsy: Onset in childhood of seizures accompanied by sweating, tearing, sialorrhea, tachycardia, hypertension, and restlessness. Cause is lesion located on floor of 3rd ventricle. Treatment is phenobarbital, carbamazepine, and surgery.

Penjdeh sore: See Aleppo boil.

pentalogy of Cantrell: Omphalocele, ectopia cordis, sternal cleft, cardiac defect, and anterior diaphragmatic defect.

Penzoldt test: Used to detect acetone; positive if blue color develops in precipitate when sample is mixed with orthonitrobenzaldehyde, then alkalinized with sodium hydroxide, and shaken with chloroform.

Penzoldt test: Used to detect glucose in urine; positive if red color develops if sample is mixed with sodium hydroxide solution and alkalinized sodium diazobenzosulfonate and shaken.

Pepper disease: See Cohen syndrome.

Pepper syndrome: Parker disease with addition of liver metastasis.

Perdrau method: Variation of Bielschowsky method for staining reticulin and collagen.

Perez reflex: Emptying of bladder, crying, and extension of head and torso elicited by holding infant in prone position and firmly tracing entire length of spine starting at sacrum and moving toward head with examiner's thumb; normally present up to 3 months of age. Absence indicates severe neuromuscular deficit.

Perez sign: Friction sound heard over sternum when arms are raised and lowered; indicates aortic aneurysm or mediastinal tumor.

Perheentupa syndrome [muscle–liver–brain–eye dwarfism (mulibrey dwarfism)]: Congenital dwarfism, thin extremities, triangular forehead, prominent neck veins, yellow spots on retina, enlarged heart and liver, and ascites. Condition is autosomal recessive and most commonly seen in Finnish persons.

Perheentupa-Visakorpi syndrome: Congenital mental retardation, difficulty feeding, nausea, vomiting, seizures, hepatosplenomegaly, hyperextensible joints, and brittle hair. Cause is defect in renal and intestinal transport of dibasic amino acids, with resulting abnormal amino nitrogen metabolism. Condition is autosomal recessive and most commonly seen in Finnish persons. Treatment is low-protein diet.

Peridiole torsiometer: Transparent overlay placed on radiographs of spine to measure rotation in scoliosis.

periodic acid–Schiff reaction: See Schiff stain.

Perkin line: Imaginary vertical line drawn on plain film through acetabular margin; used in diagnosing congenital dysplasia and dislocation of hip.

Perkoff-Slocumb syndrome: Muscle weakness with atrophy (mostly thighs) after prolonged corticosteroid administration; reverses after cessation of corticosteroids.

Perlia nucleus: Collection of cell bodies in center of oculomotor nucleus; involved in convergence abilities of eyeballs.

Perlman syndrome (Libian-Kozenitzki syndrome): Hypertrophy of Langerhans islets, bilateral kidney hamartomas, large body size at birth, fetal ascites, enlarged abdominal organs, and variable nephroblastomatosis; autosomal recessive inheritance. Death occurs in infancy.

Perls stain: Substance useful in demonstrating presence of hemosiderin.

Permount balsam: Substance used to mount histologic specimens after staining and rinsing and before coverslip is applied.

Pernio syndrome: Acute onset of chilblains on cold exposure; marked by edema, itching, blue-red discoloration, and burning pain in initial stage, which lasts approximately 1 week. Lesions become brownish for several weeks to months, and ulceration and fibrosis may develop. Cause is reaction of peripheral blood vessels to cold. Treatment is avoidance of cold and (in severe cases) nifedipine and sympathectomy.

Peroutka syndrome: Sneezing brought on by moving from dark to light environment; affects 25% of population. Condition is autosomal dominant.

Perrault syndrome: Ovarian dysgenesis, symptoms of Turner syndrome, and sensorineural deafness in females; normal development and deafness in males.

Perrin disease: Intermittent, single joint arthrosis in absence of systemic manifestations; usu. occurs in knee or occasionally ankle. Condition is most common in women, sometimes occurring synchronously with menses.

Perry syndrome: Onset of Parkinson's disease–like syndrome in 5th–6th decade with mental deterioration, insomnia, and weight loss; low serum taurine is also found. Eventual respiratory failure causes death 4–6 years after onset. Parkinson's symptoms occur late in course.

Perthes test: Method for testing patency of deep and superficial venous drainage of lower extremity; deep perforators are patent if varicose veins disappear after tourniquet is placed on involved thigh and patient ambulates.

Peter anomaly: Congenital central scarring and opacity of cornea; also with abnormality of posterior cornea and iris adhesions to cornea. Treatment is corneal transplant.

Peter Pan syndrome: High voice, pale skin, and fine hair; occurs in craniopharyngioma and other conditions.

Petersen operation: Early 20th-century surgical technique for correction of deviated septum using submucosal resection.

Petges-Cléjat syndrome: 1930s term for muscular wasting and pigmented skin areas with telangiectasia, atrophy, and calcinosis.

Petit syndrome: Irritation of sympathetic nervous system causing increased intraocular pressure, mydriasis, and abnormal retinal blood vessels.

Petit triangle hernia: Passage of intra-abdominal tissue through inferior lumbar triangle formed by latissimus dorsi, external oblique, and iliac crest; internal oblique muscle is invariably weakened.

Petragnani culture: Heat-coagulated egg, potato flour, milk, and malachite green; used to identify tubercle bacilli.

Petzetakis disease (cat-scratch fever, Debré disease, Foshay-Mollaret fever): Skin site marked by erythema, ulceration, and pustules; also with enlarged lymph nodes and fluctuant and inflamed overlying skin. Systemic symptoms are anorexia, abdominal pain, backache, chills, headache, and fever.

Originally, cause was thought to be inoculation of *Afipia felis* (gram-negative bacterium) through cat scratches and bites or penetrating splinter or thorn wounds. Diagnosis is via positive Hanger-Rose or Rice-Hyde test for *Bartonella henselae*. Disease generally resolves over several weeks to months. Antibiotics are ineffective.

Petzetakis-Takos syndrome: Superficial corneal keratitis, photophobia, blepharospasm, palpebral edema, decreased vision, and enlarged periauricular lymph nodes. Causes include insufficient vitamin A intake and poor hygiene.

Peutz-Jeghers syndrome (Hutchinson-Weber-Peutz syndrome, Touraine-Peutz syndrome): Hereditary polyposis syndrome with numerous hamartomas in stomach as well as in small and large intestine that can cause bleeding, obstruction, and intussusception; associated with characteristic pigmentation of buccal skin and also of fingers, toes, umbilical area, and forearm, which may recede at puberty. Polyps usu. occur after onset of pigment changes. Tumors of breast, ovary, uterus, and pancreas may develop; controversy exists regarding malignant potential. Condition is autosomal dominant.

Peyer patches (plaques): Aggregated nodules of lymph tissue found in mucosa and submucosa on antimesenteric border of ileum.

Peyronie disease (Buren disease): Fibrous band on dorsum of penis, which causes crooked, painful erections that interfere with sexual intercourse; lesion is common in tunica albuginea of corpora cavernosa. Condition is associated with diabetes, seizure disorder, retroperitoneal fibrosis and palmar fibromatosis, and penile trauma.

Pezzer drain: Self-retaining rubber catheter most commonly used to drain lumen of bladder or in Stamm gastrostomy.

Pfannenstiel incision: Lower abdominal wall incision widely used in obstetric and gynecologic surgery; involves transverse skin and fascia incisions with blunt dissection between rectus muscles and lateral retraction to obtain access to peritoneal cavity. Approach provides excellent cosmetic results but somewhat limited exposure and is not indicated in surgeries with known gynecologic malignancies.

Pfeiffer blood agar: Solid agar with small amount of human blood.

Pfeiffer disease: Acute infection and inflammation of cervical lymph nodes with clinical picture similar to mild infectious mononucleosis; highly contagious condition that occurs in childhood. Causes include viruses and *Toxoplasma*. Treatment of severe *Toxoplasma* infection is sulfadiazine with pyrimethamine.

Pfeiffer glandular fever: Infectious mononucleosis.

Pfeiffer syndrome: Type 5 acrocephalosyndactyly; marked by asymmetrical head due to craniosynostosis, polydactyly of digits with characteristic shortening of thumb and great toe, syndactyly of 2nd–3rd digits, wide-set eyes, and normal intelligence; autosomal dominant inheritance.

Pfeiffer type: See Noack syndrome.

Pfeiffer-Palm-Teller syndrome: Rare congenital short stature, progressive stiffness of joints, aortic stenosis, cup-shaped ears, and mask-like face.

Pfuhl sign: Increase in inspiratory flow rate in subphrenic abscess during paracentesis; decrease in rate occurs in empyema.

Phalen test: Used to diagnose carpal tunnel syndrome. Wrist is acutely flexed by examiner or (alternately) patient presses backs of hands together, forming right angles to wrists. Positive result is numbness and tingling occurring within 60 seconds in palm, index, middle, and ring fingers.

Pham sclerectomy: Procedure for treatment of glaucoma.

Phelps-Baker test: Part of hip examination given to children with cerebral palsy.

Phemister approach: Longitudinal posteromedial incision on tibial border. Used in procedures for delayed bone union.

Philadelphia chromosome: Shortened chromosome 22 (22q–) resulting from reciprocal translocation t(9;22)(q34;q11);

occurs in 90%–95% of cases of chronic myelogenous leukemia, 20% of cases of adult acute lymphocytic leukemia, and 5% of cases of pediatric acute lymphocytic leukemia. Change causes fusion of BCR gene on chromosome 22 to ABL gene on chromosome 9, disrupting proto-oncogene *c-abl* on chromosome, which encodes for tyrosine kinase ABL (part of *ras* signaling pathway).

Philadelphia cocktail: See Rivers cocktail.

Philadelphia collar: Commonly used Styrofoam neck collar for immobilizing neck; stabilizes patients in field for transport.

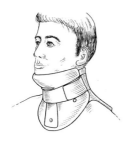

Philadelphia collar

Philip glands: Enlarged supraclavicular lymph nodes; sometimes occur in pediatric TB.

Philippine hemorrhagic fever: Hemorrhagic dengue fever.

Phillips muscle: Muscle fibers originating from radial collateral ligament and styloid process running to phalanges.

Pick body: Cytoplasmic inclusions filled with filamentous material; seen in neurons in Pick disease.

Pick disease (atrophy): Relatively rare, degenerative loss of frontal and anterior temporal neurons causing significant dementia in latter stages. Affected neurons are marked by presence of Pick bodies and assume swollen, balloon-like morphology. Initial symptoms are typically personality changes such as apathy or disregard of social decorum. Disorder is commonly misdiagnosed as Alzheimer disease.

Pick tubular adenoma (Sertoli cell tumor): Rare, benign adenoma found in testis with histopathology similar to fetal testis; can produce estrogen. Subtypes include epithelial, stromal, and stromal-epithelial.

Pickerill lines: Horizontal lines seen on surface enamel of tooth.

Pickwickian syndrome: Cyanosis, cor pulmonale, hypoventilation, polycythemia, and elevated diaphragm. Death often occurs due to pulmonary embolism. Cause is morbid obesity.

Piedmont fracture: Oblique fracture through distal radius from proximal ulnar side (in absence of ulnar fracture). Distal fragments are displaced by pronator quadratus muscle. Treatment is via open reduction.

Piehler operation (Piehler-Pluth operation): Aortic root replacement.

Pierre Robin syndrome: Treacher Collins syndrome in setting of cleft palate, micrognathia, and glossoptosis.

Pignet formula: See Black formula.

Pinard maneuver: Delivery technique in breech presentations.

Pinard sign: Indication of impending breech presentation of infant if pressure over fundus of uterus after 6th month causes sharp pain.

Pins sign: See Ewart sign.

Pinski syndrome: Mental retardation, corneal opacity, small mouth, and spastic cerebral palsy.

Pinsky-DiGeorge syndrome: Rare congenital insensitivity to pain; also with anhidrosis, mental retardation, recurrent fever, and defective lacrimation.

Piorry nucleus: Area of dullness to percussion on right posterior trunk; corresponds to area over liver.

Piotrowski sign: Exaggerated dorsal flexion and foot supination when anterior tibial muscle is percussed; seen in CNS pathology.

Pipelle instrument: Device used to obtain endometrial tissue specimens, usu. on outpatient basis.

Pipkin classification: System used to describe femoral head fracture with hip dislocation. Type 1, fracture of head caudad to fovea centralis with posterior dislocation; type 2, fracture of head cephalad to fovea centralis with posterior dislocation; type 3, type 1 or 2 fractures with additional femoral neck fracture; type 4, any of above fractures with addition of acetabular fracture.

Pippi-Salle procedure: Technique of bladder neck reconstruction most commonly used in children. Ureters are detached and reimplanted superiorly in crisscross manner, and 7×2-cm anterior vertical bladder wall flap is made with matching 7×2-cm vertical incision in trigone mucosa, with mucosal flaps raised sufficiently to suture it to mucosa of anterior flap to form cylinder. Cephalad end is then "matured" by tacking it to trigone mucosa, and anterior muscle wall is closed. If bladder enlargement is needed, portion of bowel is used to create new bladder dome.

Pirie syndrome: See Debré-Fibiger syndrome.

Pirogoff amputation (talectomy): Amputation of foot at level of ankle joint 1 cm proximal to medial malleolus, using tibiocalcaneal arthrodesis; primary indication is in children to preserve leg length and bone growth centers.

Pirquet index: Measure of nutritional status; < 0.945 is considered malnutrition.

Pirquet test: Tuberculin test in which scarification is used to administer tuberculin.

Piskacek sign: Asymmetric enlargement of cornual region of uterus in pregnancy occurring at 7–8 weeks' gestation; usu. indicates site of implantation.

Pitres sign: Scrotal numbness seen in tabes dorsalis.

Pittsburgh pneumonia agent: *Legionella micdadei;* bacterial cause of bronchopneumonia. Appearance on chest radiograph is marked by multifocal and ill-defined opacities, leading to diffuse airspace consolidations.

Planck's law: Equation $E = h\eta$, where E is quantum of energy, h is Planck's constant, and η is frequency of electromagnetic radiation in hertz.

Plimmer body: Ovoid inclusions seen in cancer cells; probably cell necrosis products.

Plugge test: Used to detect phenol; positive if odor of salicylol results and mercury is precipitated when sample is mixed with mercuric nitrate solution containing small amount of nitrous acid.

Plummer disease: Hyperfunctioning of autonomous nodule in preexisting multinoder goiter.

Plummer sign: Inability to walk up stairs or step onto chair; occurs in toxic thyroid goiter.

Plummer-Vinson syndrome: Premalignant syndrome of cervical dysphagia, upper esophageal web, spoon-shaped nails, atrophic mouth and tongue mucosa, and iron deficiency anemia; possibly related to dietary deficiency. Condition is typically seen in elderly women, most commonly in Scandinavia.

pluriformis of Retzius: Feathery lining of lateral hypoglossal eminence; represents gustatory area of cerebral cortex.

Pohl test: Used to detect presence of globulin; positive if addition of ammonium sulfate to specimen produces precipitate.

poikiloderma of Civatte (Civatte poikiloderma, Riehl syndrome): Benign pattern of hyperpigmentation and telangiectasias on neck and chest. Etiology is unknown, but condition may be related to photoallergic mechanisms, exposure to ultraviolet radiation, and menopausal hormonal alterations.

Poirier glands: Lymph nodes found on conoid ligament at upper border of thyroid gland isthmus.

Poiseuille equation: Expression that governs laminar flow of Newtonian fluids through small-diameter rigid tubes (e.g., blood flow through arteries). $Q = R^4 (P_1—P_2)/8\eta L$, where Q is flow, R is tube radius, $P_1—P_2$ is pressure drop, η is viscosity of fluid, and L is tube length.

Poisson ratio: Transverse to axial strain; dimensionless and usu. expressed as v.

Poland classification: System used to describe pediatric epiphyseal fractures. Type 1, separation across physis; type 2, separation across physis with metaphyseal fragment; type 3, separation of part of epiphysis from physis; type 4, complete separation of epiphysis from physis.

Poland syndrome: Rare non-hereditary disorder with unilaterally short 2nd–4th fingers (absence of middle phalanx), syndactyly of shortened fingers, hypoplasia of hand and forearm, absence of sternocostal head of pectoralis major on affected side, and variable absence of underlying pectoralis minor.

Poland-Moebius syndrome: Simultaneous clinical occurrence of both Poland and Moebius (Möbius) syndrome in same person. Likely cause is gene abnormality inherited in autosomal dominant fashion.

Politano-Leadbetter repair: Suprahiatal reimplantation of ureter. Intravesical ureter is mobilized, new submucosal tunnel is developed with formation of new hiatus, ureter end is spatulated and sewn into place with interrupted absorbable sutures, and old hiatus is closed.

Politzer test: Used to diagnose unilateral deafness if sound is detected in only 1 ear when vibrating tuning fork is placed in front of nose and patient swallows.

Pollacci test: Used to detect albumin in urine; positive if whitish coagulate forms when 5 g mercuric chloride, 10 g sodium chloride, and 1 g tartaric acid in 100 ml of H_2O is mixed with sample, and then 5 ml formaldehyde solution is added.

Pollitt syndrome: See Sabinas trichothiodystrophy.

Pólya operation: Type of gastrojejunostomy.

Pomeroy procedure: Method of tubal ligation.

Pomona fever: Leptospirosis; due to infection with *Leptospira interrogans* serogroup *pomona*.

Pompe disease: Defect in acid maltase metabolism leading to muscular weakness and increased glycogen deposition in heart. Infants show tongue fasciculations.

Poncet disease: Reactive polyarthritis (in absence of bacterial evidence of *Mycobacterium* in joints) in visceral or disseminated TB.

Pontiac fever: Fever, myalgia, cough, chills, headache, chest pain, confusion, and pleuritis; due to infection with *Legionella pneumophila*.

Pool-Schlesinger sign: Muscle spasm of foot and leg when thigh is flexed onto abdomen after leg extension; occurs in tetany.

Pool-Schlesinger sign: Muscle spasm of forearm, hand, and finger when extended forearm is lifted and abducted, due to tension on brachial plexus; occurs in tetany.

Popeye sign: Mass of knotted muscle halfway between elbow and shoulder; seen in biceps tendon rupture.

Porch index (communicative ability index): Test of ability to communicate using gestures, speaking, and graphs; involves 18 10-item subtests scored on 16-point scale based on accuracy, responsiveness, promptness, and completeness. Index is used to determine prognosis and therapeutic progress in left brain–damaged patients.

pores of Kahn: Microscopic openings in alveolar septum that allow direct air exchange between adjacent alveoli.

Porot-Filiu syndrome: Rare congenital seizures, bicolor iris, and variable deafness; intelligence varies from normal to mentally retarded.

Porter syndrome: Benign idiopathic pericarditis marked by chest pain radiating to shoulders that is worsened by lying flat; typically seen in young males with preceding upper respiratory infection. Treatment is rest, analgesics, and (in severe cases) steroids.

Portuguese man-of-war: Colonial marine hydroid of many specialized organisms that appear to form 1 individual; identified by iridescent float on water surface from which tentacles hang. Stings from contact with tentacles may cause severe pain, paralysis, and systemic collapse.

Posada fracture: Posterior displacement of radius and ulna, with fracture and anterior displacement of distal humerus.

postrema of Retzius: Superficial vascular structure overlying terminal end of gracilis nucleus;

associated with gustatory area of cerebral cortex.

Potain sign: Extension of dullness on right side from manubrium to 3rd costal space; sometimes seen in aortic arch dilatation.

Potain sign: High-pitched 2nd heart sound suggesting aortic arch dilatation; classically described as occurring in syphilis.

Pott disease (abscess): Infection or suppuration in spine; traditionally thought of as TB.

Pott fracture: Spiral fracture of distal fibula, avulsion of medial malleolus and ligaments, and lateral dislocation of foot.

Pott paraplegia: Clinical signs of paraplegia occurring in association with spinal TB.

Pott puffy tumor: Swelling and edema surrounding osteomyelitis of skull.

Pottenger sign: Lung or pleural inflammation, causing rigid intercostal muscles when palpated.

Pottenger sign: Increased resistance resulting from gentle palpation over solid (as opposed to hollow) organs.

Potter sequence: In utero fetal changes resulting from diminished amounts of amniotic fluid in 2nd trimester; associated with characteristic compressed facial features, limb contractures, and pulmonary hypoplasia.

Potts anastomosis: Surgical anastomosis of right pulmonary artery to right descending aorta.

Potts-Smith tissue forceps:
Commonly used tweezer-like
forceps used for grasping tissue.

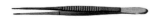

Potts-Smith tissue forceps

pouch of Douglas: Anatomic
space between rectum and bladder or uterus.

Poupart ligament: Inguinal
ligament; forms floor of inguinal
canal and runs from pubic
tubercle to anterior superior
iliac spine

Prader-Willi syndrome: Obesity, diabetes mellitus, and mental retardation; caused by break
in chromosome 15.

Praeder-Gunter syndrome:
Rare congenital lipoid hyperplasia of adrenal glands.

Prague pelvis: Spondylolisthetic pelvis; forward
displacement of 5th lumbar
vertebrae over body of sacrum.

Prasad colostomy (end-loop
colostomy): Procedure performed after segmental colectomy using GI anastomosis
stapler. Proximal end of the
colon is brought through abdominal wall, and antimesenteric end of distal colonic
staple line is then delivered
through abdominal incision.
Proximal colon is then matured
by removing suture line and
suturing bowel edges to skin,
and distal colon is then matured by removing corner staples and sewing bowel edges
to both skin and proximal
colon.

Prehn sign: Elevation of
scrotum provides relief in epi-
didymitis and orchitis but does
not improve torsional pain; used
to distinguish pain caused by epi-
didymitis or orchitis from that
caused by testicular torsion.

Preiser disease: Avascular necrosis of scaphoid bone; can occur in absence of known injury.

Present-Korelitz index: System used to describe Crohn's
disease by assessing treatment
outcomes; calculated every 3
months to determine overall
disease progression. Criteria
include use of steroids, healing
of fistulas, and amelioration of
specific signs and symptoms,
which are scored on scale of
-3 to $+3$.

Prévost sign: Deviation of
eyes toward affected hemisphere and away from affected
limbs; seen in hemiplegia.

Price-Jones curve: Frequency
distribution curve measured
by ocular micrometer; used to
plot individual diameters of
RBCs in smear.

Prieur-Trenel syndrome:
Cataracts in Sabouraud syndrome.

primitive node of Hensen:
Cranially directed invagination
of primitive groove at cephalic
end in fetus; develops into notochord.

Princeton monitor: Device
for sensing epidural pressure to
determine intracranial pressure;
uses pneumatic system, mirror,
and efferent and afferent
fiberoptic leads.

Pringle maneuver: Manual occlusion of porta hepatis to reduce blood flow to liver parenchyma; used in trauma injuries and during liver resection. Occlusion for up to 30 minutes is possible in absence of significant liver cirrhosis.

Pringle-Bourneville disease: Variant of Bourneville disease with presence of fibromas on tongue and mouth.

Prinzmetal angina: Chest pain occurring at rest and without stimulant; attacks tend to recur at same time of day. Pain correlates with ST segment elevation. Condition is most common in middle-aged women. Angina may be due to spasm of epicardial coronary arteries.

Pritchard-Walker device: Semiconstrained elbow prosthesis; used in rheumatoid arthritis.

process of Tomes: Terminal granular portion of apical end of ameloblast; formed during enamel production in developing tooth.

Prospect Hill virus: Type of hantavirus; not associated with disease in humans.

Protargol stain: Used to visualize nerve tissue; axons appear black.

Proteus syndrome: Multiple hamartomas and lipomas, macrocephaly, hyperostosis of skull, and hypertrophy of soft tissue; probable diagnosis of Joseph Merrick ("elephant man").

Proust space: Rectoprostatic space.

Prowazek body: Inclusion bodies found in pus expressed from smallpox lesions and cowpox vaccine.

Prussak space: Blind pouch off posterior malleolar recess lying between pars flaccida of tympanic membrane and malleolar neck; may fill with pus in acute otitis media.

Prussian blue (Berlin blue): Chelating agent used to treat thallium poisoning and radio-cesium poisoning; given orally via capsules over several days to weeks. Agent is not currently available for commercial use in North America.

pseudo-Babinski sign: Extension of big toe only when Babinski test is performed in poliomyelitis; due to paralysis of majority of foot muscles.

pseudo-Gaucher cell: Cell with enlarged, somewhat round, and cytoplasmic "wrinkled tissue paper" appearance similar to that of Gaucher cell; seen in thalassemia and chronic granulocytic leukemia. Accumulation of cerebroside is due to massive cell destruction and increased phagocytosis.

pseudo-Graefe sign: Lag in movement of upper lid when looking down but normal movement when looking up; occurs in Graves disease and other conditions.

Puchtler stain: Modification of Bennhold Congo red stain.

Puente disease: See Baelz disease.

Puestow procedure: Longitudinal pancreaticojejunostomy; used to relieve pain in patients with "chain of lakes" ductal anatomy.

Puretic syndrome (juvenile hyaline fibromatosis, Murray syndrome): Congenital or early childhood onset of pearly skin nodules and subcutaneous nodules with variable ulceration; associated with gingival hyperplasia. Condition leads to decreased mobility through joint contractures. Cause is abnormal glycosaminoglycan synthesis. Tumors tend to recur after resection.

Purkinje cell: Pyriform cells found in cerebellar cortex.

Purkinje fiber: Fine conduction fiber of the heart; formed from right and left bundle of His branches. Fiber runs beneath endocardium of ventricles.

Purkinje figure (shadow): Shadows thrown onto retina by oblique lighting of retinal vessels.

Purkinje system (network): Part of electrical conducting system of heart; composed of multiple Purkinje fibers.

Putnam syndrome: See Nothnagel syndrome.

Putterman-Gladstone tube: See Jones tube (modified).

Putti technique: See Abbott approach.

Putti-Platt procedure: Subscapularis and capsule imbrication; for correction of lax shoulder joint.

Puusepp reflex: Abduction of 5th toe after light stroking of lateral edge of foot; sometimes seen in extrapyramidal dysfunction.

Pyle disease: Metaphyseal dysplasia affecting mostly bones of limbs; marked by bowing deformities and metaphyseal splaying. Condition is autosomal recessive.

Quaegebeur modification: Variant of Carpentier repair of Ebstein malformation. Incompetent tricuspid valve is repaired by resecting 3/4 of large anterior leaflet and entire posterior leaflet, and remnant of anterior leaflet is then plicated to chamber wall.

Quarelli syndrome: Parkinson's disease–like symptoms following chronic exposure to carbon disulfide.

Queckenstedt test: Used to diagnose blockage of subarachnoid space above spinal puncture site and thrombosis of lateral sinus. Patient is put in recumbent position, and bilateral jugular venous compression is applied. If no pressure change occurs, thrombosis is likely present. (Lumbar manometer pressure normally rises 150 mm H_2O and falls rapidly with release.)

Queensland typhus: See Australian tick typhus.

Quelce-Salgado syndrome: See Grebe syndrome.

Quengle cast: Device applied in knee flexion contractures to effect gradual straightening of leg.

Quesada method: Radiographic positioning technique using right angle projection to view unilateral clavicle; good for imaging of comminuted fracture.

Quetelet index: Measure of body mass index; equals weight (kg)/height $(cm)^2$.

Quie-Hill syndrome: Increased serum levels of IgE, allergic rhinitis, recurrent abscesses, and eczema.

Quigley traction: Stabilization of trimalleolar and lateral malleolar fractures using overhead suspended stockinette to hold fractured ankle.

Quimby technique: Uniform pattern of seed loading in radiation treatment of prostate cancer; uses high central dose at middle of prostate with increased number of lower strength seeds.

Quincke disease (angioneurotic edema, Milton-Quincke disease): Localized pruritic swellings of skin (worse at night) and respiratory tract with distress; thought to be mediated by autonomic nervous system and emotional state. Condition is associated with nausea, vomiting, diarrhea, headache, and polyuria.

Quincke meningitis: Acute onset of aseptic meningitis.

Quincke sign (pulse): Blanching of skin at nail root when pressure is applied at tip of nail; positive for aortic regurgitation.

Quinquaud sign: Detection of trembling or worm-like sensation when fingertips touch examiner's palm after fingers are abducted, extended at interphalangeal joints, and flexed at metacarpophalangeal joints; seen in chronic alcoholism due to tremors.

Raaf catheter: Central indwelling catheter; similar to Hickman and Broviac catheters.

Rabbit syndrome: Perioral tremor caused by chronic neuroleptic administration.

Rabenhorst syndrome: Congenital narrow facies, micrognathia, malformed earlobe, ventricular septal defect, and pulmonary stenosis; unknown etiology.

Racine syndrome (premenstrual salivary syndrome): Enlargement and edema of 1 or more salivary glands 4–5 days before menses and resolving with onset.

Radovici sign: Ipsilateral facial muscle contraction caused by scratching thenar surface; seen in corticospinal tract disease, increased intracranial pressure, and latent tetany.

Raeder syndrome (cluster headache): 1–3 attacks of periorbital pain per day over several weeks, followed by pain-free interval of months; episodic type is most common. Chronic form is marked by pain attacks without pain-free interval.

Rai criteria: System used for clinical staging of chronic lymphocytic leukemia. Stage 0—lymphocytosis alone ($> 15,000/\mu l$ in peripheral blood, $> 40\%$ marrow lymphocytosis); stage I—lymphocytosis and enlarged nodes; stage II—lymphocytosis and splenomegaly and/or hepatomegaly; stage III—lymphocytosis and anemia (hemoglobin < 11 g/dl); stage IV—lymphocytosis and thrombocytopenia (platelets $< 100,000/\mu l$).

Raimiste sign: Evidence of unilateral paresis of arm; when elbow of affected arm is placed on table with examiner holding hand and forearm upright, hand flexes 130° onto forearm and exhibits flaccidity on release. Normal hands exhibit no such flexion.

Raimiste sign: Evidence of unilateral recumbent paresis of leg; when recumbent patient tries to move normal leg against resistance (either adduction or abduction), paretic leg mirrors thwarted movement.

Raji cells: Cultured lymphoblastoid cells from donor with Burkitt lymphoma; these cells express C19, C3b, C3d, and Fc of IgG receptors.

Raman spectrometer: Device used to study Raman effect of different substances; Raman signal is produced at 90° angle to direction of laser beam.

Ramirez syndrome: See Cinderella syndrome.

Ramond point: Area of tenderness on palpation between heads of sternocleidomastoid muscles; sometimes occurring in cholecystitis.

Ramond sign: Stiffness of erector spinae muscles seen in effusion and pleurisy; relaxation occurs when effusion becomes purulent.

Ramsay Hunt syndrome: Ataxic disorder with myoclonic epilepsy; autosomal recessive condition. Metabolic defect is unknown.

Ramsden eyepiece: Microscope system nearest eye; contains 2 compound lenses.

Ramsey Hunt syndrome: Ipsilateral facial paralysis secondary to herpes zoster infection in geniculate ganglion (CN VII); marked by vesicular lesions in pharynx and external ear canal. CN VIII may be involved.

Randall kidney stone forceps: Ring-handle, nonlocking forceps with slightly curved, slender shaft and open tips that are available in varying curvatures; used to grasp and remove kidney stones.

Randall plaques: Focal calcium deposits within tip of renal papillae; can project through papilla wall and act as nidus for precipitation of urinary salts.

Randolph test: Used to detect peptones in urine; positive if yellow precipitate forms when 3 drops of Millon reagent and 2 drops of saturated potassium iodide solution is added to 5 ml cold urine.

Raney alloy: Mixture with equal portions of nickel and aluminum.

Raney nickel: Nickel–aluminum–hydrogen mixture used as catalyst in hydrogenation reactions; breaks carbon–sulfur and carbon–oxygen single bonds.

Ranke complex: Calcification of healed tuberculous lesions in lung tissue and hilar lymph nodes.

Rankin hemostatic forceps: Curve-tipped, ring-handle, locking forceps; placed on vessels to control bleeding or used for tissue dissection.

Rankine thermometer: Instrument that uses Rankine scale to measure temperature.

Ranson criteria: System used to predict mortality in acute pancreatitis (following criteria vary slightly for gallstone vs. nongallstone etiology). At admission: WBC > 16,000/ml; glucose > 200 mg/dl; AST (SGOT) > 250 U/dl; age > 55 years; and LDH > 360 U/dl. At 48 hours: BUN increase > 5 mg/dl; serum calcium < 8 mg/dl; fluid deficit > 6 L; arterial Po_2 < 60 mm Hg on room air; base deficit > 4 mEq/ml; and hematocrit decrease > 10%. Presence of 1–2 criteria indicates < 1% mortality; 3–4, 15%; 5–6, 40%; and > 7, 90%–95%.

Ranvier node: Area on microscopic longitudinal section of nerve where neurolemma is seen as thin boundary of tissue pinching toward axon using hematoxylin stain; acts as short break in myelin sheath of nerve fiber.

Rapadilino syndrome: Congenital missing patellae and thumbs, stunted growth, radial hypoplasia, slender nose, and chronic diarrhea; usu. with normal intelligence.

Rappaport classification: Description of non-Hodgkin lymphoma. *I—low-grade lymphoma:* diffuse lymphocytic, well-differentiated; nodular lymphocytic, poorly differentiated; nodular mixed lymphocytic–histiocytic. *II—intermediate-grade lymphoma:* nodular histiocytic; diffuse lymphocytic, poorly differentiated; diffuse mixed lymphocytic–histiocytic; diffuse histiocytic. *III—high-grade lymphoma:* diffuse histiocytic; diffuse undifferentiated.

Rashkind balloon atrial septostomy: Procedure used to palliate transposition of great vessels. Interarterial septal defect is made by puncturing septal wall with catheter tip, inflating balloon, and pulling it back through orifice to enlarge it.

Rasin sign: See Jellinek sign.

Rassat-Moskovtchenko fistula: Dialysis fistula made by anastomosing cephalic vein to radial artery on distal wrist in "snuffbox."

Rastelli classification: System used to classify AV canal defects. Type A, none or slight bridging of left superior leaflet; type B, moderate bridging of left superior leaflet; type C, marked bridging of left superior leaflet.

Rastelli procedure: Method for repair of transposition of great vessels, pulmonary stenosis, and ventricular septal defect (VSD). Intracardiac tunnel is built, closing VSD and sending left ventricular outflow through VSD to aortic valve; palliative Blalock-Taussig shunt usu. is performed first.

Ratcliff classification: System used to describe fractures of femoral head in pediatric avascular necrosis. Type 1, involvement of entire head; type 2, segmental head involvement; type 3, fracture line runs to physis.

Rathbun syndrome: Deficiency of acid phosphatase, with wide variability in clinical presentation; see Nadler-Egan, Fraser, and Scriver syndromes.

Rathke cleft: Cleft formed from proliferation of cells during fetal development in anterior wall of Rathke pouch; may occur during childhood but regresses as adulthood approaches, leaving only few cysts.

Rathke fold: Two mesodermal folds in fetus that combine to form Douglas septum, allowing rectum to form tubular canal.

Rathke pouch: Small ectodermal diverticulum appearing in fetus at 26 days. Cells from this area produce pars anterior of hypophysis; remnants occasionally form craniopharyngiomas.

Rauber layer (primitive ectoderm): The most external of 3 layers forming embryonic disk in early embryo.

Rauchfuss triangle: See Grocco sign.

Ravelli triangle: Anatomic area in calcaneus; cysts here are well demarcated and are usu. triangular or oval.

Raven progressive matrices: Arrays used to evaluate nonverbal concept formation and intelligence in persons 6 years of age to adult.

Ray amputation: Transmetatarsal amputation.

Rayleigh law: Description of how ultrasound signal in normal tissue varies as function of frequency.

Rayleigh scattering: Pattern of sound wave reflection from particles much smaller in size than wavelength of sound (e.g., RBCs); provides physical basis behind Doppler shift used in Doppler imaging. Intensity of scattering varies with frequency to 4th power.

Rayleigh test: Method for assessment of middle and long wavelength cone function in eye. Patient is asked to match test field with wavelength of 589 nm (which appears orange-yellow) on 1 side of screen to varying mixture of color spectra (545 and 670 nm, which appear green to red) on other side.

Raymond-Foville syndrome: Variation of Brissaud-Sicard syndrome.

Raynaud disease: Intermittent spasm of small arteries and arterioles due to cold environment or emotional stress; marked by numbness, tingling, mild pain, and severe pallor of fingers, and followed by cyanosis and redness.

Raynaud phenomena: Characteristic findings of Raynaud disease occurring due to another disease process; may progress to occlusion and its sequelae, unlike the primary form of the disease.

Raz bladder neck suspension: Surgical procedure for treatment of stress urinary incontinence; has largely been replaced by pubovaginal sling procedures. Permanent helical sutures are anchored into ureteropelvic ligament, passed to retropubic space, and tied.

Réaumur thermometer: Instrument that uses Réaumur scale to measure temperature.

recess of Allison: Anatomic postcaval space bordered superiorly by right pulmonary artery, medially by superior vena cava, and inferiorly by right superior pulmonary vein.

Recklinghausen tonometer: Device used to monitor oscillatory blood pressure waveforms.

rectal column of Morgagni: Vertical folds of mucosa covering bundle of smooth muscle arranged longitudinally; found in upper anal canal.

Redlich-Fisher miliary plaques: Dark, coarse focal areas occurring in neuroglia retinaculum in brain in some cases of senile psychoses.

Reed technique: Annuloplasty for mitral incompetence that aims to leave annular circumference of 6–7 cm (mitral orifice > 2.5 cm^2). Circumference is shortened along posterior leaflet.

Reed-Sternberg cell (Dorothy Reed cell): Giant, usu. multinucleate histiocytic cell, with amphophilic cytoplasm and nucleus containing prominent nucleoli. Each cell is half mirror image of another. Presence of these cells is virtually diagnostic of Hodgkin disease.

Refsum syndrome (Kiloh-Nevin disease variant–associated retinitis pigmentosa): Ataxic disorder with retinitis pigmentosa, neuropathy, deafness, and ichthyosis; autosomal recessive condition with onset in middle childhood to adolescence. Cause is defect in phytanic acid oxidation. Screening test involves serum phytanic acid.

Rehberg test: Determination of kidney function by measuring excretion of 2 g creatinine administered in 500 ml H$_2$O.

Reichel duct: Embryologic cleft between Douglas septum and cloaca.

Reichert canal: See Hensen canal.

Reichert cartilages: Embryonic precursors of styloid processes, lesser cornua of hyoid bone, and stylohyoid liga-

ments; found on lateral sides of embryonic tympanum.

Reichl test: Used to detect protein; positive if mixture of 2 drops ferric sulfate solution, dilute sulfuric acid, and 2 drops benzaldehyde alcohol solution produces blue color.

Reid base line: Imaginary horizontal line running from lower edge of orbit through center of external auditory canal to center of occiput; used for cephalometric studies.

Reifenstein syndrome: See Gilbert-Dreyfus syndrome.

Reiger anomaly: Axenfeld anomaly in setting of iris thinning and pupil abnormality; 60% of patients develop glaucoma.

Reil triangle: Area formed by the following 3 points on axial cerebral angiogram: most anterior branch of opercular complex, most anterior part of mainstem of middle cerebral artery, and last arterial branch off opercular branch.

Reilly body: Large inclusion found in leukocytes in Hurler syndrome.

Reinke crystalloids: Normally occurring prominent cytoplasmic crystals in Leydig cells of testes and ovaries; may be interpreted as benign lesion if found in lipid cell neoplasm.

Reinke edema: Fluid accumulation causing "floppy elephant ear" in Reinke space of vocal cord; usu. associated with cigarette smoke and found in professional voice users (but not classically trained singers).

Reinke space: Superficial layer of lamina propria of vocal cords; composed of loose fibrous material and matrix and few fibroblasts.

Reinsch test: Used to detect mercury, arsenic, tellurium, antimony, some sulfur compounds, and bismuth. If copper foil is inserted into hydrochloric acid–urine solution, heated, and a gray, shiny film forms on foil, mercury is present; if gray deposit forms, arsenic or other substances are present.

Reis-Bucklers corneal dystrophy (corneal dystrophy of Bowman layer type 1, superficial variant of granular dystrophy): Rod-like opacities developing in Bowman layer and superficial stroma, resulting in significant pain, corneal erosions, and reduced vision. Condition is autosomal dominant and occurs in 1st–2nd decade. Treatment is eye drops, patching, antibiotics, and corneal transplantation.

Reisseisen muscle: Smooth muscle fibers found in smallest bronchi.

Reissner fibers: Fibers running in central canal of spinal cord.

Reissner membrane: Vestibular membrane of inner ear; forms roof of cochlear duct (scala media) and separates it from vestibular duct.

Reitan-Indiana test (aphasic screening test): Measure of word and letter deficits such as apraxia of construction and spelling, anomia, agraphia, letter and number agnosia, alexia, dysarthria, and ideokinetic apraxia.

Reiter test: Complement fixation test that detects *Treponema pallidum*.

Relton-Hall frame: Positioning frame used on operating room table for posterior approaches in spinal surgery. Device effectively decompresses abdomen but may be unstable if osteotomy is extensive. Supports of frame exert pressure on skin.

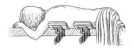

Relton-Hall frame

Renaut bodies: Pale inclusions seen in muscular dystrophy in degenerating nerve fibers.

Rendell-Baker-Soucek mask: Anesthesia face mask used in pediatric patients because of good fit around contours of cheeks and chin; also has small functional dead space.

Rendu-Osler-Weber disease: Telangiectasia and polyposis of GI tract and telangiectasia of nasopharynx and lungs; also with lesions on nailbeds and palms and increased risk of angioma. Condition is autosomal dominant.

Rennes disease: See Mason-Turner syndrome.

Rentsch press: Hand-powered piston used in external chest compression; uses baseplate positioned under patient with inverted U-shaped frame and piston connected to hand lever.

Replogle tube: Soft plastic tube with several openings at end inserted in pediatric stomach or esophageal pouches; usu. has sump apparatus.

residual body of Regnaud: Discarded organic material (lipid droplets, granules, and organelles) after tail maturation in spermatogenesis.

Rett syndrome: Ataxic disorder with autism, dementia, mental retardation, breathing dysfunction, and hand apraxia; associated with mutation in gene MECP2. Condition affects girls only, with onset in middle childhood to adolescence. Prevalence is 1 in 10,000–15,000.

Retzius cavity (prevesical space): Anatomic area between anterior bladder wall and abdominal wall; contains loose fat.

Retzius foramen: See foramen of Luschka.

Retzius veins: Vessels that run from intestinal walls to branches of inferior vena cava.

Reuss color chart: Chart with colored letters printed on different colored backgrounds; used to test color vision.

Reuss test: Used to detect atropine; positive if flowery smell (roses) is produced when specimen is mixed with oxidizing agent and sulfuric acid.

reverse Bennett fracture: Fracture/dislocation of 5th

metacarpal joint; may result in damage to deep motor branch of ulnar nerve. Subluxation is caused by traction of extensor carpi ulnaris muscle.

Revilliod sign (orbicularis sign): Evidence of hemiplegia; inability to blink eyelids on affected side without blinking eyelids on unaffected side.

Reye syndrome: Acute onset of encephalopathy, intracranial hypertension, and fatty transformation of viscera; occurs in aspirin therapy, influenza A and B, and varicella–zoster infection. Onset is usu. just as viral infection is clearing.

Reynell test: Measure of language development.

Reynold pentad: Right upper quadrant pain, fever, jaundice, mental status changes, and sepsis seen in cholangitis.

Reynolds number: Dimensionless number used to determine if flow of gas or fluid is laminar or turbulent ($Re > 2000$ for vascular system or airway). Equation: $Re = \rho DV/\eta$, where ρ is density of substance, D is diameter of tube, V is average linear velocity, and η is viscosity.

Reynolds test: Used to detect acetone; positive if black color develops when freshly prepared mercuric oxide is added to specimen and shaken and then ammonium sulfide is added.

Rezaian device: Anterior thoracic and lumbar spinal fixation device, which acts like interbody distractor with forces imparted by cellar-jack mechanism; relatively bulky, leaves little room for graft material and interferes with CT and MRI images.

Rhode Island dissectors: Small (9.5 × 38 mm), cylindrical, radiographically detectable cotton sponges used in surgery; usu. held at tip of forceps to apply blunt but gentle pressure on tissues during dissection.

Rhodesian fever: See African tick fever.

Rhodesian sleeping sickness (East African trypanosomiasis, trypanosomiasis): More severe, acute, fatal form of African sleeping sickness.

ribbon of Reil: Rostral part of medial lemniscus.

Ribes ganglion: Variably present collection of nerve cell bodies occurring close to anterior communicating artery of brain.

Rice-Hyde test: Used to diagnose catscratch disease (Petzetakis disease); involves incubation of catscratch disease antigen with WBCs.

Rich syndrome: See Lohlein syndrome.

Richardson retractor: Handheld retractor for soft tissue.

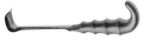

Ring-grip handle

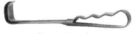

Standard handle

Richardson retractor

Richardson-Eastman retractor: Handheld, double-ended retractor for soft tissue.

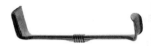

Richardson-Eastman retractor

Riches diathermy forceps: Typically used for blunt dissection in urologic procedures.

Richet aneurysm: Fusiform-type aneurysm.

Richmond bolt: Intracranial device (placed at bedside); used to measure intracranial pressure in fulminant hepatic failure and other conditions.

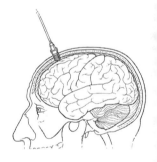

Richmond bolt

Richner-Hanhart syndrome: Type 2 tyrosinemia.

Richter hernia: Passage of antimesenteric surface of intestine within hernial sac that can manifest as partial intestinal obstruction; most commonly seen in association with femoral or inguinal hernias.

Richter syndrome (transformation): Transformation of chronic lymphocytic leukemia to diffuse large cell lymphoma; occurs in 3% of cases. Subsequent course is rapidly progressive.

Richter-Lortolary syndrome: Rare variant of Richter syndrome characterized by spontaneous regression of lymphocytosis.

Richter-Monro line: See Monro line.

Rickham reservoir: Shunt system reservoir designed for use with straight ventricular catheter; allows for CSF collection or injection of substances but cannot be flushed.

Ridley sinus: Venous plexus encircling hypophysis; formed by connections between anterior and posterior intercavernous sinuses and 2 cavernous sinuses.

Ridley syndrome: Dyspnea associated with heart failure.

Riechert frame: Stereotactic frame used in brain surgery.

Riedel lobe: Normal anatomic variation of elongated right lobe of liver, which is sometimes palpable; can be mistaken for tumor or enlarged liver.

Riedel thyroiditis (disease, struma, syndrome): Rare chronic inflammation and fibrosis of thyroid associated with hypothyroidism and tracheal compression.

Rieger anomaly: Stromal atrophy of iris occurring with Axenfeld anomaly (fat atrophy of torso and extremities); autosomal dominant condition. Glaucoma develops in 50% of cases.

Rieger syndrome: Rieger anomaly in setting of dental and skeletal defects.

Riegler test: Used to detect albumin in urine; positive if turbidity develops after 5 ml of specimen is mixed with 25 drops of 10 g beta naphthol-sulfonic acid dissolved in 200 ml H_2O.

Riegler test: Used to detect hydrochloric acid in stomach juice; positive if blue color develops when Congo red is added to sample.

Riegler test: Used to detect glucose in urine; positive if red color develops when 0.25 g sodium acetate and 0.1 g phenylhydrazine are mixed with 20 drops of specimen and boiled, and 10 ml 3% potassium hydroxide is added and entire mixture is shaken.

Riehl syndrome: See poikiloderma of Civatte.

Riesman sign: Bruit detectable via auscultation over closed eye in Graves disease.

Riesman sign: Spongy quality to eyeball under light palpation; occurs in diabetic coma.

Rieux hernia: Rare entrapment of tissue posterior to cecum.

Rift Valley fever (enzootic hepatitis): Acute onset of fever, extremity pain, and GI distress.

Cause is bunyavirus, which is mostly pathogenic in domestic animals in Africa and Middle East but can secondarily infect humans, occasionally resulting in death.

Rigler sign: Posterior projection of left ventricular contour to inferior vena cava on lateral chest radiograph caused by dilatation; occurs in isolated left atrial enlargement (mitral valve stenosis, left atrial myxoma).

Riley-Day syndrome (familial dysautonomia): Dysfunction in autonomic nervous system with hyperhidrosis, postural hypotension, and poor body temperature regulation; autosomal recessive condition seen largely in Ashkenazi Jews.

Rindfleisch fold: Pericardial folds at aortic root.

Ring prosthesis: Type of knee replacement with maximum freedom of motion of joint; requires good soft tissue stability.

Ringer lactate: See lactated Ringer's solution.

Ringertz classification: Description of primary CNS tumors.

Rinne test: Used to detects hearing loss from conduction defects. Vibrating tuning forks (256, 512, and 1024 Hz) are placed next to ear canal and then on mastoid bone. Deficit is present if sound is louder when tuning fork is on mastoid.

Riolan muscle: Cremaster muscle, which elevates testes; arises from inferior internal oblique muscle, inserts on pubic tubercle, and receives innervation from genital branch of genitofemoral nerve.

Riolan muscle: Skeletal ciliary muscle that lies close to hair follicles of eyelashes and tarsal glands; forms part of orbicularis oculi.

Riolan nosegay: Muscles originating from styloid of temporal bone.

Ripault sign: Permanent deformity in roundness of eyeball caused by palpation after death. (Palpation during life causes transient change in roundness.)

Ripstein procedure: Method used to correct rectal prolapse; based on belief that cause is intussusception of abnormally straight rectum resulting from downward forces of defecation, not pelvic floor weakness or enlarged peritoneal sac. In current modification, rectum is mobilized up to pelvic floor and down to tip of coccyx (requires opening lateral peritoneal folds), and 5-cm T-shaped Teflon or Marlex mesh is placed on posterior rectum with "arms" sutured anteriorly. Recurrence rate is 2%–16%.

Riseborough-Radin classification: System used to describe radiographic findings in distal humeral intercondylar "T" fractures. Type 1, nondisplaced fracture between capitellum and trochlea; type 2, nondisplaced "Y" or "T" fracture; type 3, separation with rotational condylar displacement; type 4, significant condylar separation with comminuted articular surface.

Risquez sign: Presence of free spirochetes in serum; seen in malaria.

Risser sign: Radiographic evidence of ossification and fusion of iliac apophysis; sign of skeletal maturity. Little progression in spine curvature occurs in scoliosis after sign appears.

Ritgen maneuver: Palm of physician's hand is placed on newborn occiput to control delivery of head, and other hand is used to exert forward pressure on chin (through perineum), which extends neck of infant; used in vertex deliveries.

Ritter-Rollet phenomenon: Increased reactivity of muscles, resulting in abduction and flexion over muscles that cause adduction and extension; elicited by electrical stimulation of motor nerve trunk of different muscle groups.

Rivalta disease: Cervicofacial actinomycosis.

Rivalta reaction (Moritz reaction): Use of acetic acid to determine if fluid is transudate or exudate.

Rivers cocktail (Philadelphia cocktail): Treatment for acute alcohol poisoning; consists of IV infusion of dextrose, insulin, and thiamine mixed in normal saline solution.

Riviere sign: Change in percussion tone during palpation over T5–T7 spinous processes in lung TB.

Rivinus duct: Minor sublingual ducts (5–15 in number).

Rivinus gland: Smallest of 3 main salivary glands located on each side of mouth; drain mucus through 10–30 sublingual ducts.

Rivinus notch (incisura tympanica, Rivinus foramen): Notch in upper part of tympanic ring (lying between greater and lesser tympanic spines of temporal bone) that is covered by flaccid part of tympanic membrane.

Robb-Persson operation: Below-knee amputation of leg using sagittal cut.

Robert formula (modified): Combination of marshmallow root, wild indigo, purple cornflower (*Echinacea*), geranium, goldenseal, poke root, comfrey, slippery elm, pancreatin, cabbage powder, and niacinamide; used for treatment of inflammatory bowel disease.

Robert ligament: Posterior meniscofemoral ligament; runs from posterior lateral meniscus superiorly and medially (behind posterior cruciate ligament) to medial femoral condyle.

Robert pelvis: Abnormal pelvic skeleton secondary to absence of alar bones of sacrum; causes smaller transverse distance.

Roberts test: Used to detect albumin in urine; positive if white film occurs at meniscus between sample and mixture of 1 part nitric acid and 5 parts saturated sulfate solution.

Robertson sign: Reddish maculopapules on arms seen in cardiac failure.

Robertson sign: Fibrillation of chest wall and left pectoralis muscle seen in impending death from cardiac failure.

Robertson sign: Palpation over truly painful area that produces pupil dilation; used to detect malingering. Absence of dilation indicates false complaint.

Robertson sign: Fullness and tension in flanks of supine patient with abdominal ascites.

Robertsonian translocation: Chromosome translocation involving any of acrocentric chromosomes (13, 14, 15, 21, and 22).

Robinson catheter: Straight, rubber catheter with hole at distal tip.

Robson grading system: Widely used modification of Flocks-Kadesky staging system to describe renal cell carcinoma. Stage 1, confined to parenchyma; stage 2, involvement of perinephric fat and/or adrenal but still confined to Gerota fascia; stage 3a, involvement of main renal vein or vena cava but no spread to regional lymph nodes; stage 3b, involvement of regional lymph nodes but no involvement of venous structures; stage 3c, involvement of regional lymph nodes and venous structures; stage 4a, involvement of adjacent organs; stage 4b, distant metastases.

Robson line: Imaginary line from umbilicus to nipple.

Rocher-Sheldon disease: See Guérin-Stern disease.

Rochester-Carmalt hemostatic forceps: Long (165–203 mm), curve-tipped, ring-handle, locking forceps; placed on vessels to control bleeding or used for tissue dissection.

Rochester-Ochsner hemostatic forceps: Long (159–254 mm,) curve- or straight-tipped, ring-handle, locking forceps; tips have 1×2 teeth. Forceps are placed on vessels to control bleeding or onto tissues to aid retraction.

Rochester-Pean hemostatic forceps: Curve- or straight-tipped, ring-handle, locking forceps; placed on vessels to control bleeding or used for tissue dissection.

Rochon-Duvigneaud syndrome: Anesthesia of upper lid and forehead, ptosis, fixed and dilated pupils, and decreased sensation in trigeminal area. Causes include tumor protruding from nose into orbit (Dejan syndrome), tumor protruding from pterygopalatine into orbit, CNS infection, or fracture of zygoma.

Rockey-Davis incision: Transverse skin incision in right lower quadrant with muscle splitting technique used in appendectomy.

Rockwell scale: Arbitrary scale measuring hardness of material by resistance to indentation from steel ball pressed on material of known force.

Rocky Mountain spotted fever: Acute infectious disease found throughout North and South America. Causative agent is *Rickettsia rickettsii*. Vector is *Dermacentor* and other ixodid ticks.

Roeder towel clamp: Sharp-tipped, perforating, ring-handle surgical instrument used to fasten drapes on sterile field. Ball stops on each tip prevent clamp from being applied too deeply.

Roenheld syndrome: Postprandial chest pain and palpitations. ECG shows sinus tachycardia, ST depression, and sometimes bradycardia 30 minutes after eating.

Roger syndrome: Small ventricular septal defect; has varying degrees of associated pulmonic stenosis and cyanosis.

Roger-Anderson external fixation: Orthopedic device used for severe proximal tibia–fibula fractures.

Rogers syndrome: Thiamine-responsive megaloblastic anemia, diabetes, situs inversus, and sensorineural deafness; autosomal recessive condition. Cause is decreased α-ketoglutarate dehydrogenase activity. Treatment is thiamine (does not correct diabetes).

Röhrer index: Measure of nutritional status; equals weight (g) $\times$ 100/height (cm)^3.

Rokitansky disease: See Budd-Chiari syndrome.

Rokitansky pelvis: Spondylolisthetic pelvis.

Rokitansky tubercle: Nodule located on inside wall of mature cystic teratoma which extends into cavity; site of attachment of hair strands. Structure can be seen when contents of cyst are evacuated.

Rokitansky-Aschoff sinuses: Buried crypts of mucosa or diverticula extending into gallbladder wall; seen in adenomyomatous hyperplasia.

Rokitansky-Cushing ulcer: See Cushing ulcer.

Rolandic area: See Brodmann area 4.

Rolando angle: Angle formed by central sulcus (Rolando fissure) and superomedial border of the cerebral hemisphere. Normal valve is 72°.

Rolando fibers: External arcuate tissue of medulla.

Rolando fissure: Central sulcus of brain running transversely on each side of cerebral hemispheres.

Rolando fracture (T-condylar fracture): Thumb fracture similar to Bennett fracture with additional fracture line at dorsal base to which abductor pollicus longus attaches.

Rolando line: Imaginary line on scalp corresponding to Rolando fissure beneath it.

Rolando tubercle: Oblong end of upper posterior area of lateral funiculus of medulla.

Rolando zone: See Brodmann area 4.

Roller central nucleus: One of nuclei found in medulla; located near raphe and between lemniscus and posterior longitudinal fasciculus.

Roller nucleus: Group of cells located around hilum of olivary nucleus.

Romano-Ward syndrome: Hereditary long QT syndrome; autosomal dominant condition.

Romanovsky stain: Used to demonstrate presence of elastin.

Romberg disease: Facial hemiatrophy with onset in 1st or 2nd decade; usu. manifests as alopecia and blanching unilaterally on scalp and face, with atrophy of subcutaneous tissue. Condition is associated with epilepsy, migraine, and brain calcification referable to involved side. Symptoms extend bilaterally in 5% of cases and occasionally involve limbs, trunk, and intra-abdominal organs.

Romberg test (sign): Used to detect cerebellar ataxia, tabes dorsalis, or labyrinthine damage; performed by having patient stand motionless with feet together and eyes closed. Positive if balance is maintained with eyes open but lost with eyes closed.

Romberg-Howship sign: Pain radiating down medial leg from thigh to knee secondary to obturator nerve compression; seen with obturator hernia.

Romberg-Wood syndrome (primary pulmonary hypertension): Syncope, angina, dyspnea, and fatigue; associated with Marfan angiitis and Raynaud phenomena. Female-to-male ratio is 5:1. Onset is infancy to old age. Death occurs 4–5 years after onset of symptoms.

Rome diagnostic criteria: Description of chronic abdominal pain and irritable bowel syndrome. Type 1—frequent or continuous for minimum 6 months; type 2—inconstant relationship with eating, defecation, or menses; type 3—activities of daily living impaired; type 4—no discernible organic etiology.

Roos test: Used to diagnose thoracic outlet syndrome. Patient sits with arm abducted to 90° and elbows flexed to 90° with shoulders braced. If patient is able to flex hands repeatedly for 3 minutes without symptoms, thoracic outlet obstruction is ruled out.

Rose-Bradford kidney: Inflamed, fibrotic kidney seen in children.

Rosemberg-Lohr syndrome: Thickening of wrist bones, coxa valga, wedged vertebrae, and thickened sella turcica; autosomal dominant condition.

Rosenbach disease: See Heberden nodes.

Rosenbaum screen (Jaeger chart): Series of reading cards shown to patient to evaluate near-distance acuity.

Rosenberg-Chutorian syndrome: See Iwashita syndrome.

Rosenfeld system: Notational description of Rh-antigen blood group.

Rosenmüller gland (node): Lacrimal gland jutting into upper eyelid.

Rosenmüller nodes: Deep inguinal lymph nodes located along femoral vein; drain into external iliac lymph nodes and collect lymph from genital area and deep tissues of leg.

Rosenthal fibers (bodies): Distinctive structures seen in juvenile pilocytic astrocytomas of optic nerve; represent areas of degeneration within astrocytic processes.

Rosenthal vein (basal vein): Vessel that originates at anterior perforated substance, runs backward and around cerebral peduncle, and drains into internal cerebral vein.

Roser-Nélaton line: See Nélaton line.

Rosetti-Hall modification: See Nissan-Rosetti procedure.

Ross bodies: Ameboid, spherical bodies in blood and fluids in syphilis.

Ross river virus: Type A arbovirus causing fever, rash, and arthralgias.

Ross-Jones test (Nonne test): Used to detect increased globulin levels in CSF. Test is positive if whitish precipitate forms when 1 ml of CSF is placed on top of 2 ml of ammonium sulfate.

Rosselli-Gulienetti syndrome: Unilateral or bilateral congenital malformation (usu. lobster-claw) of hands and feet and variable cleft palate and ectodermal dysplasia.

Rossi syndrome: See Guérin-Stern disease.

Rossolimo reflex: Reaction is performed by having patient lying supine and having foot extended and elicited by percussing ball of foot or plantar surface of big toe, stroking balls of toes, or snapping tips of toes; positive if plantar flexion of toes occurs. Reflex is seen in corticospinal tract lesions.

Roth spots: Round white spots accompanied sometimes by areas of surrounding hemorrhage; seen in retina of some patients with subacute bacterial endocarditis.

Roth syndrome: See Bernhardt-Roth sign.

Roth-Bielschowsky syndrome (pseudo-ophthalmoplegia): Paralysis of conjugate movement of eyes with vertical movements particularly affected; due to lesion in basal ganglia or tectum.

Rothman-Makai syndrome: Self-limiting condition marked by subcutaneous nodules up to 15 cm in size on front of thighs and sometimes on face and trunk; no associated systemic symptoms. Etiology is unknown.

Rothmund-Thomson syndrome (Bloch-Stauffer syndrome): Atrophy and brownish pigmentation of skin appearing on limbs, face, ears, and buttocks, with variable mental and sexual growth retardation. Female-to-male ratio is 3:1. Patients present in 1st 3–6 months after birth, and 50% develop cataracts by 4–6 years of age.

Rotor syndrome: Rare genetic disorder marked by impaired excretion by hepatocytes; autosomal recessive inheritance. Condition causes mild conjugated hyperbilirubinemia and abnormal urinary coproporphyrin excretion.

Rotter nodes: Nodes draining to level 2 central lymph nodes located behind pectoralis minor.

Rouget muscle: Circular fibers of ciliary muscle.

Rougnon-Heberden disease: See Heberden asthma.

Rouhier technique: Proximal elongation technique for superficial flexor tendons of 1st–4th fingers.

Rous virus: RNA retrovirus that causes sarcomas in chickens.

Roussy-Lévy disease: Ataxic disorder also marked by neuropathy and tremor; autosomal dominant condition. Metabolic defect is unknown. Age of onset is 6–16 years.

Roux sign: Positive for lateral pelvic fracture if there is ipsilateral widening between greater trochanter and pubic spine.

Roux syndrome: Early phase is marked by severe gastropare-

sis after subtotal gastrectomy with Roux-en-Y reconstruction. Chronic phase is marked by abdominal pain and intermittent vomiting.

Roux-en-Y procedure (anastomosis): Type of bowel anastomosis that can be used in esophago-, gastro-, hepatic, or pancreatic jejunostomy.

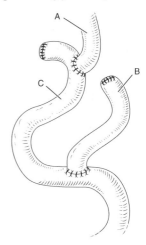

A. Esophagus
B. Closed duodenum
C. Roux-en-Y limb of jejunum

Roux-en-Y procedure

Rovsing sign: Abdominal pain in right lower quadrant on palpation in left lower quadrant; highly suggestive of appendicitis.

Rowe elimination diet: Series of 4 diets used to test for food allergy. Patients are placed on each diet for 1 week and observed for relief of symptoms. 1st 3 diets involve different combination of meats, fruits, vegetables, starches, and condiments. 4th diet is milk, tapioca, and sugar.

Rowley-Rosenberg syndrome (Busby syndrome): Growth retardation starting at 1 year of age, with motor delays, waddling gait, chronic respiratory infection, loss of subcutaneous fat, cardiomegaly, and aminoaciduria; familial recessive condition. Etiology is unknown. Death occurs by 12 years of age with full-blown syndrome.

Royer syndrome: Diabetes mellitus in association with Prader-Willi syndrome.

Royer-Wilson syndrome: Association of absent pulmonary valve and ventricular septal defect.

Rozycki syndrome: Congenital dwarfism, deafness, muscle wasting, vitiligo, and achalasia.

Rubinstein-Taybi syndrome: Mental retardation, dwarfism, underdeveloped maxilla, flattened thumbs and toes, and cardiac abnormalities, esp. patent ductus arteriosus.

Rud syndrome: Dwarfism, mental retardation, and erythroderma ichthyosiform.

Rüedi-Allgöwer classification: System used to describe subtypes of Mast-Spiegel-Pappas type 3 fracture.

Ruediger syndrome: Extremely rare congenital urethral stenosis, hypoplastic distal limbs, coarse facies, and bifid uvula. Death occurs by 1 year of age.

Ruffini endings: Nerve fibers in subcutaneous tissues that modulate warmth sensitivity.

Ruiter-Pompen disease: See Fabry disease.

Rukavinas syndrome (Indiana-type amyloidosis neuropathy, Maryland-type amyloidosis neuropathy): Peripheral neuropathy occurring in amyloidosis; associated with eye opacities, causing visual loss and scleroderma-type changes in arms and hands. Clinical picture resembles carpal tunnel syndrome with median nerve sensory deficits.

Rumel tourniquet: Commonly used technique of fastening surgical instruments in place on the operating field; involves umbilical tape encircling structure or instrument that is threaded through short piece of rubber tubing and then snugged down with hemostat to effect tightening.

Rummo syndrome: Cardioptosis.

Runge disease: See Ballantyne disease.

Runyon classification: Group 3 nonphotochromogenic microorganisms (e.g., *Mycobacterium intracellulare*).

Runyon group: 1 of 4 categories of non–TB-causing *Mycobacteria;* differentiated on basis of growth rate and pigmentation.

Russe approach (Herbert approach): Surgical approach to wrist used for exposure of scaphoid, flexor pollicus longus, and radial digital flexors. Longitudinal incision is made between radial artery and flexor carpi radialis tendon, extending onto thumb metacarpal area. Superficial branch of radial artery is ligated, and longitudinal incision is made through capsule, exposing above structures.

Russell body (fuchsin body): Plasma cell inclusions filled with surface gamma globulins.

Russell dwarf (Silver dwarf): Short stature associated with Silver-Russell syndrome.

Russell traction: Method of stabilizing hip fractures in elderly and femoral fractures in young; used to stabilize temporarily or occasionally applied for 12 weeks in nonoperative treatment. Rope and pulleys form sling to support distal thigh, and 10–15 lb of weight is used with leg in minimal flexion.

Russell viper venom clotting time (test): Coagulation test used to detect antiphospholipid antibodies (lupus anticoagulants); involves Russell viper venom extracted from pit viper. 70% of protein of venom is phospholipase A2, which activates factor X if phospholipid is present. Normal value is 24–37 seconds. Blood must be drawn in blue-topped tube.

Russell-Rees syndrome: See Carney complex.

Russell-Silver syndrome: See Partington syndrome.

Russell-Taylor nail: Type of interlocking nail, which can be placed in retrograde or antegrade manner in medullary of humerus; allows fixation of most humeral shaft fractures.

Russian forceps: Commonly used tweezer-like forceps with rounded, toothed ends for grasping fascia.

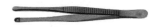

Russian forceps

Rust phenomenon: Supporting of head with hands when moving from standing to prone position or vice versa; seen in cervical bone cancer or destruction.

Rutland syndrome: Persistent respiratory problems from birth. Cause is abnormality in ciliary function (random orientation vs. parallel orientation found normally).

Rutledge classification: System used to describe extended hysterectomy. Class 1, extrafascial hysterectomy only; class 2, resection of upper 1/3 of vagina and medial 1/2 of uterosacral and cardinal ligaments; class 3, resection of upper 1/3 of vagina and entire uterosacral and cardinal ligaments (for stage 1b and 2a lesions); class 4, resection of upper 3/4 of vagina, tissue surrounding ureters, and superior vesical artery; class 5, resection of bladder and distal ureter.

Ruvalcaba syndrome
(Hunter syndrome, Sugio-Kajii
syndrome): Rare congenital mental retardation, microcephaly,
micrognathia, crooked teeth,
white forelock, pectus carinatum, kyphoscoliosis, inguinal
hernias, abnormal penile skin,
and intestinal polyps; autosomal
dominant condition.

**Ruvalcaba-Myhre-Smith
syndrome:** See Bannayan
syndrome.

Ruysch muscle: Muscular
fibers located in fundus of uterus.

Ruysch veins (posterior ciliary
veins): 4 veins that traverse
sclera and drain blood from choroid to superior ophthalmic vein.

Rye classification: Grouping
of Hodgkin disease into 4 histologic subtypes: nodular sclerosis
(40%–80%), mixed cellularity
(20%–40%), lymphocyte predominant (2%–10%), and lymphocyte
depleted (2%–15%).

Sabin vaccine: Oral vaccine
for poliomyelitis; now replaced
by IV vaccine. 3 antigenically
different live attenuated strains
grow in GI tract and cause both
local and systemic production
of antibodies. Chance of developing full-blown disease is
minute.

**Sabinas trichothiodystro-
phy** (hair-brain syndrome, Pollitt syndrome): Familial mild
mental retardation, brittle hair
and nails, and decreased fertility; autosomal recessive inheritance.

Sabolich prosthesis: Knee-
and-ankle prosthesis (weight:
~ 500 g); used with excellent

results in both above- and
below-knee amputations in
active patients.

Sabouraud agar (French
proof agar): Standard, widely
used culture medium for fungi;
contains glucose and peptone
agar at pH of 5.6.

**Sabouraud agar (Emmons
modification):** Culture medium for fungi; contains dextrose
and antibiotics.

Sachsalber disease: Hemihypertrophy of face, skull, and
internal skull structures, including foramens; more frequent on
left side. Condition is also associated with unilateral exophthalmos, vision defects, glaucoma,

and neurofibromatosis-type lesions in ipsilateral eyelid.

Sachse ureterotome: Instrument used for direct vision when performing internal urethrotomy; inserted into bladder via urethra with patient under sedation.

Sack trait: See Ehlers-Danlos syndrome type 4.

Saemlisch ulcer (pneumococcus ulcer): Suppurative ulcer found in center of cornea; cause is pneumococcus infection.

Saemlisch ulcer (Saenger macula): Inflamed, erythematous Bartholin duct opening in vulvar gonorrhea.

Saenger macula: See Saemlisch ulcer.

Saethre-Chotzen syndrome: Type 3 acrocephalosyndactyly, with congenital mental retardation, asymmetrical skull, syndactyly of 2nd and 3rd or 4th and 5th toes or fingers, convulsions, stunted growth, radioulnar synostoses, and renal anomalies. Condition is autosomal dominant, with variable penetrance and expression.

Sager splint: Splint used for traction of femoral fractures; allows stabilization while avoiding sciatica nerve pressure.

Sahlgren test: Test of color vision; detects saturation discrimination by varying grayness of visual field.

Saigon cassia: Cinnamon.

Saint Anne–Mayo system (SAMS): Classical histologic grading system for gliomas.

Grades 1 and 2 are considered low-grade; grades 3 and 4 are considered high-grade.

Saint Anthony fire: Term used in Middle Ages for ergotism caused by eating rye and other grains infested with fungus *Claviceps purpura;* marked by nausea, vomiting, confusion, coma, seizures, and extremity gangrene.

Saint Georg-Buckholz prosthesis: Type of ankle replacement.

Saint Jude valve: Artificial heart valve.

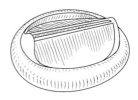

Saint Jude valve

Saint Louis encephalitis: Brain inflammation that occurs throughout U.S. Vector is *Culex* mosquito; animal hosts are horses and birds.

Saint triad: Diverticular disease, hiatal hernia, and cholelithiasis.

Saint Vitus dance: Parapsychiatric phenomenon occurring in Middle Ages; involved people who gathered near churches and sang and danced for long periods, sometimes with convulsions and loss of consciousness. Behavior is now thought to be emotional hysteria of Sydenham chorea.

Sakati-Nyhan syndrome: Acrocephalosyndactyly type 3; marked by hypoplastic tibia and abnormal fibula.

Salamon syndrome: Scant wooly hair, prominent ears, and everted lower lip.

Saldino-Mainzler syndrome: Leber congenital amaurosis in association with diffuse renal tubular atrophy and fibrosis and cone-shaped epiphyses of hands and feet (esp. middle phalanges); autosomal recessive condition.

Salgado-Quelce syndrome: See Grebe syndrome.

Salk vaccine: Inactivated IM poliovirus vaccine.

Salle procedure (Pippi Salle procedure): Bladder neck reconstruction and urethral lengthening using anterior bladder wall flap; corrects urinary incontinence in children with neurogenic bladder or bladder exstrophy.

Salleras-Ortiz disease: X-linked external ophthalmoplegia and myopia.

Salpêtrière school: Body of teachings on hysteria and 3 stages of hypnosis promulgated by Jean-Martin Charcot from La Salpêtrière psychiatric hospital; mostly superseded by later research.

Salter sling: Mechanical support used in treatment of Legg-Calvé-Perthes disease; abducts and internally rotates hip while knee is flexed.

Salzmann syndrome: Nodular corneal degeneration; forms gray opacities secondary to inflammation.

Sampaoelesi line: Line of pigment on corneal endothelium; anterior to or on Schwalbe line; diagnostic of pseudoexfoliation syndrome.

Sampson cyst (chocolate cyst, endometrial cyst): Membrane-bound collection of brownish, thick fluid caused by hemosiderin buildup following local hemorrhage; can occur after mastectomy or in ovarian endometriosis.

Sampson theory: "Regurgitation" of endometrial tissue during menses and implantation in peritoneal cavity is cause of endometriosis.

San Diego hemoglobin: High-oxygen-affinity hemoglobin resulting from replacement of valine by methiomine in $\alpha_1\beta_2$ contact area; hemoglobin levels are 16–18 g/dl.

Sander parallelogram: Illusion in which lines drawn inside parallelogram of equal length appear unequal.

Sanders-Retlaff-Kraff formula (SRK formula): Expression used to calculate intraocular lens power; equals A—2.5(AL)—0.9K, where A is lens constant (determined by manufacturer for specific lens), AL is axial length of eye in mm, and K is keratometry measurement. Approximate values are obtained by measuring contralateral cornea or from previous postoperative keratomy results using specific procedure.

Sandhoff disease (syndrome): Deficiency of hexosaminidase A and B, causing accumulation of GM_2 gangliosides in lysosomes. Disorder is characterized by loss of motor skills, macular cherry-red spot, organomegaly, and bony changes; condition is autosomal recessive. Age of onset is 6 months–6 years. Screening test is skin, conjunctival, or rectal biopsy.

Sandmann-Andra syndrome: Congenital hypohidrosis and abnormally few teeth.

Sandoz disease: Familial pulmonary fibrosis; same course as idiopathic pulmonary fibrosis but occurs at younger age. Condition is autosomal dominant, with variable expression and penetrance.

Sandström body: Parathyroid gland.

Sandwith tongue (bald tongue): Smooth surface of tongue in late-stage pellagra.

Sanfilippo syndrome (type B): Deficiency of lysosomal hexosaminidase, causing defective degeneration of heparan sulfate.

Sanfilippo syndrome (type D): Deficiency of lysosomal enzyme N-acetylglucosamine-6-sulfatase, causing defective degeneration of heparan sulfate and keratan sulfate; autosomal recessive condition.

Sanford envelopes: Small packets with slightly different weights inside used to detect small differences in weightlifting thresholds.

Sanger-Brown syndrome: Type of hereditary ataxia.

Sanger-Coulson method (dideoxy sequencing): Widely used method of DNA sequencing; uses single-stranded template DNA and short complementary primer that is annealed and extended by DNA polymerase. Reaction product is then split into 4 tubes (A, C, G, and T), each containing low concentration of indicated dideoxynucleotide along with normal deoxynucleotides. Dideoxynucleotides block further chain extension, and each tube contains mixture of chains determined by template sequence. Material in tubes is then denatured and run on acrylamide sequencing gel and bands are read.

Santavuori syndrome: Changes in visual evoked potentials.

Santorini cartilage (corniculate cartilage): Small protuberance at apex of each arytenoid cartilage anchoring arytenoid–epiglottic folds.

Santorini duct: Small, variably present accessory pancreatic duct, which lies mostly in pancreatic head and drains via minor papilla in duodenal wall; remnant of dorsal pancreatic bud. Pancreatic divisum occurs when this duct serves as main pancreatic drainage.

Santorini ligament: Crico-pharyngeal ligament; runs from cricoid lamina to midline of pharynx.

Santorini muscle: Risorius muscle, which draws corners of mouth laterally. It arises from fascia overlying masseter, inserts at skin at corners of mouth.

Sappey ligament: Thick, fibrous posterior portion of temporomandibular joint capsule.

Sappey plexus: Subareolar network of lymph vessels.

Sarfeh shunt: Small-diameter interposition portocaval shunt; acts as selective shunt to preserve hepatopetal flow to liver.

Sattler layer: Lamina containing medium-sized vessels of choroid.

Saunders-Sutton disease: Delirium tremens in chronic alcohol abusers caused by alcohol withdrawal, infection, or trauma.

Sauve-Kapandji procedure: Salvage procedure used after failed surgery of distal ulna.

Savage syndrome (resistant ovary syndrome): Continuous increased secretion of gonadotropins by pituitary. Follicles appear normal in biopsy but are not responsive to even massive doses of gonadotropins.

Savart wheel: Early device used for generating high-frequency sounds; uses hand-turned wheel capable of producing 24,000 vibrations/sec.

Savastano prosthesis: Knee replacement with maximum freedom of motion of joint; requires good soft tissue stability.

Savory dilators: Mechanical dilators with guidewire passed through esophageal stricture, with hollow tube then passed over guidewire; decreases risk of creating false passage.

Sawaguchi modification: Variation of Kasai procedure for correction of biliary atresia in infants; 1st described in 1968. Best results are obtained if procedure is performed 8 weeks after birth.

Sayre suspension apparatus: Early traction device.

Scaglietti-Dagnini syndrome: See Erdheim disease.

Scarff-Bloom-Richardson grade: Modification of Bloom-Richardson pathology system for grading breast cancer.

Scarpa fascia: Superficial fascia underlying skin and subcutaneous tissue on anterior abdominal wall made of relatively thin layer of connective tissue with generous adipose tissue; is most distinct in lower portion of abdominal wall. It provides little strength on wound closure, but approximation allows for thinner, more cosmetic scar.

Scarpa foramina: Canal located in each intermaxillary suture; contain branches of nasopalatine nerve.

Scarpa ganglion: Clustered cell bodies of vestibular nerve cells in vestibular labyrinth of ear.

Scarpa habenula: Vestigium processus vaginalis.

Scarpa nerves: Nasopalatine nerves carrying sensory and parasympathetic fibers; originates from pterygopalatine ganglion and supplies anterior hard palate and nasal septum.

Scarpa triangle (femoral triangle): Anatomic area bounded medially by medial edge of adductor longus, laterally by medial edge of sartorius, and superiorly by inguinal ligament; lies deep to fascia.

Scassellati-Sforzolini syndrome (vertical bilateral retraction): Partial or complete loss of upgaze with variable limitation of downgaze; associated with abnormalities of optic nerve, facial asymmetry, and partial lid ptosis.

Schachenmann syndrome: See Schmid-Fraccaro syndrome.

Schaefer sign: Persons are able to determine direction of plantar response by pressure applied to calf; seen in corticospinal tract lesions.

Schafer method: Artificial respiration; victim is placed prone with 1 arm positioned under forehead. Rescuer straddles patient's hips and presses vigorously on lower ribs and slowly releases; cycle is repeated every 5 seconds.

Schäffer reflex: Variably occurring 1st toe dorsiflexion in hemiplegia as result of squeezing Achilles tendon.

Schäffer syndrome: Small patches of alopecia, congenital cataracts, small head, mental retardation, dwarfism, and follicular keratosis of skin.

Schafhäutl phonometer: Early device used for measuring intensity threshold for sound involving pellet dropped from varying heights to produce known sound.

Schanz disease: Back pain and feeling of fatigue localized to lumbar spine area when patient moves from standing to prone position; caused by variety of lumbar spine conditions.

Schanz syndrome: See Albert syndrome.

Schatzker classification: System used to describe classification of tibial plateau and proximal tibial fractures. Type 1, cleavage fracture; type 2, cleavage combined with depression; type 3, central depression; type 4, medial condyle fracture; type 5, bicondylar fractures; type 6, plateau fracture dissociation of diaphysis and metaphysis.

Schatzki ring: Distal esophageal web formed by submucosal fibrosis at squamocolumnar–epithelial junction; nearly always associated with hiatal hernia. Cause is not acid reflux. Constriction is often asymptomatic; patients usu. present with dysphagia when orifice opening measures 13 mm. Dilatation is usu. curative.

Schaumann bodies: Nodular lesions occurring in sarcoidosis.

Scheele green: Greenish color of cupric salt of arsenic formed when histology specimen containing arsenic salt is washed in copper sulfate.

Scheffé method: Statistical technique used to make a posteriori comparisons in ANOVA, assuming F is significant.

Scheffé test: Statistical test for homogeneity of variance in single factor ANOVA; good for use when normal distribution in variable studied may be skewed.

Scheie disease (mucopolysaccharidosis type 1): Deficiency in α-L-iduronidase with abnormal amounts of dermatan and heparan sulfate; autosomal recessive condition. Onset of dysostosis multiplex occurs in childhood but without mental deterioration seen in Hurler disease.

Scheiner experiment: Demonstration of accommodation of eye. Patient looks through 1 of 2 pinholes punched in card at distance from each other that is less than pupil diameter; all objects outside of focal plane appear in duplicate.

Schellong-Strisower phenomenon: Clinical occurrence of drop in systolic blood pressure when moving rapidly from prone to standing position; sometimes accompanied by dizziness.

Scheuermann disease: Osteochondritis of anterior vertebral body with resulting wedge-shaped vertebrae; onset occurs at 12–13 years of age. Kyphosis with arcuate backward curvature and rounded shoulders results if 3 consecutive vertebrae are affected. Condition also involves flat thoracic area and thoracic or lumbar scoliosis. Early surgery should be performed.

Scheuermann test: Kyphosis in adolescence.

Schick test: Previously used in diagnosis of diphtheria; consists of subdermal injection of diphtheria toxin to determine degree of reactivity.

Schiff reaction: Schiff reagent used to stain aminoalcohols and adjacent hydroxyl groups red.

Schiff stain (periodic acid–Schiff stain): Schiff reagent used to demonstrate glycogen, neutral muco-type substances, reticulin, basement membranes, and some fungi and parasites (e.g., *Amoeba, Trichomonas*); also extremely useful in highlighting intracytoplasmic crystals in alveolar sarcoma.

Schiff-Sherrington phenomenon: Behavior of extremities when inhibitory response is eliminated due to spinal cord transection. When level of transection is in thoracic region, stretch response and postural reflexes in arms are exaggerated. When transection is in lumbar/sacral region, leg reflexes are exaggerated.

Schilder disease (adrenoleukodystrophy, encephalitis): Generalized white matter disorder due to demyelinization;

marked by progressive visual deficits, decreased mental status, spastic paraplegia, and variable intracranial hypertension in children and young adults. CSF shows increased total protein and cell count.

Schilder-Foix syndrome: Variable neurologic sequelae resulting from nonprogressive sclerosis of white matter due to anoxia.

Schiller test: Topical application of iodine to cervix to indicate presence of malignancy; positive result is lack of staining, because tumor cells lack glycogen.

Schiller-Duval body: Invaginated papillary structure containing a single blood vessel lined peripherally by neoplastic cells; occurs in endodermal sinus tumor.

Schilling test: 3-stage test that differentiates true pernicious anemia from blind loop syndrome; urinary excretion is measured after each stage. Stage 1—radioactive vitamin B_{12} is given; stage 2 (if there is low urine excretion after stage 1)—in low-excretion ($< 7\%$–25%), a trial of intrinsic factor is given; stage 3—tetracycline is given. (If excretion rises to normal levels, diagnosis is blind loop syndrome.)

Schimke dysplasia (immunoosseous dysplasia): Rare defective cellular immunity, progressive renal disease, and spondyloepiphyseal dysplasia; marked by short stature, triangular face, and bulbous nasal tip.

Schinz disease: Recurrent ulcers in fingers and toes; autosomal dominant condition. Similar condition also occurs in workers exposed to vinyl chloride.

Schinzel-Giedion syndrome: Rare congenital mental retardation, midface retraction, hypertrichosis, seizures, genitourinary abnormalities, and renal anomalies.

Schiötz tonometer: Handheld device placed directly on eye surface that measures intraocular pressure; deviation on scale is converted into mm Hg.

Schirmer test: Measure of reflex tear production; uses 5×35-mm filter paper strips folded at notched indentation with short end placed over lower eyelid margin. Wetness at 5 minutes (or alternately at 1 minute, with value multiplied by 3) is noted. Also, basic tear production can be measured using previously described procedure after topical anesthesia is applied to cul-de-sac and conjunctiva.

Schlatter sprain: See Osgood-Schlatter disease.

Schlemm canal: Anatomic space running circularly in deep layers of cornea.

Schlesinger law: "The mind heals itself and protects itself." Statement is applicable in psychotherapy, where patients generally do not bring into consciousness material with which they do not have the emotional resources to deal.

Schlichter test: Laboratory test most commonly used to ensure adequate antimicrobial levels in bacterial endocarditis and osteomyelitis; to be antibacterial, antibiotic must have = 1:8 dilution.

Schlieren microscopy: System for improving refractive index differences in transparent media and resolving height differences for reflected light from surface.

Schmid syndrome (metaphyseal chondrodysplasia): Collagen disease with stunted growth, coxa vara, bowleg, and waddling gait; autosomal dominant condition. Variable abnormalities in costochondral junctions also occur. Distal femoral metaphyses are more affected than proximal areas. Disorder is sometimes misdiagnosed as rickets.

Schmid-Fraccaro syndrome (Schachenmann syndrome): Cat-eye syndrome.

Schmidt syndrome: Polyglandular autoimmune syndrome type 2; characterized by lymphocyte infiltration of thyroid and adrenal glands, hypogonadism, and type 1 diabetes mellitus.

Schmidt-Lantermann clefts: Fissures that represent areas of myelin that are less contracted; seen on microscopic longitudinal view of axons as oblique incisures in myelin sheath.

Schmincke tumor: Leukemic infiltrates of basal meninges.

Schmorl nodule: Herniation of nucleus pulposus into adjoining vertebrae.

Schneider index: Measure of cardiovascular fitness based on effect of exercise on heart rate.

Schnidt hemostatic forceps: Long (184 mm), slightly curved, ring-handle, locking forceps; used on vessels to control bleeding or for tissue dissection.

Schnyder crystalline dystrophy: Relatively uncommon corneal stromal development of cholesterol crystals in ring-like, central position; associated with elevated serum cholesterol and triglycerides and genu valgum. Condition is usu. seen in Scandinavian descendents in 1st few years of life. Corneal transplantation is usu. necessary in 4th–5th decade.

Schoemaker line: Imaginary line between trochanter and anterior superior iliac spine. In normally positioned trochanter, extension of line runs above umbilicus.

Schoemaker operation: Type of gastroenterostomy.

Schoen theory of accommodation: Convexity of eye is determined by ciliary muscle by same effect as in hand squeezing rubber ball.

Schoenlein disease: Idiopathic thrombocytopenic purpura.

Schoenlein-Henoch disease: IgA nephropathy.

Scholtze disease: See Bjoerck disease.

Schreger lines (bands): See Owen lines.

Schreus disease: Small, firm yellowish nodules found on back of thighs, buttocks, and occasionally on trunk; often degenerate to keloids.

Schridde hairs: Coarse black hairs that appear in beard and on temples in patients with cancer and other cachetic disorders.

Schuchardt incision: Skin incision and dissection through tissues on either side of vagina.

Schüffner dots (Schüffner granules, Schüffner punctuation): Irregularly staining lesions (with Wright or Romanowsky stain) seen inside RBCs in patients infected with malaria caused by *Plasmodium vivax*.

Schwabach test: Diagnoses hearing loss using series of 5 tuning forks.

Schwalbe foramen (foramen of Vicq d'Azyr): Anatomic space formed by end of anterior median fissure of medulla oblongata; located at inferior edge of pons.

Schwann cells: Ectodermally derived cells that form neurilemma of peripheral nerves.

Schwann substance: Substance comprising medullary sheath.

Schwarz activator (bow activator): Orthodontic device that passively transmits force by using activated muscle to move teeth; 2 halves are connected by safety pin–type device with rubber shock absorber that opens mouth.

Schneider carmine: Carmine solution in concentrated acetic acid.

Schneiderian mucosa: Nasal mucosa.

Schneiderian papilloma (inverted papilloma:) Benign but locally invasive epithelial neoplasm arising in nasal mucosa (usu. in lateral wall) close to middle meatus or in maxillary sinus; may undergo transformation to squamous cell carcinoma.

Schobinger incision: Incision used for exposure of anterior neck structures.

Schroeder staircase: Drawing of staircase using perspective in such a way that stairs can be viewed either from above or below.

Schroeder syndrome: Congenital subluxation and dislocation of hips, knees, and shoulders and misshaped pinnae.

Schroetter syndrome: Type of focal chorea affecting larynx; results in involuntary vocal utterances.

Schrön granule: Structure found in germinal spot of ovum.

Schuetzenberger syndrome: See Barré-Liéou syndrome.

Schüller ducts: See Skene glands.

Schüller glands: Outpouchings of Gartner ducts.

Schultz-Charlton test (reaction): Test used to diagnose scarlet fever; involves subcutaneous injection of erythrogenic toxin of *Streptococcus pyogenes.*

Schultz-Dale reaction (Dale reaction): Method of detecting in vitro anaphylactic sensitization in guinea pig.

Schultze fold: Redundant amnion running from insertion site of cord into placenta into remnants of umbilical vesicle.

Schultze sign: See Chvostek sign.

Schultze sign: Local, transient depression at affected site as result of tapping of tongue; seen in tetany and myotonic dystrophy.

Schutz syndrome: See Nothnagel syndrome.

Schwabach test (absolute bone conduction test): Hearing test to determine baseline bone conduction compared to examiner (assumes normal hearing in examiner). Test is performed by closing ear canal on side to be tested using tragus and placing vibrating tuning fork on mastoid process. At moment patient cannot hear fork, examiner places fork on own mastoid bone, after closing ear canal.

Schwachman syndrome: Exocrine pancreatic insufficiency, pancytopenia, femur abnormalities, hepatic and cardiac fibrosis, and Schwalbe fissure; autosomal recessive condition. Sweat test is normal.

Schwalbe line: Normal insertion of Descemet membrane at peripheral cornea.

Schwalbe nucleus: Medial vestibular nucleus; located in midbrain.

Schwann cell: Neurolemma cell.

Schwann sheath: Outer basement membrane around peripheral nerves; forms myelin when double-wrapped around axon.

Schwartz-Jampel syndrome: Neurotonia, with intense electrical discharges for prolonged periods without waxing and waning.

Schwartze sign: Erythema and hypervascularity in otosclerosis due to formation of new stapes.

Schwarz-Lelek syndrome: Rare congenital frontal bossing of head, obliterated paranasal sinuses, and hyperostosis in skeletal girdle, with increased alkaline phosphatase; autosomal recessive condition.

Scoe syndrome: Facial anomalies, short stature, hypodontia, and plantar and palmar lesions; autosomal dominant condition.

Scoville aneurysm clip: Small metal device placed on brain aneurysms to occlude lumen.

Scoville procedure: Orbital undercutting for psychiatric treatment.

Scribanu syndrome: Onset in infancy of progressive deafness and dystonia leading to inability to ambulate and bizarre head posture; X-linked inheritance.

Death usu. occurs by adolescence.

Scribner shunt: External arteriovenous shunt once used for hemodialysis; now largely supplanted by central vein canalization for temporary or short-term dialysis access.

Scriver syndrome (pseudo-hypophosphatasia): Rare variant of Fraser syndrome (infantile hypophosphatasia) with addition of normal or increased serum alkaline phosphatase.

Seashore audiometer: Device used to measure hearing threshold; comprised of sound-producing apparatus (tuning fork or buzzer), potentiometer to vary intensity, and telephone microphone system.

Seashore test: Early musical aptitude test using phonograph record to test ability to discriminate slight variations in loudness, pitch, rhythm, time, and timbre; also tests ability to memorize tonal patterns.

Seattle Lightfoot prosthesis: Foot-and-ankle prosthesis (weight: ~ 470 g); gives excellent results when used in both above- and below-knee amputations in sedentary patients and good results when used in below-knee amputations in active patients.

Seattle Lightfoot prosthesis with ankle–foot device: Foot-and-ankle prosthesis (weight: ~ 715 g); gives excellent results when used in below-knee amputations in active patients.

Seattle model: Theory of pain experience viewed as sequential multistage process.

Sebileau hollow: Groove beneath tongue formed by sublingual glands and mucosa of the mouth.

Seeligman disease: See Carini disease.

Seelimueller sign: Pain caused by point pressure on skull in some cases of syphilis.

Segawa syndrome (progressive dystonia): Motor disturbances with childhood onset marked by diurnal variation in severity (less in morning) and relief during sleep; begins in 1 limb and extends to all, with trunk rarely affected. Condition is autosomal dominant. Treatment is L-dopa.

Séglas type: Psychomotor paranoia.

Segond fracture: Fracture of lateral tibial condyle with avulsion due to insertion of tensor fascia lata; must be differentiated from fracture tip of proximal fibula.

Séguin form board: Evaluation and training device for mentally impaired made up of geometric figures that patient inserts into cutout forms with identical shapes; is now 1 of subtests of Grace Arthur point scale and other intelligence tests.

Seidel nail: Interlocking nail used in repair of humeral fractures.

Seidel test: Use of concentrated fluorescent dye on cornea to detect leakage of aqueous fluid.

Seidlmayer syndrome: Coin-like purpuric lesions appearing in children after infections.

Seitelberger disease (variant): Sudanophilic leukodystrophy.

Seitz filter: Asbestos-based filter for microorganisms.

Seitz metamorphosing respiration: Inspiratory breath with beginning tubular bronchial murmur and finishing with cavernous quality to tone.

Selas filter: Porcelain filter for bacteria.

Seligman disease (α heavy chain disease): Type of plasma cell disorder with infiltration of lamina propria of small intestine by lymphoplasmacytoid cells that secrete shortened α chains; usu. manifests as chronic diarrhea, weight loss, and malabsorption. Resulting lymphomas range from relatively benign to malignant. Disorder is closely related to parasite-induced Mediterranean lymphoma.

Sellick maneuver (cricoid pressure): Gentle but firm pressure placed on either side of cricoid cartilage using thumb and forefinger; performed by assistant to anesthesiologist during intubation. Action causes posterior displacement of respiratory cartilages to occlude esophagus without affecting airway opening.

Selter disease: See Bilderbeck disease.

Selye syndrome: The 3 phases experienced in stressful situations. 1—alarm reaction: coping mechanisms are mobilized; 2—resistance phase: ability to deploy coping mechanisms plateaus; 3—exhaustion phase: depletion of resources and deterioration of performance occurs if stress continues.

Semliki forest virus: Arbovirus that causes fever, rash, and arthralgias.

Semmes-Weinstein monofilament: Series of small wires with different diameters used to assess loss of sensation in diabetic neuropathy (e.g., sample sizes 5.07 g, 10.0 g).

Semon sign: Decrease in mobility of vocal cords; occurs in laryngeal malignancy.

Senear-Usher syndrome: Pemphigus erythematosus.

Senegal haplotype: 1 of 4 major sickle cell haplotypes arising on chromosome 11.

Sengstaken-Blakemore tube: Thin, rubber tube inserted through nares to tamponade bleeding gastric and

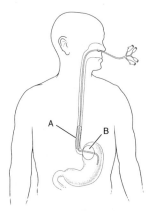

A. Esophageal balloon
B. Gastric balloon

Sengstaken-Blakemore tube

esophageal varices temporarily; has 2 inflatable balloons, each with dedicated inflation bladder, and 2 lumens for aspiration and lavage.

Sengupta technique: Procedure for proximal release of quadriceps muscle, esp. in leg contractures of infancy and childhood; involves curved incision along base of greater trochanter and longitudinally down thigh. Tensor fasciae lata and vastus lateralis are severed, vastus lateralis is released along its origin, and vastus intermedius is elevated off femoral surface. Ambulation is possible at 4 weeks.

Senn retractor: Handheld, double-ended retractor for small amounts of soft tissue or fine vascular structures.

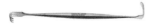

Senn retractor

Senter syndrome: See Desmond syndrome.

Seoul virus: Type of hantavirus; causes mild case of hemorrhagic fever with renal complications.

Sequin symptom (signal symptom): Involuntary muscle contractions occurring in epileptic seizures.

Serafini hernia (retrovascular hernia): Tissue that passes through femoral canal and exits posterior to femoral vessels.

Sergent-Bernard syndrome: See Addisonian crises.

Serratia: Gram-negative, facultatively anaerobic, DNAase-positive, motile rod; causes opportunistic infections of blood, urine, wounds, heart, and respiratory system in debilitated patients. Most common species is *S. marcescens.*

Serres glands: Whitish dots made up of epithelial cells found just under surface of gums in infants.

Sertoli cell: Slender, elongated cells extending from basement membrane to lumen of seminiferous tubules.

Sertoli cell adenoma: See Pick tubular adenoma.

Sertoli-Leydig tumor: Androgen-producing arrhenoblastoma; commonly manifests as mass.

Settegast position: Radiographic technique using axial projection to image vertical fractures of patella and articular surfaces of femoropatellar articulation.

Sever disease: Inflammation of heel bone at Achilles tendon insertion.

Sézary cell: Malignant circulating human T cells seen in HTLV-1–related leukemia lymphoma; nuclei are convoluted and shaped like clover leaves.

Sézary syndrome (erythroderma): Neoplastic disorder with abnormal proliferation of lymphocytes.

Shabbir syndrome: Skin erosions of face, hoarseness, and nail abnormality; autosomal recessive condition seen in Pakistan.

Shafer sign: Small clumps of pigmented cells in vitreous or anterior chamber of eye; indicative of retinal break.

Shaffer classification: Describes grading angle configuration of anterior chamber of eye.

Shaffer plate: Stainless steel arch support used in adults with flat feet.

Shafik loops: Mechanical supports placed intra-abdominally to correct rectal prolapse.

Shands dressing: Dressing with 2 layers each of cast padding and elastic bandage; used to stabilize ankle sprains and metatarsal fractures.

Shannon-Wiener measure of information: Statistical calculation of average amount of information event can contain (in bits). Equation: $H = \Sigma Pi \times \log Pi$, where Pi is probability of alternate event occurring and i is number of possible alternatives.

Sharp-Purser test: Used to detect chronic subluxation of C1 and C2; positive if slippage is felt by examiner when sitting patient tilts head forward and then backward.

sheath of Henle: Endoneurium.

sheath of Hertwig: Epithelial root sheath at base of tooth formed by outer enamel epithelium and ameloblasts.

Sheehan syndrome: Anterior pituitary failure and necrosis secondary to hemorrhage, sepsis, or shock associated with childbirth; causes amenorrhea and hypothyroidism. Treatment is replacement of corticosteroids and thyroid hormone; mineralocorticoid replacement usu. is not needed.

Sheehan syndrome: Engorgement of scalp veins, bulging fontanelle, and paralysis of upgaze seen in pediatric hydrocephalus.

Sheehan syndrome: Postpartum pituitary necrosis; marked by insufficient release of ACTH, TSH, human growth hormone, prolactin, and testosterone.

Shepherd fracture: Oblique fracture of lateral tubercle of posterior talus.

Sheppard correction: Statistical device allowing correction of standard deviation calculated from group of data with class intervals < 12.

Sheridan-Gardiner test: Visual test for young children; uses series of cards with single letters (H, O, T, V, U, X, A). Child is presented with each card and must match letter to board with all letters printed on it.

Shields syndrome: Capdepont disease in association with osteogenesis imperfecta.

Shiga bacillus: *Shigella dysenteriae.*

Shimada classification: Description of neuroblastoma

on basis of cellularity, mitosis karyorrhexis index, age, and existence of stroma (i.e., stroma-rich or stroma-poor).

Shinpo disease: See Crow-Fukase syndrome.

Shipley institute scale: Measures pathologic defects in mental functioning; uses 40-item vocabulary test and 20-item series recompletion test. Score < 100 connotes pathology.

Shirodkar operation: Cerclage technique used in pregnancy to partially close incompetent cervix. Transverse incision is made in anterior vaginal mucosa at junction of cervix, bladder is pushed cephalad, and encircling suture or mesh is placed tightly around the cervix to prevent cervical dilatation.

Shoemaker procedure: Surgical technique for removal of type 4 gastric ulcer; uses vertical extension of resection line along lesser curvature that includes all ulcer margins.

Shope papilloma: Type of wart commonly found on wild rabbits; caused by papillomavirus.

Shouldice repair (Canadian repair): Surgical repair of inguinal hernias (either direct or indirect) using 4-layered imbricated (continuous suture) repair of inguinal canal. Genital branch of genitofemoral nerve is at risk for injury. Recurrence rate is < 1% in experienced hands.

Shrapnell membrane: Upper part of tympanic membrane; outer surface is auditory canal epithelium and inner surface is mucous membrane.

Shulman syndrome: Inflammation and thickening of skin and fascia.

Shy-Drager syndrome: Degenerative disease marked by parkinsonism, impotence, postural hypotension, sweating, gastroparesis, bowel and bladder dysfunction, and lower motor neuron and pyramidal deficits. Only treatment is supportive care for postural hypotension.

Siberian ginseng: *Eleutherococcus senticosus.*

Sibson fascia: Variably present process originating off scalenus minimus and connecting to pleura cupola; makes pleura tense.

Sibson groove: Indentation occasionally seen at lower border of pectoralis major muscle.

Sibson notch: Area at left upper edge of precordial dullness where normal auscultation is surrounded by area of abnormal auscultation in acute pericardial effusions.

Siccardi syndrome: Rare condition marked by gray skin and hair, recurrent infections, lymphadenopathy, and hepatosplenomegaly; associated with defect in neutrophil activity.

Sidman avoidance: Animals receive electric shock for incorrect response and no shock for correct response; results in high, sustainable correct responses.

Siegert sign: Short, curved 5th finger; seen in trisomy 21.

Siegle otoscope: Device used to look into ear canal; uses condensed air to highlight view of tympanic membrane.

Siegrist streaks: Linear alignment of Elschnig spots in retinal pigment epithelium.

Siegrist syndrome (Siegrist-Hutchinson syndrome): Decreasing vision due to pigmentation developing in areas of choroidal vessels and exophthalmos; seen in elderly (usu. women). Condition is also associated with albuminuria.

Siemerling-Creutzfeldt disease: Leukodystrophy, hyperpigmentation of skin, and neurologic abnormalities due to loss of myelin; X-linked recessive condition. Cause is chronic adrenocortical insufficiency.

Siewert classification: System used to describe adenocarcinoma at gastroesophageal junction.

Sigmund glands: Lymph nodes located in epitrochlear area.

Sigvaris stockings: Graduated compression stockings.

Silex sign: Skin creases radiating from lips in congenital syphilis.

Sillence syndrome: Scoliosis, brachydactyly, and symphalangism ("chess pawn" finger tips); autosomal dominant condition.

Silva mind control: Imagery and relaxation techniques for purposes such as improvement of mental state and pain control; correspond to increased alpha component on EEG.

Silver-Russell syndrome: Severe intrauterine growth retardation, normal head circumference, short stature, lean body mass, facial asymmetry and dysmorphism, camptodactyly, variable hypospadias, and inguinal hernia.

Silverman needle: Long, thin needle with central trocar and outer, hollow sheath used to obtain percutaneous liver biopsy specimens.

Silverskjold disease: Aseptic necrosis of calcaneus.

Silvester method: Artificial respiration; patient is placed supine and arms are pulled over head to augment inspiration, pulled to chest level, and then pressed into chest wall to augment expiration.

Simmonds disease: Anterior pituitary failure and necrosis from any cause; marked by anorexia, weakness, emaciation, premature aging, and thyroid disturbances.

Simmons citrate agar: Bacterial medium containing citrate as only source of carbon.

Simon-Nitinol filter: Metal device placed in lower vena cava to act as mechanical barrier to prevent large pulmonary emboli.

Simond disease: See Barraquer-Simons syndrome.

Simons disease: Partial lipodystrophy.

Simpson catheter: Atherectomy catheter with positioning balloon opposite cutting window; uses guidewire inserted through peripheral artery to allow correct positioning under fluoroscopy.

Simpson directional catheter: Widely used atherectomy device with rotating cutter blade powered by cutter torque cable fastened to motor device; allows blade to shave plaque off walls and pass it to collecting chamber.

Simpson dysmorphia (bulldog dysmorphia, Golabi-Rosen syndrome, Simpson-Golabi-Behmel dysmorphia): Overprominent jaw; stubby, upturned nose; enlarged tongue; stubby fingers and hands; and short, thick torso. Inheritance is X-linked. Condition is considered an "overgrowth" syndrome with increased risk of neoplasms (e.g., Wilms tumor, neuroblastoma, hepatocellular carcinoma); also associated with cardiac arrhythmias and variable mental retardation. Defect is in gene for extracellular proteoglycan (Xq26).

Simpson forceps: Obstetrical forceps.

Sims position (left fetal position): Left lateral decubitus position with legs drawn up to torso.

Sims uterine curette: Handheld device with "open-loop" end placed inside uterus for

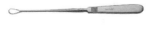

Sims uterine curette

scraping uterine cells to evaluate for cytology.

Sindbis virus: Alphavirus transmitted by mosquitoes (*Aedes, Culex,* and *Culiseta*) from birds to humans; prototype alphavirus for laboratory study. Clinical features of infection are macular rash (starting on torso and spreading to limbs), arthralgias, low-grade fever, tendonitis, headache, fatigue, and paresthesias. Virus causes Ockelbo disease (Sweden), Pogosta disease (Finland), and Karelian fever (Russia).

Sinding-Larsen-Johansson syndrome: Defective secondary ossification center of inferior patella.

Singapore ear: See Hong Kong ear.

Singer-Hastings system: Evaluation of acid–base physiology.

Singh index: Grading of trabecular patterns of femoral head and intertrochanteric region on scale of 1 to 6 (most to least osteoporotic).

Singley intestinal forceps (Tuttle intestinal forceps): Handheld forceps with both

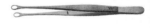

Singley intestinal forceps

ends fashioned in "open-loop" manner.

Sinsteden windmill (reversible perspective figure): Optical illusion of silhouette of windmill with vanes appearing to rotate in opposite directions as perspective is switched from looking at windmill from front and back.

sinus of Maier: Slight dilatation of upper lacrimal sac into which canaliculi empty.

sinus of Morgagni: Lateral fold of mucous membrane in larynx lying between vestibular and vocal folds.

sinus of Morgagni: See sinus of Valsalva.

sinus of Valsalva (Petit sinus, sinus of Morgagni): Small pouch in aortic wall at base of each semolina cusp.

Sipple syndrome: Multiple endocrine neoplasia type 2a (MEN-2a); marked by pheochromocytoma, medullary thyroid cancer, and parathyroid hyperplasia with hypercalcemia. Condition is autosomal dominant.

Sister Mary Joseph nodule: Periumbilical lymph node metastases.

Sisto sign: Sequelae of congenital syphilis; marked by inconsolable crying.

Sistrunk procedure: Method of resection of thyroglossal duct cyst; requires resection of duct remnants, foramen cecum, and middle part of hyoid bone.

Sisyphus dream: Psychiatric term for dream expressing frustration; from Greek myth about Sisyphus, who was condemned to keep rolling large stone up hill that rolled back down.

Sjögren hand: Visual test for young children using series of cards with hands printed with fingers pointed in different directions; child must point in same direction as hand points on card.

Sjögren syndrome: Autoimmune disease caused by antibodies against parotid duct; marked by atrophy of parotid and tear glands. Condition causes sicca syndrome and xerostomia. Disorder is common in postmenopausal women and can be seen in chronic rheumatoid arthritis and other diseases, including systemic lupus erythematosus, progressive systemic sclerosis, overlap syndrome, polymyositis/dermatomyositis, graft-versus-host disease, malignant lymphoma, chronic Hashimoto thyroiditis, and chronic active hepatitis.

Sjögren-Larsson syndrome: Ataxia, spasticity, and retinitis; autosomal recessive condition. Metabolic error is unknown. Age at onset is 6–16 years.

Skaggs-Robinson hypothesis: Ability to recall learned information is related to degree of similarity of previously learned information; more similar information results in higher degree of recall.

Skene glands (ducts, tubules): Mucus-secreting paraurethral glands whose openings lie posterior and on either side of urethral orifice in females.

Skillern fracture: Greenstick fracture of distal ulna with open distal radius fracture.

Skillman hemostatic forceps: Straight or curve-tipped, ring-handle, locking forceps; placed on vessels to control bleeding or for tissue dissection.

Skinner box: Enclosure for animal to keep it close to device (e.g., lever, bar) that offers reward for certain behavior. Animal controls device, and experimenter controls reward.

Skinner conditioning (operant conditioning): Learning by having reinforcement follow certain behaviors.

Skipper-Schabel method: Model of tumor cell kinetics suggesting that tumor cell number increases at exponential rate.

Skoda tympany (skodaic resonance): Increased resonance to percussion in upper chest wall and decreased resonance to percussion in lower chest wall.

Slocum technique: Surgical reconstruction of ligamentous injuries in medial compartment of knee; knee is flexed to 90° and incision is made 4–5 cm on medial aspect of knee. After superficial tissue is reflected posteriorly and patellar stability is checked, medial parapatellar arthrotomy to expose joint is performed, allowing for systematic exam and repair of laxities.

Slocum test: Anterior rotary drawer test.

Slocum transplant: Surgical transplant of part of patellar tendon. Medial tendon is cut away with attached osteoperiosteal layer of bone distally and placed on medial tibia.

Slocumb syndrome: See Perkoff-Slocumb syndrome.

Slosson test: Oral intelligence test of 195 items; estimates IQ and mental age.

Slot-Zielke device: Anterior fixation device for thoracic and lumbar spine used mainly for correction of kyphosis; provides compression forces only. Device has either single or dual rod construction, with Zielke screws placed through staple plates into vertebral body.

Smead-Jones technique: "Running" closure technique used to approximate abdominal fascia, rectus muscles, and anterior peritoneum; closure favored by gynecologists. Alternating different-size tissue bites are taken in "over and over" fashion; double-looped 0 Maxon suture can be used.

Smeloff-Cutter valve: Early prosthetic device used in aortic valve replacement.

Smillie nail: Small pin used to reattach small osteochondral fragments in knee injuries.

Smith antigen: Extractable nuclear antigen; presence in blood stream is 30%–40% sensitive for systemic lupus erythematosus.

Smith classification: System used to rank oligodendrogliomas on a scale of A to D.

Smith disease: See Parker disease (neuroblastoma).

Smith disease: Superior dislocation of metatarsals and medial cuneiform.

Smith fracture (reversed Colles fracture): Distal radius fractures with volar displacement of distal fragment; can be articular, nonarticular or oblique, and nonarticular. Cause is fall on dorsum of hand.

Smith maneuver: Placement of traction after externally rotating the thigh, followed by abduction, internal rotation, and adduction; used to reduce femoral neck fractures.

Smith pessary: Oblong-shaped ring inserted into vagina to correct retrodisplacement of uterus.

Smith prosthesis: Type of ankle replacement.

Smith sign (Eustace Smith sign): Indicates presence of enlarge bronchial glands if murmur can be auscultated over manubrium when patient's neck is in full extension.

Smith syndrome: See Barraquer-Simons disease.

Smith-Lemli-Opitz syndrome: See Gardner-Silengo-Wachtel syndrome.

Smith-Magenis syndrome: Rare disorder with mental retardation, chronic ear infections, self-mutilation of finger and toenails, and repetitive picking at skin. Cause is gene deletion (17p13.3).

Smith-Petersen approach (medial approach): Surgical approach used for tendon transfer procedures on ulnar aspect of hand and for Darrach procedure.

Smith-Petersen incision: Surgical approach to anterior column hip fractures.

Smith-Robinson diskectomy technique: Similar to Cloward technique, except iliac graft is fashioned precisely to evacuated intervertebral space, which allows graft to rest on posterior lip of cortical bone of adjacent bodies. High-speed drilling tools are used to harvest bone with minimal muscle dissection. Cervical collar is required for 8–12 weeks postop.

Smith-Strang syndrome (beery baby): Onset shortly after birth of loss of response to stimuli, mental deterioration, edema, and white hair; autosomal recessive condition. Infant smells strongly of stale beer. Cause is malabsorption of methionine with hydroxybutyric and phenylpyruvic acid excreted in urine. Death occurs in 1st year of life.

Sneddon-Champion syndrome (polyarteritis nodosa cutanea): Cutaneous vasculitis affecting males of all ages with painful, pink nodules on skin and variable myalgias, polyneuritis, and arthralgias; no visceral sequelae. Treatment is systemic steroids.

Snell law (law of refraction): $c_1/c_2 = $ sine θ_1/sine θ_2, where θ_1 is angle of incidence of sound approaching interface, θ_2 is angle of retraction, and c_1 and c_2 are propagation velocities of sound in media forming interface.

Snellen E chart: Direct visual testing useful in children over

2 years of age. Visual acuity is measured by showing "Es," which are printed backward and rotated, and having child point with finger in direction letter is "pointing."

Snellen reflex: Ipsilateral ear congestion when distal great auricular nerve is stimulated.

Soave operation: Definitive surgical correction of Hirschsprung disease, which is usu. performed at 6–12 months of age; involves resection of distal aganglionic bowel mucosa. Normal bowel is pulled into anal canal with delayed anastomosis to anal verge. Associated complications (more frequent than with Duhamel procedure) include rectal prolapse (25%), rectal stenosis (20%–25%), enterocolitis (20%–25%), and constipation/anastomotic leakage (5%–10%).

Sock-Barabas syndrome: See Ehlers-Danlos syndrome type 4; characterized by altered synthesis of type 3 collagen.

Soderbergh reflex: Muscular contraction after firm palpation of bones; may be seen in extrapyramidal dysfunction. Examples: flexion of fingers 3–5 when ulna is stroked downward; flexion of thumb when radius is stroked downward.

sodomy: Sexual intercourse with animals; alternate definition is anal intercourse, esp. between males.

Soemmering ring: Doughnut-shaped proliferation of lens fibers sometimes seen after cataract surgery.

Soemmering spot: See Maxwell spot.

Sofield technique: Method for correction of osteogenesis imperfecta of femur; uses multiple osteotomies, realignment of sections, and placement of medullary nails for fixation.

Somogyi effect: Rebound hyperglycemia following episode of hypoglycemia.

Soto-Hall test: See Brudzinski sign.

Sotos syndrome (cerebral gigantism): Symmetrically enlarged head, coarse facial features, congenital gigantism, mental retardation, seizures, poor motor control, and delayed speech; associated with chromosome aberration in 3p21. Condition occurs in both autosomal recessive and dominant forms.

Souques sign: Lack of leg extension when patient sitting in chair is quickly pushed over backward; seen in advanced striatal (extrapyramidal) dysfunction.

Southern blot analysis: Technique used to isolate and analyze DNA; specimen is cut into fragments by restriction enzymes and separated by electrophoresis on agarose gel.

space of Larry: Opening in diaphragm located anteriorly and just off midline through which Morgagni hernia passes.

space of Martegiani: Anatomic area located over optic nerve head.

space of Poirier: Anatomic area (between lunate and capitate) of weakness located on volar aspect of wrist between 2 "V" configurations formed by tendons; traumatic carpal dislocations most commonly occur through space.

space of Retzius: Preperitoneal space anterior to bladder.

Spahr syndrome: Type 1A metaphyseal dysplasia; marked by severe bowing of legs. Condition is autosomal recessive.

Spalding sign (Horner sign): Indication of fetal death in utero if bones of skull are seen to be overriding each other on radiography.

Spalding-Richardson operation: Procedure commonly performed in early 1900s for correction of uterine prolapse; almost never used today.

Spearman correlation coefficient: Statistical measure used to assess significance of differences between groups.

Spencer motion testing: Series of 7 motions effected by examiner to test and isolate glenohumeral motion from gross shoulder motion.

Spielmeyer stain: Iron–alum hematoxylin used to stain erythrocytes and myelin blue-black.

Spielmeyer-Vogt disease (neuronal ceroid–lipofuscinosis type 3): Abnormal accumulation of lipopigment in cells. Age of onset is 5 years, with visual deterioration progressing to psychomotor retardation and seizures. Cause is mutation on chromosome 16p 12.1. Death occurs by 3rd decade.

Spigelian hernia: Hernia at lateral border of rectus at linea semicircularis and superior to inferior epigastric vessels.

Spigelius line: Linea semilunaris.

Splendore-Almeida disease: See Almeida disease.

Splendore-Hoeppli phenomenon: Radiating eosinophilic granular material surrounding ova of schistosomiasis.

Spöndel foramen: Small opening transiently present between lower sphenoid wings and ethmoid bone in developing skull.

Spranger disease (geleophysic dwarfism): Congenital dwarfism, heart abnormalities, hepatosplenomegaly, unusually happy facies, and misshapen hands and feet; possible mucopolysaccharidoses variant. Condition is autosomal recessive. Death usu. occurs in infancy.

Sprague-Dawley rat: Commonly used experimental laboratory animal.

Sprengel deformity: Congenital abnormality of spine marked by failure of normal segmentation.

Sprinz-Nelson syndrome (Sprinz-Dubin syndrome): See Dubin-Johnson syndrome.

Spurling test: Used to detect cervical nerve root entrapment in foramina; positive is pain with neck extension and force placed on top of head.

Squire sign: Indication of basilar meningitis if pupil of eye alternately contracts and dilates.

Srb disease: Congenital aphasia and synostosis of 1st and 2nd ribs, muscle atrophy (1st and 2nd nerve supply), horned manubrium, venous blockage, and chronic pain. Treatment is surgical correction of bone deformity.

Ssabanejew-Frank operation: Method of constructing gastrostomy using section of stomach pulled up to skin and sutured in place through incision in left rectus muscle.

Stahl index: Ranking that describes lunate necrosis by height-to-width ratio of lunate. Stage 1, ratio = 45%; stage 2, ratio = 30%–44%; stage 3, ratio < 30%.

Stahl line: See Hudson-Stähli line.

Stähli pigment: See Hudson-Stähli line.

Stahr gland: Lymph node located next to facial artery.

Stamey procedure: Retropubic urethropexy using needle suspension in stress incontinence in absence of cystocele; uses cystoscope to place sutures precisely at bladder neck and knitted Dacron to reinforce tissue on each side of urethra and to prevent suture pull-out. T-shaped incision is made in anterior vaginal wall, and 2 stab wounds are made in lower abdomen. Stamey needle is then advanced into vaginal incision using fingertip control, and nylon supporting sutures are passed.

Stamey test: Measure of unilateral urine volume and *para*-aminohippurate concentration when assessing kidney.

Stamm gastrostomy: Temporary opening in stomach; performed by placing mushroom catheter through anterior stomach wall, securing with pursestring suture, and exiting skin via stab wound. Catheter should not be removed for 7–10 days to allow for peritoneal sealing.

Stanescu syndrome: Onset from birth of abnormal bone growth (osteopetrosis) resulting in small stature, stunted growth of arms and hands, narrow jaw and maxilla, and depressed frontoparietal sutures; autosomal dominant condition.

Stanford-Binet scale (test): Detailed evaluation used to provide mental age and IQ in persons from 2 years of age–adult; can be used in disabled persons if special guidelines are followed.

Stangel retrograde perfusion cannula: Small, hollow, L-shaped cannula with bulb tip; commonly used to inject dye into distal fimbriae in tubal ligation reversal to delineate previous resection.

Stannius follicle: Thymus-like lymphoid tissue in chicks.

Starling equation: Expression describing filtration of fluid across capillary membrane; net filtration = K_f[(capillary hydrostatic pressure—interstitial hydrostatic pressure) + σ(interstitial oncotic pressure—capillary oncotic pressure)]. K_f = coefficient of filtration.

Starling law: See Frank-Starling reaction.

Starr technique (plication): Method of urethral imbrication to reduce size of pediatric megaurethra; uses surgical folding plication (6–0 Lembert sutures over 12F catheter).

Starr-Edwards mitral prosthesis: Artificial heart valve with ball-valve design; requires chronic anticoagulation of patient. Heart valve lasts longer than tissue valves but is not indicated in women of child-bearing age because of teratogenic effects of warfarin (Coumadin).

Staufer syndrome: Non-metastatic hepatic dysfunction in renal cell carcinoma; affected patients have abnormal liver function tests, fevers, and leukopenia.

Stearns amentia: Amnesia and mental abnormalities caused by alcohol use; similar to delirium tremens but more severe and longer lasting.

Stecher position: Radiographic positioning technique to allow imaging of navicular bone. Prone wrist is placed flat on table with sandbag and film plate underneath hand (elevated to 20°) to bring navicular bone into right angles with x-ray.

Stefan-Boltzmann constant: 5.6699×10^{-8} W/m^2 × °K^4.

Stefan-Boltzmann law: Expression describing total radiation emitted by blackbody at all frequencies. $E = \sigma T^4$, where E is total energy, σ is Stefan-Boltzmann constant, and T is absolute temperature (°K).

Stein-Leventhal syndrome: Polycystic ovarian disease, amenorrhea, obesity, and variable hirsutism; usu. sterility results.

Steiner tumors: See Jeanselme nodules.

Steinert disease (myotonic dystrophy): Muscle wasting in setting of cataract formation.

Steinmann pin: Device inserted through femur or tibia to stabilize fractures.

Stellwag sign: Infrequent and partial blinking due to retraction of upper eyelids; occurs in exophthalmos caused by thyroid goiter.

Stenger test: Used to determine malingering in deafness.

Steno duct: See Stensen duct.

Stensen veins: See Ruysch veins.

Stenson canal (incisive canal): Channel connecting nasal fossae via a large median foramen located anteriorly on hard palate.

Stenson duct (parotid duct): Duct originating from anterior parotid gland, crossing masseter muscle 1 cm below zygoma, penetrating fat and buccinator muscle, and draining into mouth via orifice at midportion of buccal mucosa (opposite crown of 2nd upper molar); structure runs parallel to buccal branch of facial nerve, and lacerations of duct are usu. associated with paralysis in this distribution.

Stent mass: Resin used in surgery to form hard molds to fix grafts in position.

Stephen spots: See Maurer dots.

Stephenson-Gibbs reference: Placement of electrodes at right sternoclavicular junction and C7 spinous process; reduces artifacts caused by heart electrical activity on ECG.

Sterles sign: Increased pulsation of left anterior chest wall; seen in intrathoracic tumors.

Sterling sign: Adduction of normal shoulder against resistance, causing adduction of paretic arm; seen in unilateral arm paresis.

Sternberg sign: Tenderness to palpation over shoulder muscles; seen in inflammation of pleura.

Sternberg task: Test of human memory; person memorizes series of items and must determine if additional item has been included.

Stevens-Johnson syndrome (erythema multiforme): Reaction to variety of initiating factors (e.g., drugs, pregnancy, toxins) with abrupt onset of erythematous eruption of varying nature (e.g., maculopapular, vesicular, bullous); may involve all body linings and cause death. Treatment protocols closely approximate those used in burn patients.

Stewart-Morel syndrome: Episodic, chronic, progressive muscular rigidity.

Stewart-Morel-Morgagni syndrome (metabolic craniopathy): Combination of symmetrical, bilateral thickening of frontal bone and headache, obesity, virilism, and mental disease; most often occurs in middle-aged women.

Stewart-Treves syndrome: Lymphangiosarcoma; usu. occurs as postmastectomy complication within 10 years of procedure in women who had severe lymphedema in 1st year.

Sticker disease (fifth disease): Relatively benign contagious disease occurring in epidemics in children. Initial stage is onset of facial rash, followed by maculopapular rash on extremities and torso; as rash fades, distinctive lace-like pattern is evident. Condition is more clinically significant in immunocompromised patients. Cause is human parvovirus B19.

Stickler syndrome (type 1): Hypoplastic mandible, myopia, scoliosis, cleft palate, and arthritis; autosomal dominant condition. Defect is in type 2 collagen.

Stickler syndrome (type 2): Same as type 1 with absence of eye manifestations. Defect in type 9 collagen.

Stieda fracture: Fracture of medial femoral condyle with avulsion due to origin of tibial collateral ligament. Type 1, radiographic density parallel to medial femoral condyle; type 2 (occurs more frequently), delayed response to injury causing ossification next to medial femoral condyle at point where femoral shaft widens to form medial condyle.

Stierlin sign: Radiographic finding highly suggestive of intestinal TB. Absence of barium from involved bowel segment (usu. ranging from ileum to right colon) with normal-appearing adjacent bowel segments is due to hypermotility with spasm of segments.

Stifel figures: Black disks with central white spot used to locate blind spot.

Still disease: Collagen vascular disease with fever spikes in conjunction with pinkish rash on trunk; marked by increased sedimentation rate, anemia, leukocytosis, arthralgias, pleuritis, pericarditis, lymphadenopathy and splenomegaly. Treatment is aspirin and NSAIDs.

Still murmur: Midsystolic crescendo–decrescendo murmur heard in pulmonic area in children and young adults; considered benign if not accompanied by signs or symptoms of cardiac disease.

Stiller rib: Abnormally movable 10th rib on palpation.

Stilling nucleus: Group of nerve cells on ventrolateral periphery of nucleus dorsalis (Clarkes nucleus), esp. lower portion.

Stillwag sign: Infrequent blinking in Graves disease.

Stillwagon groups: Prognosis-based assessment of malignant liver tumors using 5 adverse criteria: alkaline phosphatase > 95 IU/L, AST (SGOT) > 35 IU/L, bilirubin > 1.4 mg/dl, Karnofsky status < 80%, and presence of ascites. 0–2 criteria: favorable prognosis; $\geq$ 3 criteria: unfavorable prognosis.

Stimmler syndrome: Rare congenital disorder with increased urine excretion of alanine, dwarfism, diabetes mellitus, small teeth, microcephaly, and mental retardation; autosomal recessive condition.

Stimson technique: Safe, commonly used method to reduce anterior dislocation of humerus at shoulder; requires constant observation and moni-

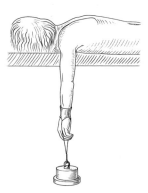

Stimson technique

toring of vital signs. Weights of 10–15 lb are applied over 20–30-minute period. If reduction is not effected after 30 minutes, humerus is rotated externally and then internally with mild force.

Stocker sign: Used to differentiate typhoid fever and meningitis caused by TB. In typhoid fever, patient takes no notice if bedclothes are removed. In tubercular meningitis, patient immediately pulls up bedclothes.

Stocker-Hol disease: See Maumenee dystrophy.

Stockholm technique: System of intrauterine application of cesium or radium (intracavitary brachytherapy) for treatment of cervical cancer. Radioactive implants are left in place for 12–36 hours 2–3 times/week for several weeks. No radium is placed in lower cervical canal.

Stokes amputation: See Gritti-Stokes amputation.

Stokes-Adams syncope: Altered mental status in aortic stenosis.

Stone intestinal anastomosis clamp: Device with metal "alligator" jaws with hinge on 1 side used to occlude bowel; closed by small, oval locking device placed over ends via Stone clamp–applying forceps.

Stone staple: 4-pronged sterile surgical staple; used most commonly for anchoring tendinous tissue to bone.

Stookey rongeur: Narrow-jawed, wide-opening rongeur; typically used to perform foraminotomy in spinal surgery.

Stoppa hernia repair: Preperitoneal, tension-free technique using prosthetic material; useful in bilateral, simultaneous repairs.

Storm Van Leeuwen chamber: Room that is free of airborne antigens; used to treat patients with allergies.

Stransky-Regala syndrome: 1940s term to describe chronic hemolytic anemia occurring in Philippines.

Strassman phenomenon: Engorgement of umbilical vein when placenta fails to detach from uterus; occurs in 3rd stage of labor.

Strassman procedure (unification): Surgical treatment of bicornuate uterus; uses transverse incision from cornu to cornu. Medial wall of each cavity is severed, and myometrium is closed in 3 layers. Vasopressin is injected into incision line before cutting to decrease bleeding.

Straub technique: Method of measuring force of eyelid closure.

Straus sign: Reaction used to differentiate central and peripheral origins of facial paralysis. When pilocarpine is injected into affected muscles, perspiration is unchanged in central etiology and altered in peripheral lesions.

Streeter bands: Amniotic bands formed from rupture of amnion that cause intrauterine necrosis and amputation or severe deformities of limbs or, less commonly, head; associated with anterior abdominal wall malformations, imperforate anus, meningomyelocele, and hypoplastic lungs.

Streeter dysplasia: Congenital bands of skin on torso or limbs.

Strome method (uvulopalatopharyngoplasty): Enlargement of oropharyngeal airspace by excising redundant soft tissues of palate and pharyngeal side walls; similar to Moran method of posterior pillar excision with addition of lateral wedge resection of palatal tissues (to reduce nasopharyngeal stenosis).

Stromeyer cephalhematocele: Subperiosteal tissue mass with communication to venous sinuses; becomes engorged with blood on strong expiratory effort.

Stromeyer hook: Device used for elevation of zygomatic arch fractures.

Strübing-Marchiafava disease: See Marchiafava-Micheli syndrome.

Strümpell reflex (Babinski pronator phenomenon, radialis sign): Closing of fingers causes dorsiflexion of wrist; seen in unilateral arm paresis.

Strümpell sign (tibialis sign): When patient is lying supine and quickly draws normal knee up to chest, paretic foot inverts and dorsiflexes, and toes may dorsiflex (normal reaction is plantar flexion); seen in unilateral leg paresis.

Strumpell-Marie disease: Rheumatoid arthritis.

Stryker needle: Device used to measure intramuscular compartment pressures when evaluating need for fasciotomy. After needle is placed, syringe handle is depressed until meniscus inside syringe moves. Value on pressure scale equals intramuscular pressure.

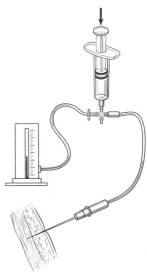

Stryker needle

Stuart-Prower factor: Factor X of clotting cascade.

Stulberg method: Measure of roundness of femoral head in Perthes disease.

Sturge-Weber syndrome:
Mental retardation, facial nevus, facial port-wine stain (usu. unilateral), seizures (often refractory), hemiparesis, meningeal calcifications, angiomatosis conversion of ovary, lungs, and GI tract, and glaucoma. Disorder is due to angiomatosis disease throughout body.

Sudan stain: Substance used to determine fat content of feces.

Sudan III stain: Component of bichromic fat stain; stains neutral fat red.

Sudeck disease (reflex sympathetic dystrophy): Often severe pain, swelling, and trophic changes to extremity; follows apparently mild trauma to extremity.

Sudeck point: Area of distal sigmoid colon between last sigmoid artery and superior rectal artery; initially thought to be at risk for ischemic colitis, but probably of minimal clinical significance.

Sugita frame: Stereotactic system used in brain surgery.

Sugiura procedure: Treatment for intractable variceal bleeds. Uses devascularization of esophagus to level of inferior pulmonary vein and devascularization of proximal 2/3 of stomach, splenectomy, selective vagotomy, and pyloroplasty or highly selective vagotomy without pyloroplasty. Left gastric (coronary) vein is preserved, hepatic function is not compromised, and no encephalopathy occurs. Operative mortality is 5%–10% if procedure is per-

formed electively and 25% if performed nonelectively. Results have been superior in Japan.

Suker sign: Defective complementary fixation when eye is moved laterally; seen in exophthalmos due to thyroid goiter.

sulcus of Reil (limiting sulcus): Sulcus that circumscribes island of Reil in floor of lateral (sylvian) fissure.

Sumner sign: Increased rigidity of abdominal muscles when iliac fossa is palpated; seen in appendicitis, nephrolithiasis, and twisted ovarian cyst.

Sundt aneurysm clip: Small metal device placed on brain aneurysms to occlude lumen.

Suresnes hemoglobin: High-oxygen-affinity hemoglobin resulting from replacement of arginine by histidine in $\alpha_1\beta_2$ contact area; hemoglobin levels are 15–16.5 g/dl.

Suruga modification: Variation of Kasai procedure for surgical treatment of biliary atresia; 1st described in 1977. Best results are obtained if procedure is performed in 1st 8 weeks of life.

Sutherland wrap: Treatment for snakebite; uses broad, constrictive wrap over bitten area and around immobilized limb, which collapses lymphatics and superficial veins.

Sutter antigen: See Kell blood group.

Sutton disease (major aphthous ulcer): Large (> 3 cm), recurrent, painful ulcers in mucosa of oral cavity, vagina, and GI tract, including anus. Cause is mucosal injury. Condition is more common in women.

Sutton disease (halo nevus): Circle of hypopigmented skin surrounding benign or malignant nevus; most commonly seen with nevi on torso.

Sutton law: Best way to diagnose condition is to "look for it where it should be."

Swan syndrome (blind spot syndrome): Physiologic adjustment of eyes that allows projection of image of nondeviating eye onto blind spot of deviating eye.

Swan-Ganz catheter: Pulmonary artery catheter commonly used to assess hemodynamic status of cardiovascular system. Placement is through Cordis catheter in internal jugular or subclavian veins; after tip is advanced to 20 cm, balloon is inflated with 2–3 ml of air, and catheter is slowly advanced through right atrium and into pulmonary vein, with characteristic waveforms given off at each location. Catheter is then slowly advanced further until inflated balloon becomes "wedged" into branch of pulmonary artery, with obliteration of pulmonary artery waveform. Once correctly positioned, preload status (central venous pressure), cardiac contractility (cardiac output and index), and afterload status (systemic vascular resistance) can be determined. Balloon must always be deflated when in place if readings are not being taken.

Swank diet: Low-fat diet used to retard progress and reduce exacerbations of multiple sclerosis; consists of < 10 g saturated fat/day, 1 tsp cod liver oil/day, and fish 3 times/week.

Swanson syndrome: Congenital insensibility to pain, mental retardation, self-mutilating behavior, and lack of sweating after physical activity; possibly related to abnormal differentiation of neural crest.

Swediauer disease: Inflammation and pain in Achilles tendon.

Swedish knee cage: Knee orthosis for support in mild-to-moderate genu recurvatum, ligament laxity, and capsular laxity; uses 3-point system of motion. Articulated version allows knee flexion but not hyperextension.

Sweeley-Klionsky disease: See Fabry disease.

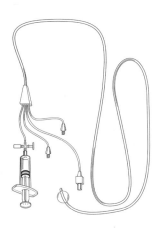

Swan-Ganz catheter

Sweet syndrome: Painful lesions on neck, torso, and limbs in setting of fever.

Swenson operation: Definitive surgical correction of Hirschsprung disease; usu. performed at 6–12 months of age. Normal ganglionic bowel is intussuscepted through abnormal bowel and out anus with resection of aganglionic bowel. Anastomosis is performed under direct vision and requires mobilization of rectum to level of levators and dissection around bladder. Good results have been reported with laparoscopic technique.

Swift disease (acrodynia): Disease of infants with erythema of trunk, nose, and extremities. Also with neurologic abnormalities and GI symptoms. Disorder is seen almost exclusively in mercury poisoning.

Swiss blue (Helvetia blue, methyl blue): Water-soluble stain used to visualize collagen (as component of Masson trichrome stain) and connective tissue (as component of Mallory technique).

Swiss tapeworm: *Diphyllobothrium madagascariensis;* human pathogen.

Swiss-type agammaglobulinemia (severe combined immunodeficiency syndrome, SCID): Rare congenital defect in both cell-mediated and humoral defenses in which vaccinations cause fatal infections and blood transfusions cause graft-versus-host disease; autosomal recessive condition.

Swube test: Application of sticky tape to perianal area for evaluation of *Enterobius*.

Sydenham chorea: Degenerative neurological disease with acute onset at 5–15 years of age; often seen in setting of infection, esp. viral encephalitis. Condition is marked by involuntary movements (increased with volition), emotional disturbances, and facial grimaces causing difficulty talking and eating, with variable presence of pseudotumor cerebri.

Syed-Noblett template: Template used to guide transperineal placement of multiple hollow 18-gauge needles into parametrial tissues for treatment of advanced cervical cancer. Iridium wires are then "afterloaded."

sylvian aqueduct (aqueduct of mesencephalon): Small-diameter opening in mesencephalon that connects 3rd and 4th ventricle.

sylvian fissure: Lateral fissure in cerebral hemisphere; deepest and most conspicuous of all brain fissures.

sylvian fossa: Embryologic invagination of lateral aspect of cerebral hemisphere during 2nd month of gestation; marks beginning of formation of sylvian fissure.

sylvian point: Point in brain topography on lateral surface of cerebral hemisphere where sylvian fissure stem divides into 3 separate branches.

Sylvian vein: Vein draining cerebral matter that runs close to sylvian (lateral) fissure and middle cerebral artery.

Syme amputation: Partial resection of foot usu. performed after severe trauma; does not require healthy plantar skin distally but is indicated for distal foot or toe infection. Procedure is contraindicated for any heel abnormality, including neuropathy. Surgery was originally described as 1-stage operation, but 2-stage Wagner modification is now most commonly performed because of better stump fitting and cosmesis. Heel pad must be anchored to bone with

reduction of soft tissue dog ears.

Syme prosthesis: Artificial foot and ankle with removable medial window to allow patient to push stump into socket; uses solid ankle cushion heel-type foot. Gait speed is decreased by 32%, and oxygen consumption is increased by 13%.

Syracuse hemoglobin: High-oxygen-affinity hemoglobin resulting from replacement of histidine by proline in 2,3-DPG–binding area; hemoglobin levels are 19–24 g/dl.

Taenzer-Unna stain: Hydrochloric acid, orcein, and methylene blue used to visualize elastic fibers; stains elastic fibers dark brown to black.

tail of Spence: Breast tissue extending into axilla, which can enlarge under hormonal stimulation; must be removed in modified radical mastectomy.

Takahara disease (acatalasia): Chronic, progressive mouth infections, sometimes leading to frank gangrene of oral cavity; caused by systemic catalase deficiency. Condition

is most commonly seen in Japan and Korea. Diagnosis is made if black-brown color results on addition of hydrogen peroxide to catalase-deficient blood. Treatment is surgery, antibiotics, and topical and systemic catalase administration.

Takatsuki disease: See Crow-Fukase syndrome.

Takayasu arteritis: Inflammatory disease of media and adventitia of thoracic aorta and branches; marked by hypertension, intermittent claudication of upper extremities, visual defects, and syncope. Presenting findings may include chronic fatigue, low-grade fever, and absent radial pulses. Laboratory tests reveal moderate leukocytosis, thrombocytosis, transient eosinophilia, and increased sedimentation rate. Condition is most common in young Asian women. In early stages, treatment is steroids. In advanced cases, bypass grafts are necessary.

Talairach system: Stereotactic system used in brain surgery.

Talma syndrome: Acquired, prolonged muscular contraction after mechanical or electrical stimulation; relaxation of muscle is delayed. Treatment is quinine and procaine.

Tamai procedure: See Gilbert repair.

Tamm-Horsfall protein: Constituent of hyaline casts; normally secreted from loop of Henle.

Tanaka modification: Variant of Kasai procedure; used to palliate biliary atresia.

Tangier disease: Abnormal cholesterol uptake by macrophages with fatty liver, hepatomegaly, orange-colored tonsils, cloudy corneas, and intermittent neurologic deficits; childhood onset is typical.

Tanner stages: System that describes development of secondary sexual characteristics in puberty. *Girls*—stage 1 (preadolescent), breast papillae elevation only and vellus pubic hair only; stage 2, breast bud elevation and sparse, slightly coarsened pubic hair; stage 3, enlargement of breast mound and darkening and curling of pubic hair; stage 4, elevation of areola and papilla to form second mound above breast tissue and adult-type pubic hair without spread to inner thighs; stage 5 (adult), rounding of breast mound with recession on areola to mound of breast tissue and spread of adult-type pubic hair to inner thighs. *Boys*—stage 1 (preadolescent), genitalia of same size and proportion as in early childhood; stage 2, reddening and coarsening of scrotal skin and slight enlargement of testes and scrotum; stage 3, growth of penis in length initially followed by some increase in breadth with further increase in size of scrotum and testes; stage 4, development of glans with further enlargement of penis; stage 5 (adult), genitalia of adult size and shape.

Tanret test: Used to detect albumin; positive if addition of Tanret reagent to sample produces white precipitate.

Tanyol sign: Downward displacement of umbilicus by ascites.

Tapia syndrome: Dysarthria and dysphagia caused by ipsilateral paralysis of vocal cord, tongue, and soft palate; due to injury or lesion affecting CNs XII and/or X.

Tardieu spots (petechiae): Subpleural ecchymosis occurring in death due to suffocation.

Tarin anterior recess (Tarin recess, Tarinus recess): Anterior portion of Tarin fossa.

Tarin fascia (Tarini fascia, Tarinus fascia): Dentate gyrus; strip of gray matter lying deep to medial edge of hippocampus.

Tarin fossa (Tarini fossa, Tarinus fossa): Groove lying between cerebral peduncles and immediately above posterior perforated substance.

Tarin posterior recess (Tarini recess, Tarinus recess): Posterior portion of Tarin fossa.

Tarin velum (Tarini velum, Tarinus velum): Inferior medullary velum; thin strip of white matter located on both sides of vermis. Medial surface forms part of lower wall of 4th ventricle and fuses anteriorly with choroid plexus and laterally with pedunculus flocculi.

Tarlov cyst (perineural cyst): Clear fluid–containing cyst that does not communicate with subarachnoid space and occurs on posterior coccygeal or sacral nerve roots; can destroy nervous tissue. Diagnosis is by MRI. Treatment is prompt excision.

Tarral-Besnier syndrome: See Devergie syndrome.

Tarrant position: Radiographic patient positioning technique useful in elderly or multiply injured patients; involves projection of clavicle (above rib cage).

Tarui disease (muscle phosphofructokinase deficiency): Type 7 glycogen storage disease; marked by exercise intolerance in childhood, hemolysis, and hyperuricemia. Deficiency is in M isoenzyme of phosphofructokinase, with complete absence in muscle and partial deficiency in blood.

Taussig-Bing disease (syndrome; incomplete transposition of the great arteries): Rare congenital condition in which aorta and pulmonary artery both arise from right ventricle; also involves ventricular septal defect below pulmonic valve and variable degree of pulmonic stenosis. Main symptom is cyanosis.

Tawara node (node of Aschoff and Tawara): See Aschoff node.

Tay spot (sign; cherry-red spot): Red circle surrounded by grayish retina found in infantile amaurotic idiocy. Condition is autosomal recessive.

Tay syndrome: Congenital ichthyosiform erythroderma, brittle hair, dysplastic nails, cataracts, ataxia, scant subcutaneous fat, and mental and growth retardation; autosomal recessive condition.

Tay-Sachs disease: Deficiency of hexosaminidase, causing accumulation of GM_2 gangliosides in lysosomes; characterized by loss of motor skills and macular cherry-red spot on slit-lamp examination. Incidence is increased in Ashkenazi Jews.

Taybi syndrome [otopalatodigital syndrome (OPD)]: Mild mental retardation, conductive deafness, elbow contracture, small stature, cleft palate, and stubby fingers and toes. Defect is in OpDI gene in Xq28.

Taybi-Lindner syndrome: Congenital abnormalities of brain (e.g., absent corpus callosum, parasagittal hemisphere defect), dwarfism, spade-like hands and feet, convulsions, and skeletal dysplasia.

Taylor orthosis: Commonly used thoracolumbosacral brace; restricts flexion and extension but requires axillary straps to be extremely tight to limit thoracic motion.

Taylor retractor: L-shaped retractor with sharp point at long end; used in spinal surgery to retract paraspinal muscles.

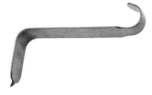

Taylor retractor

Taylor test: Variation of Schönbein test; positive for blood if addition of ether or alcohol causes blue precipitate to form purplish color.

Taylor vein patch: Elliptical vein segment sutured to roof of distal prosthetic graft that is anastomosed to native vessel; decreases effects of anastomotic intimal hyperplasia.

Teevan law: Bone fractures occur along lines of extension rather than compression.

Teichmann test: Used to detect blood; positive if hematin crystals develop when sample is mixed with salt crystals and glacial acetic acid, placed under glass, and heated and then cooled.

Telfer syndrome: Association of dominant piebald trait with neurologic impairment; also with mild-to-moderate mental retardation and variable deafness. Condition is autosomal dominant.

Tellyesnicky solution: Acid fixative composed of formalin, glacial acetic acid, 95% ethanol, and tap H_2O; used for most gynecologic surgical pathology specimens.

Temtamy syndrome (type A4 brachydactyly): Absent middle phalanges of 2nd–5th fingers and toes and mild radial clinodactyly of 4th and 5th fingers; autosomal dominant condition.

Tenckhoff catheter: Thin, hollow, Silastic tube usu. placed into peritoneal cavity for peritoneal dialysis; also occasionally used to drain ascites in patients who are not candidates for liver transplantation.

tendon of Hector: Calcaneus tendon.

tendon of Todaro: Variably present collections of small fibers (often multiple) originating in central fibrous body of right atria and ending in eustachian valve; forms 1 side of triangle of Koch. Tendon is sometimes used as anatomic landmark in electrophysiologic studies.

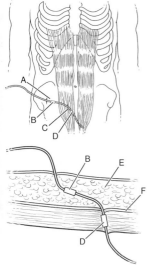

A. Subcutaneous tunnel
B. Proximal cuff
C. Incision site
D. Distal cuff
E. Subcutaneous tissue
F. Fascia

Tencknoff catheter

Tenon capsule (fascia bulbi): Fibrous tissue lining hollow in front of orbital fat; covers posterior 3/4 of eyeball and merges with sheath of optic nerve.

Tenon space: Lymph-containing space between sclera and fascia of eyeball that permits free movement of eyeball within capsule; becomes obliterated where posterior ciliary vessels and nerves perforate sclera.

Ter-Pogossian camera: Early instrument used in radionuclide imaging.

Terman test: See Stanford-Binet scale.

Terrien marginal degeneration (gutter dystrophy): Acute onset of eye pain, photophobia, excessive tearing, and hyperemia of conjunctiva; attacks last 2–7 days. Slit-lamp examination shows peripheral yellowish punctate lesions. Vision may eventually decrease after repeated attacks.

Terrien-Viel disease (Posner-Schlossman disease): Unilateral recurrent glaucoma.

Terry nails (half-and-half nails): Proximal nail bed is white with distal half pink; seen in congestive heart failure, low albumin–associated cirrhosis, and uremia.

Terry syndrome: Red-brown transverse bands on fingernails, azotemia, and cirrhosis.

Terry syndrome (retrolental fibroplasia): Visual loss, including blindness, in infants who breathe oxygen-rich air; premature infants are esp. vulnerable. (Rarely, infants who have not received oxygen therapy may also develop visual problems.)

Terry-Thomas sign: Abnormal gap between lunate and scaphoid bones seen on anterior-posterior radiograph of wrist; most common type of post-traumatic wrist instability.

Terson syndrome: Intravitreal hemorrhage; commonly seen in ruptured intracranial aneurysms.

tesla: SI unit of magnetic flux density; 1 tesla = 10,000 gauss.

tetralogy of Fallot: Congenital right ventricular hypertrophy, pulmonic stenosis, ventricular septal defect, and overriding aorta; leads to cyanosis and right-to-left shunt. Condition may also be associated with absent pulmonary artery (usu. left) and hypoplasia of ipsilateral thoracic cavity. Defect is slightly more common in males. Squatting relieves symptoms. Palliative operations are Blalock-Taussig shunt and aortopulmonary window.

Teutschlander disease (interstitial calcinosis): Abnormal calcium deposits in skin, muscle, tendon, nerves, and subcutaneous fat; viscera are rarely involved. Onset occurs in childhood or early adolescence. Condition is most common in periarticular areas. Progression to tender, painful skin over calcium deposits leads to ulcers with extrusion of chalky material. Disease is associated with collagen vascular disease and has chronic, indolent course.

Thal patch: Rotation flap of wedge of stomach fundus; used to reinforce primary suture line

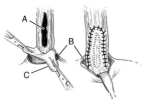

A. Perforation in
   esophagus
B. Diaphragm
C. Flap of fundus

Thal patch

in repair of perforated distal esophagus above diaphragm.

Thal procedure: Antireflux procedure using 270° gastric wrap around esophagus; less commonly performed than Nissen fundoplication.

Thanos syndrome: Mental retardation, epidermal nevus, epibulbar dermoids, bony exostoses, craniosynostosis, myopia, wide-set eyes, and kyphoscoliosis.

Thayer-Martin medium (agar): Modification of chocolate blood agar with addition of antibiotics; used to culture *Neisseria gonorrhoeae* and *N. meningitidis*.

Thebesius foramina: Multiple small openings in septal and right lateral walls of right atria.

Thebesius valve: Thin, membranous lip at edge of coronary sinus.

Theile canal (transverse pericardial sinus): Anatomic space lined by thin serous pericardium lying in front of atria and behind pulmonary trunk and aorta.

Theile gland: Small invaginations in walls of cystic duct and gallbladder neck.

Thibierge-Weissenbach disease: Calcinosis, Raynaud phenomenon, Esophageal pathology, Sclerodactyly, and Telangiectasia (CREST syndrome). Slowly progressive condition, which is more common in women; onset usu. occurs in 4th–5th decade with hand symptoms. Treatment is palliative (steroids, plasma-pheresis, azathioprine).

Thieffry-Sorrell-Dejerine syndrome: Hereditary osteolysis; also associated with hypertension, marfanoid appearance, micrognathia, scoliosis, overlapping toes, and plantar cysts. Disorder begins in childhood, with painless and progressive loss of bone in carpal and tarsal bones. Inheritance occurs in both sporadic and autosomal dominant patterns.

Thiel-Benhke corneal dystrophy (corneal dystrophy of Bowman layer type 2): Honeycomb-shaped arrangement of "squiggly" filaments developing in superficial cornea; causes pain, corneal erosion, and vision loss (usu. less severe than in Reis-Bucklers dystrophy).

Thiemann disease: Aseptic necrosis of proximal phalanges.

Thiersch operation: Procedure used for surgical correction of rectal prolapse.

Thiersch procedure: Rarely performed procedure for correction of anal incontinence; uses Dacron-impregnated Silastic sling encircling anal canal.

Thies-Schwarz disease: Onset of eruptive milia on face and neck; usu. comedos return after removal.

Thoma-Zeiss apparatus: See Abbé-Zeiss apparatus.

Thomas ampulla: Dilation of distal arterial capillaries in spleen.

Thomas heel: Heel device used in flatfoot, with curved, elevated extension used for arch support.

Thomas splint (adjustable): Device with metallic parallel rings at thigh and ankle with rods of adjustable length running between; used to stabilize fractures in field.

Thomas syndrome: Clinical manifestation of Marie-Bamberger disease in setting of hypothyroidism.

Thomas test: Failure of foot flexion with palpation of gastrocnemius/soleus muscle (with knee resting on chair and leg bent at 90°); positive in ruptured Achilles tendon.

Thomas test: Used to determine degree of flexion deformity of spine; also sometimes described in terms of detecting flexion contracture of hip. Supine patient brings 1 knee to chest and purposefully flattens lumbar spine. Bending of contralateral straight leg indicates contracture of contralateral side.

Thompson approach: Posterior surgical approach to radius. Skin incision is made from lateral epicondyle to Lister tubercle. Tissue dissection is performed at level of midshaft, proximally through deep fascia between extensor carpi radialis brevis and extensor digitorum communis, with avoidance of injury to posterior interosseous nerve. Supinator and pronator teres are incised, and abductor pollicus longus and extensor pollicis brevis are not detached from origins.

Thompson atrophy: Congenital optic atrophy marked by nystagmus and blindness; autosomal dominant condition.

Thompson line: Reddish streak on gums; sometimes seen in pulmonary TB.

Thompson test (Achilles squeeze test, Simmons test): Used to detect patency of Achilles tendon; positive for intact Achilles tendon if squeezing calf muscle causes ankle flexion.

Thomsen disease (myotonia congenita dominant inheritance): Muscle disease with stiffness and hypertrophy of muscles in absence of weakness; autosomal dominant condition. 15% of cases are due to defects in chloride channel gene (ClC-1) on chromosome 7.

Thomsen disease (preaxial polydactyly type 4): Dysplastic distal phalanges marked by central hole.

Thomson sign: See Pastia sign.

Thomson syndrome: Oculocutaneous disorder marked by skin changes identical to Rothmund disease without presence of cataracts; autosomal recessive condition.

Thoraeus filter: Radiographic filter made of tin, copper, and aluminum layers that absorbs some energy from x-ray beam used to treat deep tissues.

Thormählen test: Used to detect melanin in urine; positive if blue color develops when sample is mixed with acetic acid, sodium nitroprusside, and potassium hydroxide.

Thorn disease: Renal failure that simulates adrenocortical insufficiency; salt intake becomes less than urinary salt loss.

Thorndike tests (CAVD tests): Battery of tests that measure academic intelligence by assessing abilities in Completion, Arithmetic, Vocabulary, and Directions.

Thornton sign: Severe pain in ipsilateral flank region; seen with kidney stones.

Thornwaldt abscess: Chronic inflammation and infection of pharyngeal tissues.

Throckmorton sign: Corticospinal tract response characterized by dorsiflexion of toes; elicited by tapping over metacarpophalangeal joint of big toe, slightly medial to extensor hallucis longus tendon.

Thudichum test: Used to detect creatine; positive if red color develops when sample is mixed with dilute ferric chloride solution.

Thurman-Hillier syndrome: Congenital cardiac defect with communication between left ventricle and right atrium in membranous septum inferior to crista supraventricularis; variable location but usu. below level of tricuspid annulus. Patients are susceptible to recurrent respiratory infections, bacterial endo-carditis, and heart failure.

Thurston defect: Oral–facial–digital defect type 5; marked by median cleft of vermilion border of upper lip.

Thurston Holland fragment: Triangular metaphyseal fragment, sometimes associated with epiphysis fragment in epiphyseal separation.

Thygeson disease: Superficial punctate keratitis marked by bilateral corneal lesions; suspected viral etiology.

tic de Guinon: See Gilles de la Tourette syndrome.

Tice strain: Widely used strain of Calmette-Guérin bacillus; useful in treating some types of bladder cancer.

Tidy test: Used to detect albumin in urine; positive if white precipitate forms when sample is mixed with 15 drops of alcohol and 15 drops of phenol.

Tièche-Jadassohn nevus (blue nevus): Solitary, benign, oval, dark blue nevus with sharp border. Treatment is excision.

Tiedemann nerve: Sympathetic nerve plexus around central artery of retina.

Tieman-Jewett nail: Type of 3-flanged nail with side plate; used in hip fracture repairs.

Tietze syndrome: Painful swelling in costochondral articulations; onset usu. before 40 years of age.

Tikhoff-Linberg procedure: Surgical resection of distal clavi-cle, upper humerus, and all or part of scapula for treatment of high-grade osteosarcoma and soft tissue sarcoma of shoulder girdle and proximal humerus; contraindicated if neurovascular bundle is involved. Procedure involves elliptical incision from anterior shoulder to just proximal to antecubital fossa, with variable use of prosthesis. Postop patient usu. retains some elbow and hand function.

Tile classification: System used to describe pelvic fractures. Type A—stable, minimal displacement; type B1 (stage 1)—absence of posterior injury, symphysis pubis disruption < 2.5 cm; type B1 (stage 2)—unilateral disruption of symphysis pubis > 2.5 cm; type B1 (stage 3)—disruption of symphysis pubis > 2.5 cm, with disruption of bilateral sacrospinous and anterior sacroiliac ligament; type B2—lateral compression with posterior crush injury and anterior rami fracture; type B3 (bucket handle injury)—major anterior injury contralateral to major posterior injury; type C—fracture that is both rotational and vertically unstable.

Tiling-Wernicke disease: 1920s term for ophthalmoplegia.

Tillaux-Kleiger fracture: Fracture of distal lateral tibia; fracture line runs vertically and extends through articular surface.

Tinel sign (formication sign): Occurrence of paresthesias in palm, index, middle, or ring fingers as result of tapping over course of median nerve, with center of wrist held in supine position; used to diagnose carpal tunnel syndrome.

Tixier-Hutinel anemia: Early 1900s term for fulminant hemolysis in newborns.

Tizzoni test: Used to detect iron in tissues; positive if blue color develops when specimen is treated with 2% potassium ferrocyanide solution and 0.5% hydrochloric acid solution.

Todani modification: Variation of Alonso-Lej classification used to describe choledochal cysts. Type 1, fusiform enlargement of extrahepatic bile ducts; type 2, diverticulum off extrahepatic common bile duct; type 3, enlargement of common bile duct segment within duodenal wall (choledochocele); type 4,

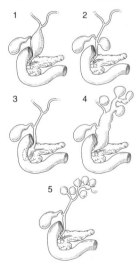

Todani modification

multiple cystic enlargements in both intra- and extrahepatic ducts; type 5, enlargement of intrahepatic ducts only.

Todd body: Eosinophilic cytoplasmic inclusions found in amphibian erythrocytes.

Todd paralysis: Post–jacksonian seizure paralysis; usu. involves same limb as preceding seizure. Condition lasts several hours to days before resolving.

Todd units: Units used to report serum titer of antistreptolysin O produced by group A streptococci; standardization often varies among laboratories.

Toglia dysostosis: Rare open skull sutures, flat nose, spadelike hands, and stubby fingers.

Tollens-Neuberg-Schwket test: Used to detect presence of uronic acid; involves variation of orcinol test.

Tolosa-Hunt syndrome: Palsy of CNs III, IV, V-1, and VI; secondary to acute idiopathic inflammation close to superior fissure, orbital sinus, and cavernous sinus. Condition also causes pain and ophthalmoplegia. Treatment is systemic corticosteroids.

Tomes granular layer: Lamina of partially calcified dentin with intermixed small globular spaces; lies immediately deep to dentinocemental junction in tooth root.

Tomes processes: Granular segment of dentinal end of ameloblast; releases enamel rod matrix.

Tommasi sign: Loss of hair on external/posterior legs; seen in men with gout.

Tommy John surgery: Transfer of a wrist tendon to replace damaged ulnar collateral ligament; most commonly performed in throwing arm of high-level baseball pitchers.

Tompkins procedure: Correction of bicornuate uterus by dividing septum along entire length and incorporating into closure; no uterine tissue is excised. Procedure is relatively avascular because incision is in midline.

Tönnis system: Grading system that describes radiographic appearance of hip dysplasia. Grade 1, mild dysplasia and subluxation; grade 2, lateral displacement of femoral head ossification center that lies inferior to superolateral edge of true acetabulum.

Topinard angle: See Broca angle.

Topinard line: Imaginary line running from center of smooth area on frontal bone between eyebrows (glabella) to most anterior point on sagittal chin contour (pogonion).

Torg syndrome: Familial multicentric osteolysis with flexion contractures of limbs and fusiform enlargement of digits; autosomal recessive condition.

Toriello syndrome (brachial arch syndrome): Mental retardation, short stature, webbed neck, bilateral deafness, microcephaly, low-set ears, variable subvalvular pulmonic stenosis, and variable cryptorchidism; X-linked inheritance.

Tornwaldt bursa (Tornwaldt cyst): See Luschka bursa.

Tornwaldt bursitis: Chronic inflammation of nasopharynx and pharyngeal recess; causes occipital headache and abscess of tonsils. Treatment is antibiotics and/or surgery.

Torres-Teixeira bodies: Cytoplasmic inclusions seen in variola minor.

Torquay test: Used to detect bile; positive if blue color changes to red when sample is mixed with 1:2000 dilution of methyl violet.

Toti operation: Procedure used to correct stenosis of lacrimal duct.

Toupay procedure: Antireflux operation using 270° wrap of gastric fundus around esophagus; less commonly performed than Nissen fundoplication.

Touraine disease: See Behçet syndrome.

Touraine syndrome: Association of retinal angioid streaks and cardiovascular pathology; considered to be part of Groenblod-Strandberg-Touraine syndrome.

Touraine syndrome (purpura telangiectasia arciformes): Variant of Majocchi disease but with fewer and larger arciform lesions.

Touraine-Solente-Gole syndrome: Primary form of osteoarthropathy marked by clubbing of fingers, new bone formation, and synovial effusions; skin becomes thickened and coarse with deep nasolabial folds. Onset occurs at puberty, and symptoms abate in adulthood.

Tourette syndrome: See Gilles de la Tourette syndrome.

Tournay sign: Unilateral pupil dilation of abducting eye; seen in extreme lateral fixation of eyes.

Touton cell: Giant multinucleated cell seen in adipose tissue with chronic resorbing inflammation; occurs in xanthogranulomatous disease.

tower of Hanoi (Burmese pyramid): Intellectual puzzle used in neuropsychological testing, esp. in cases of amnesia; evaluates nondeclarative sequence learning (planning and development of strategic approach). Aim is to move small collection of stacked disks that form pyramid completely to another pile. Disks can be placed into only 3 piles, and no disk can be placed on top of a smaller one.

Towne view: Half-axial radiographic position used in vertebral artery angiography; allows posterior cerebral arteries and superior cerebellar arteries to be projected above petrous bone.

Towne-Brocks syndrome: Imperforate anus, sensorineural deafness, hypoplastic thumbs, fusion of metatarsal bones, malformed ears, and variable hypoplastic kidney.

Townley prosthesis: Knee replacement with maximum freedom of motion of joint; requires good soft tissue stability.

Toynbee law: When otitis extends into brain parenchyma, mastoid pathology affects lateral sinuses and cerebellum, and tympanic roof pathology affects cerebrum.

Toynbee otoscope: Device for inspection of ear canal; uses narrow tube to auscultate during politzerization.

Toynbee phenomenon: Air and secretions forced into middle ear by swallowing with both mouth and nose closed.

Trantas dots: Small milky specks seen in limbus in vernal conjunctivitis.

Trapp factor: Last 2 numerals of urine specific gravity value; multiplication by 2 gives parts per thousand of solids.

Traquair scotoma: Bilateral visual field defects caused by lesions in right optic nerve and Wilbrand knee.

Traube membrane: Thin film of potassium ions formed at interface when solution of copper salt is mixed with solution of potassium ferrocyanide.

Traube sign: "Pistol shot" sound heard via stethoscope over femoral arteries; occurs in severe, chronic aortic regurgitation.

Traube-Hering-Mayer curves: Waves in CSF (frequency: 4–8/sec) occurring in synchrony with oscillating blood pressure; questionable clinical significance.

Treacher Collins syndrome (mandibulofacial syndrome): Antimongoloid slanting of palpebral fissures, notched lower eyelid, and malar flattening due to hypoplastic or absent zygomatic arch. Condition is autosomal dominant and most prevalent in Caucasians.

Treft syndrome: Rare vision loss, hearing loss, ophthalmoplegia, and myopathy; familial condition.

Trendelenburg position: Patient lies supine with head lower than pelvis ($\sim 45°$ incline).

Trendelenburg sign: Evidence of weak hip abductors (gluteus medius); performed by having patient pick up 1 leg while standing. Contralateral weakness is indicated if pelvis slants toward side of raised leg.

Trendelenburg test (retrograde filling test): Used to assess valvular competence of saphenous and communicating veins in legs; performed by elevating patient's leg to drain blood from venous system and then occluding greater saphenous system (but not femoral system) with tourniquet. Rapid filling is indication of incompetency of valves in communicating system. Sudden filling of superficial veins after patient has stood for 20 seconds and had tourniquet removed is indication of incompetency of valves in saphenous system.

Tresilian sign: Reddish appearance of Stensen duct; seen in mumps.

Tressder sign: Relief of right lower quadrant pain when patient is turned prone; seen in appendicitis.

Tretop test: Used to detect albumin in urine; positive if coagulation mass develops when small amount of 40% formalin is added to sample.

Treves fold (bloodless fold): Peritoneal fold that arises from antimesenteric edge of ileum and runs over inferior ileocecal junction and onto mesentery of appendix; contains no visible vessels. Structure forms 1 wall of inferior ileocecal fossa.

Trevor syndrome: Asymmetric overgrowth of tarsal (or less often carpal) bones; may be associated with pain, chondromas, and osteochondromas. Presentation usu. occurs in childhood, with male-to-female ratio of 3:1.

triad of O'Donoghue: Simultaneous medial meniscal tear, anterior cruciate ligament rupture, and medial collateral ligament injury.

triangle of Calot: Anatomic area formed by cystic and common bile ducts.

triangle of Killian: Area of tissue weakness lying between 2 parts of cricopharyngeal muscle.

triangle of Koch: Anatomic area on right atrial septal wall in which AV node is located; borders are anteromedial edge of coronary sinus orifice, base of septal leaflet of tricuspid valve, and tendon of Todaro.

triangle of Truesdale: Anatomic area formed at lower end of thoracic esophagus by diaphragm inferiorly, pericardium anteriorly and superiorly, and descending aorta posteriorly.

Trimadeau sign: Indication of malignancy based on shape of esophagus. If dilatation above esophageal stricture is cup-shaped, lesion is likely malignant; if dilatation is conical, lesion is likely benign and fibrotic.

triple response of Lewis: Wheal-and-flare lesion.

Troell-Junet syndrome: Toxic goiter, acromegaly, hyperostosis of skull, and variable diabetes mellitus; also usu. with pituitary adenoma. Condition is reported in women only.

Trolard net: Venous plexus surrounding hypoglossal nerve and connecting occipital sinus and longitudinal vertebral sinuses.

Trolard vein (superior anastomotic vein): Vein that connects superior sagittal sinus and superficial middle cerebral vein.

Troisier node (ganglion, sign): See Virchow node.

Tröltsch pockets: Two blind pouches that lie between tympanic membrane and free borders of anterior and posterior malleolar folds.

Trommer test: Used to detect glucose in urine; positive if orangish precipitate forms when specimen is mixed with potassium or sodium hydroxide and a few drops of dilute copper sulfate solution, and then boiled.

Trömner sign: See Hoffmann sign.

Trotter syndrome: Invasion of lateral nasopharynx and sinus of Morgagni and adjacent muscles by tumor; can occur as late development of Jacod syndrome or from tumor extending from pterygopalatine fossa. Presenting features usu. include deafness, followed by ipsilateral ear pain and pain in lower jaw, side of tongue, and side of head. Palliative treatment is radiation.

Trousseau sign: Carpopedal spasm due to hypocalcemia; elicited by placing tourniquet on affected upper extremity and inflating above systemic pressure for 3 minutes.

Trousseau spot: Engorged skin caused by digging nail into skin and dragging it across surface; seen in some cerebral lesions.

Trousseau syndrome: Coexistence of abdominal carcinoma (esp. pancreatic) and peripheral venous thrombosis or pulmonary embolism.

Trousseau test: Used to detect bile in urine; positive if green ring is formed when sample is mixed with iodine diluted with alcohol.

Trousseau tracheal dilator: Curved, blunt-tipped, ring-handle instrument used to enlarge trachea; has bivalve opening mechanism.

Trousseau-Lallemand bodies: See Bence Jones cylinders.

Troutwine profile: Proprietary psychological inventory test that assesses motivation, persistence, and commitment to accomplishing tasks; has series of 75 questions. Test is used to assess suitability for employment (and to evaluate draft prospects in NFL). Initial question is "Would you rather be a cat or a dog?"

Troyer syndrome: Spastic paraplegia, dysarthria, distal muscle wasting, and variable cerebellar signs; onset occurs in early childhood. Disorder usu. results in complete loss of ambulation by 4th decade. Condition is autosomal recessive.

Truant stain (auramine–rhodamine stain): Staining procedure used to identify mycobacteria. Specimen is heat fixed, rinsed with auramine–rhodamine solution, decolorized, rinsed with potassium permanganate, and then viewed under ultraviolet light. Organisms appear orange-yellow.

Trümmerfeld line: Line of bone degeneration in metaphyses; seen in infantile scurvy.

Truster repair: Procedure that involves aortotomy; used in patients with aortic valve incompetence and ventricular septal defect (VSD). Redundant part of cusp is sutured against aortic wall, and VSD is repaired through right ventriculotomy.

Truster rule: Used for pulmonary artery banding.

Tscherning theory of accommodation: Convexity of eye lens is determined by contraction of anterior and circular parts of ciliary muscle.

Tübinger perimeter: Device used to measure visual sensitivity quantitatively; produces static profile through any chosen meridian.

Tucker syndrome: Amyotrophic lateral sclerosis–like weakness followed by atrophy of leg muscles and proximal arm muscles. Onset occurs in 4th decade, with progression over several decades to dementia, respiratory insufficiency, and complete paresis.

Tuffier test (Hallion test): Engorgement of superficial veins in hand or foot when main artery and vein of limb is compressed in presence of aneurysm.

Tuffli-Laxova syndrome: Very rare large adrenal cyst, hypoplastic nipples, hypohidrosis, aplastic cutis, and delayed tooth eruption.

Tukey test: Statistical method that aids in determining which means are different when making multiple comparisons using ANOVA.

Tukey-Kramer test: Statistical measure used in post hoc analysis after continuous data are analyzed with ANOVA.

Tullio phenomenon: Acute loss of balance when loud

sound is made close to ear with labyrinthine fistula.

Tunbridge-Paley syndrome: Juvenile (type 1) diabetes mellitus, perceptive hearing loss, and optic atrophy; associated with other syndromes, epilepsy, and dementia. Condition is autosomal dominant.

Tuohy needle: Hollow needle with sharp, beveled end; used in spinal procedures.

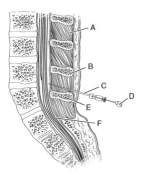

A. Ligmentum flavum
B. L4 spinous process
C. Tuohy needle
D. Stylet
E. L5 spinous process
F. Thecal sac

Tuohy needle

Tuomaala-Haapanen syndrome: Familial strabismus, nystagmus, cataracts, alopecia, hypoplastic tarsus, myopia, micrognathia, wide bridge of nose, stubby digits, and areas of skin depigmentation.

Tuomaala-Türck Turks bundle (tract): Descending cerebrotemporopontine bundle that arises in cortex of temporal lobe, runs in posterior portion of internal capsule laterally in pyramidal part of cerebral peduncle, and terminates in gray substance of pons.

Turcot syndrome: Hereditary polyposis syndrome marked by adenomas of large intestine; also associated with CNS tumors. Condition is autosomal dominant. Malignant potential is high; patients must undergo surveillance upper endoscopy at 3–5-year intervals.

Türk cell: Lymphocyte that contains greater number of basophilic particles.

Türk disease: Inability to abduct eye past midline, with simultaneous retraction; considered to be incomplete expression of Duane syndrome. Cause is degenerated external rectus muscle.

Turnbull loop stoma (modified): Procedure used to secure urinary ileal conduit to external abdominal skin in instances in which bowel lacks sufficient length or mobility or patient is morbidly obese. Knuckle of ileal loop is brought through stab wound and matured with adjacent, short blind pouch that opens cephalad to urinary stream.

Turnbull procedure: Ileostomy and "blowhole" colostomy to palliate colonic obstructions; now largely abandoned technique.

Turner cerate: Calamine ointment.

Turner sign: Flank ecchymosis; usu. due to hemorrhagic pancreatitis.

Turner syndrome: Degeneration of primordial germ cells with fibrous ovarian streaks, amenorrhea, variable short stature, and occasional telangiectasia; XO karyotype with female phenotype. Mosaic karyotypes sometimes have small uterus and ovarian cysts.

Turpin syndrome: Congenital association of vertebral abnormalities, megaesophagus and bronchiectasis, and variable presence of tracheobronchial fistula; manifests with cough, purulent sputum, and repeat respiratory infections.

Turyn sign: Pain in buttocks on dorsal bending of 1st toe; indicative of sciatica.

Tuttle proctoscope: Instrument with electric light source and mechanism for inflation of rectal ampulla to aid in insertion and exam.

Tweed triangle: Imaginary area formed by lines drawn through landmarks on lateral skull film; base of triangle is Frankfort horizontal plane.

Tween agar: Medium used to culture and identify *Candida albicans* and its chlamydospores.

Tween hydrolysis: Identification test for *Mycobacterium* based on ability to hydrolyze substrate Tween 80. Hydrolysis occurs with *M. flavescens*, *M. gastri*, *M. gordonae*, *M. malmoense*, *M. terrae* complex, and *M. triviale*. No hydrolysis occurs with *M. avium* complex, *M. serofulaceum*, *M. tuberculosis*, and *M. xenopi*.

Tween opacity: Identification test for *Mycobacterium;* used to separate *M. flavescens* (growth in 1 week) from *M. szulgai* (slow growth).

Tyndall effect: Increased scattering of light that causes "cloudiness" when viewing cellular structures under microscopy; occurs when mitochondria swell due to failure of ionic pumps to maintain normal electrolyte concentration.

Tyson test: Used to detect bile acids in urine; positive if precipitate forms when specimen is evaporated and residual matter is mixed with ether.

Tzanck test: Sampling of cells from floor of vesicular or bullous lesion; used to delineate most predominate cell type and aid in diagnosis. Presence of multinucleated giant cells indicates herpes simplex or zoster, varicella, or pemphigus.

Ueda modification: Variation of Kasai procedure for surgical treatment of biliary atresia; 1st described in 1972. Best results are obtained if procedure is performed before 8 weeks of life.

Uehlinger syndrome: See Meyenburg-Altherr-Uehlinger syndrome.

Uhthoff sign: Visual deficit occurring with exercise or increased body temperature; associated with multiple sclerosis.

Ulick syndrome: Aldosterone synthetase deficiency.

Ullrich-Feichtiger syndrome: See Fraser syndrome.

United States Army retractors: Handheld, double-ended retractors for soft tissue.

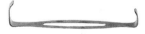

United States Army retractors

University of Wisconsin solution: Used to store organs procured from cadaveric donors for transplantation. Composed of antioxidants, hydrogen ion buffering substances, and high-energy phosphate precursors in solution; used for liver (maximum cold storage: 14–16 hours), pancreas (maximum cold storage: 12 hours), and kidney (maximum cold storage: 36 hours).

Unschuld sign: Cramping in calf; seen in early stages of diabetes.

Unsold technique: 1 of several techniques used to achieve retrobulbar anesthesia before cataract surgery; entails injection (commonly etidocaine–lidocaine mixture) with orbital muscle cone with primary eye position to lower risk of optic nerve involvement.

Urban procedure: En bloc resection for cancer; includes primary site and major regional lymph node basins.

Uriolla sign:. Small black granules found in urine secondary to hemolysis; seen in malaria.

Usher syndrome: Deafness and retinitis pigmentosa leading to blindness; caused by defect in chromosome 1 or 2.

Usher syndrome: Congenital dislocation of lenses; associated with joint stiffness, Marfan disease, and Weill-Marchesani disease.

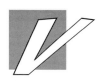

Vaandrager-type chondro-dysplasia: Lesions in metaphyses extending into adjacent diaphysis; appear as radiolucent longitudinal osteosclerotic streaks on radiographs.

Vallee disease (equine infectious anemia): Recurring fever and malaise in horses caused by virus. Inoculation and reinoculation result from bites of blood-sucking insects.

Valleix points: Tender areas along course of peripheral nerve.

Vallon-Zaber bacillus: See Welch bacillus.

Valsalva maneuver: Straining against closed glottis; decreases venous return to right heart and subsequently decreases left ventricular volume and arterial pressure. Technique may be used to help auscultate mitral valve prolapse and hypertrophic cardiomyopathy as well as to diagnose venous reflux at or above common femoral level because it produces retrograde flow signal detectable by Doppler ultrasonography.

van Buchem disease: Osteosclerosis of skull, ribs, jaw, clavicles, and thickening of skeletal bones; results in nerve compression leading to optic atrophy, facial paralysis, and deafness.

van Buren urethral sound: Metal device commonly used for urethral dilation of urethral strictures, sometimes prior to urologic operations.

van der Waals forces: Weak binding forces between atoms and molecules; result in hydrophobic bonding between nonorganic compounds.

van der Woude syndrome: See Demarquay syndrome.

van Gehuchten nucleus: Wedge-shaped structure lying on hypoglossal eminence; supplies visceral efferent fibers to vagus nerve.

van Gieson stain: Trichrome stain using iron hematoxylin to stain nuclei black; fuchsin to stain connective tissue and hyalin red; and picric acid to stain cytoplasm, muscle, amyloid, fibrin, and fibrinoid substances yellow.

van Gieson–elastic stain: Combination of van Gieson and elastic stain.

van Hoorne canal: Thoracic duct.

van Lint block: 1 of several techniques used for anesthesia in cataract surgery; does not provide akinesia of orbicularis oculi muscle. Injection is at temporal orbital margin in attempt to block zygomatic branches of facial nerve.

van Neck syndrome: Osteochondritis of ischiopubis.

Varco gallbladder forceps: Locking, ring-handled forceps with relatively fine, curved-tips used in tissue dissection.

Vater-Pacini corpuscle: See Pacinian corpuscle.

Vaughn Williams classification: Functional description of antiarrhythmic drugs. Class 1a—block sodium channels (quinidine, procainamide, disopyramide); class 1b—reduce phase 0 or maximum upstroke velocity of action potential (lidocaine, phenytoin, tocainide); class 2—block sympathetic activity (beta blockers such as propranolol); class 3—prolong duration of action potential (bretylium, amiodarone); class 4—inhibit flow of slow inward current (verapamil).

Veidenheimer resection clamp: Locking, ring-handled clamp with 30° shaft angle and tip at 90° angle with 2×3 vascular teeth; total length is 229 mm.

vein of Galen: Large vein that drains anterior cerebral branches, perforating thalamic branches of posterior cerebral arteries, branches of superior cerebellar arteries, and choroidal arteries; vessel then passes blood to straight sinus and torcular herophili. Vein is site of most common arteriovenous malformation in infancy.

vein of Labbé: Large cerebral vein that drains into transverse sinus.

vein of Mayo: Vein that overlies pylorus.

vein of Rosenthal (basilar vein): Vein that originates at level of temporal horn, running backward and around brainstem; joins internal cerebral vein and follows course similar to posterior cerebral artery.

vein of Trolard: Large superficial vein in brain that drains into petrosal sinus; anastomoses with vein of Labbé.

vein of Vieussens: Vein that drains ventral surface of right ventricle and empties into right atrium.

veins of Sappey (paraumbilical veins): Part of collateral circulation between systemic (inferior and superior epigastric veins and superior vesicle veins) and portal venous drainage; enlargement in portal venous obstruction causes caput medusae.

veins of Thebesius: Multiple small veins draining walls of heart that feed directly into heart chambers; most prominent in atria.

Veldt sore: South African term for diphtheritic desert sore; see Barcoo rot.

Velpeau dressing: Material used to fix arm in acute flexion against torso with elbow at waist and hand at chest.

Velpeau hernia (Laugier hernia:) Femoral hernia that passes superficial to femoral vessels and usu. pierces Gimbernat ligament; often requires incision of ligament to reduce hernia adequately and repair it.

Venezuelan equine encephalitis: Disease caused by type A arbovirus; occurs in southern U.S. and in Central and South America. Vector is *Culex* mosquito; animal hosts are horses and rodents.

Venus line: Principal transverse skin crease on palmar surface of wrist.

Verco sign: Small hemorrhagic areas under finger and toenails seen in patients with erythema nodosum.

Verdan zones: 8 zones of hand that correlate with prognosis of tendon laceration with fingers extended (not skin laceration site). Zone 1—repair is performed in both adults and children if injury is to profundus tendon; zone 2—in adults, repair is controversial; in children, repair is performed if injury is to profundus tendon, flexor pollicus longus, or flexor digitorum superficialis; zone 5—repair of profundus and superficial tendons is performed; zone 6—repair of only profundus tendon is performed.

Verga groove: Furrow that runs downward from lower opening of nasal duct.

Verga ventricle: Space occasionally found when undersurface of splenium and hippocampal crura do not adhere.

Verheyen stars: Small superficial veins on surface of kidney that drain surface and empty into interlobular veins.

Verhoeff procedure (enucleation): Technique for permanently removing eye from socket. For each rectus muscle, anterior adhesions between overlying Tenon capsule and muscle are lysed, with preservation of underlying muscle sheath. Muscle is then clamped at insertion point for 10 seconds and then severed with Westcott scissors; 5-mm stump is left at medial rectus insertion site.

Verhoeff stain: Material that stains elastin deep blue; used to visualize elastic fibers.

Vermel sign: Pulsations in temporal area on affected side; seen with unilateral headache in setting of hypotension.

Verner-Morrison syndrome (pancreatic cholera): Profuse watery diarrhea, hypochloremia, hypokalemia, and metabolic acidosis; likely due to pancreatic islet cell tumor that secretes vasoactive peptide.

Vernet syndrome: Paresis of CNs IX, X, and XI; usu. due to tumors or aneurysms in jugular foramen or trauma.

Vernet-Sargnon syndrome: See Collet-Sicard syndrome.

Verneuil canals: General term for system of collateral veins feeding into any main venous trunk.

Vernier acuity: Ability to detect movement of line in visual field.

Vero cells: Cell line of African green monkey kidney cells used in laboratory.

Verocay bodies: Clusters of fibrils encircled by rows of nuclei arranged in "shingled" pattern; occur in schwannomas.

Verriest test: Used to detect abnormal lightness discrimination by varying luminance of visual field.

Vesalius foramen: Small opening lying between foramen ovale and foramen rotundum in sphenoid bone; traversed by Vesalius vein as it drains into cavernosus sinus.

Vesalius vein: Small facial vein that connects pterygoid venous plexus and cavernous sinus.

Vicq d'Azyr band: See Kaes-Bekhterev line.

Vicq d'Azyr bundle: Mammillothalamic fasciculus nerve fibers running from mammillary body upward to anterior nucleus of thalamus.

vidian artery: Long, thin branch off 3rd part of internal maxillary artery; runs backward through vidian (pterygoid) canal. Artery supplies blood to roof of pharynx and gives off branches to eustachian tube and tympanum.

vidian canal: Pterygoid canal; see canal of Guidi.

vidian nerve (nerve of pterygoid canal): Nerve formed by union of deep and greater petrosal nerves; runs through vidian canal next to vidian artery.

Vieussens foramina (thebesian foramina): Openings of smallest heart veins in heart wall, which allow drainage directly into heart chambers; most common in right atrium and ventricle and scarce in left ventricle.

Vincent angina (disease, stomatitis; trench mouth): Acute, necrotizing, ulcerative gingivitis; usu. due to oral anaerobes or *Borrelia vincentii*. Disorder is marked by bleeding gingiva and fetid odor. Treatment is oral penicillin and metronidazole (Flagyl).

Vincent curtsy: Characteristic posturing of children with hyperactive bladder in attempt to prevent voiding.

Vincent organisms: *Borrelia vincentii* and *Bacteroides fusiformis;* causative agents of tropical ulcer.

Vineberg bypass: Use of internal mammary artery to bypass coronary artery blockage in end-to-side fashion.

Vineland adaptive behavior scale: Evaluation of social and adaptive skills, specifically motor and daily living skills, socialization, and communication; used in infants (1 month old) and adults.

Vinke tongs: Instrument that provides skull traction to stabilize neck injuries.

Vipond sign: Generalized lymphadenopathy in children;

occurs during incubation period of exanthematous fevers.

Virchow node: Left supraclavicular node metastases; classically considered to be due to gastric carcinoma.

Virchow oxycephaly: See Crouzon disease.

Virchow triad: 3 Risk factors for thrombosis: hypercoagulable states, endothelial defects, and stasis.

Virchow-Holder angle (Holder angle): Formed by imaginary line connecting base of anterior nasal spine and center of nasofrontal suture and imaginary line from center of nasofrontal suture to center of external auditory meatus.

Virchow-Robin space: Perivascular space.

Virtus splinter forceps: Pliers-type forceps with straight, needle-nose tip; used for grasping small objects.

Vitus dance: See Saint Vitus dance.

Vladimiroff-Mikulicz amputation (Vladimiroff-Proskauer amputation): Partial-foot amputation in which incision is made through talus and calcaneus.

Vladimiroff-Proskauer amputation: See Vladimiroff-Mikulicz amputation.

Voerner disease: Skin lesions similar to knuckle pads developing on palms and plantar surface; histologically resembles epidermolysis. Condition is autosomal dominant.

Voerner disease (nevus anemicus): Whitish patches of skin developing on chest, posterior neck, and face; autosomal dominant condition. Cause is poor blood supply.

Vogt cephalosyndactyly: See Crouzon disease.

Vogt striae: Centrally located folds in Descemet membrane seen with slit-lamp examination that disappear when pressure is applied to cornea; diagnostic sign of keratoconus.

Vogt syndrome (Nettleship cataract): White or gray "fuzzy lines" developing in variable places in cornea; marked by granular deposits in Bowman layer. Etiology is unknown. Condition is autosomal dominant.

Vogt-Koyanagi-Harada syndrome: Vitiligo (most common on face and scalp), with tinnitus, hearing loss, uveitis, and aseptic meningitis.

Voigt lines: Imaginary lines that outline distribution of peripheral nerves.

Voit nucleus: Collection of cell bodies in cerebellum lying close to dentate nucleus.

Volkmann canals: Small, centripetally oriented openings in osteonal bone that allow transport of materials to osteocytes via central Haversian canals; originate from periosteum or bone marrow. Canals cut through lamellae on bone cross-section, which distinguishes them from Haversian canals.

Volkmann contractures:
Forearm compartment syndrome caused by crush injuries, supracondylar or forearm fractures, and ischemia. Most reliable diagnostic signs are increasing pain on passive finger extension and focal tenderness over affected muscles. Treatment is wide exposure by fasciotomy and epimysiotomy with median and ulnar nerve release. Untreated fractures cause fibrosis of deep flexor compartment and severe contracture.

Volkmann deformity:
Absent/hypoplastic fibula with congenital displacement of ankle.

Volkmann fracture: Fracture of posterior lateral tibia with triangular fragment.

Volkmann paralysis: Paralysis due to ischemia of limb, usu. because of occlusion of major artery.

Volkmann retractors: Hand-held retractors with rake-like ends; available in various sizes.

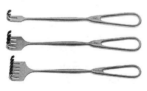

Volkmann retractors

Volkmann triangle: Bone fragment off posterior lateral tibia fracture when extending into joint.

Voltolini sign: See Heryng sign.

von Bonsdorff technique:
Inflation of sphygmomanometer cuff for 10 minutes to make arm ischemic. Cuff is then removed, and patient is asked to hyperventilate. Tetanic contractions occur earlier in ischemic arm. Condition is also seen in tetany.

von Ebner glands: Serous tubuloalveolar glands of tongue found with lamina propria and bundles of skeletal muscle fibers; has ducts that drain at base of circular furrow into fossa surrounding vallate papillae.

von Frey syndrome: See Frey syndrome.

von Gierke disease: Deficiency in lysosomal enzyme maltase with inability to metabolize glycogen; results in liver and kidney disease.

von Graefe sign: Upper eyelid that does not move downward when eyeball moves downward; seen in exophthalmos caused by thyroid goiter.

von Gudden ganglion:
Group of cell bodies lying on posterior perforated substance near superior border of pons.

von Haberer operation:
Type of gastroenterostomy.

von Hansemann cells:
Pathognomonic Michaelis-Gutmann bodies located within histiocytes seen in malacoplakia bodies.

von Hippel-Lindau disease:
Hemangioblastomas of CNS and retina, renal cysts and renal carcinoma (25%); also with

increased incidence of pancreatic islet cell tumors and pheochromocytoma. Condition is autosomal dominant and due to defect in tumor-suppressor gene (VHL) on chromosome 3.

von Mering reflex: General relaxation of abdominal muscles after eating.

von Meyenburg lesions (complexes): Small multiple, cyst-like dilated bile ducts with cuboidal epithelium and fibrous stroma, which are located in close relation to portal tracts; probably represent ductal plate malformation. Lesions belong in spectrum of congenital hepatic fibrosis and adult hepatic polycystic disease.

von Monakow fibers: Nerve fibers that run between cerebral optic tract to lenticular ganglion.

von Petrykowski syndrome: Adrenomyodystrophy.

von Recklinghausen disease (neurofibromatosis): Systemic, widespread growth (including GI tract) of neurofibromas accompanied variably by mental retardation, pachymicrogyria, extremity gigantism, hemihypertrophy, spina bifida, and meningocele; also with increased incidence of pancreatic islet cell tumors. Diagnosis requires 6 café au lait spots > 1.5 cm.

von Reuss syndrome: See Mason-Turner syndrome.

von Weber triangle: Imaginary space formed by lines connecting points corresponding to center of palmar area, 5th metatarsal head, and 1st metatarsal head.

von Willebrand disease: Clinical syndrome associated with defective or deficient von Willebrand factor; factor VIII antigen/von Willebrand factor ratio is low. Disorder causes bleeding prolonged bleeding time (esp. with concomitant aspirin use) and results in bleeding at skin and mucous membranes. PT is normal, and PTT may be prolonged or normal if factor VIII level > 30%. Platelet count and shape are usu. normal, but variant forms associated with angiodysplasia and mild thrombocytopenia are known; platelet aggregation is normal. Ristocetin-induced platelet agglutination is impaired. Condition may be either autosomal dominant or recessive.

von Willebrand factor (vWF): Coagulant protein produced by endothelial cells that is complexed to factor VIII in plasma; mediates platelet adhesion. Blood for testing is drawn in blue-top tube.

Voorhoeve disease: Osteopathia striata.

Voshell bursa: Bursa sac located just distal to joint line and lying between joint capsule and tibial collateral ligament.

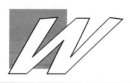

Waardenburg syndrome:
Deafness and pigment changes due to failure of melanocytes to migrate from neural crest during embryonic development; associated with defects on chromosomes 2 and 3.

Wachendorf membrane:
Embryonic structure consisting of mesodermal layer attached to front rim of iris; occasionally persists into adulthood.

Wachendorf membrane:
Plasma membrane.

Wachenheim-Reder sign:
Palpation of right iliac fossa on rectal exam, producing pain in right lower quadrant; seen in appendicitis.

Wagner classification: 5-stage categorization of diabetic foot ulcers.

Wagner disease: See David-Stickler disease.

Wagner disease: Aseptic necrosis of base of 1st metatarsal.

Wagner line: Whitish line formed by preliminary calcifications at epiphysis–diaphysis junction in bone.

Wagner modification: 2-stage procedure for midfoot amputation; see Syme amputation.

Wagstaffe fracture [LeFort fracture (of foot)]: Fracture and fragmentation of distal anterior fibula.

Waldenström classification:
Description of healing stages in Legg-Calvé-Perthes disease. Stage A1, initial stage in which epiphysis is dense with uneven margins at distal end; stage A2, fragmentation stage with epiphysis similar to multiple small granules; stage B, healing stage with revascularization and homogeneous epiphysis; stage C, growth stage with progressive ossification of deformed femoral head.

Waldenström disease:
Osteochondrosis of humeral capitellum.

Waldenström macroglobulinemia (purpura): Neoplastic disorder marked by proliferation of abnormal lymphocytes in bone marrow, with type 1 cryoglobulinemia (monoclonal proteins), anemia, increased sedimentation rate, mucosal bleeding, skin purpura, and enlarged lymph nodes.

Waldeyer fascia (rectorectal fascia): Presacral endopelvic fascia running from level of S4 downward and forward with attachment to rectum.

Waldeyer gland: Acinotubular glands located in skin at inner edge of eyelid.

Waldeyer layer: Vascular lamina of ovary.

Waldeyer line: See Farre white line.

Waldeyer tonsillar ring (Bickel ring): Circular lymphatic tissue formed by lingual and pharyngeal tonsils, two palatine tonsils, and intervening lymphoid tissue.

Waldvogel classification: Description of osteomyelitis based on etiology.

Walker appliance: See Crozat appliance.

Wallace technique (anastomosis): Surgical construction of urinary ileal conduit. Ureters are spatulated at open end for 2–3 cm and then sewn side-to-side using absorbable sutures, and patch is then anastomosed using absorbable suture to open end of bowel loop before it is brought up to abdominal wall. Advantages are ease of fashioning and wide ureteral anastomosis.

Wallenberg syndrome: Lesion in lateral medulla; usu. caused by vertebral artery thrombosis near posterior inferior cerebellar artery. Injuries occur in spinocerebellar tract (ipsilateral hemiplegia), CN V (ipsilateral loss of facial pain and temperature sensation), spinothalamic tract (contralateral loss of body pain and temperature sensation), vestibular nuclei (nystagmus), sympathetic tract (ipsilateral Horner syndrome), and nucleus ambiguus (dysphasia and dysphonia).

wallerian degeneration: Breakdown of myelin sheath to lipoid material; occurs distal to transection in nerve cell.

Walter splinter forceps: Tweezer-type forceps with straight, needle-nosed tips; used for grasping small objects.

Walthard cells: Transitional cell (urothelial) metaplasia; commonly found close to tubal serosa as 1–2 mm translucent nodules, and occasionally occur on ovaries.

Walther fracture: Hip fracture running from ischial spine to acetabulum to ischiopubis.

Wangensteen drainage: Continuous suction drainage of gastric/biliary juices through tube placed in stomach or proximal bowel; decompresses bowel obstruction or ileus.

Ward triangle: Imaginary area formed by lines of axis of femoral neck trabeculae; point of high incidence of fracture.

Warren incision: Skin incision tracing thoracomammary fold.

Warren procedure: Arthroscopic debridement of acromioclavicular joint. Burr is usually placed via anterior port, and arthroscope is placed via lateral subacromial port. Minimum of 10 mm of distal clavicle is debrided.

Warren shunt: Distal splenorenal venous anastomosis for symptomatic portal hypertension; considered a "true selective" procedure. Hepatopetal

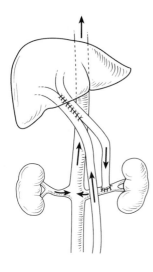

Warren shunt

flow to liver is not altered, but esophagogastric varices are decompressed. Complications include minimal incidence of postop encephalopathy but increased ascites formation.

Wartenberg sign: Slightly abducted 5th finger; sometimes seen in ulnar nerve palsy.

Wartenberg sign: Lack of free-swinging pendulum motion of arm; seen when patients with cerebellar disease ambulate.

Warthin tumor (papillary cystadenoma lymphomatosum): Second most common benign tumor of salivary glands; occurs only in parotid gland. Disorder is more common in males and is bilateral in 10% of patients.

Wasserman antibody: Serum antibody evoked by infection with *Treponema;* appears 3–6 weeks following inoculation. Quantity of antibody produced is directly proportional to number of infecting spirochetes in 1st and 2nd stages of syphilis. Antibody may be absent in latent and 3rd stages.

Waterhouse-Friderichsen syndrome: Acute bilateral destruction of adrenal glands associated with meningococcemia.

Waters view: Radiographic positioning technique that provides occipitomental view of midface; used to evaluate fractures.

Waterston classification: System used to describe esophageal atresia and tracheoesophageal fistulas in newborns. Group A, birth weight < 2500 g without associated major anomalies; group B, birth weight 1800–2500 g without associated major anomalies; group C, birth weight < 1800 g with associated major anomalies. (Presence of pneumonia moves patient into "next most severe" group.)

Waterston shunt (aortopulmonary shunt): Side-to-side anastomosis of ascending aorta to right pulmonary artery; used to treat cyanotic tetralogy of Fallot.

Watkins operation (transposition): Commonly used in early 1900s for correction of cystocele and uterine prolapse; procedure is rarely performed today. Uterus is transposed and fixed to undersurface of bladder and urethra.

Watson resection: Matched distal resection used in lieu of Darrach resection to treat unstable and painful distal radioulnar joint; preserves styloid attachment of triangular fibrocartilage complex and distal ulnar ligaments. Intact distal ulna is resected in long convex curve that "matches" opposing radial surfaces.

Watson syndrome: See Dobriner syndrome.

Watson-Jones classification: System used to describe fractures of pediatric tibial tuberosity. Type 1, superiorly displaced fragment; type 2, superiorly displaced large fragment that involves secondary center of ossification; type 3, fracture that runs posteriorly and proximally across epiphyseal plate with displacement.

Watson-Jones incision: Approach to anterior column hip fractures.

Watson-Schwartz test: Qualitative urine screening test used in acute porphyria; positive if red color develops when urine sample with porphobilinogen is added to Erlich reagent in acidified solution.

Waugh prosthesis (UCI prosthesis): Knee replacement with maximum freedom of motion; requires good soft tissue stability.

Way classification: System used to describe injuries to extrahepatic bile ducts during laparoscopic cholecystectomy. Class 1, incomplete transection; class 2, strictures caused by clip or cautery damage; class 3, complete transection of common or lobar duct; class 4, injury to right hepatic duct when mistaken for cystic duct.

Webber-Ferguson incision: Skin incision over lower medial eyelid for exposure for resection of lacrimal sac tumors.

Weber gland: Mucus-secreting glands of tongue.

Weber ligament (transverse ligament of knee): Connective tissue fibers running from anterior margin of lateral meniscus to anterior margin of medial meniscus.

Weber line: Hypothetical line separating Australian zone from Asian zone in Australia; important in epidemiology of infectious diseases (e.g., Ross River virus does not occur west of this line).

Weber protocol: Exercise tolerance test procedure; best used in patients with decreased cardiac reserve or disability.

Weber sign: Hemiplegia of 1 side; occurs with oculomotor nerve paralysis on contralateral side.

Weber syndrome: Ipsilateral CN III palsy with contralateral hemiparesis; due to injury in medial basal midbrain and cerebral peduncle. Condition is often caused by occlusion of proximal posterior cerebral artery.

Weber test: Hearing test used to detect sensorineural hearing loss. Vibrating tuning fork is placed on scalp in midline; deficit is present if sound is louder in normal ear than in diseased ear.

Weber tubercle: Lesser tubercle of humerus; serves as attachment point of subscapular muscle.

Weber-Christian disease (systemic nodular panniculitis): Extensive inflammation of skin, joints, and internal organs; relapsing and remitting in nature, but usu. recovery occurs eventually.

Weber-Ferguson approach: Technique used for subtotal maxillectomy or total maxillectomy with orbital preservation. First, incision is made running from ipsilateral nasal vestibule laterally to base of nasal columella and transversely to midline of upper lip, splitting upper lip in zigzag fashion. Then a horizontal gingival buccal incision is made. (Both infra- and supraorbital incision extensions can be made.) Facial flap is retracted laterally in subperiosteal plane, with preservation of infraorbital nerve.

Weber-Vasey technique (traction–absorption wiring technique): Procedure used to repair fractures to olecranon; involves 2 pins placed longitudinally through fracture, with figure-of-8 wiring system that secures segments.

Webster flap: Cheek advancement flap for lower lip reconstruction. Slightly curved, full-thickness incision of one-half length of defect is made laterally on side of defect, and 2nd, smaller, parallel incision is made. Rectangular tissue flap is advanced with sliding technique, and adjacent inner lip mucosa is rotated to form new lip surface.

Webster sutures: Fine PDS sutures placed subcutaneously to produce pronounced skin eversion when closing wound; usu. combined with 6–0 nylon to effect epidermal closure. Used in scar revision in areas where there is active underlying muscle (frontalis, orbicularis oculi, or upper lip).

Wechsler Intelligence Scale for Children-Revised (WISC-R): Group of tests that evaluate children 6–16 years of age; highlights specific strengths or deficiencies.

Wechsler Preschool and Primary Scale of Intelligence-Revised (WPPSI-R): Group of tests that evaluate children 3–6 1/2 years of age using verbal and performance scales; highlights developmental strengths and deficiencies in children at or close to normal levels.

Wechsler-Bellevue scale: Test of mentation that measures verbal and nonverbal performance (i.e., drawing, puzzle assembly, arranging blocks, copying, digit symbol, and picture story arrangement).

Weck laser: Device used to make radial incisions on fimbriae for correction of hydrosalpinx (rapid continuous firing mode).

Wegener granulomatosis:
Necrotizing granulomatous vasculitis of lungs, glomerulonephritis, and disseminated vasculitis; marked by pulmonary infiltrates and cavitation, hematuria, proteinuria, skin papules and ulcerations, sinusitis, nasal septal perforations, pancarditis, and neuropathy. Leukocytosis, anemia, and hypergammaglobulinemia are characteristic, and sedimentation rate is increased. Cytoplasmic antinuclear antibody (cANCA) test is usu. positive.

Wegner disease: See Parrot pseudoparalysis.

Wegner sign: Discolored appearance seen in widened epiphysis in fatal, congenital syphilis.

Weibel-Palade body: Cytoplasmic laminated groupings of microtubules specific for vascular endothelial cells; visible only with electron microscopy.

Weigert fibrin stain:
Bichromic stain using nuclear fast red to stain nuclei red and Lugol solution and crystal violet to stain fibrin and bacteria blue.

Weigert law: Destruction of substance or element in organic world is usu. overproduced during process of regeneration and/or repair.

Weigert stain: Substance used to demonstrate presence of elastin.

Weigert-Meyer rule: Principle that describes relative position of the ureteral orifices in patients with complete ureteral duplication. Ureteral orifice of upper pole ureter lies caudal and medial to lower pole ureteral orifice.

Weigert-Pal method:
Method using mordanted sections and hematoxylin that stains gray matter nerve fibers. Myelinated fibers stain purple-blue, and nonmyelinated fibers stain light blue.

Weil basal layer: Lamina composed of thin fibrils in ground substance found just deep to odontoblastic layer that is incorporated into matrix during dentinogenesis.

Weilby reconstruction:
Digital pulley reconstruction to optimize transforming tendon excursion into finger flexion.

Weill sign: Hypoexpansion of subclavicular area of thoracic cage on affected side in infantile pneumonia.

Weill-Marchesani syndrome: Short fingers, short stature, microspherophakia, subluxed lens, and myopia; not associated with mental retardation.

Weinberg vagotomy retractor (Joe's hoe): Handheld retractor with weighted shaft.

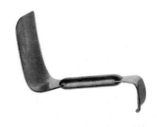

Weinberg vagotomy retractor

Weingartner forceps: Hawk-billed instrument used for grasping in ear canal.

Weir Mitchell disease (erythromelalgia, Gerhardt disease, Mitchell disease): Rare paroxysmal pain, swelling, erythema, and sweating in extremities (usu. feet); due to hypersensitivity of pain fibers in skin to warmth and dependent position. Treatment is rest, elevation, and cold.

Weismann theory (germ plasm): Tenet that genetic characteristics are passed to offspring through germ line with no contribution from somatic cells.

Weismann-Netter-Stuhl syndrome: Mental retardation, dwarfism, bowleg, and dural calcification.

Weiss disease (storage pool platelet deficiency, SPPD): Hereditary defect in platelet function caused by deficiency in platelet adenine nucleotides in either α or δ dense granules; associated with moderate hemorrhagic sequelae and pulmonary hypertension.

Weiss reflex: Elliptical reflection to nasal side of disk on funduscopic exam; sometimes seen in myopia.

Weiss ring: Ring-shaped posterior vitreous face often seen in patients after posterior vitreous detachment.

Weiss sign: See Chvostek sign.

Weitbrecht cartilage: Variably present pad of fibrocartilage found in articular space of acromioclavicular joint.

Weitbrecht foramen: Space in shoulder joint capsule that runs beneath subscapularis muscle; it carries synovial membrane.

Weitbrecht ligament (cord, oblique cord of elbow): Small fibrous band running from lateral edge of ulnar tuberosity to radius (just distal to tuberosity).

Welch abscess: Walled-off purulent collection that contains gas; often caused by *Clostridium perfringens*.

Welch bacillus (Achalme bacillus, Vallon-Zaber bacillus): *Clostridium perfringens*.

Well procedure: Technique for correction of complete rectal prolapse performed by fully mobilizing rectum and dividing lateral stalks; seldom performed because of septic complications. Sterile Ivalon sponge is wrapped around posterior 3/4 of rectum and attached to presacral fascia.

Wells modification: Variation of Stenger test for detection of deafness in 1 ear in malingering patient. Malingering patient reports no hearing in supposedly damaged ear until tuning fork is very close to ear. Patient with true deafness of 1 ear reports hearing (from good ear) when tuning fork is at considerable distance.

Wenckebach heart block: Second-degree AV heart block, type 1, with progressive PR-interval elongation in front of

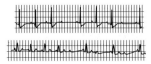

Wenckebach heart block

"dropped" P waves; usu. due to abnormality at AV node.

Wenger program: Early, progressive return to activity after MI; aim is going from bed rest in cardiac care unit to climbing 2 flights of stairs in 14 days (without ischemia, arrhythmia, or congestive heart failure). Program has significant psychological benefits.

Wenger-Cooper deficiency: Rare congenital deficiency of β mannosidase with buildup of disaccharides; features include mental retardation, respiratory infections, and labile emotions. Condition is autosomal recessive.

Werdnig-Hoffmann disease: Neuromuscular disease caused by neuron destruction; marked by hypotonia in newborns, proximal muscle weakness, areflexia, and tongue fasciculations at birth. Condition is autosomal recessive.

Werlhof disease: Idiopathic thrombocytopenic purpura.

Wermer syndrome: Multiple endocrine neoplasia type 1 (MEN-1); characterized by parathyroid, pituitary, and pancreatic islet cell tumors ("3 Ps"). Islet cell tumor is usually insulinoma or gastrinoma, causing Zollinger-Ellison syndrome. Condition is autosomal dominant.

Werner suppression test: Measure of long-acting thyroid stimulator (LATS); aids in diagnosis of subtle cases of Graves disease.

Wernicke aphasia (receptive aphasia): Rapid, voluble speech with correct inflection and articulation but with incomprehensible meaning (paragrammatism). Naming, writing, and reading comprehension are impaired due to lesion in left temporal lobe. Cardinal sign is defective listening comprehension.

Wernicke area (center): Posterior 1/3 of left superior temporal gyrus.

Wernicke encephalopathy: Lethargy, confusion, ataxia, ophthalmoplegia, and nystagmus; caused by thiamine deficiency (usu. in setting of chronic alcohol abuse). Disorder almost always occurs with Korsakoff syndrome.

Wernicke second motor speech area (field, zone): Posterior superior temporal gyrus (abutting transverse temporal gyri), supramarginal gyrus, and angular gyrus.

Wernicke sign: Contraction of iris when light stimulus is applied to 1 side of retina; light has no effect when directed to other side of retina. Sign occurs in hemianopia.

West African trypanosomiasis: See Gambian sleeping sickness.

Westergren scale: Reference units used to report erythrocyte sedimentation rate; normal values: < 25 mm/hr if < 50 years of age; < 30 mm/hr if > 50 years of age.

Westermark sign: Loss of pulmonary vascular markings distal to lesion in pulmonary embolus visible on chest radiograph; may be segmental, lobar, or involve entire lung field.

Western equine encephalomyelitis: Viral disease found in southern Canada, U.S., and Argentina. Vector is *Culex* mosquito; animal hosts are horses and birds.

Westphal nucleus: See Edinger-Westphal nucleus.

Westphal pupillary reflex (Galassi reflex, Gifford reflex, Westphal-Piltz reflex): Attempt to close eyelids that are forcibly held apart; pupil contracts and then dilates.

Westphal sign: Loss of knee jerk reflex in patients with gait ataxia.

Weyer disease: Congenital condition marked by multiple areas of intestinal atresia.

Weyers syndrome: Congenital nail dysplasia, conical teeth, short limbs, polydactyly, and cleft of mandibular symphysis; autosomal dominant condition.

Wharton ducts: Ducts of submandibular gland. Orifices drain into mouth at base of tongue, and lingual nerve runs over these structures.

Whipple disease: Unusual systemic disease involving tissues that have large glycoprotein-containing macrophages and *Tropheryma whippleii*, which are small, rod-shaped, gram-positive, non–acid fast organisms. Disorder marked by variable occurrence of abdominal pain, diarrhea, weight loss, intestinal malabsorption, CNS involvement, hyperpigmentation, lymphadenopathy, anemia, arthralgias, pericarditis, pleuritis, and visual deterioration. Abdominal manifestations in small intestine and mesenteric lymph nodes include granulomatous inflammation, fatty degeneration, and chyle stasis. Biopsy of mucosa of duodenum or jejunum provides best tissue for diagnosis. Antibiotic treatment varies widely but should probably include 3rd-generation cephalosporin and/or TMP-SMZ for 6–12 months.

Whipple triad: Fasting hypoglycemia (blood sugar < 50 mg/dl) with associated symptoms (e.g., syncope, diaphoresis) relieved by glucose administration; seen in insulinoma.

White classification: System that categorizes diabetes mellitus in pregnancy. Class A—gestational diabetes with glucose intolerance occurring during pregnancy, may be managed with insulin or diet alone; class B—onset ≥ 20 years of age or < 10 years' duration, insulin-dependent; class C, onset at 10–19 years of age or 10–19 years' duration; class D—onset < 10 years of age, > 20 years' duration, or presence of hypertension or mild retinopathy; class F—renal disease; class H—coronary artery disease; class R—proliferative retinopathy; class T—after renal transplantation. (Class E is no longer used.)

white line of Toldt: Lateral peritoneal reflections of ascending and descending colon.

Whitfield disease: Onset in older women of aching legs (after standing), edema, and eruption of painful nodular lesions after trauma or exposure to cold; associated with TB and vasculitis.

Whiting incision: Additional incision made from center of mastoid wound toward occipital protuberance in mastoid operations with complication of infected sinus thrombosis; enlarges operative field.

Whitman frame: Device that causes extension of spine, esp. if cast is to be applied.

Whitman plate: Stainless steel arch support used in flatfoot in children.

Whittaker test: Invasive pressure study after antegrade puncture of collecting system used in evaluation of hydronephrosis; rarely performed today. Readings are taken at increasing flow rates; normally, flow rates up to 10 ml/sec result in no increase in pressure.

Wichmann asthma: See Kopp asthma.

Wickham retractor: Self-retaining body wall retractor that can be shaped to fit habitus; often used in kidney surgery that involves flank incision.

Widal test: Used to detect typhoid fever; measures presence of agglutinating antibodies to H or O antigens.

Widmar reaction: Indicative of appendicitis if temperature in right axilla is higher than in left axilla.

Widowitz sign: Bulging eyeballs and lagging eye movements seen in paralysis/paresis caused by diphtheria.

Wieacker-Wolff syndrome: Mild mental retardation; congenital foot contractures; slowly progressive distal muscle atrophy; and loss of coordination of tongue, face, and eye muscles. Inheritance is X-linked.

Wiedemann syndrome (Lenz syndrome): Thalidomide-induced birth defects (esp. at 23–36 days' gestation), which vary from minor thumb abnormalities to complete absence of upper arms. Condition also involves hydrocephalus, skull abnormalities, cleft palate, meningomyelocele, capillary hemangioma of face, and internal organ malformation, usu. with normal intelligence.

Wieder tongue depressor: L-shaped, handheld retractor

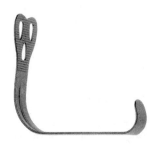

Wieder tongue depressor

with flattened end used to hold tongue away from surgical field.

Wieder treatment: Therapy for eustachian strictures, using filiform bougies for mechanical enlargement. After blowing cocaine solution and lubricating oil into ear, bougies are manipulated until 1 passes. Other 2 are then passed along side, left for several minutes, and withdrawn.

Wiegert ligament: Area of attachment of eye lens to area of condensation of vitreous; lies immediately central to insertion of fibers of posterior zonula.

Wiegert stain: Iron hematoxylin stain.

Wiener system: Notational description of Rh antigen blood group.

Wiktor stent: Flexible, balloon-expandable (single tantalum wire, zigzag-shaped), intravascular stent; possibly useful in peripheral vascular applications.

Wilbrand knee: Looping retinal ganglion cell axons at junction of optic nerve and optic chiasm, which are crossed inferonasal fibers that extend anteriorly with contralateral posterior optic nerve for short distance prior to continuation in optic tract. Posterior optic nerve lesion affecting these fibers can cause superior quadrantic visual field defect in contralateral eye.

Wilcoxon rank sum test: Quantitative statistical test for hypothesis about population medians; nonparametric equivalent of t-test.

Wilde forceps: Long, slender grasping instrument (serrated or mouse-toothed tip) used in ear canal.

Wilder sign: Occurrence of slight twitch when gaze is moved medially or laterally; sometimes seen in early Graves disease.

Wilder stain: Reticulin stain helpful in differentiating epithelial from nonepithelial tumors.

Wildermuth ear: Congenitally deformed ear with obliterated helix and prominent anthelix.

Wildervanck syndrome: Rare association of Klippel-Feil sequence, Duane anomaly, and conduction or sensorineural deafness; occurs in 1% of deaf children.

Wilkie disease: Mechanical compression of duodenum against spinal column by superior mesenteric artery; occurs with acute weight loss, immobilization in body cast, correction of spine curvature using rods, and prolonged recumbency. Diagnosis is made using upper GI contrast dye study.

Wilkins-Bergada syndrome: Hypoplasia of testes and penis, hypospadias, and low testosterone levels; testes may be in inguinal canal. Sex assignment in patients (46,XY) can be problematic.

Willet disease: See Dorph disease.

Willett forceps: Obstetrical forceps.

Williams orthosis: Lumbosacral brace using lever action

and abdominal support for control of extension, lumbar lordosis, and moderate lateral control; allows flexion.

Williams procedure: Surgical creation of neovagina; 1st described for congenital agenesis and now most commonly used for failed McIndoe procedure or damage after radiotherapy. Technique involves reapproximation of labial tissue, with skin flaps folded over and sutured in midline. Resulting "kangaroo pouch" may require progressive dilation.

Williams sign: Dullness percussed in 2nd intercostal space with ipsilateral pleural effusion.

Williams splinter forceps: Ring-handled forceps with curved, needle-nosed tips; used for grasping small objects.

Williams syndrome: Idiopathic hypercalcemia of infancy with elfin facies, mental retardation, and supravalvular aortic stenosis. Gene mutation is at 7q11.

Williams-Campbell syndrome: Congenital absence of bronchial annular cartilage; marked by early childhood onset of pneumonia, cough, and bronchiectasis. Treatment is fluidization of secretions and antibiotics.

Williamson sign: Much lower blood pressure in leg as opposed to arm on same side; occurs in pneumothorax or pleural effusions.

Willis cords: Fibrous bands crossing superior sagittal (longitudinal) sinus in brain.

Wilms tumor: Renal tumor (most common neoplasm of urinary tract in children); may be associated with other abnormalities (15%) such as aniridia, hemihypertrophy, or visceromegaly. Condition is thought to be secondary to loss of tumor suppressor gene on chromosome 11.

Wilson disease: Kayser-Fleischer rings of cornea, cirrhosis, and psychiatric disturbances; autosomal recessive condition. Cause is abnormal copper transport.

Wilson fracture: Fracture of proximal middle phalanx.

Wilson lead (central terminal): Common negative pole with resistance of 50,000 Ω; used in unipolar lead configuration in ECG.

Wilson muscle: Sphincter muscle of urethra.

Wilson technique: Tranvenous Fogarty balloon catheter occlusion of iatrogenic brachiocephalic fistula to innominate artery.

Wimberger sign: Bilateral proximal tibial erosions; seen on radiography in congenital syphilis.

Winkelmann syndrome: See Crosti reticulosis.

Winkler body: Spherical inclusion found in syphilitic lesions.

Winslow pancreas: Uncinate portion of pancreas.

Winterbottom sign: Enlargement of posterior cervical

lymph nodes in African trypano-somiasis.

Wintrich sign: Change in percussion sound in lung cavities when mouth is closed and then opened.

Wintrobe scale: Reference units for erythrocyte sedimentation rate; normal value is 0–20 mm/hr.

Wirsung duct: Main pancreatic duct in 90% of individuals, which starts in tail of organ and runs nearer posterior surface, becoming largest in head (3 mm), where it turns obliquely downward to drain into duodenum at ampulla of Vater; contains 20 secondary branches.

Wiskott-Aldrich syndrome: Abnormal platelet function, thrombocytopenia, eczema, repeated infections, and increased risk of lymphoma and leukemia; usu. fatal in childhood. Inheritance is X-linked recessive.

Wistar rat: Albino variant of *Rattus norvegicus.*

Wistar-Kyoto rat: Normotensive control strain to Aiko-Okamato rat used in study of essential hypertension in humans.

Witt anemia: See Faber anemia.

Witz test: Used to detect hydrochloric acid in gastric juice; positive if addition of 1:48 aqueous solution of methyl violet causes color change from blue to green.

Wolfe-Kawamoto technique: Procedure for taking iliac bone graft. Center iliac wedge is removed, with reapproximation of outer pieces with intact muscular and periosteal attachments.

Wolff law: Bone formation and remodeling occurs in direction of forces acting on it.

Wolff reagent: Solution containing distilled H_2O, absolute alcohol, concentrated hydrochloric acid, and phosphotungstic acid.

Wolff-Parkinson-White disease: Usu. asymptomatic cardiac disease with AV bypass fibers that conduct in antegrade direction; majority of accessory pathways conduct in left free wall. Types are dependent on direction of initial delta wave on ECG. Type A—ventricular activation occurs 1st in inferior-posterior region of left ventricle, with anteriorly directed delta wave and variably appearing Q-wave in leads II, II, and aVF; type B—ventricular activation occurs 1st in inferior-posterior region of right ventricle, with delta wave directed posteriorly and to left with negative initial deflection and rS or qS pattern in V_1; type C—ventricular activation occurs 1st in posterior-lateral region of left ventricle, with positive delta wave in V_1 and negative or isoelectric delta wave in leads V_5 and V_6.

wolffian body (mesonephros): Transitory embryonic structure found in developing urogenital tract, which develops as projection off dorsal abdominal wall; genital ridge forms on this.

Wölfler operation: Type of gastrojejunostomy.

Wolfram syndrome: Congenital diabetes mellitus and diabetes insipidus; also associated with hydroureter, optic atrophy, and deafness.

Wolfring glands: Accessory lacrimal ducts that lie above tarsal plate.

Wolfson disease: Spinal metastasis causing irritation to nerve roots with pain, increased alkaline phosphatase, and increased sedimentation rate.

Wollaston doublet: 2 plano-convex lenses used to correct chromatic aberrations in microscope lens system.

Wolman disease: Defect in acid cholesterol ester hydrolase function with infantile onset, mild mental retardation, hepatomegaly, and adrenal calcification; autosomal recessive condition.

Wonderlic test: Type of mental ability test originally used to screen for industrial employment. Test is now also used to evaluate candidates for NFL draft.

Wood's lamp: Ultraviolet lamp that generates 360-nm wavelength light, which is produced by mercury vapor source passed through nickel oxide filter. Certain tissues appear in characteristic manner when viewed under lamp because of absorption and emission of energy (e.g., tissue colonized with *Pseudomonas* appears light blue).

Wood sign: Fixed eyes, relaxed orbicularis muscle, and divergent strabismus; seen in deep anesthesia.

Woodbury test: Used to detect alcohol in urine; positive if green color is produced when 1 ml of sulfuric acid and crystal of potassium dichromate is added to sample.

Woodcock-Johnson Psycho-educational battery: Academic achievement test used from 3 years of age to adult; provides standard scores and percentiles in reading, written languages, mathematics, and general tasks for each age and grade level.

Woods-Pendleton disease: Abrupt onset of loss of control of muscles of equilibrium; also with torsion spasms, athetosis, hearing loss, and lethargy. Disorder is possibly related to toxic injury to globus pallidus or substantia nigra.

Woods-Schaumberg disease: Slowly progressive ataxia, extrapyramidal rigidity, distal muscle weakness, and nuclear ophthalmoplegia; childhood onset. Histology shows degeneration of pons, spinocerebellar tract, substantia nigra, dentate nucleus, and anterior horn cells.

Woodworth personal data sheet: Earliest known self-report inventory, which asks 116 questions to probe for psychiatric symptoms; used in mass screening of soldiers in World War I.

Woodworth-Mathews personal data sheet: Early self-report inventory developed for use in children.

Woringer-Kolopp disease (pagetoid verticulosis): Rare isolated, slowly expanding plaque occurring on distal leg, with minimal symptoms; possible variant of Alibert-Bazin disease. Treatment is surgical removal and low-dose radiotherapy.

wormian bone: Bony fragment of temporal bone found in each parietal notch.

Worth amblyoscope: Early, handheld instrument with movable tubes to allow any degree of divergence or convergence.

Worth syndrome (endosteal hyperostosis): Thickening and overgrowth of mandible, forehead, and skull; onset in late childhood. Disorder is usu. benign and may cause headaches and cranial nerve symptomatology (auditory, optic, facial). Inheritance is autosomal dominant.

Worth test: Used to detect grossly impaired vision; performed by rolling 5 successively smaller balls (1 1/2–5 in.) and asking patient to retrieve them.

Wratten filter: Optical filter with 2 glass plates and organic dye–gelatin compound in between.

Wright hemostatic: Substance used to stop bleeding in dental procedures; consists of mixture of gelatin and formaldehyde solution.

Wright maneuver: Positive for thoracic outlet syndrome if lifting arm overhead obliterates radial pulse.

Wright method: Technique for evaluating platelet aggregation; involves measuring platelet binding capacity to wall of slowly turning cylinder.

Wright prosthesis: Knee replacement with maximum freedom of motion of joint; requires good soft tissue stability.

Wright respirometer: Early portable instrument used to measure resting minute ventilation by having exhaled breath pass through weirs to turn rotor at rate known to be proportional to minute ventilation.

Wright-Leishman stain: Substance that stains Cabot ring bodies red.

Wrisberg cartilages (cuneiform cartilages): Small protuberances found in each arytenoid-epiglottic fold; lie anterior to Santorini cartilages.

Wrisberg nerve (glossopalatine nerve): Largely sensory root of facial nerve, which also contains some parasympathetic fibers; arises in geniculate ganglion. Fibers comprise chorda tympani that supplies palate, anterior tongue, and some taste buds.

Wrisberg nerve: Medial cutaneous nerve of arm carrying sensory fibers; originates from medial cord of brachial plexus and supplies skin on posterior and medial arm.

Wullstein tympanoplasty:
Procedure involving destruction of malleus, incus, crura of stapes, and tympanic membrane with footplate of stapes remaining intact; allows footplate to be exposed to sound energy and round window membrane to be blocked from sound energy. Operation requires normal, intact mucous membrane in cavum minor.

Wunderlich hematoma:
Traumatic injury to kidney parenchyma through compression or contusion; associated with hematuria, variable degree of shock, and palpable mass.

Wundt color sphere: Paradigm that saturation, hue, and brightness can be arranged on 3-D sphere.

Wundt gravity phonometer: Audiometer that detects hearing threshold. Steel balls are dropped onto hard wood from different heights to produce calibrated sound.

Wundt-Lamansky law: Line of vision in frontal plane moves in straight line when looking along vertical or horizontal plane but in curved path when looking in all other directions.

Wyburn-Mason syndrome:
Congenital arteriovenous aneurysm of midbrain and retina, variable mental retardation, variable psychosis, and vascular facial nevi. Symptoms of hemorrhage usu. develop in 3rd decade, with vomiting, headache, and unilateral loss of vision.

Yamanaka-Hobbs modification: Description of anomalies of coronary arteries. *Benign anomalies*—separate origin of left anterior descending artery and left circumflex artery from left sinus of Valsalva, origin of left circumflex artery from right sinus of Valsalva or right coronary artery, absent left circumflex artery with maximally dominant right coronary artery and ectopic origin of left main trunk or right coronary artery from posterior sinus of Valsalva, small coronary fistulae, intercoronary communication, and ectopic coronary artery origin from ascending aorta. *Potentially life-threatening anomalies*—origin of left main trunk from pulmonary artery (Bland-

White-Garland syndrome, origin of right coronary artery from left sinus of Valsalva, origin of left anterior descending artery from right sinus of Valsalva, origin of right coronary artery from pulmonary artery, and origin of left coronary artery from right sinus of Valsalva.

Yankauer curet: Instrument used to strip mucous membrane from eustachian tube in chronic otorhinorrhea.

Yankauer suction device: Curved, hollow tube that is commonly used to "suck" blood or fluid out of operating field.

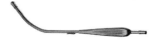

Yankauer suction device

Yankauer suction tube: Instrument consisting of external silver catheter and soft flexible internal bougies that are slowly advanced until tip is observed at tympanic membrane; used to dilate eustachian strictures.

Yasargil aneurysm clip: Spring clip used to obliterate intracranial aneurysm with small ringlet that acts as alignment guide; belongs to alpha class of design with "cross-leg" mechanism.

Yeomans rectal biopsy forceps: Long (368–457 mm), 90°, ring-handled device used to obtain small tissue specimens from rectal canal; available with rotating and nonrotating oblong basket jaw.

Yergason sign: Pain on resistance to supination; occurs in 50% of cases of bicipital tenosynovitis.

Yesudian syndrome: Congenital mental retardation, scaly skin, excessive splitting of hair, and increased levels of amino acids in serum and urine; autosomal recessive condition.

York-Mason procedure (modified): Technique for repair of vesicorectal fistula; does not require diverting colostomy in mechanically and antibiotically prepped bowel. Patient is placed in prone position with buttocks reflected and taped laterally. Sagittal incision is made from posterior anal verge to coccyx with separation and tagging of muscle layers (including complete thickness of posterior rectal wall) for correct reapproximation. Fistula is then excised with separate closures of bladder and rectum (2-layered closures) and overlying muscle fibers reapproximated.

Younge-Dees-Leadbetter procedure: Technique for bladder neck tubulization that commonly uses patch of bowel wall (remaining on its mesentery); can be used in correction of bladder exstrophy.

Yvon coefficient: Urea-to-phosphate ratio in urine.

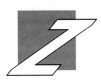

Zackay syndrome: Rare familial mental retardation, stunted growth, small head, and skeletal abnormalities.

Zahn disease (pseudoinfarct of liver): Occlusion of small branches of hepatic veins caused by dilatation of neighboring sinusoids; does not cause parenchymal necrosis. Condition is sometimes seen after splenectomy.

Zahorsky disease: See Mikulicz aphthae.

Zamboni disease: Tachycardia, tachypnea, frothy sputum and bilateral perihilar infiltrate seen on chest radiograph; occurs in ice skaters exposed to nitrogen oxides in fumes of ice-resurfacing machines. Condition spontaneously resolves in 2–3 days.

Zambusch syndrome (guttate morphea): See Hallopeau syndrome (type 1).

Zang space (lesser supraclavicular fossa): Space behind clavicle lying between 2 tendons of sternocleidomastoid muscle.

Zange-Kindler syndrome: Space-occupying lesion at cisterna magna causing blockage of CSF flow; marked by mental deterioration, headaches, optic disk bulging, nausea, and vomiting.

Zanoli-Vecchi syndrome: Convulsions occurring after spinal surgery caused by blood entering brain ventricles. Treatment is supportive with diazepam.

Zappert chamber: Type of counting chamber for quantification of cells and blood particles.

Zappert syndrome: Acute onset of cerebellar ataxia often following infection (e.g., scarlet fever, chickenpox, measles). Course is highly variable and ranges from complete recovery to residual mental deterioration to death.

Zaufal sign: Saddle nose deformity.

Zeek disease: Hypersensitivity angiitis with involvement of pulmonary arteries, hypertension, and ear infection. Condition is similar to Kussmaul-Maier disease but does not involve muscular wall arteries. Disorder is marked by variable presence of bifurcations and predilection for lung involvement.

Zeiss glands: Sebaceous glands attached to hair follicles of eyelashes.

Zeissel layer: Lies between tunica muscularis mucosae and tela submucosa layers in stomach.

Zellweger syndrome: Congenital generalized defect of peroxisome with psychomotor retardation, retinopathy, liver disease, and severely reduced levels of docosahexanoic acid (DHA). Recent treatments include exogenous administration of DHA and ethyl ether.

Zenker diverticulum (pharyngoesophageal diverticulum): Pulsion diverticula (mucosa and submucosa only) found in cervical esophagus in posterior midline between fibers of inferior pharyngeal constrictors and just proximal to cricopharyngeus; key defect is dysfunction of cricopharyngeus muscle. Common presenting features are regurgitation of putrid food, halitosis, aspiration, pneumonia, and dysphagia. Treatment is excision or tacking via left neck incision to allow dependent drainage of contents. Condition usu. occurs after 50 years of age.

Zickel classification: System used to describe subtrochanteric fracture. Type 1A, fracture running from superior to lesser trochanter to lower lateral shaft; type 1B, longer fracture running from superior to lesser trochanter; type 1C, transverse fracture running inferior to lesser trochanter to near isthmus.

Ziegler disease: Nonbacterial endocarditis associated with chronic disease, malignancy, and cachexia; valve growths may embolize peripherally, causing symptoms of arterial blockage. Condition is some-times associated with fever and systolic murmur.

Ziehen-Oppenheim disease (Schwalbe-Ziehen-Oppenheim disease): Slowly progressive torsion-type body movements; onset occurs in childhood. Patients usu. present with unilateral foot inversion, and eventually, condition involves entire extrapyramidal system. Autosomal variation is more severe and seen in Jews; autosomal dominant inheritance more benign. Treatment involves multimodality therapy (l-dopa, surgery, biofeedback), with disappointing results.

Ziehl-Neelsen stain: Bichromic stain using hemalum to stain nuclei blue and carbofuchsin to stain acid-fast rods and leprosy bacilli red.

Zielke device: Anterior fixation device made of stainless steel and used for thoracic and lumbar spine in scoliosis; similar to Dwyer device, except with threaded rod instead of cable for gradual, controlled application of compressive force.

Zieman test: Used to diagnose presence of groin hernia if bulging is felt when patient coughs and examiner places index finger on internal ring, middle finger on external ring, and ring finger on saphenous orifice.

Zieve syndrome: Jaundice, hemolytic anemia, and hyperlipidemia seen in heavy and chronic alcohol intake.

Zigmond chamber (orientation chamber): Apparatus used

to determine ability of cells (usu. neutrophils) to orient in chemoattractant gradient; has 2 wells with cells in one and chemoattractant in other. Scoring is based on determining orientation of cells as they diffuse or by actually filming their movement.

Zimmer mesher: Roller-type device used to mesh skin grafts to increase surface area before applying to recipient site; allows surface area expansion of 1.5:1–9:1.

Zimmer method: Radiographic technique using latero-medial projection to image both sternoclavicular articulations.

Zimmerman arch: Variably present embryonic structure between 4th aortic and pulmonary arches; may develop into anomalous vascular structures.

Zinn circle (central artery of retina): Branch of ophthalmic artery; enters through optic papilla and branches into nasal, inferior and temporal branches.

Zinsser-Cole-Engman syndrome (Cole-Rauschkalb-Toomey syndrome): Nail degeneration with shedding and paronychia followed by reticular skin pigmentation and atrophy, telangiectasia, macular rash on soles and palms, erosions on conjunctiva and mucosa, mouth tumors, testicular atrophy, and mental deterioration; onset occurs in childhood. Early death from carcinoma results.

Ziprkowski-Adam syndrome: Congenital deafness occurring in setting of complete albinism; autosomal recessive condition.

Ziprkowski-Margolis syndrome: Association of congenital sensorineural deafness and oculocutaneous albinism; affects only males due to X-linked inheritance pattern.

Zoellner-Clancy technique: Surgical procedure used to correct recurrent dislocation of peroneal tendon; involves J-shaped incision posterior to lateral malleolus. Peroneus brevis and longus tendons are reflected anteriorly, and bone is removed from posterior fibula to deepen groove. Tendons are then returned to their anatomic position and secured with periosteal flap.

Zollinger-Ellison disease: Hypersecretion of acid leading to severe ulcer disease; due to gastrinoma in duodenum or head of pancreas. Presenting features may include diarrhea or jejunal or duodenal ulcer. Condition occurs sporadically and in association with MEN-1 (Wermer syndrome).

Zondek-Bromberg-Rozin syndrome: Rare hyperhypothalamus functioning with increased production of TSH, estrogens, and lactation hormones; condition causes excessive uterine bleeding, hyperthyroidism, and galactorrhea. Disorder occurs only in parous women. Treatment is partial ablation of hypothalamus.

zonule of Zinn (Zinn membrane, Zinn tendon): Suspensory ligament of lens. Reduction of tension via contraction of ciliary muscles causes lens to become more convex.

Zucker catheter: Fairly stiff catheter used for right heart catheterization; has side holes and electrode near tip that allows optional cardiac pacing and simultaneous recording of intracardiac pressures as well as ECG.

Zucker rat: Morbidly obese rat extensively used as animal model for non–insulin-dependent diabetes mellitus; also exhibits severe hypertriglyceridemia and cholesterolemia.

Zuckerkandl line: Anterior wall of sphenoid.

Zuelzer disease: Recurrent pain in testis caused by injury to pudendal nerve.

Zuelzer-Ogden disease: 1940s term for association of infection, vitamin C deficiency, and megaloblastic anemia.

Zunich syndrome (neuro-ectodermal syndrome): Mental retardation, migratory ichthyosiform rash, conductive-type deafness, seizures, coloboma, cleft palate, and congenital heart abnormalities; autosomal recessive condition.

Appendix I.
LIST OF ALTERNATE ORDER EPONYM NAMES

Note: The names in boldface type indicate where the definition of the entry is found in the main text. For example, Abbott-Miller tube is one alternate order for Miller-Abbott tube, which appears in the "M" entries.

Abbott-**Miller** tube
Adam-**Ziprkowski** syndrome
Adams-**Fisher** syndrome
Adams-**Lance** syndrome
Adams-**Morgagni**-Stokes syndrome
Adams-**Stokes** syncope
Addison-**Hunter** disease
Adie-**Holmes** syndrome
Adson-**Anderson** scalp retractor
Aird-**Flynn** syndrome
Alajouanine-**Foix** syndrome
Alajouanine-**Guillain**-Garcin syndrome
Albright-**Forbes** syndrome
Albright-**Lightwood** disease
Albright-**McCune** syndrome
Aldrich-**Wiskott** syndrome
Allen-**Corner** test
Allgöwer-**Rüedi** classification
Almeida-**Lutz**-Splendore disease
Almeida-**Splendore** disease
Amalric-**Diallinas** syndrome
American-**French**-British classification
Anderson-**Glenn** repair
Anderson-**Roger** fixation
Andra-**Sandmann** syndrome
Andre-**Fitch** syndrome
Anthony-**Lance** syndrome

Antley-**Bixler** syndrome
Arnold, **bifurcate** deep ligaments of
Arnold, **bigeminate** ligaments of
Arrillaga-**Ayerza** disease
Aschoff-**Rokitansky** sinuses
Assman-**Henck** syndrome
Aubineau-**Lenoble** syndrome
Auerbach-**Friedreich** syndrome
Augier-**Bessauds**-Hilmand syndrome
Azan-**Mallory** stain
Bacall-**Bogart** syndrome
Baehr-**Löhlein** lesion
Baker-**Phelps** test
Baker-**Rendell**-Soucek mask
Bamberger-**Marie** disease
Bannwarth-**Garin**-Bujadoux disease
Barabas-**Sock** syndrome
Bárány-**Nylen** test
Barnes-Lloyd-**Jones** and Roberts classification
Barré-**Guillain** syndrome
Barr-**Epstein** virus
Barr-**Jackson** disorder
Batson-**Carmody** operation
Batten-**Holthouse** syndrome
Bauer-**Kirby** stain
Baumgarten-**Cruveilhier** syndrome

Bazin-**Alibert** disease
Beasley-Cohen Danlos-**Ehlers** type
Beath-**Harris** footprinting mat
Beath-**Harris** procedure
Bechterew-**Mendel** reflex
Beer-**Löw** position
Behçet-**Adamantiades** syndrome
Behçet-**Halushi** syndrome
Bekhterev-**Kaes** line
Bellevue-**Wechsler** scale
Belot-**Mouchet** syndrome
Bending-**Charleston** brace
Benhke-**Thiel** dystrophy
Benz-**Mercedes** sign
Berg-**Cotton** syndrome
Bergada-**Wilkins** syndrome
Bernard-**Sergent** syndrome
Bertolotti-**Gruner** syndrome
Besant-**Lewis** syndrome
Besnier-**Tarral** syndrome
Bevan-**Cross** reagent
Bickel-**Fanconi** disease
Biedl-**Bardet** syndrome
Biedl-Moon-**Laurence** syndrome
Bielschowsky-**Roth** syndrome
Biermer-**Ehrlich** disease
Binet-**Stanford** scale
Bing-**Taussig** disease
Bird-**Duncan** sign
Biskis-**Finkel**-Jinkins virus
Blackfan-**Diamond** syndrome
Blakemore-**Sengstaken** tube
Blanc-**Bonnet**-Dechaume syndrome
Blass-**Londsdale** syndrome
Blaus-**Jabs** syndrome
Bloom-Richardson-**Scarff** grade
Blum-**Gougerot** disease
Bock **Otto** hand
Boeck-**Besnier** disease
Bolthauser-**Joubert** syndrome
Boltzmann-**Stefan** constant
Boltzmann-**Stefan** law
Bost-**Abbott**-Saunders arthrodesis

Bottcher-**Charcot** crystalloids
Bourne-**Barnett** nitrate
Bourneville-**Pringle** disease
Bradford-**Rose** kidney
Braun-**Böhler** frame
Brenner-**Jacob** model
Bridge-Good-**Berendes** disease
British-**French**-American classification
Brock-**Bessey**-Lowry unit
Brocks-**Towne** syndrome
Brodwell-**Jacobsen** syndrome
Brooke-**Morrow** acne
Browder-**Lund** method
Brown-**Allen** criteria
Brown-**Hines** test
Brown-**Sanger** syndrome
Browne-**Crichton** sign
Browne-**Denis** splint
Brunhes-**Chavany** syndrome
Brunhes-**Fritzsche**-Chavany syndrome
Buckholz-**Saint Georg** prothesis
Bucklers-**Reis** corneal dystrophy
Bucy-**Klüver** syndrome
Bugg-**Conrad** trapping
Bujadoux-**Garin**-Bannwarth disease
Bunnell-**Paul** test
Bunnell-**Paul**-Davidsohn test
Burchard-**Liebermann** reaction
Burford-**Graham**-Mayer syndrome
Burk-**Lineweaver** equation
Burn-**Baraitser** syndrome
Calvé-**Legg**-Perthes disease
Campanacci-**Jaffe** syndrome
Canada-**Cronkhite** syndrome
Carmalt-**Rochester** hemostatic forceps
Carol-**Godfried**-Prick-Prakken syndrome
Carrel-**Dakin** fluid
Carteaud-**Gougerot** syndrome
Castaigne-**Achard** method
Castaneda-**Codman** kit

Chaix-**Favre** syndrome
Champion-**Sneddon** syndrome
Charlton-**Schultz** test
Chase-**Albright** resection
Chastang-**Gatellier** approach
Chavany-Brunhes-**Fritzsche** syndrome
Chavany-**Foix**-Marie syndrome
Cheney-**Hajdu** syndrome
Chiari-**Arnold** malformation
Cholewa-**Itard** sign
Chotzen-**Saethre** syndrome
Christian-**Hand**-Schüller disease
Christian-**Weber** disease
Chutorian-**Rosenberg** syndrome
Ciocalteau-**Folin** reagent
Clancy-**Zoellner** technique
Clark-**Linch** syndrome
Clayton-**Hoffman** procedure
Cléjat-**Petges** syndrome
Cléret-**Leaunois** syndrome
Cloquet-**Bilhaut** procedure
Closs-**Danbolt** disease
Coenen-**Henle** test
Cogan-**Bielschowsky**-Lutz syndrome
Cohen-Danlos-**Ehlers** type Beasley
Cohen-**Malamud** disease
Cohn-**Krackow** technique
Coldman-**Goldie** hypothesis
Cole-**Hopkins** test
Cole-**Huppert** test
Cole-**Liebermann** syndrome
Cole-**Zinsser**-Engman syndrome
Coller-**Astler** classification
Coller-**Astler** classification (modified)
Colles-**Ace** fixator
Collins **Treacher** syndrome
Congo-**Crimean** hemorrhagic fever
Conn-**Fajans** standards
Connor-**Bhattacharyya** syndrome
Connor-**Holmgren** syndrome

Conwell-**Key** classification
Cooke-**Gordon** syndrome
Coombs and **Gell** classification
Coombs-**Carey** murmur
Cooper-**Wenger** deficiency
Cornil-**Lhermitte**-Quesnel syndrome
Coscia-**Aebi**-Etter fixation
Costero-**Barroso**-Moguel silver method
Cotton-**Bouveret** syndrome
Coulson-**Sanger** method
Courmont-**Arloing** test
Crandall-**Bjornstad** syndrome
Creutzfeldt-**Siemerling** disease
Crile-**Barnes** hemostatic forceps
Critchley-**Adie** syndrome
Critchley-**Ferguson** ataxia
Crosti-**Gianotti** syndrome
Crouzon-**Apert** syndrome
Curtis-**Fitz**-Hugh syndrome
Cushing-**Bailey** disease
Cushing-**Rokitansky** ulcer
Cutter-**Smeloff** valve
D'Alonzo-**Anderson** classification
Dagnini-**Scaglietti** syndrome
Dake-**Fontaine** stent
Dakin-**Carrel** fluid
Dally-**Bell** dislocation
Dameshek-**Estren** syndrome
Danielli-**Davson** model
Danlos-**Ehlers** syndrome types 1–11
Danlos-**Ehlers** Beasley-Cohen type
Danlos-**Ehlers** Friedman-Harrod type
Danlos-**Ehlers** Hernandez type
Danlos-**Ehlers** Viljoin type
Davidoff-Masson-**Dyke** syndrome
Davidsen-**Arlt** syndrome
Davidson-**Barach** tent
Davies-Colley-**Cyriax** syndrome
Davis-**Lloyd** stirrups

Davis-**Rockey** incision
Dawe and **Kalamchi** classification
Dawley-**Sprague** rat
Day-**Riley** syndrome
De La Paz-**Cannon** syndrome
Dechaume-Blanc-**Bonnet** syndrome
Dees-**Younge**-Leadbetter procedure
Degos-**Dowling** syndrome
Del Castillo-**Ahumada** syndrome
Del Castillo-**Argonz** syndrome
DeLee-**Clanton** algorithms
Dervin-**Banks** rod
Deseze-**Laquesna** angle
DeToni-**Fanconi** syndrome
Diamond-**Blackfan** syndrome
Diamond-**Gardener** syndrome
Diethrich-**Codman** kit
DiGeorge-**Pinsky** syndrome
Dighton-**Adair** syndrome
Dimmer-**Biber**-Haab dystrophy
Doering-**Hallerman** syndrome
Doisy-**Allen** test
Doisy-**Allen** unit
Donnan-**Gibbs** effect
Donovan-**Leishman** body
Dorfman-**Chanarin** syndrome
Doubilet-**Fishman** test
Doudoroff-**Entner** pathway
Down **Langdon** syndrome
Downey-**Jacob** disease
Dox-**Czapek** agar
Drachman-**Fischer**-Sargent syndrome
Drager-**Shy** syndrome
Drash-**Denys** syndrome
Drbohlar-Locke-**Boeck** medium
Dreifuss-**Emery** syndrome
Drennan-**Levine** angle
Dreyfus-**Gilbert** syndrome
Drigalski-**Conradi** agar
Driscoll-**Lucey** syndrome
Dube-**Birt**-Hogg syndrome
Dubois-**Aub** table

Dubousset-**Cotrel** instrumentation
Dubow-**Bailey** technique
Duchenne-**Aran** disease
Dujardin-**Goeminne** syndrome
Dukes-**Filatov** disease
Duperrat-Werther-**Gougerot** syndrome
Dutemps-**Dupuy** operation
Duval-**Schiller** body
Duvernay-**Graber** procedure
Duvigneaud-**Rochon** forceps
Duvigneaud-**Rochon** syndrome
Eastman-**Richardson** retractor
Ebstein-**Armanni** kidney
Ebstein-**Pel** fever
Edwards-**Carpentier** prosthesis
Edwards-**Levine** classification
Edwards-**Starr** prosthesis
Efron-**Paine** syndrome
Egan-**Nadler** syndrome
Ellison-**Zollinger** disease
Emery-**Fried** syndrome
Engelmann-**Camurati** syndrome
Engman-**Zinsser**-Cole syndrome
Epstein-**Faulk**-Jones syndrome
Epstein-Jones-**Faulk** syndrome
Erb-**Duchenne** syndrome
Erb-**Goldflam** disease
Erdheim-**Chester** disease
Erdheim-**Gsell** disease
Eriksson-**Forsius** syndrome
Ernst-**Babes** bodies
Etter-Coscia-**Aebi** fixation
Evans-**Long** rat
Evelyn-**Malloy** method
Evens-**François** syndrome
Exner-**Call** vacuole
Falls-**Haney** syndrome
Falls-**Nettleship** syndrome
Fanconi-**Bickel** syndrome
Favre-**Gamna** bodies
Favre-**Goldman** disease
Feichtiger-**Ullrich** syndrome
Feil-**Klippel** syndrome
Ferguson-**Hill** rectal retractor

Ferguson-**Webber** incision
Ferguson-**Weber** approach
Ferrand-**Darier** syndrome
Fibringer-**Debré** syndrome
Filatow-**Dukes** disease
Filiu-**Porot** syndrome
Finney-**Grondahl** operation
Fischer-**Ace** frame
Fisher-**Herbert** classification
Fisher-Lucas-**Abbott** procedure
Fisher-**Miller** syndrome
Fisher-**Redlich** plaques
Fitz-**Balser** disease
Flaujeac-**Fitzgerald**-Williams factor
Flaujeac-**Fitzgerald**-Williams trait
Fleischel-**Aubert** paradox
Fleischer-**Kayser** rings
Flint-**Austin** murmur
Flint-**Austin** respiration
Foix-**Marie** sign
Foix-**Schilder** syndrome
Foley-**Adams** disorder
Fordyce-**Fox** disease
Forest-**Kyasanur** disease
Forssman-Lehman-**Boerjeson** syndrome
Foville-**Raymond** syndrome
Fowler-**Anderson** procedure
Fraccaro-**Parenti** syndrome
Fraccaro-**Schmid** syndrome
François-**Hallerman**-Streiff syndrome
Frankel-**Bordier** sign
Fraumeni-**Li** syndrome
Friedman-Harrod Danlos-**Ehlers** type
Frei-**Hoffman** test
Friderichsen-**Waterhouse** syndrome
Frommel-**Chiari** syndrome
Fryns-**Lujan** syndrome
Fuchs-**Dalen** nodules
Fuchs-**Foerster** spots
Fukase-**Crow** syndrome
Furst-**Ostrum** syndrome
Gallais-**Apert** syndrome

Gallante-**Miller** prosthesis
Gallwey-**Ferriman** scale
Galton-**Edelman** whistle
Gamble-**Darrow** syndrome
Gandy-**Gamna** bodies
Garcin-**Guillain**-Alajouanine syndrome
Gardiner-**Sheridan** test
Garland-White-**Bland** syndrome
Gass-**Irving** syndrome
Gastaut-**Lennox** syndrome
Gaussel-**Grasset**-Hoover sign
Gellhorn-**Emmert** pessary
Gengou-**Bordet** agar
Gengou-**Bordet** bacillus
Gerold-**Baller** syndrome
Gibbon-**Bailey** rib contractor
Gibbon-**Mayo** heart–lung machine
Gibbs-**Stephenson** reference
Gibson-**Andersch** test
Giedeon-**Langer** syndrome
Giedion-**Schinzel** syndrome
Giemsa-Grünwald-**May** stain
Gill-**Abbott** osteotomy
Giovannetti-**Giordano** diet
Gladstone-**Putterman** tube
Goldberg-**Berger** disease
Goldberg-**Frykman** procedure
Goldner-**Mason** stain
Gole-**Touraine**-Solente syndrome
Golgi-**Holmgren** canal
Gomori-**Grocott** solution
Good-**Berendes**-Bridge disease
Gopalan-**Grierson** syndrome
Gorlin-**Glass** syndrome
Gottron-**Arndt** syndrome
Gouw-**Letts**-Vincent syndrome
Graham-**Arkless** syndrome
Grand-**Edgarton** procedure
Gray-**Arieti** disease
Greenfield-**Kimray** filter
Gregoir-**Lich** procedure
Griffith-**Bazex** syndrome
Griffith-**Ma** technique
Griffiths-**Abrams** nomogram
Grof-**Jendrassik** method

Groh-**Gross**-Weippl syndrome
Gronenouw-**Fuchs** syndrome
Gross-**Ladd** syndrome
Gruber-**Martin** anastomosis
Grünwald-**May**-Giemsa stain
Gubler-**Millard** syndrome
Guérin-**Calmette** bacillus
Gulienetti-**Rosselli** syndrome
Gunn **Marcus** phenomenon
Gunn **Marcus** pupil
Gunter-**Praeder** syndrome
Gutmann-**Michaelis** bodies
Haab-Dimmer-**Biber** dystrophy
Haapanen-**Tuomaala** syndrome
Hadfield-**Clarke** syndrome
Hadorn-**Albright** syndrome
Haeckerman-**Laimer** area
Hall-**Relton** frame
Hall-**Rosetti** modification
Hall-**Soto** test
Hanhart-**Richner** syndrome
Hansen-**Asboe** disease
Hansen-**Lauge** classification
Hare-**Hickey** test
Harrington-**Kostuick**
    instrumentation
Harris-**Goodenough** drawing
    test
Harris-**Houston** syndrome
Harrod-Danlos-**Ehlers**-
    Friedman type
Hartlage-**DiMauro** disease
Hasselbach-**Henderson**
    equation
Hastings-**Singer** system
Hauser-Rokitansky-Kuster-
    Mayer syndrome
Haustrate-**François** syndrome
Haxthausen-**Blegvad** syndrome
Hayward-**Juberg** syndrome
Healy-**Blackett** position
Heberden-**Rougnon** disease
Hecht-**Beals** syndrome
Hegglin-**Fanconi** disease
Hegglin-**May** anomaly
Heise-**Crane** syndrome
Heller-**Doehle** disease
Hellwig-**Kersting** tumor

Henoch-**Schoenlein** disease
Henseleit-**Krebs** cycle
Hering-**Traube**-Mayer curves
Hernandez Danlos-**Ehlers** type
Hernandez-**Gomez**-Lopez
    syndrome
Herxheimer-**Jarisch** reaction
Heyman-**Herndon** procedure
Higashi-**Chédiak** disease
Hill-**Lowenberg** syndrome
Hill **Prospect** virus
Hillier-**Thurman** syndrome
Hilmand-Augier-**Bessauds**
    syndrome
Hinton-**Mueller** agar
Hirschfield-**Birsch** syndrome
Hobbs-**Yamanaka** modification
Hochwart-**Frankl** syndrome
Hoeppli-**Splendore**
    phenomenon
Hoffman-**Charcot**-Marie-Tooth
    disease
Hoffman-**Werdnig** disease
Hofstee-**Eadie** equation
Hogg-Dube-**Birt** syndrome
Hol-**Stocker** disease
Holland **Thurston** fragment
Holmes-**Hootnick** syndrome
Holt-**Juberg** syndrome
Hoover-**Grasset**-Gaussel sign
Horan-**Nance** syndrome
Horowitz-**Neer** classification
Horsfall-**Tamm** protein
Hortega-**Foot** stain
Houtsmuller-**De Hass** syndrome
Howard-**Kenny** splint
Howship-**Romberg** sign
Hreidarsson-**Hoyeraal**
    syndrome
Hudson-**Ewald** forceps
Huebner-**Nierhoff** syndrome
Huenermann-**Conradi**
    syndrome
Huët-**Pelger** anomaly
Huët-**Pelger** pseudoanomaly
Hugh-**Fitz**-Curtis syndrome
Hunt-**Ramsay** syndrome
Hunt-**Tolosa** syndrome

Hunter-**Addison** disease
Hunziker-**Laugier** syndrome
Hutchins-**Anderson** procedure
Hutinel-**Tixier** anemia
Huttenlocher-**Alpers** syndrome
Hyde-**Rice** test
Hyman-**Gelfard** disease
Ibrahim-**Beck** syndrome
Indiana-**Reitan** test
Iwanoff-**Blessig** syndrome
Jacob-**Lortat**-Degós syndrome
Jadassohn-**Tièche** nevus
Jakob-**Creutzfeldt** disease
Jalaguier-Kammerer-**Battle** incision
Jamieson-**Killian** diverticulum
Jampel-**Schwartz** syndrome
Jansky-**Bielschowsky** syndrome
Jarisch-**Bezold** reflex
Jeanselme-**Lutz** nodules
Jefferson-**Foix** syndrome
Jeghers-**Peutz** syndrome
Jensen-**Birch** syndrome
Jersild-**Huguier** syndrome
Jessner-**Cole** syndrome
Jewett-**Tieman** nail
Jinkins-**Finkel**-Biskis virus
Joanny-**Leri** syndrome
John **Tommy** surgery
Johnson-**Dubin** syndrome
Johnson-**Stevens** syndrome
Johnson-**Woodcock** battery
Jolly-**Howell** bodies
Jones-**Bence** albumosuria
Jones-**Bence** cylinders
Jones-**Bence** proteins
Jones-**Ellis** technique
Jones-**Faulk**-Epstein syndrome
Jones-**Henderson** chondromatosis
Jones-**Krackow**-Thomas technique
Jones-**Price** curve
Jones-**Smead** technique
Jones-**Watson** classification
Jones-**Watson** incision
Joseph-**Machado** disease

Judet-**Letournel** classification
Junet-**Troell** syndrome
Kalamachi-**Achterman** classification
Kammerer-**Battle**-Jalaguier incision
Kapandji-**Sauve** procedure
Karrer-**Gasser** syndrome
Kasabach-**Merritt** syndrome
Kauffman-Lignac-**Abderhalden** syndrome
Kaufman-**Franceschetti** disease
Kaufman-**McCarey** medium
Kaufman-**McKusick** syndrome
Kawamoto-**Wolfe** technique
Kay-Stansel-**Damus** technique
Kellie-**Monro** doctrine
Kelly-**Paterson** syndrome
Kendall-**Graham** test
Kennedy-**Foster** syndrome
Kennedy-**Kelly** plication
Kerr-**Munro** incision
Kershner-**Adams** disease
Kertesz-**Falls** syndrome
Keuls-**Newman** test
Khetarpal-**Chandra** syndrome
Kindberg-**Loehr** syndrome
Kindler-**Zange** syndrome
Kirklin-**Carman** sign
Kite-**Hoke** procedure
Kivlin-**Krause** syndrome
Kleiger-**Tillaux** fracture
Kleihauer-**Bethke** test
Klein-**Franceschetti** syndrome
Klingenstein-**Dudley** disease
Klionsky-**Sweeley** disease
Kolopp-**Woringer** disease
Korelitz-**Present** index
Kornsweig-**Bassen** syndrome
Kozenitzki-**Libian** syndrome
Kraff-**Sanders**-Retlaff formula
Kramer-**Tukey** test
Krantz-**Marshall**-Marchetti procedure
Kraupa-**Fuchs** syndrome
Kreysig-**Heim** sign
Kuhnt-**Junius** syndrome

Künkel-Slater-**Bearne** syndrome

Kuster-Rokitansky-Hauser-**Mayer** syndrome

Kyoto-**Wistar** rat

Laehmung-**Foville** syndrome

Lallemand-**Trousseau** bodies

Lamansky-**Wundt** law

Lambert-**Eaton** syndrome

Lamy-**Maroteaux** syndrome

Landis and **Gibbon** test

Landsteiner-**Donath** phenomenon

Lang-**Frost** operation

Langenbeck-**Kocher** approach

Langer-**Beemer** syndrome

Lantermann-**Schmidt** clefts

Lapine-**Chassard** position

Larsen-**Sinding**-Johansson syndrome

Larssen-**Helweg** syndrome

Larsson-**Sjögren** syndrome

Lavastine-**Laignel**-Viard syndrome

Lawler-**Jackson** syndrome

Laxova-**Tuffli** syndrome

Layer-**Knoblock** syndrome

Leadbetter-**Politano** repair

Leadbetter-**Younge**-Dees procedure

Leclef-**Denys** phenomenon

Lefèvre-**Papillon** syndrome

Lége-**Papillon** and Psaume syndrome

Lehman-**Boerjeson**-Forssman syndrome

Leishman-**Wright** stain

Lemli-**Smith**-Opitz syndrome

Leri-**Marie** syndrome

Lerman-**Means** sign

Lester-**Martin** agar

Leventhal-**Stein** syndrome

Levin-**Jarcho** syndrome

Levin-**Kleine** syndrome

Levy-**Creyx** syndrome

Levy-**Lhermitte** syndrome

Lévy-**Roussy** disease

Lewis-**Holstein** fracture

Leyden-**Charcot** crystals

Leydig-**Sertoli** cell

Liebermann-**Cole** syndrome

Liéou-**Barré** syndrome

Lignac-**Abderhalden**-Kauffman syndrome

Linberg-**Tikhoff** procedure

Linder-**Albert** bone sectioning

Lindner-**Taybi** syndrome

Lindqvist-**Fahraeus** effect

Lindzey-**Allport**-Vernon study of values

Lisser-**Escamilla** syndrome

Littler-**Eaton** reconstruction

Lloyd-Barnes-**Jones** and Roberts classification

Lobstein-**Ekman** syndrome

Locke-**Boeck**-Drbohlar medium

Loeffler-**Klebs** bacillus

Loewenthal-**Grebe**-Myle syndrome

Lohlein-**Baehr** lesion

Lohr-**Rosemberg** syndrome

Londe-**Fazio** disease

Lopez-**Gomez**-Hernandez syndrome

Lopresti-**Essex** fracture

Lorand-**Laki** factor

Lortolary-**Richter** syndrome

Loutit-**Hayem**-Widal syndrome

Lowry-Brock-**Bessey** unit

Lucas-**Abbott** technique

Lucas-**Abbott**-Fisher procedure

Luc-**Caldwell** operation

Luder-Sheldon-**Fanconi** disease

Luft-**Ernster** syndrome

Luque-**Espildora** syndrome

Lurie-**Garcia** syndrome

Lutz-Cogan-**Bielschowsky** syndrome

Lyon-Meltzer test

MacLean-**Papez** theory

MacNab-**Andrade** procedure

MacNeal-**Novy** blood agar

Madlener-**Kelling** procedure

Magendie-**Bell** law

Magendie-**Hertwig** position

Magenis-**Smith** syndrome

Maia-**Freire** syndrome
Mainzler-**Saldino** syndrome
Majewski-**Lenz** syndrome
Makai-**Rothman** syndrome
Maloney-**Hurst** dilators
Mancall-**Adams**-Victor
  syndrome
Mancall-Richardson-**Åström**
  syndrome
Mann-**Dixon** sign
Marchesani-**Weill** syndrome
Marchetti-**Marshall**-Krantz
  procedure
Marchiafava-**Bignami** disease
Marchiafava-**Strübing** disease
Marfan-**Dennie** syndrome
Marg-**MacKay** tonometer
Margolis-**Ziprkowski** syndrome
Marie-**Foix**-Chavany syndrome
Marie-**Strumpell** disease
Marie-Tooth-Hoffman-**Charcot**
  disease
Marshall-**Jewett** system
Marsidi-**Juberg** syndrome
Martin-**Chick** tests
Mason-**Koch** dressing
Mason-**Wyburn** syndrome
Mason-**York** procedure
Masson-**Barre** syndrome
Masson-**Dyke**-Davidoff
  syndrome
Masson-**Fontana** stain
Masson-**Fontana** technique
Mathews-**Woodworth** data
  sheet
Mauch-**Henschke** device
Maxwell-**Goldberg**-Morris
  syndrome
Mayer-**Fleming** flap
Mayer-**Graham**-Burford
  syndrome
Mayer-**Traube**-Hering curves
Mayo–**Saint Anne** system
Mazzoni-**Golgi** corpuscles
McIntosh-**Marshall** technique
McKeever-**Meyers** classification
Meara-**Dowling** epidermolysis
Meary-**Hibb** angle

Medin-**Heine** disease
Mees-**Aldrich** lines
Meier-**Kaplan** method
Meige-**Nonne**-Milroy syndrome
Mendel-**Bechterew** reflex
Menten-**Michaelis** equation
Merritt-**Kasabach** syndrome
Merzbacher-**Pelizaeus** disease
Messenbaugh-**Amspacher**
  osteotomy
Meyer-**Weigert** rule
Meyerhof-Parnas-**Embden**
  pathway
Meyers-Schwickerath-**Fraser**
  syndrome
Meztger-**Fischgold** line
Michälsson-**Juhlin** syndrome
Micheli-**Marchiafava** syndrome
Miescher-**Lutz** disease
Mikulicz-**Heineke** pyloroplasty
Millar-**Allison** classification
Milroy-**Nonne**-Meiger syndrome
Miura-**Cooperman** syndrome
Moebius-**Leyden** type
Moebius-**Poland** syndrome
Moguel-Costero-**Barroso** silver
  method
Mollaret-**Foshay** fever
Monro-**Richter** line
Montgomery-**Ockuly** syndrome
Moon-Biedl-**Laurence**
  syndrome
Moore-**Austin** arthroplasty
Moore-**Hohl** classification
Moore-**Pélouse** test
Moos-**Chimani** test
Mooser-**Neill** body
Morel-**Oppenheim**-Scholz
  syndrome
Morel-**Stewart** syndrome
Morel-**Stewart**-Morgagni
  syndrome
Morgagni-**Stewart**-Morel
  syndrome
Morris-**Goldberg**-Maxwell
  syndrome
Moskovtchenko-**Rassat** fistula
Mowat-**Galloway** syndrome

Muir-**Passy** valve
Müller-**formol** fixative
Müller-**Geiger** counter
Mummery-**Lockhart** excision
Munk-**Haim** syndrome
Munsell-**Farnsworth** test
Mustian-**Farmer** syndrome
Myhre-**Ruvalcaba**-Smith syndrome
Myle-**Grebe**-Loewenthal syndrome
Nageotte-**Babinski** syndrome
Najjar-**Crigler** syndrome
Neel-**Bing** syndrome
Neelsen-**Ziehl** stain
Neemeh-**Lemieux** syndrome
Neetens-**François** syndrome
Nélaton-**Roser** line
Nelson-**Sprinz** syndrome
Netter-**Weismann**-Stuhl syndrome
Neuberg-**Tollens**-Schwket test
Neugenbauer-**Karsch** syndrome
Neuhausser-**Boucher** syndrome
Nevin-**Kiloh** syndrome
Nielson-**Lange** syndrome
Nitinol-**Simon** filter
Noblett-**Syed** template
Nyhan-**Lesch** syndrome
Nyhan-**Sakati** syndrome
Nystrom-**Hessel** pins
Ochsner-**Rochester** hemostatic forceps
Oh-**Froimson** technique
Oliver-**Adams** syndrome
Opitz-**Dicker** syndrome
Opitz-Lemli-**Smith** syndrome
Oppenheim-**Ziehen** disease
Oppler-**Boas** bacillus
Oram-**Holt** syndrome
Orthuys-**Delleman** syndrome
Oseretsky-**Lincoln** scale
Osler-**Rendu**-Weber disease
Ourgaud-**Jayle** syndrome
Overstreet-**Gordon** syndrome
Pal-**Weigert** method
Palade-**Weibel** body
Paley-**Tunbridge** syndrome

Palm-**Pfeiffer**-Teller syndrome
Pankovich-**Abraham** technique
Pankovich-**Hall** procedure
Papas-**Bartsocas** syndrome
Pappas-**Mast**-Spiegel classification
Parker-**Patterson** technique
Parkinson-**Wolff**-White syndrome
Parnas-**Embden**-Meyerhof pathway
Partsch-**Miehlke** syndrome
Pasini and Pierini, **atrophoderma** of
Patau-**Edwards** syndrome
Pean-**Rochester** hemostatic forceps
Pendleton-**Woods** disease
Persson-**Robb** operation
Petersen-**Smith** approach
Petersen-**Smith** incision
Pfizer-**Mason** virus
Pic-**Bard** disease
Pick-**Lubarsch** disease
Pick-**Niemann** disease
Pierini and Pasini, **atrophoderma** of
Pierquin-**Laquerrier** position
Pilling-**Ossoff** microlaryngoscope
Pin-**Hsieh** syndrome
Pindborg-**Andersen** syndrome
Pogossian-**Ter** camera
Politano-**Leadbetter** procedure
Polyz **Oregon** prosthesis
Pompen-**Ruiter** disease
Porter-**Dormandy** syndrome
Potter-**Doege** syndrome
Power-**Goodall** modification
Prager-**Aronson** procedure
Prakken-**Godfried**-Prick-Carol syndrome
Pratt-**Chambers** syndrome
Pratt-**Jackson** drain
Prick-**Godfried**-Prakken-Carol syndrome
Prowazek-**Greefe** body
Prower-**Stuart** factor

Psaume and **Papillon**-Lége syndrome
PULSES-**Barthel** index
Purser-**Sharp** test
Putti-**Platt** procedure
Quelce-**Salgado** syndrome
Querol-**Forestier**-Rotes spondylosis
Quesnel-**Lhermitte**-Cornil syndrome
Race-**Fisher** hypothesis
Race-**Fisher** system
Racouchot-**Favre** syndrome
Radin-**Riseborough** classification
Radovici-**Marinesco** sign
Rahe-**Holmes** scale
Ralston-**Colonna** approach
Ramstedt-**Fredet** operation
Ransley-**Cantwell** technique
Rawson-**Abbott** tube
Reder-**Wachenheim** sign
Reed-**Dorothy** cells
Reenstierna-**Ito** test
Rees-**Jackson** circuit
Rees-**Russell** syndrome
Reese-**Cogan** syndrome
Regala-**Stransky** syndrome
Rehder-**Holzgreve**-Wagner syndrome
Rehman-**Nadbath** technique
Reichmann-**Goldstein** syndrome
Reitan-**Halstead** battery
Remondini-**Osebold** syndrome
Retlaff-**Sanders**-Kraff formula
Retzius **postrema**
Reynals-**Duran** factor
Reynier-**Nager** syndrome
Ricci-**Cacchi** disease
Rich-**Hamman** syndrome
Richardson-**Åstroöm**-Mancall syndrome
Richardson-**Scarff**-Bloom grade
Richardson-**Spalding** operation
Richner-**Lutz** syndrome
Richter-**Clough** disease

Richter-**Monro** line
Rieger-**Axenfeld** anomaly
Riggs-**Hall** syndrome
Riordan-**Haddad** arthrodesis
Roberts and **Jones**-Barnes-Lloyd classification
Robertson **Argyll** pupils
Robertson-**Neal** litter
Robin **Pierre** syndrome
Robinson-**Skaggs** hypothesis
Robinson-**Smith** diskectomy
Robson-Mayo intestinal forceps
Rochain-**Bartshci** syndrome
Rock-**Garcia** curette
Roessle-**Hanot** syndrome
Rokitansky-Kuster-Hauser-**Mayer** syndrome
Rollet-**Ritter** phenomenon
Romberg-**Howship** sign
Rosales-**Mancall** syndrome
Rosch-**Gianturco** Z-stent
Rosen-**Golabi** syndrome
Rosenberg-**Rowley** syndrome
Rosenheim-**Acree** test
Rosenthal-**Melkersson** syndrome
Rosenthal-**Muenzer** triad
Rossetti-**Nissen** procedure
Rotes-**Forestier**-Querol spondylosis
Rothman-**Makai** lipogranulomatosis
Roussy-**Darier** syndrome
Roussy-**Lévy** syndrome
Roy-**Friedman** syndrome
Rueter-**Becker** syndrome
Ruiter-**Gougerot** syndrome
Russell-**Silver** syndrome
Ruttan-**Harding** test
Sachs-**Ghon** bacillus
Sachs-**Hill** fracture
Sachs-**Tay** syndrome
Sacks-**Libman** disease
Saldino-**Langer** syndrome
Salle-**Pippi** procedure
Sanders-**Holzbach** syndrome
Sargent-**Fischer**-Drachman syndrome

Steritek-**Ladd** system
Stevenson-**Beare** cutis gyratum
Stickler-**David** disease
Stieda-**Koehler** disease
Stieda-**Pellegrini** syndrome
Stokes-**Adams** syncope
Stokes-**Adams** syndrome
Stokes-**Cheyne** nystagmus
Stokes-**Cheyne** respiration
Stokes-**Gritti** amputation
Stokes-**Morgagni**-Adams
    syndrome
Stoloff-**Kugel** disease
Stoner-Kelly-**Barbour** medium
Stovin-**Hughes** syndrome
Strang-**Smith** syndrome
Straussler-Scheinker-
    Gerstmann syndrome
Streiff-François-**Hallerman**
    syndrome
Strisower-**Schellong** phenome-
    non
Strümpell-**Bekhterer** syndrome
Strümpell-**Marie** disease
Stuhl-**Weismann**-Netter
    syndrome
Suit-**Fletcher** radiotherapy
Sutton-**Saunders** disease
Sweet-**Gordon** stain
Szymanowski-**Kuhnt** procedure
Tabatznik-**Berk** syndrome
Takos-**Petzetakis** syndrome
Taussig-**Blalock** procedure
Tay-**Hutchinson** syndrome
Taybi-**Rubinstein** syndrome
Taylor-**Jebsen** test
Taylor-**Russell** nail
Teixeira-**Torres** bodies
Teller-**Pfeiffer**-Palm syndrome
Terrier-**Courvoisier** syndrome
Their-**Franceschetti** syndrome
Thevenard-**Foix** syndrome
Thiemer-**Krüger** hypothesis
Thiers-**Achard** syndrome
Thomas-**Andre** sign
Thomas-**Krackow**-Jones
    technique
Thomas-**Terry** sign

Thoms-**Allis** tissue forceps
Thomson-**Rothmund** syndrome
Tommasi-**Jeune** syndrome
Tooth-Hoffman-**Charcot**-Marie
    disease
Toriello-**Kapur** syndrome
Torre-**Muir** syndrome
Tourette **Gilles** syndrome
Trélat-**Leser** sign
Trenaunay-**Klippel** syndrome
Trenel-**Prieur** syndrome
Treves-**Stewart** syndrome
Tribondeau-**Bergonié** law
Trillat-**Elmslie** transplant
Tronow-**Kulenkampff**
    syndrome
Tuekel-**Goekay** syndrome
Tuerler-**Fanconi** syndrome
Turnbull-**Jennison** modification
Turner-**Aufranc** prosthesis
Turner **Grey** sign
Turner-**Hefke** sign
Turner-**Parsonage** syndrome
Uddin-**Mobin** filter
Unna-**Taenzer** stain
Upmark-**Ask** kidney
Urbach-**Oppenheim** syndrome
Usher-**Senear** syndrome
Vainsel-**Guibaud** syndrome
Van Bogaert-**Dow** syndrome
Van Creveld-**Ellis** syndrome
Van Leeuwen **Storm** chamber
Vaquez-**Babinski** syndrome
Vaquez-**Osler** disease
Vasey-**Weber** technique
Vecchi-**Zanoli** syndrome
Vernet **Gil** incision
Vernon-**Allport** study of
    values
Vernon-Lindzey-**Allport** study
    of values
Victor-Adams-**Banker** disease
Victor-Mancall-**Adams**
    syndrome
Viel-**Terrien** disease
Viljoin Danlos-**Ehlers** type
Vincent-**Letts**-Gouw syndrome
Vinson-**Plummer** syndrome

Appendix II.
EPONYMS LISTED BY SUBJECT

Note: This appendix contains a listing of eponyms by subject in the following categories:

A: Anatomic Locations
B: Anatomic Structures
C: Embryology Terms
D: Oncology Terms
E: Radiology Terms
F: Reflexes, Signs, and Tests

ANATOMIC LOCATIONS

Addison line
Addison planes
Addison point
Aeby plane
Alsberg angle
Alsberg triangle
angle of His
angle of Louis
angle of McRae
angle of Rolando
area of Laimer
Assézat triangle
Baer point
Bamberger area
Barker point
Barnes curve
Baumann angle
Béclard triangle
Betz cell area
Blumensaat line
Boas point
Bolton point
Bolton triangle
Brewer point
Broadbent registration point

Broca angle
Broca convolution
Broca diagonal band
Broca fissure
Broca motor area
Broca parolfactory area
Brodmann areas
Bryant line
Bryant triangle
Budge center
Burns space
Calot triangle
Cantlie line
Cantrell line
Chamberlain line
Chauffard point
circles of Weber
Cobb method
Colles space
Cotunnius space
curve of Carus
Czermak space
Daubenton angle
de Mussy point
Desjardins point
Diogenes cup

Disse space
Dorr ratio
Douglas line
Douglas pouch
Downs Y axis
Duhot line
Ebstein angle
Einthoven triangle
Ellis line
Erb point
Farabeuf triangle
Feiss line
Fick angle
Fischgold line
Fontana space
foramen of Bochdalek
foramen of Magendie
foramen of Monro
foramen of Pacchionius
foramen of Rivini
foramen of Vesalius
foramen of Winslow
fossa of Rosenmueller
Fruchard orifice
Gerhardt triangle
Gottinger line
Griffith point
Guyon canal
Hannover canal
Helmholtz line
Henke space
Hensen canal
Heschl gyri
Hesselbach triangle
Heuter line
Hibb-Meary angle
Hilgenreiner angle
Hilgenreiner lines
His perivascular space
Holder angle
Hueter line
island of Reil
Jackson safety triangle
Jacquart angle
Kanavel spaces
Kanavel triangle
Kaplan line
Kiesselbach area

Killian area
Kohler line
Konstram angle
Laimer-Haeckerman area
Landzert fossa
Langer lines
Lanz point
Laquesna-Deseze angle
Larrey cleft
Larrey spaces
Laurin angle
lesser fossa of Scarpa
Lesshaft space
Levine-Drennan angle
Leydig cylinders
Lietaud trigone
Lisfranc joint
Little area
Lovibond angle
Luschka fossa
Macewen triangle
Magendie foramen
Magendie spaces
Malgaigne triangle
master knot of Henry
McBurney point
McGregor line
Meckel caves
Mehta angle difference
Meynert commissure
Michaelis rhomboid
Monro line
Monro-Richter line
Moyer line
Munro point
Nance leeway space
Ogston line
Panum area
Pascal triangle
Pawlik triangle
Perkin line
Piorry nucleus
pouch of Douglas
Proust space
Ramond point
Rauchfuss triangle
Ravelli triangle
recess of Allison

Reid base line
Reinke space
Retzius cavity
Retzius foramen
Robson line
Rolandic area
Rolando angle
Rolando fissure
Rolando line
Scarpa triangle
Schlemm canal
Schoemaker line
Schwalbe foramen
Sibson notch
space of Larry
space of Martegiani
space of Poirier
space of Retzius
Sudeck point
sulcus of Reil
sylvian point
Tarin anterior recess
Tarin fascia
Tarin fossa
Tarin posterior recess
Tenon space
Topinard line
triangle of Calot
triangle of Killian
triangle of Koch
triangle of Truesdale
Tweed triangle
Valleix points
Verdan zones
Vesalius foramen
vidian nerve
Vieussens foramina
Virchow-Robin space
Voight lines
Voit nucleus
Volkmann canals
von Weber triangle
Ward triangle
Wernicke area

ANATOMIC STRUCTURES

Abbott artery
Abernethy fascia

accessory ligament of Henle
    (lateral)
accessory ligament of Henle
    (medial)
accessory portal system of
    Sappey
Achilles tendon
Acrel ganglion
Adamkiewicz cell
Adam's apple
Albini nodules
Albinus muscle
Albrecht bone
Alcock canal
Amici disk
Amussat valves (gallbladder)
Amussat valves (urethra)
Andernach ossicles
Andersch ganglion
Andersch nerve
angle of Louis
antrum of Willis
apophysis of Ingrassia
apophysis of Rau
apparatus of Goormaghtigh
aqueduct of Cotunnius
aqueduct of Sylvius
Arantius ligament
Arantius nodule
Arantius ventricle
arc of Riolan
arcade of Frohse
arcade of Struthers
arch of Corti
Arlt sinus
Arnold canal
Arnold ganglion
Arnold head
Arnold ligament
Arnold nerve
arterial circle of Viussens
arteries of Mueller
artery of Adamkiewicz
artery of Huebner
artery of Percheron
artery of Zinn
ascending veins of Rosenthal
Aschoff node

Aschoff nodule
Aselli gland
Auerbach plexus
Baillarger stripes
Ball valves
band of Schreger
Barkow ligament (elbow)
Barkow ligament (foot)
Bartholin duct (mouth)
Bartholin duct (vagina)
Bartholin glands
Batson plexus
Bauhin valve
Bechterew bundle
Bechterew nucleus
Béclard nucleus
Bell muscle
Bell nerve
Bellini ducts
Bellini ligament
Bekhterev nucleus
Benninghoff arcades
Bérard ligament
Béraud valve
Berger space
Bergmann fibers
Bernard duct
Bernard glandular layer
Berry ligament
Bertin bones
Bertin columns
Bertin ligament
Betz cells
Bezold ganglion
Bichat fissure
Bichat ligament
Bidder ganglion
bifurcate deep ligaments of
    Arnold
Bigelow septum
Billroth cords
Birbeck granules
Blandin ganglion
Blandin glands
Blumenau nucleus
Blumenbach clivus
Blumenbach process
Bochdalek ganglion

Bock ganglion
Bock nerve
Boettcher cells
Botallo duct
Botallo ligament
Böttcher cells
Bourgery ligament
Bowman capsule
Bowman glands
Bowman layer
Bowman space
Bowman tube
Boyd perforating veins
Boyer bursa
Breschet bones
Breschet canals
Breschet hiatus
Breschet sinus
Breschet veins
Broca convolution
Broca motor area
Broca parolfactory area
Brodel white line
Brodie bursa
Brodie ligament
Brodmann areas
Browing vein
Bruch membrane
Brücke lines
Brücke muscle
Brunn membrane
Brunner glands
Buck fascia
Bünger bands
Burdach column
Burdach fissure
Burns ligament
Burns space
Burow vein
Burr cells
bursa of Achilles tendon
Cajal cell
Cajal nucleus
Caldani ligament
Calori bursa
Campbell ligament
Camper fascia
canal of Arantius

canal of Corti
canal of Cotunnius
canal of Guidi
canal of Hering
Carcassone ligament
Carcassone perineal ligament
Casser ligament
cells of Cajal
cells of Corti
cells of Hensen
cells of Martinotti
cells of van Gehuchten
central canal of Stilling
Charcot-Böttcher crystalloids
Chassaignac tubercle
Chiari net
Chievitz layer
Chievitz organ
Chopart joint
circle of Willis
circles of Haller
circles of Weber
circular structure of Santorini
Civinini ligament
Civinini process
Clado anastomosis
Clado ligament
Clara cell
Clarke column
Claudius cell
Cleland ligaments
Clevenger fissure
Cloquet canal
Cloquet ganglion
Cloquet ligament
Cloquet node
Cloquet septum
Cockett perforating veins
Cohnheim artery
Cohnheim field
Colles fascia
Colles ligament
Colles space
column of Bertin
column of Clarke
Cooper fascia
Cooper ligament
Cooper suspensory ligament

corpus luysii
Corti ganglion
Corti membrane
Corti tunnel
Coschwitz duct
Cotunnius nerve
Cotunnius space
Cowper fascia
Cowper glands
Cowper ligament
criminal nerve of Grassi
Crooke cells
Cruveilhier ligament (hand)
Cruveilhier ligament (knee)
Cruveilhier plexus
crypts of Fuchs
crypts of Haller
Curvier ducts
Custer cell
Cyon nerve
Darkschewitsch fibers
Darwin tubercle
Davidoff cells
Debove membrane
Deiters cells
Deiters nucleus
Demours membrane
Denonvilliers fascia
Denonvilliers ligament
Denucé ligament
Descemet membrane
Diogenes cup
Disse space
Dobie globule
Dobie line
Dodd perforating veins
Donné bodies
Dorendorf canal
Dorothy Reed cell
Douglas ligament
Douglas line
Douglas pouch
duct of His
duct of Vater
ducts of Cuvier
Duncan folds
Duverney foramen
Duverney glands

Eberth glands
Eberth line
Edinger-Westphal nucleus
Egger line
Ehrenritter ganglion
eustachian tube
fallopian aqueduct
fallopian ligament
fallopian tube
Fananas cell
Farre white line
Ferrein ligament
Ferrein tube
fibers of Winslow
Flechsig tract
Fleischmann bursa
Flemming center
Flint arcade
Floegel layer
Flood ligament
fold of Marshall
folds of Hoboken
Folius muscle
Foltz valve
Fontana space
foramen of Bochdalek
foramen of Magendie
foramen of Monro
foramen of Pacchionius
foramen of Rivini
foramen of Vesalius
foramen of Winslow
fossa of Rosenmueller
Fothergill sign
Foville fasciculus
Frankenhäuser ganglion
frenum of Morgagni
Frommann lines
Froriep ganglion
Fruchard orifice
Galeati glands
Galen loop
Galen nerve
Galen veins
Gall body
Gallaudet fascia
ganglion of Valentine
ganglion of Wrisberg

Gantzer muscle
Gartner duct
Gasserian ganglion
Gavard muscle
Gay glands
Gegenbaur cell
Gerdy fibers
Gerdy ligament
Gerdy loop
Gerdy tubercle
germinal epithelium of
    Waldeyer
Gerota fascia
Gierke cell
Gierke corpuscle
Gimbernat ligament
Giraldes organ
gland of Zeis
glands of Wolfring
glaserian fissure
glenoid ligament of Cruveilhier
glenoid ligament of Macalister
Gley cell
Gley gland
Glisson capsule
Golgi-Mazzoni corpuscles
Goll column
Goll fasciculus
Goll fibers
Goll tract
Goormaghtigh cells
Gottstein fibers
Gowers tract
Graafian follicle
Grandy corpuscle
Grayson ligament
Gudden commissure
Guérin fold
Guérin glands
Guérin sinus
Guérin valve
Günz ligament
Guthrie muscle
Guyon canal
Haglund disease
Haller aberrant duct
Haller arches
Haller duct

Haller habenula
Haller layer
Haller membrane
Hannover canal
Harder glands
Hartigan foramen
Hartmann pouch
Häsner valve
Hassall corpuscle
Haversian canals
Haversian system
Heidenhain cells
Helmholtz ligament
Helvetius ligament
Helweg bundle
Henke space
Henle ampule
Henle elastic membrane
Henle fenestrated membrane
Henle fiber layer
Henle glands
Henle layer
Henle ligament
Henle loop
Henle membrane
Hensen canal
Hensen cell
Hensen line
Hensen node
Hensing ligament
hepatic funiculus of Rauber
Hering nerve
Herxheimer fibers
Heschl gyri
Hesselbach ligament
Heubner artery
Hey ligament
Highmore antrum
Highmore body
Hilton muscle
Hilton white line
Hirschfeld canal
His bundle
His perivascular space
His tubercle
Hoboken valve
Hofbauer cells
Hoffmann duct

Holden line
Horner muscle
Hortega cell
Houston muscle
Houston valves
Howship lacuna
Hudson-Stähli line
Hueck ligament
Huguier canal
Huguier sinus
Humphry ligament
Hunter canal
Hunter ligament
Hunter line
Huschke foramen
Huschke ligament
Huschke valve
Hutchinson notch
Huxley layer
hydatid cyst of Morgagni
Hyrtl loop
islets of Langerhans
Jackson membrane
Jacob membrane
Jacobson canal
Jacobson cartilage
Jacobson nerve
James fibers
Jarjavay muscle
joints of Luschka
Jung muscle
Kaes-Bekhterev line
Kanavel spaces
Keith node
Kent bundles
Kerckring valves
Kirk arcade
Kohlrausch folds
Kohlrausch veins
Kohn pores
Kölicker membrane
Kommerell diverticulum
Korff fibers
Kovalevsky canal
Koyter muscle
Krause end bulb
Krause gland
Krause membrane

Krause valve
Krukenberg veins
Kugel artery
Kuhnt intermediary tissue
Kuhnt postcentral vein
Kupffer cell
Küttner ganglion
Labbé vein
Ladd band
Landsmeer ligaments
Landström muscle
Landzert fossa
Langer lines
Langer muscle
Langley nerves
Lanterman clefts
Larrey cleft
Larrey spaces
laryngeal cartilage of Luschka
Laumonier ganglion
Leber corpuscle
Leber plexus
Lee ganglion
lesser fossa of Scarpa
Leydig cell
Leydig duct
Lieberkuhn crypts
Liebermeister grooves
ligament of Scarpa
limbal palisades of Vogt
line of Gennari
lines of Park
lines of Retzius
liquor of Scarpa
Lisch nodules
Lisfranc joint
Lisfranc tubercle
Lissauer tract
Lister tubercle
Littre glands
Lobstein ganglion
Loewenthal disease
loop of Henle
lower tubercle
Lumsden center
Luschka bursa
Luschka cartilage
Luschka fossa

Luschka tubercle
Luschke crypts
Luse bodies
Luys body
Macdowel frenum
Magendie foramen
Magendie spaces
Mahaim bundles
Maissiat band
Malassez rest
Malgaigne triangle
malpighian corpuscle
Marchand adrenals
Marshall fold
Marshall oblique vein
Martin-Gruber anastomosis
master knot of Henry
Mauthner membrane
Meckel cartilage
Meckel caves
Meckel diverticulum
Meckel ganglion
Meckel tubercle
Meibomian glands
Meissner corpuscle
Meissner plexus
Mercier bar
Merkel muscle
Merkel tactile cell
Meyer sinus
Meynert commissure
Meynert fasciculus
Meynert layer
Moll glands
Monro bursa
Montgomery glands
Montgomery tubercles
Morgagni foramen of tongue
Morgagni glands
Morgagni hydatid
Morgagni lacunae
Morgagni nodule
Morgagni tubercle
Muller cells
Müllerian duct
muscle of Muller
Nélaton fold
Nélaton line

nerve of Latarjet
nerve of Luschka (ethmoid)
nerve of McCrea
nerve of Willis
nerves of Lancisi
nerves of Luschka (spine)
Neubauer artery
Nissl body
Nitabuch layer
node of Rouvier
Nuck canal
Nuel spaces
Ochsner muscle
Odland body
Ollier layer
Onuf nucleus
organ of Corti
organ of Giraldès
organ of Rosenmüller
organ of Zuckerkandl
Owen lines
pacchionian bodies
Pacinian corpuscles
Paneth cell
Pappenheimer body
parietal vein of Santorini
Perlia nucleus
Peyer patches
Phillips muscle
Pickerill lines
pluriformis of Retzius
Poirier glands
pores of Kahn
postrema of Retzius
pouch of Douglas
Poupart ligament
Proust space
Purkinje cell
Purkinje fiber
Purkinje system
Ranvier node
recess of Allison
rectal column of Morgagni
Reinke space
Reisseisen muscle
Reissner membrane
residual body of Regnaud
Retzius cavity

Retzius foramen
Retzius veins
ribbon of Reil
Ribes ganglion
Ridley sinus
Riedel lobe
Rindfleisch fold
Riolan muscle (eye)
Riolan muscle (testes)
Riolan nosegay
Rivinius duct
Rivinius gland
Rivinius notch
Robert ligament
Rolando fibers
Rolando fissure
Rolando tubercle
Roller central nucleus
Rosenmüller gland
Rosenmüller node
Rosenthal vein
Rotter nodes
Rouget muscle
Ruffini endings
Ruysch muscle
Ruysch veins
Sandström body
Santorini cartilage
Santorini duct
Santorini ligament
Santorini muscle
Sappey ligament
Sappey plexus
Sattler layer
Scarpa fascia
Scarpa ganglion
Scarpa habenula
Scarpa nerves
Scarpa triangle
Schlemm canal
Schmidt-Lantermann clefts
Schneiderian mucosa
Schrön granule
Schüller ducts
Schüller glands
Schultze fold
Schwalbe foramen
Schwalbe line

Schwalbe nucleus
Schwann cells
Schwann sheath
Sebileau hollow
Serres glands
Sertoli cell
sheath of Henle
sheath of Hertwig
Shrapnell membrane
Sibson fascia
Sibson groove
Sigmund glands
sinus of Maier
sinus of Morgagni
sinus of Valsalva
Skene glands
space of Larry
space of Martegiani
space of Poirier
space of Retzius
Spigelius line
Stahr gland
Steno duct
Stensen duct
Stensen veins
Stenson canal
Stilling nucleus
sulcus of Reil
sylvian aqueduct
sylvian fissure
sylvian fossa
sylvian vein
tail of Spence
Tarin anterior recess
Tarin fascia
Tarin fossa
Tarin posterior recess
Tarin velum
Tawara node
tendon of Hector
tendon of Todaro
Tenon capsule
Tenon space
Thebesius valve
Theile gland
Thomas ampulla
Tiedemann nerve
Tomes processes

Treves fold
triangle of Calot
triangle of Killian
triangle of Koch
triangle of Truesdale
Trolard net
Trolard vein
Tröltsch pockets
van Gehuchten nucleus
van Hoorne canal
vein of Galen
vein of Labbé
vein of Mayo
vein of Rosenthal
vein of Trolard
vein of Vieussens
veins of Sappey
veins of Thebesius
Venus line
Verga groove
Verga ventricle
Vesalius foramen
Vesalius vein
Vicq d'Azyr bundle
vidian artery
vidian canal
vidian nerve
Vieussens foramina
Volkmann canals
von Ebner glands
von Gudden ganglion
von Monakow fibers
Voshell bursa
Wagner line
Waldeyer fascia
Waldeyer gland
Waldeyer layer
Weber gland
Weber ligament
Weber tubercle
Weil basal layer
Weitbrecht cartilage
Weitbrecht foramen
Weitbrecht ligament
Wernicke area
Westphal nucleus
Wharton ducts
white line of Toldt

Wiegert ligament
Wilbrand knee
Willis cords
Wilson muscle
Winslow pancreas
Wirsung duct
Wolfring glands
wormian bone
Wrisberg cartilages
Wrisberg nerve (arm)
Wrisberg nerve (face)

EMBRYOLOGY TERMS

Ammon fissure
anus of Rusconi
Baer cavity
Baer law
Balbiani body
Barr body
Buerger disease
Béclard nucleus
Béclard sign
Bergmeister papilla
Blessig groove
Brachet fold
corpus of Oken
Douglas septum
Haller isthmus
His bursa
His canal
Kerckring center
Langhans layer
Mall ridge
Pander layer
primitive node of Hensen
process of Tomes
Rathke cleft
Rathke fold
Rathke pouch
Rauber layer
Reichel duct
Reichert canal
Reichert cartilages
Spöndel foramen

ONCOLOGY TERMS

Abernethy sarcoma
Abrikossoff tumor

Agnell rule
Ames test
Amsterdam criteria
Ann Arbor classification
Antoni patterns
Askin tumor
Auer rod
Bageshaw chemotherapy
    (modified)
Bailey-Cushing disease
Bangle body
Bazex-Griffith syndrome
Bednar tumors
Bergkvist classification
Bethesda system
Billroth disease
Bloom-Richardson grade
Blumer shelf
Borrmann classification
Brenner nodules
Breslow method
Brill-Symmers disease
Broders classification (lip)
Broders classification (stomach)
Broders index
Brodie disease
Burkitt lymphoma
Buschke-Löwenstein tumor
Castleman disease
Chung classification
Clark levels
Clarke body
Codman tumor
Contarini syndrome
Cotswolds classification
Crosti reticulosis
Deelman effect
Denys-Drash syndrome
di Guglielmo syndrome
Eaton-Lambert syndrome
Ewing sarcoma
Farre tubercles
French-American-British
    classification
Gleason grade
Gleason score
Godwin tumor
Goldie-Coldman hypothesis

Gompertzian growth
Gordon test
Grabstald staging
Haagensen criteria
Haagensen test
Haggitt system
Halban disease
Halsted theory of breast cancer
Harding-Passey melanoma
Hodgkin sarcoma
Hodgkin staging laparotomy
Homer-Wright rosettes
Hürthle adenoma
Hürthle carcinoma
Hürthle cell
Hutchinson freckle
Hutchinson sign
Irish node
Jarcho syndrome
Jensen disease
Jewett-Marshall system
Jewett-Whitmore classification
Krukenberg tumor
Kaposi sarcoma
Kernohan grade
Kirkland classification
Klatskin tumor
Kupffer cell sarcoma
Küstner sign
Lauren classification
Lennert lymphoma
Leydig cell tumor
Li-Fraumeni cancer syndrome
Mallory leukemia
Manchester classification
Manchester technique
MD Anderson system
Merkel cell tumor
Mott body
Mostofi system
Naegeli leukemia
Nevin system
Nigro protocol
Okuda groups
Paget disease (breast)
Paget dieseae (perineum)
Paris technique
Parker disease

parvilocular tumors of Schiller
Patey mastectomy
Peutz-Jeghers syndrome
Pick tubular adenoma
Quimby technique
Rai criteria
Raji cells
Rappaport classification
Ringertz classification
Robson grading system
Rosenthal fibers
Saint Anne–Mayo system
Scarff-Bloom-Richardson grade
Schiller-Duval body
Schmincke tumor
Schneiderian papilloma
Schridde hairs
Sertoli-Leydig tumor
Sézary cell
Sézary syndrome
Shimada classification
Siewert classification
Sipple syndrome
Sister Mary Joseph nodule
Smith classification
Stillwagon groups
Stockholm technique
Tice strain
Turcot syndrome
Verocay bodies
von Hippel-Landau disease
von Recklinghausen disease
Warthin tumor
Wermer syndrome

RADIOLOGY TERMS

Albert position
Alexander position
Alfven instability
Alfven waves
Anger camera
angle of Boogaard
Ashhurst sign
Barkhof criteria
Baumann angle
Bennett angle
Bergman sign
Bloch equations

Blumensaat line
Böhler angle
Bohr magneton
Bosniak classification
Bragg peak
Brett syndrome
Brewerton view
Brodie abscess
Brown-Dodge method
Carr-Purcell-Meiboom-Gill technique
Carr-Purcell pulse sequence
Chang algorithm
Chaoul tube
Chassard-Lapiné position
Cleaves position
Cobb angle
Cobb method
Cole sign
Compton effect
Coolidge tube
Correra line
Coutard law
Crookes space
Davis line
Dawson fingers
Didiee projection
Dolan lines
Downs analysis
Downs Y axis
Eklund modification
Fairbanks changes
Fazekas criteria
Felson silhouette sign
Fisk position
Fleischner atelectasis
Fleischner sign
forssel sinus
Frankel line
Frauenhofer zone
Fresnel zone
Fuchs method (modified)
Garth view
Ghon tubercle
Graham test
Grashey view
Hampson unit
Hampton line

Hann filter
Harris lines
Haudek niche
Henning sign
Hill-Sachs lesion
Hill-Sachs lesion (reversed)
Holzknekt space
Hopman hump
Hounsfield unit
Hughston view
Isherwood positions
Judet views
Kager triangle
Kantor string sign
Kerley B lines
Kurzbauer position
Laquerrier-Pierquin position
Law position
Lawrence position
Lilienfeld position
Looser zone
Lorenz position
Löw-Beer position
Lückenschädel deformity
Lysholm method
Mach bands
Monod sign
Pearson technique
Quesada method
Reil triangle
Roux sign
Settegast position
Stecher position
Tarrant position
Tönnis system
Towne view
Waters view

REFLEXES, SIGNS, AND TESTS

Aaron sign
Abadie sign (Graves disease)
Abadie sign (syphilis)
Abeshouse triad
Abrahams sign (gallbladder)
Abrahams sign (TB)
Abrams reflex (heart)
Abrams reflex (lung)

Abrams treatment
Achilles bulge sign
Achilles reflex
Achilles squeeze test
Adams test
Addis test
Adson maneuver
Adson maneuver (modified)
Alder sign
Allen maneuver
Allen test
Allis sign
Amoss sign
Anderson grind test
André Thomas sign (cerebellar lesion)
André Thomas sign (hand)
Andre Thomas sign (trapezius)
Anghelescu sign
Apley scratch test
Apley sign
Apley test
Archibald sign
Arroyo sign
Aschner inverted phenomenon
Aspinall progressive tests
Astwood test
Auenbrugger sign
Aufrecht sign
Auspitz sign
Austin Flint murmur
Austin Flint respiration
Babinski pronator phenomenon
Babinski reflex
Babinksi reinforcement sign
Babinski sign (platysma)
Babinski sign (S1 pathology)
Babinski thigh reflex
Babinsky-Weil test
Babkin reflex
Baccelli sign
Bachman test
Baillarger sign
Bainbridge reflex
Bakody sign
Ballance sign (left lateral decubitus position)
Ballance sign (palpation)

Ballet sign
Ballotment sign
Bamberger sign (extremity)
Bamberger sign (heart)
Bancroft sign
Bárány maneuver
Barkman reflex
Barlow sign
Barré sign (iris)
Barré sign (paresis)
Baruch sign
Bastedo sign
Battle sign
Beau lines
Beaumés sign
Beccaria sign
Bechterew sign (hemiparesis)
Bechterew sign (syphilis)
Bechterew test
Bechterew-Mendel reflex
Beck triad
Béclard sign
Beevor sign (paralysis)
Beevor sign (umbilicus)
Bekhterev deep reflex
Bekhterev reflex (abdominal wall)
Bekhterev reflex (eye)
Bekhterev reflex (facial)
Bekhterev sign
Bekhterev test
Bell phenomenon (eyelid)
Bergman triad
Bernhardt sign
Bethea sign
Bezold sign
Bezold-Jarisch reflex
Biederman sign
Biernacki sign
Bikele sign
Bing sign
Bing test
Bird sign
Bittorf reaction
Blackburne ratio
Blatin sign
Blumberg sign
Boas sign

Bohler sign
Bonnet sign
Borchardt triad
Borsieri sign
Boston sign
Bouillaud disease
Bouvier maneuver
Boyce sign
Boyes test
Bozzolo sign
Bragard sign
Brain reflex
Brissaud reflex
British test
Broadbent sign (left atrium)
Broadbent sign (pericardium)
Broadbent test
Brockenbrough sign
Brodie sign
Brudzinski sign (face)
Brudzinksi sign (knees)
Bryant sign
Bryson sign
Buerger sign
Burton line
Cantelli sign
Cardarelli sign
Carducci test
Carey-Coombs murmur
Carman sign
Carnett sign
Carvallo sign
Casoni test
Castellino sign
Cattaneo sign
Cegka sign
Chaddock sign (foot)
Chaddock sign (hand)
Chadwick sign
Charcot sign
Charcot triad (bile system)
Charcot triad (multiple
  sclerosis)
Chauffard sign
Chimani-Moos test
Chvostek sign
Clapton line
Clark sign

Clarke sign
Claude sign
Claybrook sign
Cleeman sign
Cloquet sign
Codman sign
Coleman test
Collier sign
Comby sign
Comolli sign
Coopernail sign
Cope sign
Corrigan sign
Courvoiser sign
Coutard law
Cowen sign
Cozen test
Crafts test
Craig test
crescent sign of Caffey
Crichton-Browne sign
Cruveilhier sign
Cruveilhier-Baumgarten sign
Cullen sign
Cushing triad
Dagnini reflex
Dalrymple sign
D'Amato sign
Dance sign
Darier sign
Davidsohn sign
Dawbarn sign
de la Camp sign
Déjérine sign
Delbet sign
Delmege sign
Demarquay sign
Demianoff sign
Dennie line
Desault sign
D'Espine sign
Destot sign
Dew sign
Dix-Hallpike maneuver
Doppler effect
Drawer sign
Drummond sign
Duchenne sign

Dugas test
Duncan sign
Dunphy sign
Dupuytren sign
Duroziez sign
Earle sign
Egawa sign
Einhorn string test
Elliot sign (eye)
Elliot sign (syphilis)
Ellis line
Elsberg test
Elson middle slip test
Ely sign
Enroth sign
Epley manuever
Erben reflex
Erhard test
Erichsen sign
Erni sign
Escherich sign
Eustace Smith sign
Ewart sign
Ewing sign
Faber test
Faget first sign
Faget second sign
Fairbanks test
Fajersztajn sign
Farnsworth test
Farnsworth-Munsell test
Feagin test
Federici sign
Ferguson reflex
Filiipovitch sign
Finkelstein test
Flack test
Fowler maneuver
Fowler test
Fox sign
Fränkel sign
Fränkel test
Franz sign
Friderichsen test
Friedrich sign
Froment sign
Frund sign
Fürbringer sign

Gaenslen sign
Gage sign
Galant reflex
Galassi phenomenon
Galeazzi sign
Gallavardin effect
Garel sign
Gault test
Gianelli sign
Gibbon and Landis test
Gibson murmur
Gifford sign
Gilbert sign
Gilchrest sign
Gillet test
Glasgow sign
Godfrey test
Goggia sign
Goldstein sign
Goldthwait sign
Gonda sign
Goodell sign
Gordon reflex
Gordon sign
Gorlin sign
Gottron sign
Gowers sign (iris)
Gowers sign (standing)
Graefe sign
Graefe test
Graham-Steell murmur
Grancher sign
Granger sign
Grasset-Gaussel phenomenon
Grasset-Gaussel-Hoover sign
Greene sign
Grey Turner sign
Griesinger sign
Griffith sign
Grisolle sign
Grocco sign (chest)
Grocco sign (liver)
Grossman sign
Guilland sign
Gunn dot
Gunn sign (eyelid)
Gunn sign (hypertension)
Guyon sign

Haagensen test
Haenel sign
Hall sign
Hallpike maneuver
Halsted maneuver
Hamilton test
Hamman sign
Hatchcock sign
Hawkins impingement sign
Hefke-Turner sign
Hegar sign
Heim-Kreysig sign
Heimlich maneuver
Helbings sign
Henle-Coenen test
Hertwig-Magendie position
Heryng sign
Heuter sign
Hibbs test
Higouménakis sign
Hill sign
Hirschberg sign (foot)
Hirschberg sign (thigh)
Hirschberg test
Hitzelberger sign
Hitzig test
Hochsinger sign
Hoehne sign
Hoffmann sign
Holzknekt sign
Homan sign
Hoover sign (heel)
Hoover sign (inspiration)
Horn sign
Horner sign
Horsley sign
Hoyne sign
Huchard sign (lung)
Huchard sign (pulse rate)
Hueter sign
Hughston drawer sign
Hughston plica test
Huntingdon sign
Hutchinson sign (herpes)
Hutchinson sign (melanoma)
Hutchinson sign (syphilis)
Huygens principle
Jaccoud sign

Jackson sign (asthma)
Jackson sign (TB)
Jacquemir sign
Jansen test
Jeanne sign
Jeliffe method
Jellinik sign
Jendrassik maneuver
Jendrassik sign
Jobe test
Joffroy sign
Kanavel sign
Karplus sign
Kashida sign
Keen sign
Kehr sign
Kellock sign
Kelly sign
Kenawy sign
Kerandel sign
Kergaradec sign
Kernig sign
Kernohan notch sign
Kerr sign
Kestenbaum sign
Kleinman shear test
Klemm sign
Kliest sign
Klippel-Weil sign
Knapp streaks
Knies sign
Kocher maneuver
Kocher sign
Kohnstamm phenomenon
Korányi sign
Korotkoff sounds
Krimsky test
Krisowski sign
Kussmaul sign
Küstner sign
Lachman test
Lafora sign
Langoris sign
Laplace law
Lasègue sign (anesthesia)
Lasègue sign (sciatica)
Laugier sign
Leichtenstern sign

Lennhoff index
Lennhoff sign
Leri sign
Leser-Trélat sign
Lesieur sign
Levine sign
Lhermitte sign
Lichtheim sign
Lichtman test
Linder sign
Litten sign
Livierato sign
Lloyd sign
Lomadtse sign
Lombard effect
Lombardi sign
Lorenz sign
Love test
Lovett test
Löwenberg sign
Lucas sign
Ludloff sign
Macewen sign
Magendie sign
Magnan sign
Mahler sign
Maisonneuve sign
Mann sign
Mannkopf sign
Marcus Gunn phenomenon
Marcus Gunn pupil
Marfan sign
Marie sign
Marie-Foix sign
Marinesco-Radovici sign
Markle sign
Mayer reflex
Mayne sign
McBurney sign
McDonald sign
McGinn-White syndrome
McMurray test
Mean sign
Means-Lerman sign
Mees line
Meltzer sign
Mendel-Bechterew reflex
Mennell sign

Mercedes-Benz sign
Meunier sign
Mexican hat sign
Mills maneuver
Minor sign
Mirchamp sign
Möbius sign
Moniz sign
Moro response
Morton test
Mosler sign
Müller sign
Munson sign
Murat sign
Murphy sign
Musset sign
Myerson sign
Neer sign
Negro sign
Neri sign
Neuhauser sign
Nicoladoni sign
Nikolsky sign
Nothnagel sign
Nylen-Bárány test
Ober test
Oppenheim reflex
Oppenheim sign
Ortolani sign
Parrot sign
Pastia sign
Patrick test
Payr sign
Pende sign
Perez reflex
Perez sign
Pfuhl sign
Phelps-Baker test
Pinard sign
Pins sign
Piotrowski sign
Piskacek sign
Pitres sign
Plummer sign
Pool-Schlesinger sign (foot)
Pool-Schlesinger sign (hand)
Popeye sign

Potain sign (aortic arch
dilatation)
Potain sign (syphilis)
Pottenger sign (lung)
Pottenger sign (organs)
Prehn sign
Prévost sign
pseudo-Babinksi sign
pseudo-Graefe sign
Puusepp reflex
Queckenstedt test
Quincke sign
Quinquaud sign
Radovici sign
Raimiste sign
Ramond sign
Rasin sign
Revilliod sign
Reynold pentad
Riesman sign (bruit)
Riesman sign (diabetes)
Rigler sign
Ripault sign
Risquez sign
Risser sign
Riviere sign
Robertson sign (arms)
Robertson sign (chest wall)
Robertson sign (flanks)
Romberg sign
Romberg-Howship sign
Roos test
Rosselli-Gulienetti syndrome
Rossolimo reflex
Rovsing sign
Rust phenomenon
Sahlgren test
Saint triad
Sandwith tongue
Schaefer sign
Schäffer reflex
Schirmer test
Schultze sign (cheek)
Schultze sign (tongue)
Schwabach test
Schwartze sign
Seelimueller sign
Seidel test

Sellick maneuver
Semon sign
Shafer sign
Siegert sign
Silex sign
Sisto sign
Snellen reflex
Soderbergh reflex
Souques sign
Spurling test
Squire sign
Stellwag sign
Sterles sign
Sterling sign
Sternberg sign
Stierlin sign
Stillwag sign
Stocker sign
Straus sign
Strümpell reflex
Strümpell sign
Suker sign
Sumner sign
Tanyol sign
Tardieu spots
Tay spot
Terry-Thomas sign
Thomas test (hip)
Thomas test (spine)
Thompson line
Thompson test
Thomson sign
Thornton sign
Throckmorton sign
Tinel sign
Tommasi sign
Tournay sign
Traube sign
Trendelenburg sign
Trendelenburg test
Tresilian sign
Tressder sign
Trimadeau sign
Troisier sign
Trousseau sign
Tullio phenomenon
Turner sign
Turyn sign

Uhthoff sign
Unschuld sign
Uriolla sign
Verco sign
Vermel sign
Vipond sign
Voltolini sign
von Graefe sign
von Mering reflex
Wachenheim-Reder sign
Wartenberg sign (arm)
Wartenberg sign (finger)
Wegner sign
Weill sign

Weiss ref
Wernicke sign
Westermark sign
Westphal sign
Widowitz sign
Wilder sign
Williamson sign
Wimberger sign
Winterbottom sign
Wintrich sign
Wood sign
Worth test
Wright maneuver